SPELLRIGHT
A Medical Word Book

Jane Rice, RN, CMA-C
Medical Assisting Program Director
Coosa Valley Technical Institute
Rome, Georgia

A combined alphabetic listing of medical words, drugs, lab tests, surgical operations, and terms with a special section devoted to medical abbreviations

APPLETON & LANGE
Norwalk, Connecticut/San Mateo, California

Copyright © 1991 by Appleton & Lange
A Publishing Division of Prentice Hall

91 92 93 94 / 10 9 8 7 6 5 4 3 2 1

Prentice-Hall International (UK) Limited,London
Prentice-Hall of Australia Pty. Limited, Sydney
Prentice-Hall Canada Inc., Toronto
Prentice-Hall Hispanoamericana, S.A., Mexico
Prentice-Hall of India Private Limited, New Delhi
Prentice-Hall of Japan, Inc., Tokyo
Pearson Education Asia Pte. Ltd., Singapore
Editora Prentice-Hall do Brasil, Ltda., Rio de Janeiro

Library of Congress Cataloging-in-Publication Data

Rice, Jane
    SPELLRIGHT / by Jane Rice.
        p. cm.
    "A Medical word book."
    ISBN 0-8385-6290-6
    1. Medicine--Terminology. 2. English language--Orthography and spelling. I. Title.
    [DNLM: 1. Nomenclature.   W 15 R496ma]
R123.R525 1990
610'.14--dc20
DNLM/DLC
for Library of Congress

                                                    89-18602
                                                    CIP

PRINTED IN THE UNITED STATES OF AMERICA

Contents

Dedicated to

Charles Larry Rice

I could use 90,000 words to describe you, and all the help
that you give me, but I only need two words
"Amor Semper."

Preface

The purpose of this book is to provide a current and convenient spelling reference that is both quick and easy to use. This book contains over 90,000 medical words, drugs, and abbreviations. In *SPELLRIGHT*, all entries are in alphabetic order; therefore, the correct spelling of whatever you are looking for is always at your fingertips.

This reference provides the scope and depth of content unavailable in other texts. The lising of medical words contains everything from **A** (Aaron's sign) to **Z** (zymotic). Drugs are listed according to their trade name,which is in bold type and, where possible, the generic name is provided in parentheses. Example: **A.P.L.** (chorionic gonadotropin). This method of entry provides a user with rapid verification of the spelling of most trade and generic drug names in one easy look.

SPELLRIGHT provides two methods for looking up an abbreviation:

1. In the main body of the text, the abbreviation follows the word entry and is enclosed in parentheses. Example:

    above elbow (AE)

2. Over 6,000 abbreviations are included in a special section in the back of the text. The abbreviation is given in bold type with its meaning (or meanings) directly across from it. Example:

    AA   Alcoholics Anonymous; amino acid; achievement age; authorized absence; auto accident; active assistive; arm ankle (pulse ratio); acetic acid; ascending aorta; amino-acetone; alveolar-arterial

    S Surgical nomenclature
    P Practical and current entries
    E Easy-to-use format
    L Lists of over 6,000 abbreviations
    L Laboratory terminology
    R R$_x$ for all medical spelling needs
    I ICD and CPT vocabulary
    G Generic names of drugs
    H Handy book size
    T Trade names of drugs

Jane Rice

Acknowledgments

I would like to thank Marion K. Welch, Jamie Sokol, Karen Davis, and Kathy Gionet. Also I thank Sara Marshall, my friend and neighbor, for helping me input the "P" words.

Listing of Medical Words

A

A.P.L. (chorionic
  gonadotropin)
A-200 Pyrinate
  (pediculicide shampoo)
A-Hydrocort
  (hydrocortisone sodium
  succinate)
A/T/S (erythromycin)
Aaron's sign
abacterial
abaissement
abarticular
abasia
abate
abatement
Abbe's operation, rings
Abbe-Estlander repair,
  lip
Abbokinase (urokinase for
  injection)
Abbott-Miller tube
Abderhalden-Kaufmann-
  Lignac syndrome
abdomen (abd)
abdominal
abdominal aorta
abdominal cavity
abdominal hysterectomy
  (AH)
abdominalgia
abdominocentesis
abdominogenital
abdominohysterectomy
abdominohysterotomy
abdominoperineal
abdominoplasty

abdominoscopy
abdominoscrotal
abdominothoracic
abdominouterotomy
abdominovaginal
abdominovesical
abducens
abducens muscle
abducens nerve
abducent
abducent nerve
abduct
abduction
abductor
Abercrombie's syndrome
Abernethy's operation
aberrancy
aberrant
aberratio
aberration
abetalipoproteinemia
abevacuation
abeyance
abionarce
abiosis
abiotic
abiotrophy
abirritant
abirritation
ablactation
ablate
ablatio
ablation
ablepharia
ablepharous
ablepsia

abluent
ablutomania
abnormal (AB)
abnormalities
abnormality
abnormity
ABO + Rh typing
ABO blood typing
abocclusion
abolition, language
aboral
abort
aborter, habitual or
  recurrent
abortifacient
abortion (AB)
abortion, by aspiration
  curettage
abortion, by dilation and
  curettage
abortion, hysterectomy
abortion, hysterotomy
abortion, insertion
  intra-amniotic
  injection (saline)
abortion, insertion
  laminaria
abortion, insertion
  prostaglandin
  suppository
abortion, therapeutic
abortionist
abortive
abortus
aboulomania
above elbow (AE)
above knee (AK)
abrachia
abrachiatism
abrachiocephalia
abrachiocephalus
abradant
abrade
Abrami's disease
Abramov-Fiedler
  myocarditis
abrasion
abrasive

abreaction
Abrikossov's tumor
abrism
abruptio placenta
abruptio placentae
abscess
abscission, cornea
absence
absorb
absorbable
absorbable hemostat
absorbance
absorbent
absorptiometer
absorption
abstinence
abstraction
Abt-Letterer-Siwe
  syndrome
abulia
abulomania
Aburel operation
abuse
abutment
acalcerosis
acalcicosis
acalculia
acanthiomeatal line (AML)
acanthocheilonemiasis
acanthocyte
acanthocytosis
acanthoid
acanthokeratodermia
acantholysis
acanthoma
acanthosis
acapnia
acarbia
acardia
acardiacus
acardiotrophia
acariasis
acaridiasis
acarinosis
acarodermatitis
acaroid
acarophobia
acarus

acatalasemia
acatalasia
acatamathesia
acataphasia
acatastasia
acathectic
acathexis
acathisia
accelerated
  idioventricular rhythm
  (AIVR)
acceleration
accentuation
acceptor
accessory
accessory nerve
accessory sinuses
accident
accidental
accommodation (A)
accouchement force
accreta placenta
accretio cordis
accretions on teeth
accumulation secretion,
  prostate
Accurbron (theophylline)
Accutane (isotretinoin)
Ace bandage
acephalia
acephalic monster
acephalism
acephalobrachia monster
acephalocardia
acephalocardius
acephalochiria
acephalochirus monster
acephalogaster
acephalostomus monster
acephalothorax
acephalus
acetabular
acetabular augmentation
acetabulectomy
acetabuloplasty
acetabulum
acetaldehyde
acetamide

acetaminophen
acetaminophen toxicology
  test
Acetaminophen Uniserts
  (rectal suppositories)
acetate
acetic acid
acetoacetic acid
acetone
acetone, ketone bodies
  test
acetonemia
acetonglycosuria
acetonuria
acetous
acetyl
acetylation
acetylcholine
acetylcholine receptor
acetylcholinesterase
acetylene (C_2H_2)
acetylsalicylic acid
  (ASA)
acetylsalicylic acid,
  phenacetin, caffeine
  (APC)
acetylsalicylic acid,
  phenacetin, caffeine
  with codeine (APC-C)
acetyltransferase
AcG (factor 5)
achalasia
Achard-Thiers syndrome
ache
acheilia
acheiria
achievement quotient (AQ)
achievement ratio (AR)
Achilles tendon
achillobursitis
achillodynia
achillorrhaphy
achillotenotomy
achillotomy
achlorhydria
achlorhydric
achloroblepsia
achloropsia

acholia
acholuria
acholuric jaundice
achondrogenesis
achondroplasia
achrestic anemia
achroma
achromacyte
achromate
achromatic
achromatin
achromatism
achromatopsia
achromia
achromotrichia
Achromycin (tetracycline HCl)
achylia
achymosis
Aci-Jel (therapeutic vaginal jelly)
acid
acid clearing test
Acid Mantle Creme
acid peel
acid perfusion studs
acid phosphatase (ACP) test
acid phosphate
acid reflux test
acid-base balance
acid-base ratio (A/B)
acid-fast (AF)
acid-fast bacilli (AFB)
acidemia
acidifier
acidity
acidocytopenia
acidocytosis
acidopenia
acidophil
acidosis
aciduria
aciniform
acinitis
acinus
acladiosis
aclasis

acleistocardia
Aclovate (alclometasone dipropionate)
aclusion
acme
acmesthesia
acne
acne scarring dermabrasion
acnegenic
acneiform
acnitis
acomia
aconuresis
Acosta's disease
acousia
acousma
acoustic
acoustic nerve
acoustic reflex decay
acousticophobia
acoustics
acquired
acquired immunodeficiency syndrome (AIDS)
acragnosis
acrania
Acremonium
acrid
acroagnosis
acroanesthesia
acroarthritis
acroasphyxia, chronic
acrobrachycephaly
acrobystitis
acrocephalopolysyndactyly
acrocephalosyndactyly
acrocephaly
acrochondrohyperplasia
acrocyanosis
acrodermatitis
acrodermatosis
acrodynia
acrodysplasia
acrohyperhidrosis
acrohypothermy
acrokeratosis verruciformis

acromastitis
acromegaly
acromelalgia
acromicria
acromikria
acromioclavicular (AC)
acromioclavicular joint
acromiohumeral
acromion
acromionectomy
acromioplasty
acromioscapular
acromiothoracic
acronyx
acropachy
acropachyderma
acroparalysis
acroparesthesia
acropathology
acropathy
acrophobia
acroposthitis
acroscleriasis
acroscleroderma
acrosclerosis
acrosphacelus
acrosphenosyndactylia
acrospiroma, eccrine
acrostealgia
acrosyndactyly
acrotic
acrotrophodynia
acrylic acid
Acthar (corticotropin)
Actidil (triprolidine
HCl)
Actidose with Sorbitol
(activated charcoal
suspension)
Actidose-Aqua (activated
charcoal suspension)
Actifed
actinic
actinic dermatitis
Actinobacillus
actinocutitis
actinodermatitis
actinogenesis

Actinomyces
Actinomycetales
actinomycosis
actinoneuritis
actinotherapy
(ultraviolet light)
activator
active range of motion
(AROM)
activities of daily
living (ADL)
actomyosin
acuity
acupressure
acupuncture
acusection
acute (ac)
acute cardiovascular
disease (ACVD)
acute lymphoblastic
leukemia (ALL)
acute myelocytic leukemia
(AML)
acute myocardial
infarction (AMI)
acute necrotizing
ulcerative gingivitis
(ANUG)-trench mouth
acute physiology and
chronic health
evaluation (APACHE)
acute respiratory disease
(ARD)
acute respiratory failure
(ARF)
Acutrol sutures
acyanoblepsia
acyanopsia
acystia
acystinervia
acystineuria
adactylia
adactylism
adactyly
Adair's forceps
Adair-Dighton syndrome
Adalat (nifedipine)
Adam's apple

adamantine
adamantinoblastoma
adamantinoma
adamantoblastoma
Adams' operation
Adams' position
Adams-Stokes syndrome
Adapin (doxepin HCl)
adaptation
addict
addiction
Addis count
Addison's disease
Addison-Biermer anemia
Addison-Gull disease
addisonian crisis
addisonism
additive
adducent
adduct
adduction
adductor
Adeflor Chewable
(fluoride with
vitamins)
Aden fever
adenalgia
adenasthenia gastrica
adenectomy
adenectopia
adenitis
adenoacanthoma
adenoameloblastoma
adenoblast
adenocarcinoma
adenocele
adenocellulitis
adenochrondroma
adenocyst
adenocystoma
adenocyte
adenofibroma
adenofibrosis
adenohypophysis
adenoidectomy
adenoiditis
adenoids
adenolipomatosis

adenolymphitis
adenolymphoma
adenoma
adenomalacia
adenomatome
adenomatosis
adenomatous
adenomyoma
adenomyometritis
adenomyosarcoma
adenomyosis
adenopathy
adenopharyngitis
adenophlegmon
adenosalpingitis
adenosarcoma
adenosclerosis
adenosine
adenosine diphosphate
(ADP)
adenosine monophosphate
(AMP)
adenosine triphosphatase
(ATPase)
adenosis
adenotome
adenotonsillectomy
adenovirus
adentia
adherent
adhesiolysis
adhesion
adhesiotomy
adhesive
adiastole
Adie's syndrome
adipectomy
Adipex-P (phentermine
HCl)
adipoid
adipolysis
adiponecrosis neonatorum
adiposa dolorosa
adiposalgia
adipose
adiposis
adipositis
adiposity

adiposogenital dystrophy
Adipost (phendimetrazine
 tartrate)
adiposuria
adjacent
adjunct
adjustment
adjuvant therapy
administer
administration,
 antibiotics
administration,
 antitoxins
administration, antivenin
administration, bacillus
 Calmette-Guerin (BCG)
administration, Bender
 Visual-Motor Gestalt
 test
administration, Benton
 Visual Retention test
administration, botulism
administration,
 chemotherapeutic agent
administration,
 chemotherapy
administration,
 diphtheria
administration,
 diphtheria-tetanus-
 pertussis (DTP)
administration, gamma
 globulin
administration, gas
 gangrene
administration, immune
 sera
administration,
 intelligence test or
 scale
administration, measles-
 mumps-rubella (MMR)
administration, Memory
 Scale
administration, Minnesota
 Multiphasic Personality
 (MMP)

administration, passive
 immunization agent
administration,
 poliomyelitis
administration,
 psychologic test
administration, RhoGam
administration, scarlet
 fever
administration, Stanford-
 Binet
administration, tetanus
administration, Wechsler
adnexa
adnexitis
adnexopexy
adolescence
adolescent
adrenal
adrenal angiography
adrenal cortex
adrenal cortical hormone
 (ACH)
adrenal glands
adrenal medulla
adrenal venography
adrenalectomy
Adrenalin (epinephrine)
adrenaline
adrenalinemia
adrenalinuria
adrenalism
adrenalitis
adrenalopathy
adrenalorrhaphy
adrenergic
adrenitis
adrenocortical hormone
adrenocorticotropic
 hormone (ACTH)
adrenoleukodystrophy
adrenomegaly
adrenotropic
Adriamycin (doxorubicin
 HCl)
**Adriamycin, Blenoxane,
 Velban, and DTIC-Dome
 (ABVD)**

Adrucil (fluorouracil)
Adson's forceps
adsorbent
adtorsion
adult respiratory
   distress syndrome
   (ARDS)
adulteration
adult-onset diabetes
   mellitus (AODM)
adutorsion
Advance (nutritional
   beverage with iron)
advanced flap
advancement
adventitious
Advil (ibuprofen)
Aedes
aerated
aeration
aeriform
Aerobacter
aerobe
Aerobid (flunisolide)
Aerochamber (aerosol
   holding chamber)
aerodynamics
aerogram
aerography
Aerolate Liquid
   (theophylline,
   anhydrous)
Aeromonas
aerophagia
aerophobia
aerophore
Aeroplast dressing
aeropleura
Aeroseb-Dex
   (dexamethasone)
Aeroseb-HC
   (hydrocortisone)
aerosol
aerospace medicine
Aerosporin (polymyxin B
   sulfate)
aerotitis
Aesculapius

aesthesiometer
aesthetics
afebrile
affect
affection
affective
affective disorders
afferent
affiliation
affinity
afflux
afibrinogenemia
Afrin (oxymetazoline)
against medical advice
   (a.m.a.)
agalactia
agalorrhea
agamic
agammaglobulinemia
agar
Agar diffusion method
   (antibiotic
   sensitivity)
agathanasia
age (A)
agenesis
agenosomia
agent
Agent Orange
agerasia
agglomerate
agglutinable
agglutinant
agglutination
agglutinin
agglutinogen
aggression
agitation
agitographia
aglossia
aglossostomia
aglutition
aglycemia
aglycosuric
agnathia
Agnew-Verhoff incision
agnosia
agonist

agony
agoraphobia
agraffe
agranulocyte
agranulocytosis
agranuloplastic
agraphia
agromania
Ahlfeld's sign
AIDS-related complex
(ARC)
ailment
air conduction (AC)
air hunger
akaryocyte
akathisia
Akerlund deformity
akinesia
Akineton (bigeriden HCl)
ala
alalia
alanine aminotransferase
(ALT)
alar
alba
Alba-Lybe (appetite
stimulant and sorbitol)
Alba-Temp 300
(acetaminophen)
Albafort (iron and B
complex)
Albamycin
Albee operation
Albers-Schönberg disease
Albert's disease
Albert operation
Albert's suture, position
albicans
Albini's nodules
albinism
albino
albinuria
Albright's disease
albumin (alb)
albumin test
albumin-globulin ratio
(A/G)

Albuminar-5 (albumin
[human])
Albuminar-25 (albumin
[human])
albuminaturia
albuminimeter
albuminoid
albuminoreaction
albuminorrhea
albuminosis
albuminuria
Albutein 5% (albumin
[human])
Alcaligenes
Alcock's canal
alcohol
alcohol (isopropyl)
alcohol (methyl)
alcohol injection
alcohol syndrome, fetal
alcohol toxicology test
alcoholic
alcoholic psychosis
Alcoholics Anonymous (AA)
alcoholism
alcoholomania
alcoholometer
Aldactazide
(spironolactone with
hydrochlorothiazide)
Aldactone
(spironolactone)
aldehyde
Aldoclor (methyldopa-
chlorothiazide)
aldolase (ALD)
Aldomet (methyldopa)
Aldoril (methyldopa-
hydrochlorothiazide)
aldose
aldosterone
aldosterone test
aldosteronism
Aleppo boil
aleukocytosis
Alexander operation
Alexander-Adams operation
alexia

alexipyretic
Alfenta (alfentanil HCl)
algae
algesia
algolagnia
algolagnist
algometer
algophobia
algor
algos
algospasm
alicyclic
alien
alienate
alienation
alignment
aliment
alimentary
alimentary canal
alimentation
alimentotherapy
alinement
Alka-Mints
Alka-Seltzer
alkalemia
alkali
alkaline (alk)
alkaline phosphatase
   (ALP, alk phos)
alkalinity
alkalinuria
alkalization
alkalize
alkaloid
alkaloid drug screen
alkene
Alkeran (melphalan)
alkyl
alkylating agent
alkylation
allachesthesia
Allarton's operation
Allbee C-800 plus Iron
   Tablets
Allbee C-800 Tablets
Allbee With C Caplets
Allen's clamp, trocar
Allen-Doisy test

Allen-Doisy unit
Allerest
allergen
allergen immunotherapy
allergenic
allergic
allergist
allergy
allergy testing
allesthesia
Allingham's operation,
   speculum, ulcer
Allis' forceps
Allis-Ochsner forceps
Allison's suture
allochroism
allograft
allograft application
allokinesis
alloplasty
alloy
Alm's retractor
Almoor operation
aloe
alopecia
alpha cells
Alpha Keri (moisture rich
   body oil)
Alpha Plus (urea cycle
   intermediates)
alpha rays
alpha-1 antitrypsin
alpha-1-antitrypsin
   determination
alpha-adrenergic blocking
   agent
alpha-adrenergic receptor
alpha-fetoprotein (AFP)
alpha-globulins
alpha-rhythm
alphaREDISOL
   (hydroxocobalamine)
alphaREDISOL(vitamin B_{12})
Alphatrex (betamethasone
   dipropionate)
Alport's syndrome
Alramucil (psyllium
   hydrophilic mucilloid)

Altemeier operation
ALternaGEL (aluminum
hydroxide)
alternans
Alternaria
alternating days (alt
dieb)
alternating hours (alt
hor)
alternating nights (alt
noc)
alternating current (AC)
Alu-Tab
Aludrox (alumina and
magnesia)
alum
alum-precipitated toxoid
(APT)
aluminum
aluminum, blood
aluminum hydroxide
Alupent (metaproterenol
sulfate)
Alurate (aprobarbital)
Alurate Elixir
(aprobarbital)
alveobronchitis
alveolar
alveolar mucosa
alveolar nerve
alveolar nitrogen
equilibration
alveolar ridge
alveolectomy
alveoli
alveolitis
alveolodental
alveololingual
alveoloplasty
alveolotomy
alveolus
alymphocytosis
Alzheimer's disease
amalgam
amalgamator
amanita
amarthritis
amastia

amaurosis
amazia
Ambenyl (cough syrup)
Ambenyl-D (decongestant
cough formula)
ambidextrous
ambient
ambilateral
ambiopia
ambisexual
ambivalence
amblyaphia
amblyopia
ambon
Ambu bag
ambulance
ambulatory (AMB)
Amcap
Amcill
Amcort
ameba
amebiasis
amebic
amebic dysentery
amebicide
ameboid
ameboid movement
ameburia
amelia
amelioration
ameloblastoma
amelodentinal
amelus
Amen (medroxyprogesterone
acetate)
amenorrhea
amentia
American Cancer Society
(ACS)
americium (Am)
ametria
ametropia (Am)
Amicar (aminocaproic
acid)
amicrobic
amidase
Amidate (etomidate)
amide

amidin
amikacin sulfate
Amikin (amikacin sulfate)
amimia
amine
amino acid
Amino-Cerv
aminoacetic acid
aminoacidemia
aminoacidopathies
aminobenzene
aminobenzoic acid
aminocaproic acid
aminoglutethimide
aminoglycoside level test
aminoglycosides
aminohippurate, para
  (PAH)
aminohippurate sodium
aminohippurate test
aminohippuric acid,
  sodium
Aminolete (crystalline
  amino acid formulation)
aminolevulinic acid (ALA)
aminolevulinic acid test
aminolysis
Aminomine (excitatory
  neurotransmitters and
  L-glutamine)
aminopeptidase, cystine
aminopeptidase, leucine
Aminophyllin
  (aminophylline)
Aminoplex (crystalline
  amino acid formulation)
aminopurine
Aminosine (arginine-free
  amino acid formulation)
Aminostasis (branched
  chain amino acid
  formulation)
Aminotate (glycogenic
  amino acid formulation)
Aminoxin (pyridoxal-5'-
  phosphate)
Amipaque (metrizamide)
amitosis

amitotic
amitriptyline
  hydrochloride
Ammon operation
ammonia (NH_3)
ammonia test
ammoniemia
ammonium
amnesia
amniocentesis
amniography
amnioinfusion
amnion
amniorrhea
amniorrhexis
amnioscope
amnioscopy
amniotic
amniotic cavity
amniotic fluid
amniotic fluid analysis
amniotic sac
amniotome
amniotomy
amnitis
amobarbital
amoeba
amoralia
amorphism
amorphous
amount (amt)
amoxapine
amoxicillin
Amoxil (amoxicillin)
ampere
amphetamine
amphetamine screen
amphiarthrosis
Amphibia
amphicyte
amphidiarthrosis
amphitheater
amphocyte
amphoric
ampicillin
amplifier
amplitude
ampul

ampule (amp)
ampulla
ampullitis
amputation
amputation, abdominopelvic
amputation, above-elbow (AE)
amputation, above-knee (AK)
amputation, ankle
amputation, arm through carpals
amputation, arm through elbow
amputation, arm through forearm
amputation, arm through humerus
amputation, arm through shoulder
amputation, arm through wrist
amputation, arm upper
amputation, Batch-Spittler-McFaddin
amputation, below-knee (BK)
amputation, Boyd
amputation, Callander's
amputation, carpals
amputation, cervix
amputation, Chopart's
amputation, clitoris
amputation, Dieffenbach
amputation, Dupuytren's
amputation, ear, external
amputation, elbow
amputation, finger
amputation, foot
amputation, forearm
amputation, forefoot
amputation, forequarter
amputation, Gordon-Taylor
amputation, Gritti-Stokes
amputation, Guyon
amputation, hallux
amputation, hand

amputation, hindquarter
amputation, hip
amputation, humerus
amputation, interscapulothoracic
amputation, interthoracoscapular
amputation, King-Steelquist
amputation, Kirk
amputation, knee
amputation, Larry
amputation, leg
amputation, Lisfranc
amputation, lower limb
amputation, Mazet
amputation, metacarpal
amputation, metatarsophalangeal
amputation, midtarsal
amputation, nose
amputation, penis
amputation, Pirogoff's
amputation, root (tooth)
amputation, S.P. Rogers
amputation, shoulder
amputation, Sorondo-Ferre
amputation, supracondylar
amputation, supramalleolar
amputation, Syme's
amputation, thigh
amputation, thumb
amputation, toe
amputation, transcarpal
amputation, transmetatarsal
amputation, upper limb
amputation, wrist
amputee
amuck
Amussat's operation
amychophobia
amyelencephalia
amyelia
amyeloneuria
amyelotrophy
amygdalohippocampotomy

amygdalolith
amygdalopathy
amygdalotome
amygdalotomy
amylase
amylase, serum test
amylase, urine test
amylin
amyloid
amyloid disease
amyloid kidney
amyloid nephrosis
amyloidosis
amylolytic
amylose
amyocardia
amyosthenia
amyotonia
amyotrophic
amyotrophic lateral
  sclerosis (ALS)
Amytal (amobarbital)
amyxia
amyxorrhea
ANA-Kit (insect sting
  treatment kit)
anabasis
anabiosis
anabiotic
anabolism
anabolite
anacatharsis
anacidity
Anacin (aspirin)
anacrotic
anacrotic pulse
anacrotism
anadicrotic
anadicrotism
anadidymus
anadipsia
anadrenalism
Anadrol-50 (oxymetholone)
anaerobic
anagen
anakusis
anal
anal canal

analgesia
analgesic
analgia
analogous
analogue
analogy
Analpram-HC
analysis
analysis of variance
  (ANOVA)
analyze
analyzer
Anamid
anamnestic
anaphia
anaphoria
anaphrodisia
anaphylactic
anaphylactic shock
anaphylaxis
anaplasia
anaplastic
Anaprox (naproxen sodium)
anasarca
anaspadias
Anaspaz (L-hyoscyamine
  sulfate)
anastole
anastomose
anastomosis
anastomosis, accessory-
  facial nerve
anastomosis, accessory-
  hypoglossal nerve
anastomosis, aorta
  (descending)-pulmonary
  (artery)
anastomosis, aorta-renal
  artery
anastomosis, aorta-
  subclavian artery
anastomosis, aortoceliac
anastomosis,
  aorto(ilio)femoral
anastomosis,
  aortomesenteric
anastomosis, appendix

anastomosis,
arteriovenous
anastomosis, artery
(suture of distal to
proximal end)
anastomosis, artery with
bypass graft
anastomosis, artery with
excision of vessel
anastomosis, artery with
revision
anastomosis, bile ducts
anastomosis, bladder to
intestine
anastomosis, bladder with
ileum
anastomosis, bladder with
isolated segment of
intestine
anastomosis, bladder with
open loop of ileum
anastomosis, bowel
anastomosis,
bronchotracheal
anastomosis,
carotid-subclavian
artery
anastomosis, caval-
mesenteric vein
anastomosis, caval-
pulmonary artery
anastomosis,
cervicoesophageal
anastomosis,
colohypopharyngeal
anastomosis, common bile
duct
anastomosis, common
pulmonary trunk and
left atrium
anastomosis, cystic bile
duct
anastomosis, cystocolic
anastomosis, epididymis
to vas deferens
anastomosis,
esophagocolic

anastomosis,
esophagocolic with
antesternal or
antethoracic
anastomosis,
esophagocolic with
interposition
anastomosis,
esophagocologastric
anastomosis,
esophagoduodenal
anastomosis,
esophagoenteric
anastomosis,
esophagoesophageal
anastomosis,
esophagogastric
anastomosis, esophagus
with colon
anastomosis, esophagus
with gastrectomy
anastomosis, esophagus
with jejunum
anastomosis, esophagus
with small bowel
anastomosis,
facial-accessory nerve
anastomosis, facial-
hypoglossal nerve
anastomosis, fallopian
tube
anastomosis, for renal
dialysis
anastomosis, gallbladder
to hepatic ducts
anastomosis, gallbladder
to intestine
anastomosis, gallbladder
to pancreas
anastomosis, gallbladder
to stomach
anastomosis, hepatic duct
anastomosis, hypoglossal-
accessory nerve
anastomosis, hypoglossal-
facial nerve

anastomosis, ileal loop
to bladder
anastomosis, ileoanal
anastomosis, inferior
vena cava and portal
vein
anastomosis, internal
mammary artery to
coronary artery
anastomosis, internal
mammary artery to
double vessel
anastomosis, internal
mammary artery to
myocardium
anastomosis, intestine
(large-to-anus)
anastomosis, intestine
(large-to-rectum)
anastomosis, intestine
(small-to-anus)
anastomosis, intestine
(small-to-rectal stump)
anastomosis, intestine
(small-to-small)
anastomosis, intrahepatic
anastomosis,
intrathoracic vessel
anastomosis, kidney
(pelvis)
anastomosis, lacrimal sac
to conjunctiva
anastomosis, left-to-
right (systemic-
pulmonary artery)
anastomosis, lymphatic
(channel; peripheral)
anastomosis, mesenteric-
caval
anastomosis, mesocaval
anastomosis, nasolacrimal
anastomosis, nerve
(cranial; peripheral)
anastomosis, pancreas to
bile duct
anastomosis, pancreas to
gall bladder

anastomosis, pancreas to
intestine
anastomosis, pancreas to
jejunum
anastomosis, pancreas to
stomach
anastomosis, pleurothecal
(with valve)
anastomosis, portacaval
anastomosis, portal vein
to inferior vena cava
anastomosis, pulmonary
artery and superior
vena cava
anastomosis, pulmonary
vein and azygos vein
anastomosis, pulmonary-
aortic (Pott's)
anastomosis, pulmonary-
innominate artery
(Blalock)
anastomosis, pulmonary-
subclavian artery
(Blalock-Taussig)
anastomosis,
pyeloileocutaneous
anastomosis,
pyeloureterovesical
anastomosis, rectum,
rectal
anastomosis, renal vein
and splenic vein
anastomosis, renoportal
anastomosis,
salpingothecal
anastomosis, splenic to
renal vein
anastomosis, splenorenal
anastomosis,
subarachnoid-peritoneal
anastomosis,
subarachnoid-ureteral
anastomosis, subclavian-
aortic
anastomosis, superior
vena cava to pulmonary
artery

anastomosis, systemic-
pulmonary artery
anastomosis, thoracic
artery to coronary
artery
anastomosis, thoracic
artery to myocardium
anastomosis, ureter to
bladder
anastomosis, ureter to
colon
anastomosis, ureter to
ileal pouch
anastomosis, ureter to
ileum
anastomosis, ureter to
intestine
anastomosis, ureter to
skin
anastomosis,
ureterocalyceal
anastomosis, ureterocolic
anastomosis, urethra
(end-to-end)
anastomosis, vas deferens
anastomosis, veins
(mesenteric to vena
cava)
anastomosis, veins
(portal to inferior
vena cava)
anastomosis, veins
(splenic and renal)
anastomosis, ventricle,
ventricular
anastomosis,
ventriculocaval
anastomosis,
ventriculomastoid
anastomosis,
ventriculopleural
anastomosis, vesicle
anatomic
anatomical position
anatomist
anatomy
Anavar (oxandrolone)

Anbesol (antiseptic
anesthetic)
Ancef (cefazolin sodium)
anchorage
ancillary
Ancobon (flucytosine)
anconad
anconeus
anconitis
Ancylostoma
Ancylostomatidae
ancylostomiasis
ancyroid
Andernach's ossicles
Andersen's disease
Anderson operation
Andral's decubitus
Andrews' operation
andriatrics
Andro 100
androgen
androgenic
androgynoid
android
Android-5
(methyltestosterone
[tabs])
Android-10
(methyltestosterone
[tabs])
Android-25
(methyltestosterone
[buccal])
Android-F
(fluoxymesterone)
andrology
andromorphous
androphobia
androstane
androsterone
anecdotal evidence
Anectine (succinylcholine
chloride)
Anel's operation
Anel's probe
anemia
anencephalus
anencephaly

anergia
aneroid
Anestacon (lidocaine HCl)
anesthesia
anesthesiologist
anesthesiology
anesthetic
anesthetist
anesthetization
anesthetize
anetoderma
aneurysm
aneurysmectomy
aneurysmoplasty
aneurysmorrhaphy
aneurysmorrhaphy, with
 anastomosis
aneurysmorrhaphy, by
 clipping
aneurysmorrhaphy, by
 coagulation
aneurysmorrhaphy, by
 electrocoagulation
aneurysmorrhaphy, by
 excision or resection
aneurysmorrhaphy, with
 filipuncture
aneurysmorrhaphy, with
 graft replacement
aneurysmorrhaphy, Matas'
aneurysmorrhaphy, by
 methyl methacrylate
aneurysmorrhaphy, by
 suture
aneurysmorrhaphy, by
 wiring
aneurysmorrhaphy, by
 wrapping
aneurysmotomy
angel dust (PCP)
Angelucci's syndrome
angiasthenia
angiectasis
angiectomy
angiectomy, abdominal
 artery
angiectomy, abdominal
 vein

angiectomy, aorta
angiectomy, graft
 replacement
angiectomy, head and neck
angiectomy, intracranial
angiectomy, lower limb
 (artery; vein)
angiectomy, thoracic
 vessel
angiectomy, upper limb
 (artery; vein)
angiectomy, with
 anastomosis
angiectopia
angiitis
angina pectoris
anginal
anginiform
anginoid
anginophobia
angioataxia
angioblast
angioblastoma
angiocardiogram
angiocardiography
angiocardiography, carbon
 dioxide (negative
 contrast)
angiocardiography,
 combined right and left
 heart
angiocardiography, left
 heart
angiocardiography, right
 heart
angiocardiography,
 selective
angiocardiography, vena
 cava
angiocardiokinetic
angiocardiopathy
angiocarditis
angiocavernous
angiocholecystitis
angiocholitis
angiocrine
angiodystrophia
angioedema

angioendothelioma
angiofibroma
angiogenesis
angiogenic
angioglioma
angiogram
angiograph
angiography
angiography, basilar
angiography, brachial
angiography, by
  ultrasound
angiography, carotid
angiography, celiac
angiography, cerebral
angiography, coronary
angiography, eye
  (fluorescein)
angiography, femoral
angiography, heart
angiography, intra-
  abdominal
angiography, intracranial
angiography,
  intrathoracic vessels
angiography, lower
  extremity
angiography, neck
angiography, placenta
angiography, pulmonary
angiography, renal
angiography, transfemoral
angiography, upper
  extremity
angiography, veins
angiography, vertebral
angiohyalinosis
angiohypertonia
angiohypotonia
angioid
angioid streaks
angiokeratoma
angiokinetic
angioleukitis
angiolipoma
angiolith
angiology
angiolymphitis

angiolysis
angioma
angiomalacia
angiomatosis
angiomegaly
angiometer
angiomyocardiac
angiomyolipoma
angiomyoma
angiomyoneuroma
angionecrosis
angioneurectomy
angioneuromyoma
angioneurotic
angioneurotic edema
angioneurotomy
angionoma
angioparesis
angiopathology
angiopathy
angiophakomatosis
angioplasty
angiopoiesis
angiopressure
angiorrhaphy
angiorrhexis
angiosarcoma
angiosclerosis
angioscope
angioscopy
angioscotoma
angiosialitis
angiospasm
angiostaxis
angiostenosis
angiostrophy
angiosynizesis
angiotelectasis
angiotenic
angiotensin
angiotensin-converting
  enzyme (ACE)
angiotitis
angiotome
angiotomy
angiotomy, abdominal
  (artery; vein)
angiotomy, aorta

angiotomy, head and neck
angiotomy, intracranial
angiotomy, lower limb
  (artery; vein)
angiotomy, thoracic
angiotomy, upper limb
  (artery; vein)
angiotonic
angiotonin
angiotribe
angiotripsy
angiotrophic
angitis
angle
angor
angor animi
angstrom unit
angular
angulation
anhemolytic
anhepatia
anhidrosis
anhidrotic
anhydrase
anhydration
anhydremia
Anhydron (cyclothiazide)
anhydrous
anile
aniline
anima
animal
animation
animatism
animus
anion
anionic
aniridia
anisochromatic
anisocoria
anisocytosis
anisogamy
anisokaryosis
anisomastia
anisomelia
anisometropia
anisopia
anisotonic

ankle
ankyloblepharon
ankylochilia
ankylodactylia
ankyloglossia
ankylopoietic
ankylosed
ankylosis
ankylostoma
ankylotome
annectent
Annelida
annexa
annexitis
annexopexy
annular
annuloplasty
annulorrhaphy
annulus
anococcygeal
anodal
anodal closure
  contraction (ACC)
anodal opening
  contraction (AOC)
anodal opening sound
  (AOS)
anode
anodmia
anodontia
anodyne
anodynia
anoesia
anoetic
anomaloscope
anomaloscopy
anomalous
anomalous venous return
  repair
anomaly
anomia
anonychia
Anopheles
anophoria
anopia
anoplasty
Anoplura
anopsia

anorchidism
anorchism
anorectal
anorectal manometry
anorectal wall biopsy
anorectic
anorectoplasty
anorexia
anorexia nervosa
anorexigenic
anorganic
anorgasmy
anorthography
anorthopia
anorthosis
anoscope
anoscopy
anosigmoidoscopy
anosmatic
anosmia
anospinal
anostosis
anotia
anotropia
anovaginal
anovarism
anovesical
anovular
anoxemia
anoxia
anoxic
ansa
Anson-McVay operation
Anspor (cephradine)
Antabuse (disulfiram)
antacid
antagonist
antasthmatic
ante cibum (a.c.)
ante mortem
ante partum
antebrachium
antecardium
antecedent
antecubital
antecurvature
antefebrile
anteflect

anteflexion
antegrade
antelocation
antemetic
antenatal
Antepar
antepartal
anterior (ant, A)
anterior and posterior
  (A&P)
anterior chamber surgery
anterior pituitary
  extract (APE)
anteroexternal
anteroinferior
anterointernal
anteroposterior
anterosuperior
anteversion
anteverted
anthelmintic
Anthemis
anthocyanin
Anthomyia
anthophobia
Anthra-Derm (anthralin)
anthracemia
anthracene
anthracia
anthracoid
anthracosis
anthrax
anthropobiology
anthropogeny
anthropology
anthropometric
anthropometry
anthropopathy
anthropophilic
anthropozoonoses
anti-acetylcholine
  receptor antibody test
anti-DNA binding antibody
anti-DNA binding test
anti-G suit
anti-icteric
anti-immune
anti-infectious

anti-inflammatory
anti-isolysin
anti-Parkinson
anti-Rh immunoglobulin
  testing (RhoGAM type)
antiadrenergic
antiagglutinin
antiamebic
antiamylase
antianaphylaxis
antiandrogen
antianemic
antiantibody
antiantitoxin
antianxiety
antiarrhythmic
antibacterial
antibiogram
antibiosis
antibiotic
antibody
antibody deficiency
  syndrome (ADS)
antibrachium
anticardium
anticarious
anticatarrhal
anticathode
anticholinergic
anticholinesterase
anticipate
anticoagulant
anticodon
anticomplement
anticonvulsant
anticus
anticytotoxin
antidepressant
antidiabetic
antidiarrheal
antidiuretic
antidiuretic hormone
  (ADH)
antidiuretic substance
  (ADS)
antidotal
antidote
antidysenteric

antiembolic filter, vena
  cava
antiemetic
antienzyme
antiepileptic
antifebrile
antifibrinolysin
antifungal
antigalactic
antigen
antigen-antibody reaction
antigenic
antigenotherapy
antiglobulin
antigonorrheic
antihemolysin
antihemophilic
antihemophilic factor
  (AHF)
antihemophilic globulin
  (AHG)
antihemorrhagic
antihidrotic
antihistamine
antihypercholesterolemic
antihypertensive
antihypnotic
antilepsis
antileptic
antilethargic
antilipemic
Antilirium (physostigmine
  salicylate)
antiluetic
antily
antilymphocyte globulin
  (ALG)
antilymphocytic serum
  (ALS)
antilysin
antilysis
antilytic
antimalarial
antimanic
antimetabolite
antimetropia
antimicrobial
antimicrobial level

antimicrosomal antibody
test
Antiminth (pyrantel
pamoate)
antimitochondrial and
antismooth muscle test
antimitotic
antimonial
antimony
antinauseant
antineoplastic
antinephritic
antineuralgic
antineuritic
antinion
antinuclear
antinuclear antibody test
(ANA)
antiodontalgic
antiovulatory
antioxidant
antioxidation
antiparalytic
antiparasitic
antipepsin
antiperistalsis
antiperspirant
antiphobic treatment
antiplasmin
antiplastic
antiplatelet
antiprostaglandin
antiprotozoal
antipruritic
antipsychotic
antipyic
antipyretic
antipyrine
antirheumatic
antiscorbutic
antiseborrheic
antisecretory
antisepsis
antiseptic
antiserum
antisocial
antispasmodic

antistreptolysin O titer
(ASO)
antithyroglobulin
antibody test
antithyroglobulin test
antithyroid microsomal
test
antitoxin
antitropin
antituberculosis
antitussive
antivenin
Antivenin (Crotalidae)
Polyvalent (serum
globulins)
Antivenin (latrodectus
mactans)
Antivert (meclizine HCl)
antiviral
antrectomy
antrectomy, mastoid
antrectomy, maxillary
antrectomy, maxillary
(radical)
antrectomy, pyloric
antrocele
Antrocol
antronasal
antrophore
antroscope
antroscopy
antrostomy
antrotomy
antrotomy, Caldwell-Luc
(maxillary sinus)
antrotomy, exploratory
(nasal sinus)
antrotomy, intranasal
antrotomy, intranasal
(radical)
antrotomy, intranasal
with external approach
antrotomy, maxillary
(external)
antrotomy, maxillary
(radical)
antrotomy, maxillary
(simple)

antrotomy, maxillary with removal of membrane lining
antrotomy, with Caldwell-Luc approach
antrotomy, with removal of membrane lining
antropathy
antrum
antrum window operation
Anturane (sulfinpyrazone)
anuclear
anulus
anuresis
anuria
anus
Anusol-HC Cream
Anusol-HC Suppositories
anvil
anxiety
anxiolytic
aorta
aortal
aortectasia
aortectomy
aortic
aortic anomalies
aortic balloon pump
aortic insufficiency (AI)
aortic murmur
aortic regurgitation
aortic semilunar valve
aortic stenosis
aortic valve
aorticopulmonary window operation
aortitis
aortoceliac bypass graft
aortocoronary bypass
aortofemoral bypass graft
aortofemoral-popliteal bypass graft
aortogram
aortography
aortoiliac bypass graft
aortoiliac embolectomy
aortoiliac thrombectomy

aortoiliac thromboendarterectomy
aortoiliofemoral bypass graft
aortolith
aortomalacia
aortopathy
aortoplasty
aortopulmonary window
aortorenal bypass graft
aortorrhaphy
aortosclerosis
aortostenosis
aortotomy
aothrectomy, knee
apareunia
apathetic
apathic
apathy
apepsia
Apert's syndrome
aperture
apex
apexcardiogram
apexcardiogram (with ECG lead)
apexograph
Apgar score
aphagia
aphakia
aphasia
apheresis
aphonia
aphrasia
aphrenia
aphrodisia
aphrodisiac
aphthae
aphthongia
aphylactic
apiaotomy
apical-aortic conduit
apicectomy
apicetomy, lung
apicetomy, petrous pyramid
apicetomy, tooth (root)

apicetomy, tooth (root)
with root canal therapy
apicoectomy
apicolocator
apicolysis
apicostomy
apicostomy, alveolar
apinealism
apituitarism
aplasia
aplastic
aplastic anemia
Aplisol (tuberculin
purified protein
derivative, diluted)
Aplitest (tuberculin
purified protein
derivative)
apnea
apneumatic
apneusis
apobiosis
apocamnosis
apocope
apocrine
apodal
Apogen
apolipoprotein
immunoassay
Apomorphine hydrochloride
aponeurology
aponeurorrhaphy
aponeurosis
aponeurositis
aponeurotome
aponeurotomy
apophysis
apophysitis
apoplexia
apoplexy
apoptosis
aporepressor
apostasis
apothanasia
apothecaries
apothecary
apparatus
appendage

appendalgia
appendectomy
appendicectomy
appendices
appendicitis
appendicocecostomy
appendicolysis
appendicopathy
appendicostomy
appendicotomy
appendicular skeleton
appendix
apperception
apperceptive
appetite
appetizer
applanation
appliance
application
application, anti-shock
trousers
application, arch bars
(orthodontic)
application, arch bars
for immobilization
(fracture)
application, Barton's
tongs (skull)
application, Bryant's
traction
application, Buck's
traction
application, caliper
tongs (skull)
application, cast
(fiberglass)
application, cast
(plaster)
application, cast
(plastic)
application, cast (spica)
application, cervical
collar
application, clamp,
cerebral aneurysm
(Crutchfield;
Silverstone)

application, Cotrel's
 traction
application, crown
 (artificial)
application, Crutchfield
 tongs (skull)
application, Dunlop's
 traction
application, elastic
 stockings
application, electronic
 gaiter
application, forceps,
 with delivery
application, gallows
 traction
application, graft
application, gravity
 (G-) suit
application, intermittent
 pressure device
application, Lyman Smith
 traction
application, MAST
 (military anti-shock
 trousers)
application, Minerva
 jacket
application, neck support
 (molded)
application, obturator
 (orthodontic)
application, orthodontic
 appliance (wiring)
application, periodontal
 splint (orthodontic)
application, plaster
 jacket
application, pressure
 dressing
application, pressure
 dressing (Gibney
 bandage)
application, pressure
 dressing (Robert Jones'
 bandage)

application, pressure
 dressing (Shanz
 dressing)
application, prosthesis
 for missing ear
application, Russell's
 traction
application, skeletal
 traction
application, skin
 traction
application, spinal with
 Crutchfield tongs
application, spinal
 traction with caliper
 tongs
application, spinal
 traction with halo
 device
application, spinal with
 synchronous insertion
application, spinal with
 Vinke tongs
application, splint, for
 immobilization
 (plaster)
application, splint, for
 immobilization
 (pneumatic; tray)
application, Thomas'
 collar
application, Thomas'
 splint
application, traction
 (adhesive tape-skin)
application, Unna's paste
 boot
application,
 vasopneumatic device
application, Velpeau
 dressing
application, wound
 dressing
applicator
Appolito's operation
apposition

approach
approximal
approximate
apraxia
Apresazide (hydralazine
HCl and
hydrochlorothiazide)
Apresoline HCl
(hydralazine HCl)
Apresoline-Esidrix
(hydralazine HCl and
hydrochlorothiazide)
aprobarbital
apron
aptitude
aptyalism
AquaMEPHYTON
(phytonadione)
aquanaut
aquaphobia
Aquaphor (petrolatum,
mineral oil, mineral
wax, wool wax alcohol)
Aquaphyllin
(theophylline,
anhydrous)
Aquasol A (vitamin A)
Aquatar (therapeutic tar
gel)
aquatic
aqueduct
aqueous
aqueous humor
**Ar-Ex Hypo-Allergenic
Cosmetics**
Arachnida
arachnitis
arachnoid
arachnoid villi
arachnoiditis
Aralen Hydrochloride
(chloroquine HCl)
Aralen Phosphate
(chloroquine phosphate)
Aramine (metaraminol
bitartrate)
Aran-Duchenne disease
Arantius' body, nodule

arbor vitae
arborescent
arborization
arboviruses
arc
arc lamp
arcade
arcate
arch
architis
archocele
arciform
Arco-Lase (broad pH
spectrum digestant)
Arco-Lase Plus (broad pH
spectrum digestant)
arcus
ardent
ardor
area
Arelen phosphate
arenation
arenaviruses
areola
areola reconstruction
areolar glands
areolar tissue
areolitis
areometer
Arfonad (trimethaphan
camsylate)
Argasidae
argema
arginine
argon (Ar)
Argyll-Robertson pupil
Argyll-Robertson suture
Arias-Stella reaction
Aristocort
(triamcinolone)
Aristocort A
(triamcinolone
acetonide)
aristogenics
Aristospan (triamcinolone
hexacetonide)
Arlidin (nylidrin HCl)
Arlt's suture

arm
Arm-A-Med (isoetharine inhalation solution)
Arm-A-Med (metaproterenol sulfate inhalation)
Arm-A-Vial (sterile water, sodium chloride)
Armour Thyroid (thyroid)
armpit
Armsby's operation
aromatic
arrachement
arrectores pilorum
arrest
arrest, bone growth (epiphyseal)
arrest, bone growth (femur)
arrest, bone growth (fibula)
arrest, bone growth (humerus)
arrest, bone growth (radius)
arrest, bone growth (ulna)
arrest, bone growth (tibia)
arrest, bone growth by stapling
arrest, cardiac, induced (anoxic)
arrest, circulatory induced (anoxic)
arrest, hemorrhage (control)
arrhythmia
arrhythmic
arsenic (As)
arsenic testing
arsenical
arsenicism
arsine
Arslan operation
arsphenamine
Artane (trihexyphenidyl HCl)
artefact

arterectomy
arterial
arterial blood gases (ABGs)
arterial non-invasive peripheral diagnostic studies
arteriectasia
arteriectomy
arteriectomy, abdominal
arteriectomy, with anastomosis
arteriectomy, aorta
arteriectomy, with graft replacement
arteriectomy, head and neck
arteriectomy, intracranial
arteriectomy, lower limb
arteriectomy, thoracic
arteriectomy, upper limb
arteries
arterioatony
arteriocapillary
arteriogram
arteriography
arteriography, aorta
arteriography, basilar
arteriography, brachial
arteriography, carotid
arteriography, contrast
arteriography, coronary
arteriography, coronary double catheter (Ricketts and Abrams)
arteriography, coronary double catheter technique (Judkins)
arteriography, coronary single catheter (Sones)
arteriography, Doppler (ultrasonic)
arteriography, femoral
arteriography, fluoroscopic
arteriography, head and neck

arteriography, intra-
abdominal
arteriography,
intrathoracic
arteriography, lower
extremity
arteriography, placenta
arteriography, pulmonary
arteriography,
radioisotope
arteriography, renal
arteriography, retrograde
arteriography, superior
mesenteric artery
arteriography,
transfemoral
arteriography, ultrasound
arteriography, upper
extremity
arteriole
arterioles
arteriolith
arteriolitis
arteriology
arteriolonecrosis
arteriomotor
arterionecrosis
arteriopathy
arterioplasty
arteriopressor
arteriorrhaphy
arteriorrhexis
arteriosclerosis
arteriosclerotic
arteriosclerotic
cardiovascular disease
(ASCVD)
arteriosclerotic heart
disease (AHD)
arteriospasm
arteriotome
arteriotomy
arteriotomy, abdominal
arteriotomy, aorta
arteriotomy, head and
neck
arteriotomy, intracranial
arteriotomy, lower limb

arteriotomy, thoracic
arteriotomy, upper limb
arteriovenostomy
arterioversion
arteritis
artery
arthralgia
arthrectomy
arthrectomy, ankle
arthrectomy, elbow
arthrectomy, foot and toe
arthrectomy, hand and
finger
arthrectomy, hip
arthrectomy,
intervertebral disc
arthrectomy, semilunar
cartilage
arthrectomy, shoulder
arthrectomy, spine
arthrectomy, wrist
arthredema
arthritic
arthritis
arthritism
arthrobacterium
arthrocentesis
arthroclasia
arthrodesis
arthrodesis, ankle
arthrodesis, carporadial
arthrodesis,
cricoarytenoid
arthrodesis, elbow
arthrodesis, finger
arthrodesis, foot
arthrodesis, hip
arthrodesis, lumbosacral
arthrodesis, McKeever
arthrodesis,
metacarpocarpal
arthrodesis,
metacarpophalangeal
arthrodesis, midtarsal
arthrodesis, pantalar
arthrodesis, sacroiliac
arthrodesis, shoulder
arthrodesis, spinal

arthrodesis, subtalar
arthrodesis, tarsometatarsal
arthrodesis, tibiotalar
arthrodesis, toe
arthrodesis, triple
arthrodesis, wrist
arthrodynia
arthroendoscopy
arthrogram
arthrography
arthrogryposis
arthrolith
arthrology
arthrolysis
arthromeningitis
arthrometer
arthroneuralgia
Arthropan
arthropathology
arthropathy
arthrophyte
arthroplasty
arthroplasty, ankle
arthroplasty, carpals
arthroplasty, Carroll and Taber
arthroplasty, cup (hip)
arthroplasty, Curtis
arthroplasty, elbow
arthroplasty, finger(s)
arthroplasty, foot
arthroplasty, Fowler
arthroplasty, hand
arthroplasty, hip
arthroplasty, Kessler
arthroplasty, knee
arthroplasty, metacarpophalangeal joint
arthroplasty, shoulder
arthroplasty, temporomandibular
arthroplasty, toe
arthroplasty, wrist
arthropod
Arthropoda
arthropyosis

arthrorheumatism
arthrorrhagia
arthrosclerosis
arthroscope
arthroscopy
arthroscopy, ankle
arthroscopy, elbow
arthroscopy, finger
arthroscopy, foot
arthroscopy, hand
arthroscopy, hip
arthroscopy, knee
arthroscopy, shoulder
arthroscopy, toe
arthroscopy, wrist
arthrotome
arthrotomy
arthrotomy, with arthrography
arthrotomy, with arthroscopy
arthrotomy, injection of drug
arthrotomy, removal of prosthesis
articular
articulate
articulation
artifact
artificial
artificial insemination (AI)
artificial insemination by husband (AIH)
artificial insemination donor (AID)
artificial insemination homologous (AIH)
artificial kidney
artificial pace maker
artificial respiration
artificial rupture of membranes (ARM)
arytenoidectomy
arytenoidopexy
as desired (ad lib)
Asai operation
asbestos

asbestosis
Asbron G Elixir
Asbron G Inlay-Tabs
ascariasis
ascaricide
Ascaris
Aschheim-Zondek test (AZT)
Aschner's phenomenon, reflex, sign
Aschoff bodies, cells, nodules
ascites
Ascoli's reaction test
Ascomycetes
ascorbic acid (vitamin C)
Ascriptin with Codeine
ascus·
asemia
Asendin (amoxapine)
asepsis
aseptic
aseptic technique
asexual
ash
Ashford's mammilliplasty
Asiatic cholera
asocial
asoma
asonia
asparagine
Asparagus
aspartame
aspartate aminotransferase (AST)
aspect
aspergillin
aspergillosis
Aspergillus
aspermatic
aspermatism
aspermatogenesis
aspermia
asphyxia
asphyxiant
asphyxiate
asphyxiation
aspidium

aspirate
aspiration
aspiration, abscess
aspiration, anterior chamber, eye
aspiration, aqueous humor, eye
aspiration, ascites
aspiration, Bartholin's gland
aspiration, biopsy
aspiration, bladder
aspiration, bone marrow
aspiration, breast
aspiration, bronchus
aspiration, bursa
aspiration, calculus, bladder
aspiration, cataract with phacoemulsification
aspiration, cataract with phacofragmentation
aspiration, chest
aspiration, cisternal
aspiration, craniobuccal pouch
aspiration, craniopharyngioma
aspiration, cul-de-sac
aspiration, curettage, uterus
aspiration, cyst
aspiration, diverticulum, hypopharyngeal
aspiration, endotracheal
aspiration, extradural
aspiration, eye
aspiration, fallopian tube
aspiration, fascia
aspiration, gallbladder
aspiration, hematoma
aspiration, hydrocele
aspiration, hygroma
aspiration, hyphema
aspiration, hypophysis
aspiration, intracranial space

aspiration, joint
aspiration, kidney
aspiration, liver
aspiration, lung
aspiration, middle ear
aspiration, muscle
aspiration, nail
aspiration, nasal sinus
aspiration, nasotracheal
aspiration, orbit
aspiration, ovary
aspiration, percutaneous
aspiration, pericardium
aspiration, pituitary
aspiration, pleural
   cavity
aspiration, prostate
aspiration, Rathke's
   pouch
aspiration, seminal
   vesicle
aspiration, seroma
aspiration, skin
aspiration, soft tissue
aspiration, spermatocele
aspiration, spinal
   (puncture)
aspiration, spleen (cyst)
aspiration, subarachnoid
   space (cerebral)
aspiration, subcutaneous
   tissue
aspiration, subdural
   space (cerebral)
aspiration, tendon
aspiration, testis
aspiration, thymus
aspiration, thyroid
aspiration, trachea
aspiration, tunica
   vaginalis
aspiration, vitreous
aspirator
aspirin
asplenia
assault
assay
assessment

assessment, fitness to
   testify
assessment, mental status
assessment, nutritional
   status
assessment, personality
assessment, temperament
assessment, vocational
assimilate
assimilation
assistance
assistance, cardiac
assistance, cardiac with
   extracorporeal
   circulation
assistance, hepatic,
   extracorporeal
assistance, respiratory
   (endotracheal)
assistance, respiratory
   (mechanical)
association
assonance
astasia
astatine (At)
asteatosis
aster
asternal
asteroid
asthenia
asthenic
asthenometer
asthenope
asthenopia
asthenoxia
asthma
asthmatic
astigmatism (Ast)
astigmatometer
astigmatoscope
astigmatoscopy
astragalectomy
Astramorph PF (morphine
   sulfate)
astrict
astringent
astroblast
astroblastoma

astrocyte
astrocytoma
astroglia
asyllabia
asylum
asymmetrical tonic neck
  reflex (ATNR)
asymmetrogammagram
asymmetry
asymptomatic
asyndesis
asynovia
asyntaxia
asystole
Atabrine Hydrochloride
  (quinacrine HCl)
atactic
Atarax (hydroxyzine HCl)
ataraxia
atavism
ataxia
ataxiagram
ataxiagraph
ataxiameter
ataxiamnesia
ataxic
atelectasis
atelencephalia
atelia
atelocephaly
atelocheilia
ateloencephalia
ateloglossia
atelomyelia
athelia
atherogenic index
atheroma
atheromatosis
atheromatous
atheronecrosis
atherosclerosis
athetoid
athetosis
athlete's foot
Athrombin-K
athymia
athyreosis
athyroidemia

Ativan (lorazepam)
atlas
atlas-axis arthrodesis
atmosphere (atm)
atocia
atom
atomic
atomic number (at. no.)
atomic number (Z)
atomization
atomizer
atonic
atonicity
atony
atopic
atopy
atoxic
Atrac-Tain (therapeutic
  moisturizing cream)
atraumatic
atremia
atresia
atria
atrial
atrial baffle procedure
atrial fibrillation
atrial septal defect
atrial septectomy
atrichia
atrichosis
atriocommissuropexy
atrioplasty
atrioseotoplasty
atrioseptopexy
atrioseptostomytatriotome
atriotomy
atrioventricular (AV)
atrioventricular bundle
atrioventricular canal
  repair
atrioventricular node
atrioventriculostomy
atrium
Atrohist Sprinkle
  (antihistamine and
  decongestant)
Atroloc suture
Atromid-S (clofibrate)

atrophia
atrophic
atrophy
atropine sulfate
Atropisol
Atrovent (ipratropium
  bromide)
attachment
attachment, eye muscle
attachment, pedicle flap
attachment, pharyngeal
  flap
attachment, retina
attack
attendant
attention deficit
  disorder
attenuant
attenuate
attenuated
attenuation
Attenuvax (measles virus
  vaccine)
attic
atticitis
atticoantrostomy
atticoantrotomy
atticotomy
attitude
attraction
attrition
atypical
audible
audile
audioanesthesia
audiogenic
audiogram
audiologic function tests
audiologist
audiology
audiometer
audiometry
audiphone
audition
auditive
audito-oculogyric reflex
auditory
auditory canal

Auenbrugger's sign
Auerbach's plexus
Aufrecht's sign
augment
augmentation
augmentation, acetabular
augmentation, bladder
augmentation, breast
augmentation, buttock
augmentation, chin
augmentation, genioplasty
augmentation, mammoplasty
augmentation, outflow
  tract
augmentation, vocal
  cord(s)
Augmentin (amoxicillin/
  clavulanate potassium)
augnathus
aula
aura
aural
aural glomus tumor
aural polyp
Auralgan (antipyrine,
  benzocaine and
  glycerin)
Aureomycin
  (chlortetracycline HCl)
auriasis
auricle
auricular
auriculectomy
auriform
auris
auris sinistra (AS), left
  ear
auriscope
aurist
aurotherapy
auscultate
auscultation
auscultation and
  percussion (A&P)
Austin Flint murmur
Australian antigen
autacoid
autarcesis

autechoscope
autism
autoactivation
autoagglutination
autoagglutinin
autoallergy
autoamputation
autoanalysis
Autoanalyzer
autoantibodies, thyroid
autoantibody
autoantigen
autoantitoxin
autoblast
autocatalysis
autocatharsis
autoclasis
autoclave
autocytolysis
autodermic
autodigestion
autodiploid
autodrainage
autoerotism
autogenesis
autogenous
autograft
autohemagglutination
autohemic
autohemolysis
autohemotherapy
autoimmune disease
autoimmune hemolytic
  anemia (AIHA)
autoimmunity
autoimmunization
autoinfection
autoinfusion
autoinoculation
autointoxication
autoisolysin
autokinesis
autokinetic
autolesion
autologous
autolysin
autolysis

automated chemistry tests
automated data processing
  (nuclear medicine)
automated laboratory
  testing
automatic
automatism
autonomic
autonomic nervous system
autonomous
autonomy
autopathy
autophil
autophobia
autophony
autoplasty
Autoplex T (anti-
  inhibitor coagulant
  complex)
autopsy
autosmia
autosomatognosis
autosome
autostimulation
autosuggestibility
autotherapy
autotransfusion
autotransplant
autotransplantation
autotransplantation,
  adrenal tissue
autotransplantation,
  kidney
autotransplantation, lung
autotransplantation,
  ovary
autotransplantation,
  pancreatic tissue
autotransplantation,
  parathyroid tissue
  (heterotopic)
autotransplantation,
  parathyroid tissue
  (orthotopic)
autotransplantation,
  thyroid tissue
  (heterotopic)

autotransplantation,
  thyroid tissue
  (orthotopic)
autotransplantation,
  tooth
autovaccination
autovaccine
AV fistula repair
Avail (calcium,
  multivitamin and
  minerals for women)
AVC (sulfanilamide)
Avellis' paralysis
  syndrome
aversion therapy
aviation medicine
avidin
avirulent
avitaminosis
Avitene (microfibrillar
  collagen hemostat)
Avogadro's law
Avogadro's number
avoidance
avoirdupois measure
avulsion
avulsion, nerve (phrenic)
avulsion, nerve
  (sympathetic)
Axenfeld's suture
axenic
axial
axial skeleton
axilla
axillary (ax)
axillary artery
  embolectomy
axillary nerve injection
axillary vein
  thrombectomy
axillary-axillary bypass
  graft
axillary-brachial artery,
  repair

axillary-brachial
  embolectomy
axillary-femoral bypass
  graft
axillary-femoral-femoral
  bypass graft
axio-occlusal
axiobuccal
axioincisal (AI)
axiolabial
axiomesial
axiopulpal
axis
axolysis
axometer
axon
Ayerst Epitrate
  (epinephrine
  bitartrate)
Ayerza's syndrome
Aygestin (norethindrone
  acetate)
Azactam (aztreonam)
azalein
azidothymidine (AZT)
Azima battery
Azlin (azlocillin)
Azmacort (triamcinolone
  acetonide)
azo compounds
Azo Gantrisin
  (sulfisoxazole and
  phenazopyridine HCl)
azoic
azoospermia
Azorean disease
azote (Az)
azotemia
Azotobacter
azoturia
Azulfidine
  (sulfasalazine)
azure lunulae
azygography
azygos

B

B & O Supprettes
(belladonna and opium)
B cells
B-A-C (butalbital,
aspirin and caffeine)
B-C-Bid (B complex with
vitamin C)
b-CAPSA I Vaccine
(Haemophilus b
polysaccharide vaccine)
B-cell evaluation
B-lymphocytes (B cells)
B-scan
Babbitt metal
Babcock's operation
Babcock's test
Babès-Ernst granules
Babesia
babesiosis
Babinski's reflex
Babinski's sign
baby
Baby Anbesol (anesthetic
gel)
bacca
bacciform
Bachelor of Medical
Science (BMS)
Bachelor of Science (BS)
Baciguent (antibiotic
ointment)
Bacillaceae
bacillar
bacillary
bacille Calmette-Guérin
(BCG)
bacillemia
bacilli
bacilliform
bacillophobia
bacillosis
bacilluria

Bacillus
bacillus, abortus
bacillus, acid-fast
bacillus, Bang's
bacillus, Bordet-Gengou
bacillus, cereus
bacillus, cholerae
bacillus, comma
bacillus, diphtheria
bacillus, Döderlein's
bacillus, Ducrey's
bacillus, Flexner's
bacillus, Friedländer's
bacillus, gas
bacillus, Hansen's
bacillus, Klebs-Loeffler
bacillus, Koch-Weeks
bacillus, licheniformis
bacillus, melaninogenicus
bacillus, Morax-Axenfeld
bacillus, Pfeiffer's
bacillus, Shiga
bacillus, Sonne
bacillus, tubercle
bacillus, typhoid
back
backache
backbone
backflow
background radiation
bacteremia
bacteria
bacterial antagonism
bacterial resistance
bacterial smear
bactericidal
bactericide
bacterid
bacteriemia
bacterioagglutinin
bacteriocidal
bacteriocin
bacteriocinogen
bacterioclasis
bacteriogenic
bacteriohemagglutinin
bacteriohemolysin
bacterioid

bacteriologic
bacteriological
bacteriologist
bacteriology
bacteriolysin
bacteriolysis
bacteriolytic
bacteriophage
bacteriophagia
bacteriophytoma
bacterioprecipitin
bacterioprotein
bacteriopsonin
bacteriosis
bacteriostasis
bacteriostatic
bacteriotoxic
bacteriotropin
bacteristatic
bacterium
bacteriuria
bacteroid
Bacteroides
Bactine
Bactrim (trimethoprim and
  sulfamethoxazole)
baculiform
Baffle, atrial or
  interatrial
Baffle technique
bag, of waters
bagassosis
baker
baker leg (knock-knee;
  genu valgum)
Baker's cyst
BAL in Oil Ampules
  (dimercaprol)
balance, acid-base
balance, analytical
balance, electrolyte
balance, fluid
balance, nitrogen
balanic
balanitis
balanoblennorrhea
balanocele
balanoplasty

balanoposthitis
balanopreputial
balanorrhagia
balanorrhea
balantidial
balantidiasis
Balantidium
balanus
baldness
Baldy-Webster operation
Balkan frame
Balke test
ball
ball, of foot
ball, of hair
ball, of thumb
Ball operation
ball, thrombus
ball-and-socket joint
ball-valve action
ballism
ballismus
ballistics
ballistocardiography
ballistocardiograph
balloon pump, intra-
  aortic
balloon systostomy
  (atrial)
balloon
balloon angioplasty
balloon atrial septectomy
balloon counterpulsation
balloon insertion, intra-
  aortic
balloon occlusion
balloon pulmonary
  valvotomy
ballooning
ballottable
ballottement
balm
Balmex
Balneol (perianal
  cleansing lotion)
balneology
balneotherapeutics
balneotherapy

Balnetar (water-
dispersible emollient
tar)
balsam
Balser's fatty necrosis
bamboo spine
Bancap HC (hydrocodone
bitartrate and
acetaminophen)
Bancroft's filariasis
band
bandage
bandage, abdomen
bandage, Ace
bandage, amputation-stump
bandage, ankle
bandage, axilla
bandage, back
bandage, Barton's
bandage, breast
bandage, butterfly
bandage, buttocks
bandage, capeline
bandage, chest
bandage, circular
bandage, cohesive
bandage, cravat
bandage, crucial
bandage, demigauntlet
bandage, ear
bandage, elastic
bandage, Esmarch's
bandage, eye
bandage, figure-of-eight
bandage, finger
bandage, foot
bandage, forearm
bandage, four-tailed
bandage, Fricke's
bandage, Galen's
bandage, Garretson's
bandage, groin
bandage, hand
bandage, head
bandage, heel
bandage, hip
bandage, Hippocrates'
bandage, Hueter's

bandage, immovable
bandage, impregnated
bandage, knee
bandage, knotted
bandage, leg
bandage, Maissonneuve's
bandage, many-tailed
bandage, Martin's
bandage, neck
bandage, oblique
bandage, plaster
bandage, postoperative
bandage, pressure
bandage, protective
bandage, quadrangular
bandage, recurrent
bandage, reversed
bandage, roller
bandage roller
bandage, rubber
bandage, scultetus
bandage, shoulder
bandage, spica
bandage, spiral reverse
bandage, suspensory
bandage, T.
bandage, tailed
bandage, Theden's
bandage, toe
bandage, triangular
bandage, Velpeau's
banding, pulmonary artery
Bandl's ring
bandly leg (bowleg; genu
varum)
bank
bank, blood
bank, sperm
Bankart operation
Banti's syndrome
Banting, Sir Frederick
Grant
bar, median
baragnosis
barber's itch
barbiturate
barbiturate toxicology
test

barbotage
barbula hirci
Bardenheurer operation
baresthesia
baresthesiometer
bariatrics
barium enema (BE,BaE)
barium meal
barium sulfate
barium swallow
barium test
bark
Barlow's disease
barognosis
baroreceptor
baroreflexes
baroscope
barosinusitis
barospirator
barotaxis
barotitis
barotrauma
barotropism
Barr bodies, test
Barr body
barrel chest
barren
barrier
barrier, blood-brain
Barsky operation
Bartholin's cyst
Bartholin's ducts
Bartholin's glands
bartholinitis
Barton, Clara
Bartonella
bartonellosis
Bartter's syndrome
Baruch's law
baryglossia
barylalia
baryphonia
basad
basal
basal energy expenditure
   (BEE)
basal ganglia
basal lamina

basal metabolic rate
   (BMR)
basal metabolism
basal ridge
basal temperature chart
Basaljel (basic aluminum
   carbonate gel)
base
baseball finger
Basedow's disease
baseline
basement lamina
basement membrane
baseplate
basial
basiarachnoiditis
basic
Basic Preventive
   (multiple vitamin-
   mineral-trace elements)
basic salt
basicranial axis
Basidiomycetes
basifacial axis
basihyal
basilar
basilar membrane
basilateral
basilemma
basilic
basilic vein
basiloma
basioccipital bone
basion
basiotripsy
basiphobia
basirhinal
basis
basisphenoid
basket
basket cells
Basle Nomina Anatomica
   (BNA)
basocyte
basophil
basophil count, direct
basophile
basophilia

basophilic
basophilism
basophilism, pituitary
basophobia
bass deafness
Bassett operation
Bassini's operation
bastard
Batch-Spittler-McFadden
  operation
bath
bath, acid
bath, air
bath, alcohol
bath, alkaline
bath, alum
bath, antipyretic
bath, aromatic
bath, astringent
bath, bed
bath, bland
bath, blanket
bath, box
bath, bran
bath, brine
bath, bubble
bath, carbon dioxide
bath, cold
bath, colloid
bath, continuous
bath, contrast
bath, earth
bath, emollient
bath, foam
bath, foot
bath, full
bath, glycerin
bath, herb
bath, hip
bath, hot
bath, hot air
bath, hyperthermal
bath, kinetotherapeutic
bath, lukewarm
bath, medicated
bath, milk
bath, mud
bath, mustard

bath, Nauheim
bath, needle
bath, neutral
bath, neutral sitz
bath, oatmeal
bath, oxygen
bath, paraffin
bath, powdered borax
bath, saline
bath, sauna
bath, seawater
bath, sedative
bath, sheet
bath, shower
bath, sitz
bath, sponge
bath, starch
bath, steam
bath, stimulating
bath, sulfur
bath, sun
bath, sweat
bath, therapeutic
bath, towel
bath, vapor
bath, whirlpool
bathophobia
bathroom privileges (BRP)
bathyanesthesia
bathycardia
bathyesthesia
bathyhyperesthesia
bathyhypesthesia
battered child syndrome
battery
Baudelocque's diameter
Baudelocque's method
Baumé scales
bay
Bayer Aspirin
  (acetylsalicylic acid)
Bayes' theorem
bayonet leg
Bazin's disease
BCG immunization
BCG Vaccine (tuberculosis
  immunizing agent)
bdellometer

beaded
beads, rachitic
beaker
beam
bearing down
beat
beat, apex
beat, capture
beat, ectopic
beat, escape
beat, forced
beat, premature
Beau's lines
Bechterew's reflex
Beck operation
Beck-Jianu operation
Beclovent (beclomethasone
  dipropionate)
Beconase (beclomethasone
  dipropionate)
Beconase AQ
  (beclomethasone
  dipropionate,
  monohydrate)
bed
bed, air
bed, air-fluidized
bed, capillary
bed, circular
bed, float
bed, flotation
bed, fracture
bed, Gatch
bed, hydrostatic
bed, metabolic
bed, nail
bed, open
bed, recovery
bed, surgical
bed, tilt
bed, water
bed blocking
bed blocks
bedbug
bedfast
bedlam
Bednar's aphthae
bedpan

bedrest
bedridden
bedsore
bedwetting (enuresis)
Beelith (magnesium oxide
  and pyridoxine HCl)
Beer's operation
bee sting
beeswax
beeturia
before meals (a.c.)
behavior
behavior modification
behaviorism
Behçet's syndrome
bejel
Bekesy audiometry
Bekhterev's reflex
bel
belch
belching
belenmoid
Bell, Sir Charles
Bell's law
Bell's nerve
Bell's palsy
Bell-Magendie's law
bell-metal resonance
Belladenal
Belladenal-S
Bellergal-S
Bellini's tubules
Bellocq's cannula
belly
belly ache
belly button
belonephobia
belonoid
belonoskiascopy
below elbow (BE)
below knee (BK)
Belsey IV procedure
Belsey operation
Beminal 500 (vitamin B
  complex with vitamin C)
Ben-Gay (analgesic
  product)

Benadryl (diphenhydramine HCl)
Bence Jones protein
Bender gestalt visual motor test
Bender Visual-Motor Gestalt
bends
Benedict's solution
Benedict's test
Benedikt's syndrome
Benemid (probenecid)
Benenenti operation
benign
benign prostatic hypertrophy (BPH)
Bennett double-ring splint
Bennett fracture
Bennett quadriceps plasty
Bennett respirator
Benoquin (monobenzone)
Bensulfoid Lotion
Bensulfoid Tablets and Powder
bentonite
Bentyl (dicyclomine HCl)
Benzac (benzoyl peroxide)
5 Benzagel (benzoyl peroxide)
10 Benzagel (benzoyl peroxide)
Benzamycin (erythromycin-benzoyl peroxide)
benzene (C_6H_6)
benzestrol
benzidine
benzin
benzine
benzoate
benzodiazepine
benzoic acid
benzoin
benzol
benzyl
beolocator
Beraud's valve
berdache

beriberi
Berke operation
Berkefeld filter
berkelium (Bk)
Bernard's aneurysm
Bernard's duct
Bernard's glandular layer
Bernstein test (perfusion test)
Berocca Parenteral Nutrition (vitamins)
Berocca Plus Tablets (vitamins and minerals)
Berocca Tablets (vitamins)
Bertin, columns of
Bertin's ligament
berylliosis
beryllium (Be)
bestiality
beta
beta cells
beta particles, rays
beta subunit
beta-2 microglobulin
beta-adrenergic blocking agent
beta-adrenergic receptor
beta-glucosidase
beta-lactamase resistance
betacism
Betadine (povidone-iodine)
Betatrex (betamethasone valerate)
betatron
Betoptic (betaxolol HCl)
Betz cells
bezoar
bezoar, balloon
biarticular
Biavax (rubella and mumps virus vaccine)
bibasic
bibliomania
bibliotherapy
bibulous
bicameral

bicapsular
bicarbonate (HCO_3)
bicarbonate excretion
bicarbonate loading test
bicellular
biceps
biceps, brachii
biceps, femoris
biceps reflex
Bichat, Marie François X
Bichat's canal
Bichat's fat ball
Bichat's fissure
Bichat's ligament
Bichat's tunic
bichloride of mercury
  ($HgCl_2$)
Bicillin C-R (penicillin
  G benzathine and
  penicillin G procaine)
Bicillin L-A (penicillin
  G benzathine)
bicipital
Bicitra (sodium citrate
  and citric acid)
BiCNU (carmustine [BCNU])
biconcave
biconvex
bicornate
bicornis
bicornis uterus
bicoronal
bicorporate
bicuspid
bicuspid tooth
bicuspidization of heart
  valve (aortic)
bicuspidization of heart
  valve (mitral)
bicycle dynamometer
bicycle ergometer
bicycle exercise test
bidet
biduous
Bielschowsky disease
bifacial
bifemoral bypass graft
bifid

bifid digit
bifid spine
bifid tongue
bifocal
bifocal glasses
bifurcate
bifurcated
bifurcation
bifurcation, bone
Bigelow operation
bigemina
bigeminal
bigeminal pulse
bigeminum
bigeminy
bilabe
bilateral
bilateral symmetry
bilateralism
bile
bile acids
bile acids, blood
bile duct
bile pigments
bile salts
Bilezyme (bile acids and
  digestive enzymes)
Bilharzia
bilharzial
bilharziasis
bilharzic
biliary
biliary calculus
biliary colic
biliary tract
bilicyanin
biliflavin
bilifulvin
bilifuscin
biligenesis
biligenetic
biligenic
bilihumin
bililite therapy
bilineurine
bilious
bilious fever
biliousness

biliprasin
bilirachia
bilirubin
bilirubin, indirect test
bilirubin, total and
  direct test
bilirubin, urine
bilirubinate
bilirubinemia
bilirubinuria
biliuria
biliverdin
billion
Billroth I operation
Billroth II operation
bilobate
bilobular
bilocular
Biltricide (praziquantel)
bimalleolar ankle
  fracture
bimanual
bimaxillary
bimodal
binary
binary acid
binary digit
binary gas
binaural
binder
binder, abdominal
binder, chest
binder, double-T
binder, obstetrical
binder, Scultetus
binder, T.
binder, towel
binocular
binocular microscopy
binocular vision
binomial
binotic
binovular
binuclear
binucleate
bioassay
bioastronautics
bioavailability

Biocal 250
biocatalyst
biochemical marker
biochemistry
biochemorphology
biocide
bioclimatology
biocolloid
biodegradable
biodegradation
biodynamics
bioelectronics
bioenergetics
biofeedback
biofeedback,
  psychotherapy
biofeedback training
biogenesis
biogenetic
biogenic amines
biokinetics
biologic
biologic half-life
biological
biological degradation
biological rhythms
biological warfare
biologically false
  positive (BFP)
biologicals
biologist
biology
bioluminescence
biolysis
biolytic
biomass
biome
biomechanics
biomedical
biomedical engineering
biometeorology
biometrics
biometry
biomicroscope
bion
bionergy
bionics
bionomics

bionomy
bionosis
biophagism
biophagy
biophotometer
biophysics
bioplasm
biopsy (Bx)
biopsy, cone
biopsy, excisional
biopsy, incisional
biopsy, needle
biopsy, punch
biopsy, sternal
biopterin
biorhythms
bios
bioscience
bioscopy
biospectrometry
biospectroscopy
biosphere
biostatics
biostatistics
biosynthesis
Biot's breathing
biota
biotaxis
biotaxy
biotelemetry
biotics
biotin
biotomy
biotoxin
biotransformation
biotype
biovular twins
bipara
biparasitic
biparental
biparietal
biparous
bipartite patella
biped
bipenniform
biperforate
biperiden hydrochloride
Biphetamine (amphetamine)

bipolar
biramous
bird breeder's lung
birefractive
birefringent
birth, multiple
birth canal
birth certificate
birth, complete
birth control
birth, cross
birth defect
birth, dry
birth injury
birth, live
birth palsy
birth, premature
birth rate
birthing room deliveries
birthmark
bis in die (twice a day;
 b.i.d.)
bisacromial
Bischoff laminectomy
Bischoff operation
biscupid valve
bisection
bisection, hysterectomy
bisection, ovary
bisection, stapes foot
 plate
Bisenberger operation
bisexual
bisferious
bisiliac
bismuth (Bi)
bismuth poisoning
bismuth subcarbonate
bismuth, subgallate
bismuth, subnitrate
bistoury
bisulfate
bite
bite, balanced
bite, close
bite, closed
bite, end-to-end
bite, open

bite, over
bite, under
bite-wing radiograph
bitelock
bitemporal
biteplate
bites
biting insect antigen
Bitot's spots
bitrochanteric
bitter
bituminosis
biuret
biuret test
bivalent
bivalving (cast)
biventer
biventral
bizygomatic
Bjerrum's screen
Bjerrum's sign
black
black death
black eye
black lung
black measles
black vomit
black widow
blackhead (comedo)
blackout
blackwater fever
bladder
bladder, atony of
bladder, autonomous
bladder drill
bladder, exstrophy of
bladder, hypertonic
bladder, irritable
bladder, nervous
bladder, neurogenic
bladder, spastic
bladder training
bladder, urinary
bladder worm
Blalock operation
Blalock-Hanlon operation
Blalock-Taussig operation
blanch

bland
bland diet
Blandin's glands
blanket, hypothermia
Blascovic operation
blast
blastema
blastid
blastocele
blastochyle
blastocoele
blastocyst
blastocyte
blastocytoma
blastoderm
blastodermic vesicle
blastodisk
blastogenesis
blastokinin
blastolysis
blastoma
blastomere
blastomerotomy
Blastomyces
Blastomyces brasiliensis
Blastomyces dermatitidis
blastomycete
blastomycin
blastomycosis
blastomycosis, keloidal
blastomycosis, North
    American
blastomycosis skin test
blastomycosis, South
    American
blastopore
blastospore
blastula
Blatta
Blatta germanica
Blatta orientalis
bleaching powder
bleb
bleeder
bleeder's disease
bleeding
bleeding, arterial
bleeding, breakthrough

bleeding, occult
bleeding time
bleeding time test
bleeding, venous
blennadenitis
blennemesis
blennogenic
blennogenous
blennoid
blennometritis
blennophthalmia
blennorrhagia
blennorrhea
blennorrhea, inclusion
blennorrhea, neonatorum
blennostasis
blennostatic
blennothorax
blennuria
Blenoxane (bleomycin
  sulfate)
blepharadenitis
blepharal
blepharectomy
blepharedema
blepharism
blepharitis
blepharitis, angularis
blepharitis, ciliaris
blepharitis, marginalis
blepharitis, parasitica
blepharitis, squamosa
blepharitis, ulcerosa
blepharoadenitis
blepharoadenoma
blepharoatheroma
blepharochalasis
blepharochromhidrosis
blepharoclonus
blepharoconjunctivitis
blepharodiastasis
blepharoncus
blepharopachynsis
blepharopathia
blepharophimosis
blepharoplast
blepharoplasty
blepharoplegia

blepharoptosis
blepharopyorrhea
blepharorrhaphy
blepharorrhea
blepharospasm
blepharosphincterectomy
blepharostat
blepharostenosis
blepharosynechia
blepharotomy
blind
blind rehabilitation
  therapy
blind spot
blindness, amnesic color
blindness, color
blindness, cortical
blindness, day
blindness, eclipse
blindness, hysterical
blindness, letter
blindness, night
blindness, psychic
blindness, snow
blindness, transient
blindness, word
blink
blink reflex
blister
blister, blood
blister, fever
blister, fly
bloated
Blocadren (timolol
  maleate)
block, air
block, atrioventricular
block, caudal
block, celiac ganglion or
  plexus
block, dissection
  (breast)
block, dissection
  (bronchus)
block, dissection
  (larynx)
block, dissection (lymph
  nodes)

block, dissection (neck)
block, dissection (vulva)
block, ear
block, epidural, spinal
block, field
block, gasserian ganglion
block, heart
block, intercostal nerves
block, intrathecal
block, nerve (cranial;
  peripheral)
block, neuromuscular
block, paravertebral
block, paravertebral
  stellate ganglion
block, sinoatrial
block, spinal
block, spinal nerve root
block, stellate
  (ganglion)
block, subarachnoid,
  spinal
block, sympathetic nerve
block, trigeminal nerve
block, ventricular
blockade
blocking
blocking factor
blood (Bld)
blood alcohol
  concentration (BAC)
blood, autotransfusion
blood bank
blood cell
blood cell casts
blood clot
blood clot lysis time
blood, clotting of
blood component
blood, cord
blood corpuscles
blood count
blood crossmatch
blood crossmatching
blood, defibrinated
blood donor
blood, duodenal, gastric
  contents

blood dust
blood flow study,
  Doppler-type
blood gas analysis
blood gases
blood group (ABO)
blood loss study, GI
blood, occult
blood osmolality
blood patch, spine
  (epidural)
blood platelets
blood poisoning
blood, precipitin test
blood pressure (BP,B/P)
blood pressure, central
blood pressure, diastolic
blood pressure, direct
  measurement of
blood pressure, indirect
  measurement of
blood pressure, mean
blood pressure monitor
blood pressure, negative
blood pressure, normal
blood pressure, systolic
blood shunting
blood, sludged
blood smear
blood sugar (BS)
blood test
blood transfusion
blood type and cross-
  matching test
blood typing
blood, unit of
blood urea nitrogen (BUN)
blood vessels
blood viscosity
blood volume
blood warmer
blood withdrawal
  (sampling)
blood-brain barrier
bloodless
bloodletting
bloodshot
bloodstream

bloody sweat
bloody weeping
blotch
Blount operation
blowfly
blowout fracture
blowpipe
Blubor (astringent
  soaking solution)
blue
blue baby
bluebottle flies
Blumberg's sign
Blumenbach's clivus
blush
Blyth's test
Boari operation
Boas' point
Bochdalek's ganglion
Bodo
body
body, acetone
body, amygdaloid
body, aortic
body, asbestosis
body, Barr
body, basal
body, carotid
body cast
body cavities
body, chromaffin
body, ciliary
body, coccygeal
body composition
body fluid
body, foreign
body, geniculate, lateral
body, geniculate, medial
body, Hensen's
body image
body, inclusion
body, ketone
body language
body, malpighian
body, mammillary
body mechanics
body, medullary
body, olivary

body, pacchionian
body, perineal
body, pineal
body, pituitary
body plethysmography
body, polar
body, postbranchial
body, psammoma
body, restiform
body section radiography
body snatching
body strapping
body, striate
body substance isolation
  (BSI)
body surface area (BSA)
body, trachoma
body type
body, vertebral
body, vitreous
body, wolffian
bodies, Aschoff
bodies, chromophilous
bodies, Donovan
bodies, Leishman-Donovan
bodies, Negri
bodies, Nissl
Boeck's sarcoid
Boerhaave syndrome
Bohler reduction
boil
boiling
boiling point
bolometer
bolus
bombardment
bombesin
bond
bonding, mother-infant
bone
bone age
bone age studies
bone, ankle
bone autograft
bone, breast
bone, brittle
bone, cancellous
bone, cartilage

bone, cavalry
bone cell
bone, collar
bone, compact
bone conduction hearing
  device
bone, cotyloid
bone, cranial
bone cyst
bone density studies
bone, dermal
bone, endochondral
bone graft
bone imaging
bone, incarial
bone, innominate
bone, intracartilaginous
bone, ivory
bone length studies
bone, marble
bone marrow
bone marrow aspiration
bone marrow biopsy
bone marrow transplant
bone, membrane
bone, perichondrial
bone, periosteal
bone, ping pong
bone, replacement
bone, sesamoid
bone, spongy
bone survey
bone, sutural
bone, thigh
bone, wormian
bonelet
Bonine (meclizine HCl)
Bonney operation
Bontril PDM
  (phendimetrazine
  tartrate)
bony
booster
boot
borate
borated
borax
borborygmus

border
border brush
Bordet-Gengou bacillus
Bordetella
Bordetella pertussis
boredom
boric acid (H_3BO_3)
boric acid poisoning
borism
Bornholm disease
boroglycerin
boroglycerol
boron (B)
Borrelia
Borrelia duttonii
Borrelia recurrentis
Borrelia vincentii
Borthen operation
boss
bosselated
Bost operation
Boston arm
Bosworth operation
Botallo's duct
botfly
both ears (AU)
both eyes (OU)
botryoid
botuliform
botulin
botulinic acid
botulism
bouba
Bouchut's respiration
Bouchut's tubes
bougie
bouillon
bouquet
bourdonnement
boutonniere
boutonniere deformity
boutons terminaux
bovine
bowel
bowel movement (BM)
bowleg (genu varum)
Bowman's capsule
Bowman's glands

Bowman's membrane
box splint
box-note
boxing
Boyd operation
Boyer's bursa
Boyer's cyst
Boyle's law
Bozeman-Fritsch catheter
brace
brachia
brachial
brachial artery
brachial cleft cyst
brachial plexus
brachial veins
brachialgia
brachialis
brachiocephalic
brachiocrural
brachiocubital
brachiocyllosis
brachioradialis
brachium
brachium, conjunctivum
brachium, pontis
Bracht maneuver
brachybasia
brachycardia
brachycephalic
brachycephalous
brachycheilia
brachydactylia
brachygnathia
brachymetropia
brachymorphic
brachyphalangia
brachystasis
brachytherapy
Bradford frame
bradyacusia
bradyarrhythmia
bradycardia
bradycrotic
bradydiastole
bradyecoia
bradyesthesia
bradyglossia

bradykinesia
bradykinin
bradylalia
bradylexia
bradylogia
bradyphagia
bradyphrasia
bradyrhythmia
bradyspermatism
bradysphygmia
bradystalsis
bradytachycardia
bradytocia
bradyuria
braille
brain
brain death
brain echogram
brain edema
brain fever
brain sand
brain scan
brain stem
brain swelling
brain tumor
Brain's reflex
brainstem auditory evoked
    potential (BAEP)
brainstem evoked response
    recording (BERR)
brainstem magnetic
    resonance imaging
    (BMRI)
brainstorm
brainwashing
bran
branch
branchial
branchial arches
branchial clefts
branchial grooves
branchial muscles
branchiogenic
branchiogenous
branchioma
branchiomeric
Brandt-Andrews maneuver
brandy

Branhamella (Neisseria)
  catarrhalis
brash
brass poisoning
Brauer operation
brawny induction
Braxton Hicks sign
break
breakage syndromes,
  chromosome analysis
breakbone fever
breast
breast, chicken
breast feeding
breast pump
breast self-examination
  (BSE)
breath
breath hydrogen test
breathing, asthmatic
breathing, bronchial
breathing, cog-wheel
breathing, continuous
  positive-pressure
breathing, intermittent
  positive-pressure
breathing, shallow
breatholyzer
breech
breech extraction
breech presentation
breeze
Breeze Mist (foot powder)
bregma
bregmatic
bregmocardiac reflex
brei
Breisky's disease
Brenner's tumor
Brethaire (terbutaline
  sulfate)
Brethancer (spacer
  inhaler)
Brethine (terbutaline
  sulfate)
Bretylol (bretylium
  tosylate)
Brevibloc (esmolol HCl)

brevicollis
Brevicon (norethindrone
  and ethinyl estradiol)
brevilineal
Brevital Sodium
  (methohexital sodium)
Brexin E.X.
  (pseudoephedrine HCl
  and guaifenesin)
Brexin
  L.A.(chlorpheniramine
  maleate,
  pseudoephedrine HCl)
Bricanyl (terbutaline
  sulfate)
Bricker operation
bridge
bridgework
bridgework, fixed
bridgework, removable
bridle
Bright's disease
brim
brisement
Brisement operation
Brissaud's reflex
Bristow operation
British antilewisite
  (BAL)
British Medical
  Association (BMA)
British Pharmacopoeia
  (BP)
British thermal unit
  (BTU)
brittle diabetes
broach
broad ligament
Broadbent's sign
Broca's area
Brock operation
Brockman operation
Brodie abscess
bromelains
Bromfed (brompheniramine
  maleate and
  pseudoephedrine HCl)
bromhidrosis

bromide
bromide poisoning
bromides
bromidrosiphobia
bromidrosis
bromine (Br)
brominism
bromism
bromoderma
bromoiodism
bromomania
bromomenorrhea
bromopnea
Brompton's cocktail
bromsulphalein (BSP)
bronchadenitis
bronchi
bronchial
bronchial brush biopsy
bronchial crises
bronchial glands
bronchial tree
bronchial tubes
bronchial washing
bronchiarctia
bronchiectasis
bronchiloquy
bronchiocele
bronchiogenic
bronchiole
bronchiolectasis
bronchiolitis
bronchiolus
bronchiospasm
bronchiostenosis
bronchitis
bronchitis, acute
bronchitis, chronic
bronchitis, plastic
bronchitis, putrid
bronchitis, vegetal
bronchium
bronchoadenitis
bronchoalveolar
bronchoblennorrhea
bronchocele
bronchoconstriction
bronchodilatation

bronchoedema
bronchoesophageal
bronchofiberscope
bronchogenic
bronchogram
bronchography
Broncholate CS (codeine phosphate, ephedrine HCl, guaifenesin)
Broncholate Softgels (ephedrine HCl and guaifenesin)
broncholith
broncholithiasis
bronchomotor
bronchomycosis
bronchopathy
bronchophony
bronchoplasty
bronchoplegia
bronchopleural
bronchopneumonia
bronchopulmonary
bronchopulmonary lavage
bronchorrhagia
bronchorrhaphy
bronchorrhea
bronchoscope
bronchoscopy
bronchosinusitis
bronchospasm
bronchospirochetosis
bronchospirometer
bronchospirometry
bronchostaxis
bronchostenosis
bronchostomy
bronchotomy
bronchotracheal
bronchovesicular
bronchus
Brondecon (oxtriphylline and guaifenesin)
Bronkodyl (theophylline, anhydrous)
Bronkosol (isoetharine)
brontophobia
bronzed skin

brood capsule
broth
brow
brow persentation
Brown-Séquard's paralysis
Brown-Séquard's syndrome
Browne (-Denis) operation
brownian movement
Brucella
brucella agglutinins
brucellar
brucellin
brucellosis
brucellosis skin test
Bruch's membrane
brucine
Bruck's disease
bruise
bruissement
bruit
Brunner's glands
Brunschwig operation
brush border
Brushfield spots
brushing
Brusque esophageal
  dilation
bruxism
Bryant's traction
bubo
bubo, axillary
bubo, indolent
bubo, inguinal
bubo, pestilential
bubo, venereal
bubonadenitis
bubonic plaque
bucardia
bucca
buccal
buccal cavity
buccal fat pad
buccal glands
buccinatolabialis
buccinator
buccoaxiocervical
buccocervical
buccoclusal

buccodistal
buccogingival
buccolabial
buccolingual
buccomesial
buccopharyngeal
buccopulpal
buccoversion
buccula
Bucet (butalbital and
  acetaminophen)
Buck's extension
Buck's traction
buckling, scleral with
  implant
buckling, scleral with
  resection
buckling, scleral with
  tamponade
buckling, scleral with
  vitrectomy
buckling, scleral with
  vitreous implant
bucks studies
Bucky diaphragm
Bucladin-S Softab
  (buclaizine HCl)
bucnemia
bud
budding
Buerger's disease
buffalo hump
buffer
Bufferin (buffered
  aspirin)
buffy coat
bug, assassin
bug, bed
bug, kissing
bug, red
bulb
bulb, aortic
bulb, duodenal
bulb, of the eye
bulb, hair
bulb, olfactory
bulb, terminal, of Krause
bulb, of the urethra

bulb, of the vestibule
bulbar
bulbar paralysis
bulbiform
bulbitis
bulbocavernosus
bulboid
bulbomimic reflex
bulbonuclear
bulbospongiosum
bulbospongiosum reflex
bulbourethral gland
bulbous
bulbus
bulimia
bulimic
bulla
bulla, ethmoidalis
bulla, ossea
bullet wound
bullous
Bumex (bumetanide)
Buminate 5% (albumin
  [human])
bundle, Arnold's
bundle, atrioventricular
bundle branch block
bundle of His
bundle of Turck
bundle, Schultze's
bunion
bunionectomy
bunionette
Bunnell operation
Bunsen burner
buphthalmia
buphthalmos
Buprenex (buprenorphine
  HCl)
bur
Burdach's tracts
buret
burette
Burgess operation
Burhenne technique
Burkitt's lymphoma
burn
burn, acid

burn, alkali
burn, brush
burn, chemical
burn dressing
burn, electric
burn, of eye
burn, fireworks
burn, first degree
burn, flash
burn, gunpowder
burn, radiation
burn, respiratory
burn, second degree
burn, thermal
burn, third degree
burn, X-ray
Burnett's syndrome
burning foot syndrome
burnisher
Burow's solution
burr
burr holes
burrow
bursa
bursa, Achilles
bursa, adventitious
bursa, olecranon
bursa, omental
bursa, patellar
bursa, pharyngeal
bursa, subacromial
bursae
bursal
bursalis
bursalogy
bursectomy
bursitis
bursocentesis
bursolith
bursopathy
bursotomy
bursula, testium
Burton's line
burying of fimbriae in
  uterine wall
Buspar (buspirone HCl)
butane

Butazolidin
  (phenylbutazone)
Butesin Picrate (butamben
  picrate)
Butisol Sodium
  (butabarbital sodium)
butt
butterfly
butterfly rash
buttocks
button
button suture
buttonhole
butylene (C_4H_8)
butyraceous
butyrate
butyric acid
butyrin
butyroid
butyrometer
butyrous
by mouth (PO)
bypass
bypass, aorta-carotid-
  brachial
bypass, aorta-iliac-
  femoral
bypass, aorta-renal
bypass, aorta-subclavian-
  carotid
bypass, aorta-superior
  mesenteric
bypass, aortocarotid
bypass, aortoceliac
bypass, aortocoronary
bypass, aortofemoral
bypass, aortofemoral-
  popliteal
bypass, aortoiliac
bypass, aortoiliofemoral
bypass, aortomesenteric
bypass, aortopopliteal
bypass, aortorenal
bypass, aortosubclavian
bypass, arterial
bypass, axillary-brachial
bypass, axillary-femoral

bypass, cardiopulmonary
bypass, carotid to
  subclavian artery
bypass, common hepatic-
  common iliac-renal
bypass, coronary artery
bypass, femoral-femoral
bypass, femoroperoneal
bypass, femoropopliteal
bypass, gastric
bypass,
  gastroduodenostomy
bypass, gastroenterostomy
bypass, gastrogastrostomy
bypass grafts
bypass, heat-lung
bypass, high gastric
bypass, ileo-jejunal
bypass, iliofemoral
bypass, ilioiliac
bypass, internal mammary-
  coronary artery
bypass, intrathoracic
bypass, jejunal-ileum
bypass, peripheral artery
bypass, popliteal-tibial
bypass, pulmonary
bypass, renal artery
bypass, shunt (intestine)
bypass, shunt (stomach)
bypass, splenorenal
bypass, subclavian-
  axillary
bypass, subclavian-
  carotid
bypass, subclavian-
  subclavian
bypass, terminal ileum
bypass, vascular
bypass, Y graft to renal
  arteries
Byrd respirator
bysma
byssinosis
byssocausis
byssoid

C

C bar
C substance
C-Reactive Protein (CRP)
c-terminal
Cabot's ring bodies
cacanthrax
cacao
cachectic
cachet
cachexia
cachexia, cancerous
cachexia, hypophysiopriva
cachexia, lymphatic
cachexia, malarial
cachexia, pituitary
cachexia, strumipriva
cachinnation
cacochylia
cacodylate
cacoethes
cacogenesis
cacogenic
cacogeusia
cacoplastic
cacorhythmic
cacosmia
cacotrophy
cacumen
cadaver
cadaveric
cadaverine
cadaverous
cadence
cadmiosis
cadmium (Cd)
caduca
caduceus
caelotherapy
café au lait spot
Cafegot (ergotamine
tartrate and caffeine)
Cafergot P-B

caffeine
caffeine and sodium
benzoate
caffeine and sodium
salicylate
caffeine, citrate
caffeine poisoning
caffeinism
Caffey, John
Caffey's disease
Caffey's syndrome
cage, Faraday
cage, thoracic
cainotophobia
caisson disease
caked breast
Cal-Bid (calcium with
vitamin C and D)
Cal-Plus (high potency
calcium)
calage
calamine
calamus scriptorius
Calan (verapamil HCl)
calcaneal
calcanean
calcanectomy
calcaneoapophysitis
calcaneocuboid
calcaneodynia
calcaneofibular
calcaneonavicular
calcaneoscaphoid
calcaneotibial
calcaneum
cacoethes
cacogenesis
cacogenic
cacogeusia
cacoplastic
cacorhythmic
cacosmia
cacotrophy
cacumen
cadaver
cadaveric
cadaverine
cadaverous

cadence
cadmiosis
cadmium (Cd)
caduca
caduceus
caelotherapy
café au lait spot
Cafegot (ergotamine
  tartrate and caffeine)
Cafergot P-B
caffeine
caffeine and sodium
  benzoate
caffeine and sodium
  salicylate
caffeine, citrate
caffeine poisoning
caffeinism
Caffey, John
Caffey's disease
Caffey's syndrome
cage, Faraday
cage, thoracic
cainotophobia
caisson disease
caked breast
Cal-Bid (calcium with
  vitamin C and D)
Cal-Plus (high potency
  calcium)
calage
calamine
calamus scriptorius
Calan (verapamil HCl)
calcaneal
calcanean
calcanectomy
calcaneoapophysitis
calcaneocuboid
calcaneodynia
calcaneofibular
calcaneonavicular
calcaneoscaphoid
calcaneotibial
calcaneum
calcaneus
calcaneus fracture
calcanodynia

calcar
calcar, avis
calcar, femorale
calcar, pedis
calcareous
calcareous deposits
  removal
calcarine
calcariuria
calcaroid
calcemia
Calcet (calcium)
Calcibind (cellulose
  sodium phosphate)
calcic
calcicosis
Calciferol
  (ergocalciferol,
  vitamin D)
calciferous
calcific
calcific tendinitis
calcification
calcification, arterial
calcification, metastatic
calcification,
  Monckeberg's
Calcigard 250 (acidified
  calcium citrate)
calcigerous
Calcimar (calcitonin)
calcination
calcine
calcinosis
calcinosis, circumscripta
Calciparine (heparin
  calcium)
calcipectic
calcipenia
calcipexis
calcipexy
calciphylaxis
calciprivia
calcitonin
calcium (Ca)
calcium antagonists
calcium carbide (CaC_2)
calcium carbonate ($CaCO_3$)

calcium channel blockers
calcium channel blockers
  test
calcium chloride (CaCl$_2$)
calcium cyclamate
calcium disodium edetate
**Calcium Disodium
  Versenate** (calcium
  disodium edetate)
calcium gluconate
calcium glycerophosphate
calcium hydroxide
  (Ca(OH)$_2$)
calcium lactate
calcium levulinate
calcium mandelate
calcium oxalate (CaC$_2$O$_4$)
calcium oxide (CaO)
calcium pantothenate
calcium phosphate,
  precipitated
calcium saccharin
calcium, serum test
calcium sulfate
calcium, total serum
calcium tungstate
calciuria
calcophorous
calcospherite
calculary
calculated date of
  confinement (CDC)
calculi
calculifragous
calculogenesis
calculosis
calculous
calculus
calculus, biliary
calculus, dental
calculus, hemic
calculus, pancreatic
calculus, renal
calculus, salivary
calculus, urinary
calculus, vesical
CaldeCORT
  (hydrocortisone)

Calderol (calcifediol)
Caldesene (medicated baby
  powder and ointment)
Caldwell operation
Caldwell-Luc operation
calefacient
Calel-D (calcium and
  vitamin D)
calf
caliber
calibration
calibration, urethra
calibrator
caliceal
calicectasis
calicectomy
calices
caliculus gustatorius
caliculus ophthalmicus
caliectasis
californium (Cf)
caligo
caliper
calipers
calisthenics
calix
Callander operation
Calliphora vomitoria
callisection
callomania
callosal
callositas
callosity
callosomarginal
callosum
callous
callus
callus, definitive
callus, provisional
calmative
Calmette's reaction
calmodulins
calomel
calor
calorescence
Calori's bursa
caloric
caloric study

caloric test, vestibular
function
caloric vestibular test
caloricity
calorie-large (C, Cal)
calorie-small (c, cal)
calorifacient
calorific
calorigenic
calorimeter
calorimeter, bomb
calorimeter, respiration
calorimetry
caloripuncture
calory
Calphosan (calcium
glycerophosphate/
calcium lactate)
Caltrate 600 (calcium)
**Caltrate 600 + Iron &
Vitamin D** (calcium,
iron and vitamin D)
Caltrate 600 + Vitamin D
(calcium and vitamin D)
calvaria
Calvé-Perthes disease
calvities
calx chlorinata
calx sulfurata
calx usta
calx viva
calycectomy
calyces
calyciform
calyco-ileoneocystostomy
calycotomy
*Calymmatobacterium
granulomatis*
calyx
**Cama Arthritis Pain
Reliever**
camera
camera anterior bulbi
camera posterior bulbi
Camey enterocystoplasty
camisole
camomile

Camoquin Hydrochloride
(amodiaquine HCl)
Campbell operation
Campho-Phenique (cold
sore gel)
camphor
camphor poisoning
camphorated
camphorated oil
camphoromania
campimeter
campimetry
campospasm
camptocormia
camptodactylia
camptomelic dwarfism
camptospasm
Campylobacter
Campylobacter fetus
Campylobacter jejuni
Canadian Medical
Association (CMA)
Canadian Nurses'
Association (CNA)
Canadian Nurses'
Association Testing
Service (CNATS)
Canadian Physiotherapy
Association (CPA)
canal
canal, adductor
canal, Alcock's
canal, alimentary
canal, alveolar, inferior
canal, anal
canal, auditory, external
canal, auditory, internal
canal, birth
canal, carotid
canal, central
canal, cervical
canal, cochlear, spiral
canal, condylar
canal, craniopharyngeal
canal, facial
canal, femoral
canal, gastric
canal, haversian

canal, hyaloid
canal, hypoglossal
canal, incisive
canal, infraorbital
canal, inguinal
canal, intestinal
canal, lacrimal
canal, mandibular
canal, maxillary
canal, medullary
canal, nasolacrimal
canal, Nuck's
canal, nutrient
canal, obturator
canal, optic
canal, pharyngeal
canal, portal
canal, pterygoid
canal, pterygopalatine
canal, pudendal
canal, pulp
canal, root
canal, sacral
canal, Schlemm's
canal, spinal
canal, spiral, cochlear
canal, spiral, of the
  modiolus
canal, uterine
canal, uterocervical
canal, uterovaginal
canal, vaginal
canal, vertebral
canals, alveolar
canals, dental
canals, ethmoidal
canals, semicircular,
  bony
canals, semicircular,
  membranous
canals, Volkmann's
canalicular
canaliculi, lacrimal
canaliculodacryo-
  cystostomy
canaliculoplasty
canaliculorhinostomy
canaliculus

canalis
canalization
canaloplasty, external
  auditory meatus
canavanine
cancellated
cancelli
cancellous
cancellous bone
cancellus
cancer (CA)
cancer cell
cancer clusters
cancer grading and
  staging
cancericidal
cancerigenic
cancerogenic
cancerophobia
cancerous
cancra
cancriform
cancroid
cancrum
candela
candicidin
Candida
Candida albicans
candidiasis
Candistat 300 (caprylic
  acid supplement)
candle
candle power (CP)
candy striper
cane
cane sugar
canescent
canine
canities
canker
cannabis
cannibalism
cannula
cannulate
cannulation
cannulation, ampulla of
  Vater
cannulation, antrum

cannulation,
  arteriovenous
cannulation, artery
cannulation, caval-
  mesenteric vein
cannulation, cisterna
  chyli
cannulation, eustachian
  tube
cannulation, lacrimal
  apparatus
cannulation, lymphatic
  duct
cannulation, nasal sinus
cannulation, pancreatic
  duct
cannulation, renoportal
cannulation, sinus
  (nasal)
cannulation, splenorenal
cannulation, thoracic
  duct
cannulization
canthal
cantharidal
cantharides
Cantharis
Cantharone (cantharidin
  collodion)
Cantharone Plus
canthectomy
canthi
canthitis
canthocystostomy
cantholysis
canthopexy
canthoplasty
canthorrhaphy
canthotomy
canthus
Cantil (mepenzolate
  bromide)
cap
cap, cradle
cap, knee
capacitance
capacitation
capacitor

capacity
Capastat Sulfate
  (capreomycin sulfate)
capeline
Capgras' syndrome
capillarectasia
Capillaria
Capillaria philippinensis
capillariasis
capillariography
capillaritis
capillaropathy
capillaroscopy
capillary
capillary attraction
capillary permeability
capillaries
capillaries, arterial
capillaries, bile
capillaries, blood
capillaries, lymphatic
capillaries, venous
capillus
capital
**Capital and Codeine
  Suspension**
  (acetaminophen and
  codeine)
capitate
capitation fee
capitatum
capitellum
Capitrol (antibacterial
  cream shampoo)
capitula
capitular
capitulum
capitulum, fibulae
capitulum, humeri
capitulum, mallei
capitulum, stapedis
Caplan's syndrome
capnophilic
capotement
Capoten (captopril)
Capozide (captopril
  hydrochlorothiazide)
capping

capsicum
capsid
capsitis
capsomer
capsul
capsula articularis
capsula bulbi
capsula fibrosa
  perivascularis
capsula glomeruli
capsula lentis
capsulae
capsular
capsular contracture
  release
capsulation
capsule, articular
capsule, auditory
capsule, bacterial
capsule, Bowman's
capsule, cartilage
capsule, Glisson's
capsule, glomerular
capsule, lens
capsule, nasal
capsule of kidney
capsule of Tenon
capsule, optic
capsule, otic
capsule, renal
capsule, suprarenal
capsule,
  temporomandibular joint
capsulectomy
capsulitis
capsulo-iridectomy
capsulociliary
capsulodesis
capsulolenticular
capsuloplasty
capsulorrhaphy
capsulotome
capsulotomy
captopril
capture
capture, ventricular
caput
caput gallinaginis

caput medusae
caput succedaneum
car sickness
Carafate (sucralfate)
caramel
carbachol
carbamazepine
carbamide $(CO(NH)_2)$
carbaminohemoglobin
carbarsone
carbenicillin indanyl
  sodium
carbidopa
carbinoxamine maleate
Carbocaine (mepivacaine
  HCl)
Carbocaine Hydrochloride
  (mepivacaine HCl)
**Carbocaine with Neo-
  Cobefrin** (mepivacaine
  HCl and levonordefrin)
carbohydrate (CHO)
carbohydrate loading
carbolic acid
carbolism
carbolize
carboluria
carbon (C)
carbon dioxide (CO_2)
carbon dioxide combining
  power
carbon dioxide inhalation
carbon dioxide poisoning
carbon dioxide solid
  therapy
carbon dioxide test
carbon monoxide (CO)
carbon monoxide poisoning
carbon tetrachloride
carbon tetrachloride
  (CCl_4)
carbon tetrachloride
  poisoning
carbon-14 (^{14}C)
carbonate
carbonate of soda
carbonemia
carbonic

carbonic acid
carbonic anhydrase
carbonize
carbonuria
carbonyl
Carbowax (polyethylene
  glycols)
carboxyhemoglobin
carboxyhemoglobin test
carboxyl
carboxylase
carboxylation
carboxylic acids
carboxylmethylcellulose
  sodium
carbuncle
carbuncular
carbunculosis
carbunculus
carbutamide
carcass
carcinelcosis
carcinoembryonic antigens
  (CEA)
carcinogen
carcinogenesis
carcinogenic
carcinoid
carcinoid syndrome
carcinolysis
carcinolytic
carcinoma
carcinoma, alveolar cell
carcinoma, basal cell
carcinoma, bronchogenic
carcinoma, chorionic
carcinoma, cylindrical
carcinoma, embryonal
carcinoma, epidermoid
carcinoma, giant cell
carcinoma, glandular
carcinoma in situ
carcinoma, lipomatous
carcinoma, medullary
carcinoma, melanotic
carcinoma, oat cell
carcinoma, scirrhous
carcinoma, squamous-cell

carcinomatophobia
carcinomatosis
carcinophilia
carcinosarcoma
carcinosarcoma, embryonal
carcinosis
cardamom
cardamon
Cardarelli's sign
cardia
cardiac
cardiac arrest
cardiac arrhythmia
cardiac atrophy
cardiac blood pool
  imaging
cardiac care unit (CCU)
cardiac catheterization
cardiac compensation
cardiac cycle (CC)
cardiac evaluation panel
cardiac failure
cardiac flow study,
  imaging
cardiac hypertrophy
cardiac insufficiency
cardiac massage
cardiac monitor
cardiac output (CO)
cardiac output monitoring
  and diagnostic unit
  (COMDU)
cardiac plexus
cardiac reflex
cardiac regurgitant index
cardiac reserve
cardiac shunt detection
cardiac transplantation
cardiac tumor resection
cardiac wound repair
cardialgia
cardiaortic
cardiasthenia
cardiasthma
cardiectasia
cardiectasis
cardiectomy
cardiectomy, donor

cardiectomy/
  pneumonectomy, donor
Cardilate (erythrityl
  tetranitrate)
cardilysin
cardinal
cardio-omentopexy
cardioaccelerator
cardioactive
cardioangiography
cardioaortic
cardioassist-method
cardiocatheterization
cardiocele
cardiocentesis
cardiochalasia
cardiocirrhosis
cardiodiaphragmatic
cardiodilator
cardiodynamics
cardiodynia
cardioesophageal
cardioesophageal reflux
cardiogenesis
cardiogenic
cardiogenic shock
cardiogram
cardiograph
cardiographic
cardiography
cardiohepatic
cardiohepatomegaly
cardioinhibitory
cardiokinetic
cardiokymography
cardiolipin
cardiolith
cardiologist
cardiology
cardiolysis
cardiomalacia
cardiomegaly
cardiometer
cardiomotility
cardiomyoliposis
cardiomyopathy
cardiomyopathy, alcoholic
cardiomyopexy

cardiomyotomy
cardionecrosis
cardionecteur
cardionector
cardionephric
cardioneural
cardioneurosis
cardiopathy
cardiopericardiopexy
cardiopericarditis
cardiophobia
cardiophone
cardioplasty
cardioplegia
cardiopneumatic
cardiopneumograph
cardiopneumopexy
cardioptosis
cardiopulmonary
cardiopulmonary arrest
cardiopulmonary
  resuscitation (CPR)
cardiopuncture
cardiopyloric
Cardioquin (quinidine
  polygalacturonate)
cardiorenal
cardiorrhaphy
cardiorrhexis
cardioschisis
cardiosclerosis
cardioscope
cardioscopy
cardiospasm
cardiosphygmograph
cardiosplenopexy
cardiostenosis
cardiosymphysis
cardiotachometer
cardiotherapy
cardiotomy
cardiotonic
cardiotyrotoxicosis
cardiovalvulitis
cardiovalvulotomy
cardiovalvulotome
cardiovascular (CV)
cardiovascular reflex

cardiovascular stress
  test
cardiovascular system
  (CVS)
cardiovasology
cardioversion
cardioverter
carditis
carditis, Coxsackie
Cardizem (diltiazem HCl)
Cardrase (ethoxzolamide)
Cari-Tab (fluoride,
  vitamins A, D and C)
caries
caries, arrested
caries, bottle mouth
caries, dental
caries, necrotic
caries, radiation
caries, rampant
caries sicca
caries, spinal
carina nasi
carina tracheae
carina urethralis
carinae
carinate
cariogenesis
carious
carisoprodol
Carisoprodol Compound
  (aspirin and
  carisoprodol)
carminative
Carmol 10 (urea lotion)
Carmol HC (hydrocortisone
  acetate)
carmustine
carnal
carnal knowledge
carneous
carnification
carnitine
Carnitor (levocarnitine)
carnivore
carnivorous
carnophobia
carnose

carnosine
carnosity
carotenase
carotene
carotenemia
carotenoid
carotenosis
carotic
caroticotympanic
carotid
carotid arteriography
  injection
carotid artery
carotid body
carotid bypass graft
carotid embolectomy
carotid phonoangiograph
  (CPA)
carotid phonoangiography
carotid pulse
carotid sinus
carotid sinus injection
carotid siphon
carotid-carotid bypass
  graft
carotid-cavernous repair
carotid-subclavian bypass
  graft
carotidynia
carotin
carotinase
carotinemia
carpal
carpal bone
carpal tunnel
carpal tunnel syndrome
carpale
carpectomy
carphenazine maleate
carphologia
carphology
carpometacarpal
carpometacarpal joint
carpopedal
carpopedal spasm
carpoptosis
carpus
carrageen

carragheen
Carrel-Dakin treatment
carrier
carrier, active
carrier, convalescent
carrier, genetic
carrier, healthy
carrier, incubatory
carrier, intermittent
carrier, passive
carrier-free
Carrion's disease
Carroll and Taber
  arthroplasty
cartilage
cartilage, articular
cartilage, costal
cartilage, fibrous
cartilage, hyaline
cartilage, semilunar
cartilage, thyroid
cartilage, yellow
cartilaginification
cartilaginoid
cartilaginous
cartilago
caruncle
caruncle, lacrimal
caruncle, sublingual
caruncle, urethral
caruncula
caruncula, hymenales
carver
carver, amalgam
carver, wax
cascade
case
case control
case control study
case history
caseate
caseation
Casec (calcium caseinate)
casefinding
casein
caseinogen
caseous
Casoni's reaction

cassette
cast
cast, blood
cast, body
cast, bronchial
cast, epithelial
cast, fatty
cast, fibrinous
cast, granular
cast, hyaline
cast, pseudo
cast, pus
cast, urinary
cast, uterine
cast, waxy
Castellani Paint
casting
Castle's intrinsic factor
castor oil
castrate
castrated
castration
casualty
casuistics
cat
CAT scan
cat scratch disease
cat scratch fever
cat's eye pupil
cat's eye reflex
cat-cry syndrome
catabasis
catabatic
catabolic
catabolin
catabolism
catabolite
catacrotic
catacrotism
catadicrotic
catadicrotism
catadioptric
catagen
catagenesis
catalase
catalepsy
cataleptic
cataleptiform

cataleptoid
catalysis
catalyst
catalytic
catalyze
catalyzer
catamenia
catamenial
catamnesis
cataphasia
cataphora
cataphoresis
cataphoria
cataphoric
cataphrenia
cataphylaxis
cataplasia
cataplasis
cataplasm
cataplectic
cataplexia
cataplexy
Catapres (clonidine HCl)
Catapres-TTS (clonidine [transdermal])
cataract
cataract, capsular
cataract, hypermature
cataract, immature
cataract, lenticular
cataract, morgagnian
cataract, overripe
cataract, radiation
cataract, ripe
cataract, senile
cataractogenic
catarrh
catarrhal
catatonia
catatonia, Stauder's
catatonic
catatricrotic
catatricrotism
catatropia
catchment area
catecholamines
catelectrotonus

Catemine (catecholamine precursor)
catenating
catenoid
caterpillar sting
catfish sting
catgut
catgut, chromic
catharsis
cathartic
cathepsins
cathepsis
catheresis
catheter (cath)
catheter, arterial
catheter, cardiac
catheter, central
catheter, central venous
catheter, condom
catheter, double-channel
catheter, elbowed
catheter, eustachian
catheter, female
catheter fever
catheter, Foley
catheter, indwelling
catheter, intra-aortic
catheter, intravenous
catheter, Karman
catheter, male
catheter, pacing
catheter, prostatic
catheter, pulmonary artery
catheter, self-retaining
catheter, suprapubic
catheter, Swan-Ganz
catheter, Tenckhoff peritoneal
catheter, triple-lumen
catheter, vertebrated
catheter, winged
catheterization
catheterization, arteriovenous
catheterization, artery
catheterization, bladder
catheterization, bronchus

catheterization, cardiac
catheterization,
  eustachian tube
catheterization, for
  retrograde pyelogram
catheterization, heart
catheterization, hepatic
  vein
catheterization, inferior
  vena cava
catheterization,
  lacrimonasal duct
catheterization,
  laryngeal
catheterization,
  nasolacrimal duct
catheterization,
  pancreatic cyst
catheterization, renal
  vein
catheterization,
  suprapubic
catheterization, Swan-
  Ganz
catheterization,
  umbilical vein
catheterization, ureter
catheterization, urethra
catheterization, vein
catheterize
cathexis
cathodal
cathode
cathode stream
cathode-ray tube (CRT)
cathodic
cation
catlin
catoptric
catoptrophobia
Cattell operation
Caucasian
caucasoid
cauda
cauda epididymidis
cauda equina
cauda helicis
cauda pancreatis

cauda striati
caudad
caudal
caudate
caudation
caudocephalad
caul
cauliflower ear
causalgia
cause, antecedent
cause, determining
cause, predisposing
cause, proximate
cause, remote
cause, ultimate
caustic
cauterant
cauterization
cauterization, anus
cauterization,
  Bartholin's gland
cauterization, broad
  ligament
cauterization, canaliculi
cauterization, cervix
cauterization, chalazion
cauterization, chemical
cauterization, choroid
  plexus
cauterization,
  conjunctiva
cauterization, cornea
cauterization, ear,
  external
cauterization, electrical
cauterization,
  endometrial implant
cauterization, entropion
cauterization, esophagus
cauterization, eyelid
cauterization, fallopian
  tube
cauterization,
  hemorrhoids
cauterization, iris
cauterization, lacrimal
  gland

cauterization, lacrimal
  punctum
cauterization, larynx
cauterization, liver
cauterization, lung
cauterization, meibomian
  gland
cauterization, nose, for
  epistaxis
cauterization, ovary
cauterization, palate
  (bony)
cauterization, pannus
  (superficial)
cauterization, rectum
cauterization, round
  ligament
cauterization, sclera
cauterization, skin
cauterization,
  subcutaneous tissue
cauterization, tonsillar
  fossa
cauterization, urethra
cauterization,
  uterosacral ligament
cauterization, uterotubal
  ostia
cauterization, uterus
cauterization, vagina
cauterization, vocal
  cords
cauterization, vulva
cauterize
cautery
caution
cava
caval
cavalry bone
cavern
cavernitis
cavernoma
cavernoscopy
cavernositis
cavernostomy
cavernotomy, kidney
cavitary
cavitation

cavitis
cavity, abdominal
cavity, alveolar
cavity, amniotic
cavity, articular
cavity, body
cavity, buccal
cavity classification
cavity, cotyloid
cavity, cranial
cavity, dental
cavity, glenoid
cavity, oral
cavity, pelvic
cavity, pericardial
cavity, peritoneal
cavity, peritoneal,
  lesser
cavity, pleural
cavity preparation
cavity, pulp
cavity, Rosenmüller's
cavity, serous
cavity, splanchnic
cavity, tympanic
cavity, uterine
cavography
cavum
cavum abdominis
cavum conchae
cavum mediastinale
cavum medullare
cavum oris
cavum pelvis
cavum septi pellucidi
cavum trigeminale
cavum tympani
cavum uteri
cavus
cavus foot
cayenne pepper
Ce-Vi-Sol (vitamin C)
cebocephalus
cecal
cecetomy
Cecil operation
cecitis
Ceclor (cefaclor)

cecocolopexy
cecocoloplicopexy
cecocolostomy
cecofixation
cecoileostomy
cecopexy
cecoplication
cecoptosis
cecosigmoidostomy
cecostomy
cecotomy
cecum
Cedilanid (lanatoside C)
Cedilanid-D (deslanoside)
Cee NU (lomustine [CCNU])
Cefadyl (cephapirin
  sodium)
cefamandole nafate
Cefizox (ceftizoxime
  sodium)
Cefobid (cefoperazone
  sodium)
Cefol Filmtab (B-complex,
  folic acid, vitamin E
  and C)
Cefotan (cefotetan
  disodium)
cefoxitin sodium
Celbenin (methicillin
  sodium)
Celestone (betamethasone)
Celestone Phosphate
  (betamethasone sodium
  phosphate)
Celestone Soluspan
celiac
celiac artery
celiac disease
celiac plexus
celiectomy
celiocentesis
celiocolpotomy
celioenterotomy
celiogastostomy
celiogastrotomy
celiohysterectomy
celiohysterotomy
celioma

celiomyalgia
celiomyomectomy
celiomyomotomy
celiomyositis
celioparacentesis
celiopathy
celiorrhaphy
celiosalpingectomy
celioscope
celioscopy
celiotomy
celitis
cell
cell, acidophil
cell, acinar
cell, adipose
cell, adventitial
cell, band
cell bank
cell, basal
cell, basket
cell, basophil
cell, bipolar
cell, blast
cell block and
  Papanicolaou smear
cell, castration
cell, centroacinar
cell, cleavage
cell, columnar
cell, cone
cell count
cell, cuboid
cell culture
cell cycle
cell, daughter
cell division
cell, endothelial
cell, epithelial
cell, ethmoidal
cell, fat
cell, ganglion
cell, giant
cell, glia
cell, goblet
cell, Golgi's
cell growth cycle
cell, gustatory

cell, HeLa
cell, horizontal
cell, hybridoma
cell, interstitial
cell, juxtaglomerular
cell kill
cell kinetics
cell, Kupffer's
cell, L.E.
cell, littoral
cell, lutein
cell mass
cell, mast
cell membrane
cell, mother
cell, mucous
cell, myeloma
cell, nerve
cell, Niemann-Pick
cell, olfactory
cell organelle
cell, oxyntic
cell, parent
cell, pigment
cell, prickle
cell, Purkinje's
cell, pus
cell, pyramidal
cell receptor
cell, red
cell, reticular
cell, Rieder
cell, rod
cell, segmented
cell, sensory
cell, Sertoli
cell, sickle
cell, signet-ring
cell, somatic
cell, spider
cell, squamous
cell, stellate
cell, stipple
cell, target
cell, tart
cell, taste
cell, totipotent
cell, Touton giant

cell, Türk's irritation
cell, Tzanck
cell, undifferentiated
cell, visual
cell wall
cell, wandering
cell, white
cells, alpha
cells, argentaffin
cells, beta
cells, Betz
cells, capsule
cells, chief
cells, chromaffin
cells, clue
cells, foam
cells, granule
cells, Hurthle
cells, islet
cells, mastoid
cells, microglia
cells, nature killer
cells, neuroglia
cells, phalangeal
cells, plasma
cells, primordial
cells, Reed-Sternberg
cells,
    reticuloendothelial
cells, rosette
cells, Rouget
cells, satellite
cells, septal
cells, Sternberg-Reed
cells, sympathicotrophic
cells, sympathochromaffin
cells, zymogenic
cell-free
cell-mediated immunity
    (CMI)
cellobiose
cellophane
cellucidal
cellula
cellular
cellular immunity
cellulase
cellulifugal

cellulipetal
cellulitis
cellulofibrous
celluloneuritis
cellulose
cellulotoxic
celology
celom
celoma
Celontin Kapseals
(methsuximide)
celoschisis
celoscope
celosomia
celozoic
Celsius scale
cement.
cementicle
cementitis
cementoblast
cementoclast
cementogenesis
cementoid
cementoma
cementum
cemetoclasia
cenesthesia
cenesthesic
cenesthopathia
cenesthopathy
cenosis
cenosite
cenotic
cenotophobia
cenotype
censor
center, apneustic
center, auditory
center, autonomic
center, Broca's
center, burn
center, cardioaccelerator
center, cardioinhibitory
center, chondrification
center, ciliospinal
center, community health
center, deglutition
center, epiotic

center, feeding
Center for Disease
Control (CDC)
center, germinal
center, gustatory
center, higher
center, lower
center, medullary
center, micturition
center, motor cortical
center, neighborhood
health
center, nerve
center, ossification
center, pneumotaxic
center, psychocortical
center, reflex
center, respiratory
center, satiety
center, speech
center, suicide
prevention
center, taste
center, temperature
center, thermoregulatory
center, trophic
center, vasoconstrictor
center, vasodilator
center, vasomotor
center, visual
center, Wernicke's
center, word
center's, defecation
center's, heat-regulating
centesis
centigrade (C)
centimeter (cm)
centimeter-gram-second
(CGS)
centinormal
centipede
centipoise
centrad
central
central auditory function
test
central axis depth dose
central core disease

central I.V. line
central inhibitory state
  (CIS)
central line
central nervous system
  (CNS)
central ray (CR)
central slip repair,
  extensor tendon
central sulci
central supply (CS)
central supply room (CSR)
central venous catheter
central venous pressure
  (CVP)
centraphose
Centrax (prazepam)
centre
centriciput
centrifugal
centrifugal force
centrifuge
centrilobular
centriole
centrioles
centripetal
centrocyte
centrodesmus
centrolecithal
centromere
centrophose
centrosclerosis
centrosome
centrosphere
centrostaltic
centrum
Centrum (multivitamin-
  multimineral)
centrum semiovale
centrum tendineum
Cepacol (anesthetic
  lozenges [troches])
Cepacol
  (mouthwash/gargle)
Cepacol (throat lozenges)
Cepastat (lozenges)
cephalad
cephalalgia

cephalalgic
cephalea
cephaledema
cephalhematocele
cephalhematoma
cephalic
cephalic index
cephalitis
cephalocaudal pattern of
  development
cephalocele
cephalocentesis
cephalodynia
cephaloglycin
cephalogram
cephalogyric
cephalohemometer
cephalomenia
cephalomeningitis
cephalometrics
cephalometry
cephalomotor
cephalone
cephalonia
cephalopathy
cephalopelvic
cephaloplegia
cephalorhachidian
cephaloridine
cephaloscope
cephalosporin
cephalothoracic
cephalothoracopagus
cephalotome
cephalotomy
cephalotomy, fetus
cephalotrypesis
cephapirin sodium
Cephulac (lactulose)
ceptor
ceptor, chemical
ceptor, contact
ceptor, distance
ceramics, dental
ceramide
ceramide,
  oligosaccharides
ceramodontia

cerate ceratum
ceratocele
ceratotome
cercaria
cercaricide
cerclage
cerclage, uterine cervix
Cercomonas
cercomoniasis
cercus
cerea flexibilitas
cereals
cerebellar
cerebellifugal
cerebellipetal
cerebellitis
cerebellopontine angle
  tumor
cerebellospinal
cerebellum
cerebral
cerebral anoxia
cerebral artery
cerebral blood flow study
cerebral cortex
cerebral cortical scar
  excision
cerebral evoked
  potentials
cerebral hemispheres
cerebral hemorrhage
cerebral neurostimulator
  electrode
cerebral palsy (CP)
cerebral palsy feeder
cerebral seizure focus
cerebration
cerebrifugal
cerebripetal
cerebritis
cerebroid
cerebromalacia
cerebromedullary
cerebromeningitis
cerebropathy
cerebrophysiology
cerebropontile
cerebropsychosis

cerebrosclerosis
cerebroscope
cerebroscopy
cerebrose
cerebroside
cerebrosidosis
cerebrosis
cerebrospinal
cerebrospinal axis
cerebrospinal fever
cerebrospinal fluid (CSF)
cerebrospinal ganglia
cerebrospinal nerves
cerebrospinal puncture
cerebrosuria
cerebrotomy
cerebrovascular accident
  (CVA)
cerebrum
Cerespan (papaverine HCl)
cerium (Ce)
ceroid
ceroma
ceroplasty
Cerose-DM (cough/cold
  preparation with
  dextromethorphan)
certifiable
certification
certified medical
  transcriptionist (CMT)
certified nurse-midwife
  (CNM)
certified occupational
  therapy assistant
  (COTA)
certified registered
  nurse anesthetist
  (CRNA)
certified respiratory
  therapy technician
  (CRTT)
Cerubidine (daunorubicin
  HCl)
ceruloderma
ceruloplasmin
cerumen
Cerumenex Drops

ceruminal
ceruminolysis
ceruminolytic agent
ceruminosis
ceruminous
ceruminous glands
ceruse
cervical
cervical cap
cervical cystic hygroma
cervical mucus
  penetration test
cervical mucus test
cervical nerves
cervical plexus
cervical plexus injection
cervical rib
cervical ribs
cervical smear
cervical spinal nerves
cervical spine
cervical spondylosis
cervical sympathectomy
cervical vertebrae
cervicectomy
cervices
cervicitis
cervicobrachial
cervicocerebral
  angiography
cervicocolpitis
cervicocranial
  arthrodesis
cervicodynia
cervicofacial
cervicoplasty
cervicothoracic
cervicovaginitis
cervicovesical
cervix
cervix, uteri
cervix, vesicae
Cesamet (nabilone)
cesarean hysterectomy
cesarean section (c-
  section, CS)
cesarean section,
  classical

cesarean section,
  corporeal
cesarean section,
  extraperitoneal
cesarean section, fundal
cesarean section,
  laparotrachelotomy
cesarean section, Latzko
cesarean section, low
  cervical
cesarean section, lower
  uterine segment
cesarean section,
  peritoneal exclusion
cesarean section,
  supravesical
cesarean section,
  transperitoneal
cesarean section, upper
  uterine segment
cesarean section, vaginal
cesarean section, Waters
cesarean-obtained
  barrier-sustained
  (COBS)
cesarotomy
cesium (Cs)
cesium-137
cesspool
Cestan-Chenais syndrome
Cestoda
cestode
cestodiasis
cestoid
Cestoidea
Cetacaine
Cetacort (hydrocortisone)
Cetamide (sulfacetamide
  sodium)
Cetane (ascorbic acid)
Cetaphil (skin cleanser)
Cetylcide
cetylpyridinium chloride
Cevi-Bid (vitamin C)
Cevi-Fer (hematinic with
  vitamin C)
Chaddock's reflexes
chafe

chafing
Chagas' disease
chain
chaining
chair, birthing
chalasia
chalazion
chalcosis
chalice cell
chalicosis
chalinoplasty
challenge
chalone
chamber, altitude
chamber, anterior
chamber, aqueous
chamber, Boyden
chamber, hyperbaric
chamber, low pressure
chamber, posterior
chamber, pulp
chamber, vitreous
chamomile
chancre
chancre, hard
chancre, simple
chancre, soft
chancre, true
chancroid
chancrous
Chandler operation
change, fatty
change of life
channel
chapped
character
character, acquired
character, anal
character analysis
character, dominant
character, primary sex
character, recessive
character, secondary sex
character, sex-
  conditioned
character, sex-linked
characteristic
characteristic radiation

charbon
charcoal
Charcot's joint
Charcot-Leyden crystals
Charcot-Marie-Tooth
  disease
Charcot's triad
charge, customary and
  reasonable
charlatan
charlatanry
Charles operation
Charles' law
charleyhorse
Charnley operation
chart
charta
charting
chartula
chasma
chaude-pisse
chauffage
chaulmaugra
chaulmoogra oil
chaulmugra
Chaussier's areola
chavicine
Cheatle-Henry operation
check
check bite
check-up
Chediak-Higashi syndrome
cheek
cheek retractor
cheekbone
cheilectomy
cheilectropion
cheilitis
cheilitis, actinica
cheilitis, exfoliativa
cheilitis, glandularis
cheilitis, venenata
cheilognathopalatoschisis
cheilophagia
cheiloplasty
cheilorrhaphy
cheiloschisis
cheilosis

cheilostomatoplasty
cheilotomy
cheirognostic
cheirology
cheirospasm
chelate
chelating agent
chelation
cheloid
chemabrasion
chemexfoliation
chemical
Chemical Abstract Service
  (CAS)
chemical bond
chemical cauterization
chemical change
chemical compound
chemical element
chemical peel
chemical peel, skin
chemical reflex
chemical warfare
chemically pure (CP)
chemiluminescence
chemise
chemist
chemistry
chemistry, analytical
chemistry, biological
chemistry, general
chemistry, inorganic
chemistry, nuclear
chemistry, organic
chemistry, pathological
chemistry, pharmaceutical
chemistry, physical
chemistry, physiological
chemobiotic
chemocauterization
chemocauterization
  corneal epithelium
chemocautery
chemoceptor
chemocoagulation
chemodectoma
chemodectomy
chemoluminescence

chemolysis
chemoneurolysis
chemonucleolysis
chemonucleolysis,
  intervertebral disk
chemopallidectomy
chemopeel, skin
chemoprophylaxis
chemopsychiatry
chemoreceptor
chemoreceptor trigger
  zone (CTZ)
chemoreflex
chemoresistance
chemosensitive
chemosensory
chemoserotherapy
chemosis
chemosmosis
chemosterilant
chemosurgery
chemosynthesis
chemotactic
chemotaxis
chemotaxis assay
chemothalamectomy
chemotherapeutic index
  (CI)
chemotherapy
chemotic
chemotropism
Chenix (chenodiol)
chenopodium oil
Cheracol D (cough
  formula)
Cheracol Plus (head
  cold/cough formula)
cherophobia
cherry-red spot
cherubism
chest
chest, emphysematous
chest, flail
chest, flat
chest, pigeon
chest prominences and
  depressions
chest regions

chest thump
chest x-ray (CXR)
chestnut, horse
Chevalier-Jackson
  operation
Chevron bunion procedure
Chexit
Cheyne-Stokes Respiration
  (CSR)
Chiari procedure
Chiari's deformity
Chiari-Frommel syndrome
chiasm
chiasma
chiasma, optic
chickenpox
chief complaint (CC)
chiggers
chigo
chigre
chikungunya virus
chilblain
child
child abuse
child neglect
Child operation
childbed
childbed fever
childbirth
childbirth, natural
childbirth, prepared
childproof
Children's Tylenol
  (acetaminophen)
chilectropion
chilitis
chill
chill, nervous
chiloangioscopy
Chilomastix mesnili
chilotomy
chimera
chimney sweeps' cancer
chimpanzee
chin
chin jerk
chin reflex
China clay

Chinese restaurant
  syndrome
chip
chiragra
chiralgia
chirismus
chirognostic
chirokinesthesia
chiromegaly
chiroplasty
chiropodist
chiropody
chiropractic
chiropractor
chirospasm
chirurgery
chirurgia
chirurgiae magister (CM)
chisel
chi-square
chitin
chitinous
Chlamydia
chlamydia smear
chloasma
chloasma, gravidarum
chloasma, idioptahic
chloasma, symptomatic
chloasma, traumaticum
chloasma, uterinum
Chlor-3 (potassium
  chloride, sodium
  chloride, magnesium
  chloride)
chloracne
Chlorafed
  (chlorpheniramine
  maleate;
  pseudoephedrine HCl)
chloral
chloral hydrate
chloral hydrate poisoning
chlorambucil
chloramines
chloramphenicol
Chloraseptic Liquid
  (phenol and sodium
  phenolate)

Chloraseptic Lozenges
(benzocaine-based
topical anesthetic)
chlorate
chlorbutanol
chlorbutol
chlorcyclizine
hydrochloride
chlordane
chlordantoin
chlordiazepoxide
hydrochloride
chloremia
Chloresium
chlorhexidene gluconate
chlorhydria
chloride
chloride poisoning
chloridemia
chloridimeter
chloriduria
chlorinated
chlorinated hydrocarbons
chlorinated lime
chlorination
chlorine (Cl)
chlorine preparations
chlorite
chlormerodrin Hg 197
chlormerodrin Hg 203
chloroazodin
chlorobutanol
chloroform ($CHCl_3$)
chloroformism
chloroleukemia
chloroma
Chloromycetin
(chloramphenicol)
Chloromycetin Ophthalmic
(chloramphenicol)
Chloromycetin Otic
(chloramphenicol)
Chloromycetin Palmitate
(chloroamphenicol
palmitate)
**Chloromycetin Sodium
Succinate**
chloropenia

chloropenic
chlorophane
chlorophenothane
chlorophyll
chloropia
chloroplast
chloroplastid
chloroprivic
chloroprocaine
hydrochloride
chloropsia
chloroquine hydrochloride
chloroquine phosphate
chlorosis
chlorothiazide sodium
chlorothymol
chlorotic
chlorotrianisene
chlorpheniramine maleate
chlorphenoxamine
hydrochloride
chlorpromazine
chlorpromazine poisoning
chlorpropamide
chlorprothixene
chlorquinaldol
chlortetracycline
hydrochloride
chlorthalidone
chlorzoxazone
choana
choanal atresia repair
choanoid
choke
choke-saver
choked disk
chokes
choking
choking on food
cholagogue
Cholan-DH (dehydrocholic
acid)
cholangiectasis
cholangio-enterostomy
cholangiocarcinoma
cholangioenterostomy
cholangiogastrostomy
cholangiogram

cholangiography
cholangiojejunostomy
cholangiole
cholangiolitis
cholangioma
cholangiopancreatography
cholangiostomy
cholangiotomy
cholangitis
cholanopoiesis
cholate
cholecalciferol
cholecyst
cholecystagogue
cholecystalgia
cholecystangiography
cholecystectasia
cholecystectomy
cholecystenterorrhaphy
cholecystenterostomy
cholecystic
cholecystnephrostomy
cholecystocecostomy
cholecystocholangiogram
cholecystocolostomy
cholecystocolotomy
cholecystoduodenostomy
cholecystoenterostomy
cholecystogastrostomy
cholecystogram
cholecystography
cholecystoileostomy
cholecystojejunostomy
cholecystokinin
cholecystolithiasis
cholecystolithotripsy
cholecystomy
cholecystopancreatostomy
cholecystopathy
cholecystopexy
cholecystoptosis
cholecystorrhaphy
cholecystostomy
cholecystotomy
choledochal
choledochal cyst
choledochal stent
  placement

choledochectasia
choledochectomy
choledochitis
choledochoduodenostomy
choledochoenterostomy
choledochography
choledochojejunostomy
choledocholith
choledocholithiasis
choledocholithotomy
choledocholithotripsy
choledochopancreatostomy
choledochoplasty
choledochorrhaphy
choledochoscopy
choledochostomy
choledochotomy
choledochus
Choledyl (oxtriphylline)
choleic
cholelith
cholelithiasis
cholelithic
cholelithotomy
cholelithotrity
cholemesis
cholemia
cholepathia
choleperitoneum
cholepoiesis
cholera
cholera immunization
choleragen
cholerase
choleresis
choleretic
choleric
choleriform
cholerigenic
cholerigenous
cholerine
choleroid
choleromania
cholerophobia
cholescintigraphy
cholestasia
cholestatic
cholesteatoma

cholesteremia
cholesterin
cholesterinemia
cholesterinuria
cholesterohydrothorax
cholesterol (Ch,Chol)
cholesterolemia
cholesteroluria
cholesterosis
cholestyramine resin
choletelin
choletherapy
choleuria
choleverdin
cholic acid
choline
choline salicylate
cholinergic
cholinergic fibers
cholinesterase
cholinoceptive
cholinolytic
cholinomimetic
cholochrome
chologenic
cholohemothorax
chololith
chololithiasis
cholorrhea
Choloxin (dextrothyroxine
  sodium)
choluria
choncha auriculae
choncha bullosa
choncha, nasal
choncha sphenoidalis
chonchotome
chonchotomy
chondral
chondralgia
chondralloplasia
chondrectomy
chondric
chondrification
chondrigen
chondrin
chondritis
chondro-osseus

chondro-osteodystrophy
chondroadenoma
chondroangioma
chondroblast
chondroblastoma
chondrocalcinosis
chondroclast
chondrocostal
chondrocranium
chondrocyte
chondrodermatitis
  nodularis chronica
  helicis
chondrodynia
chondrodysplasia
chondrodystrophy
chondroendothelioma
chondroepiphysitis
chondrofibroma
chondrogen
chondrogenesis
chondrogenic
chondroid
chondroitin
chondrolipoma
chondrology
chondrolysis
chondroma
chondromalacia
chondromatosis
chondromatous
chondromucin
chondromucoid
chondromucoprotein
chondromyoma
chondromyxoma
chondromyxosarcoma
chondropathology
chondropathy
chondroplasia
chondroplast
chondroplasty
chondroporosis
chondroproteins
chondrosarcoma
chondrosin
chondrosis
chondrosternal

chondrosternoplasty
chondrotome
chondrotomy
chondroxiphoid
Chondrus
Chopart's amputation
chorda
chorda dorsalis
chorda gubernaculum
chorda obliqua
chorda tympani
chorda umbilicalis
chorda vocalis
chordae tendineae
chordal
Chordata
chordee
chorditis
chorditis nodosa
chordoma
chordotomy
chorea
chorea, acute
chorea, Bergeron's
chorea, chronic
chorea, electric
chorea, epidemic
chorea, gravidarum
chorea, Henoch's
chorea, hereditary
chorea, Huntington's
chorea, hyoscine
chorea, mimetic
chorea, minor
chorea, posthemiplegic
chorea, senile
chorea, Sydenham's
choreal
choreic
choreiform
choreoathetoid
choreoathetosis
choreomania
choreophrasia
chorioadenoma
chorioadenoma destruens
chorioallantois
chorioamnionitis

chorioangioma
choriocapillaris
choriocarcinoma
choriocele
chorioepithelioma
choriogenesis
chorioid
chorioma
choriomeningitis
choriomeningitis,
  lymphocytic
chorion
chorion frondosum
chorion laeve
chorionepithelioma
chorionic
chorionic gonadotropin
chorionic plate
chorionic
  somatomammotropin
chorionic villi
chorionic villus
chorionic villus sampling
  (CVS)
chorionitis
chorioretinal
chorioretinitis
chorista
choristoma
choroid
choroid plexus
choroidal fluid
  aspiration
choroideremia
choroiditis
choroiditis, anterior
choroiditis, areolar
choroiditis, central
choroiditis, diffuse
choroiditis, exudative
choroiditis, guttata
  senilis
choroiditis, metastatic
choroiditis, suppurative
choroiditis, Tay's
choroidocyclitis
choroidoiritis
choroidopathy

choroidoretinitis
choromania
Christian Science
Christian-Weber disease
Christmas disease
Christmas factor (CF)
chromaffin
chromaffin cells
chromaffin reaction
chromaffin system
chromaffinoma
chromaffinopathy
Chromagen
Chromagen OB
chromaphil
chromate
chromatic
chromatid
chromatin
chromatin body test
chromatin-negative
chromatinolysis
chromatinorrhexis
chromatism
chromatogenous
chromatogram
chromatographic sugars
chromatography
chromatography,
  adsorption
chromatography, column
chromatography, gas
chromatography, gas-
  liquid
chromatography, high-
  performance liquid
chromatography, paper
chromatography, partition
chromatography, thin
  layer
chromatoid
chromatokinesis
chromatolysis
chromatometer
chromatophil
chromatophilic
chromatophore
chromatopsia

chromatoptometry
chromatosis
chromaturia
chromesthesia
Chrometrace (chromic
  chloride injection)
chromhidrosis
chromicize
chromidiosis
chromidium
chromidrosis
chromium (Cr)
chromium poisoning
chromoblast
chromocenter
chromocrinia
chromocystoscopy
chromocyte
chromocytometer
chromodacryorrhea
chromogen
chromogenesis
chromogenic
chromolipoid
chromolysis
chromomere
chromometer
chromometry
chromomycosis
chromoparic
chromopectic
chromopexic
chromophane
chromophil
chromophile
chromophilic
chromophilous
chromophobe
chromophobia
chromophore
chromophoric
chromophose
chromophytosis
chromoplasm
chromoplastid
chromoprotein
chromopsia
chromoptometer

chromoradiometer
chromoscope
chromoscopy
chromosome
chromosome, accessory
chromosome analysis
chromosome, bivalent
chromosome, Philadelphia
chromosome, sex
chromosome, somatic
chromosome, X
chromosome, Y
chromosomes, banded
chromosomes, giant
chromotherapy
chromotoxic
chromotrichia
chromoureteroscopy
chronaxie
chronaximeter
chronic
chronic ambulatory
  peritoneal dialysis
  (CAPD)
chronic bacterial
  prostatitis (CBP)
chronic brain syndrome
  (CBS)
chronic granulomatous
  disease
chronic obstructive lung
  disease (COLD)
chronic renal failure
  (CRF)
chronic ulcerative
  colitis (CUC)
chronicity
chronobiology
chronognosis
chronograph
chronological
chronoscope
chronotaraxis
chronotropic
chronotropism
chronotropism, negative
chronotropism, positive
Chronulac (lactulose)

chrysarobin
chrysiasis
chrysoderma
chrysotherapy
Chvostek's sign
chylangioma
chyle
chylemia
chylifacient
chylifaction
chylifactive
chylification
chyliform
chylocele
chyloderma
chylology
chylomediastinum
chylomicron
chylopericardium
chyloperitoneum
chylophoric
chylopneumothorax
chylopoiesis
chylorrhea
chylothorax
chylous
chyluria
chymase
chyme
chymopapain
chymosin
chymotrypsin
Cibacalcin (calcitonin-
  human)
Cibalith-S (lithium
  citrate)
cibisotome
cibophobia
cibus (cib)
cicatricial
cicatricial lesion
  excision
cicatricotomy
cicatrix
cicatrizant
cicatrization
cicatrize
cicutism

cigarette
ciguatera
ciguatoxin
cilia
cilia, immotile, syndrome
ciliariscope
ciliarotomy
ciliary
ciliary apparatus
ciliary arteries
ciliary body
ciliary ganglion
ciliary glands
ciliary muscle
ciliary nerves, long
ciliary nerves, short
ciliary processes
ciliary reflex
Ciliata
ciliate
ciliated
ciliated epithelium
ciliectomy
ciliogenesis
ciliospinal
ciliospinal center
ciliospinal reflex
ciliostatic
ciliotomy
ciliotoxicity
cilium
cilosis
cimbia
cimetidine
Cimex lectularius
cimicosis
cinch, for scleral
  buckling
cinch, ocular muscle
cinching, for scleral
  buckling
cinching, ocular muscle
cinchona
cinchonism
cinchophen
cinclisis
cincture sensation
cine recording

cineangiocardiography
cineangiocardiography,
  radionuclide
cinecystourethrogram
cinefluorography
cinematics
cinematoradiography
cinemicrography
cineplastic prosthesis
cineplastics
cineplasty
cineraceous
cineradiograph
cineradiography
cinerea
cinereal
cineritious
cineurography
cingulotomy
cingulum
cingulumotomy
cinnamon
Cinobac (cinoxacin)
cinoxacin
CinQuin (quinidine
  sulfate)
cion
Circ-O-Lectric bed
circa (c)
circadian
circinate
circle of diffusion
circle of Willis
circuit
circular
circulation
circulation, bile salts
circulation, blood
circulation, collateral
circulation, coronary
circulation,
  extracorporeal
circulation, fetal
circulation, lymph
circulation, portal
circulation, pulmonary
circulation rate
circulation, systemic

circulation time
circulation, venous
circulatory
circulatory assist
circulatory collapse
circulatory failure
circulatory overload
circulatory system
circulus
circumarticular
circumcision
circumcision, ritual
circumclusion
circumcorneal
circumduction
circumference
circumferential
circumflex
circuminsular
circumlental
circumnuclear
circumocular
circumoral
circumoral pallor
circumorbital
circumpolarization
circumrenal
circumscribed
circumstantiality
circumvallate
circumvallate papillae
circumvascular
cirrhosis, alcoholic
cirrhosis, atrophic
cirrhosis, biliary
cirrhosis, cardiac
cirrhosis, fatty
cirrhosis, hypertrophic
cirrhosis, infantile
cirrhosis, macronodular
cirrhosis, metabolic
cirrhosis, micronodular
cirrhosis, obstructive
  biliary
cirrhosis, primary
  biliary
cirrhosis, syphilitic
cirrhosis, toxic

cirrhosis, zooparasitic
cirrhotic
cirsectomy
cirsoid
cirsomphalos
cirsotome
cirsotomy
cis
cisplatin
cissa
cistern
cisterna
cisterna chyli
cisterna subarachnoidalis
cisternal
cisternal puncture
cisternography
cisvestitism
Citanest (prilocaine HCl)
Citelli's syndrome
Citracal (calcium
  citrate)
citrate
citrate solution
citrated
citric acid
citric acid cycle
citric acid test
Citrocarbonate (antacid)
citronella
citrovorum factor (CF)
citrulline
citrullinemia
citrullinuria
cladosporiosis
Cladosporium
Claforan (cefotaxime
  sodium)
Clagett operation
clairvoyance
clamp and cautery,
  hemorrhoids
clamp, rubber-dam
clamping, aneurysm
clamping, blood vessel
clang
clap
clapotage

clapotement
clapping
Clapton's lines
clarificant
clarification
Clark's rule
Clarke, Jacob A.L.
Clarke's bodies
Clarke's column
Clarke-Hadfield syndrome
clasmatocyte
clasmatodendrosis
clasmatosis
clasp
clasp-knife rigidity
classification, plant or
   animal
clastic
clastogenic
clastothrix
Claude's syndrome
claudication,
   intermittent
claudication, venous
Claudius' cells
Claudius' fossa
claustrophilia
claustrophobia
claustrum
clausura
clava
clavate
clavicle
clavicle, dislocation of
clavicle, fracture of
clavicotomy
clavicular
claviculectomy
clavus
claw finger
claw toe
clawfoot
clawhand
Clayton gas
Clayton operation
clean room
clean-catch method
cleaning, ultrasonic

cleaning, wound
Clear Eyes (lubricating
   eye redness reliever)
clearance
clearance, bladder
clearance, pelvic
clearance, prescalene fat
   pad
clearance, renal pelvis
clearance, ureter
clearing agent
Clearsil
   (sulfur/resorcinol)
cleavage
cleavage cell
cleavage lines
cleft, alveolar
cleft, branchial
cleft cheek
cleft, facial
cleft hand
cleft hand repair
cleft lip repair
cleft palate repair
cleft sternum
cleft tongue
cleftfoot
cleftlip
cleftpalate
cleidocostal
cleidorrhexis
cleidotomy
clemastine fumarate
clenching
Cleocin (clindamycin HCl)
Cleocin HCl (clindamycin
   HCl)
Cleocin Pediatric
   (clindamycin palmitate
   hydrochloride)
Cleocin Phosphate
   (clindamycin phosphate)
Cleocin T (clindamycin
   phosphate)
cleptomania
click
clidinium bromide
client

climacteric
climatology, medical
climatotherapy
climax
clindamycin hydrochloride
clinic (CL)
clinical
clinical analysis
clinical judgment
clinical nurse specialist
  (CNS)
clinical pathology
clinical thermometer
clinical trial
clinician
clinician, nurse
clinicopathologic
clinicopathologic
  conference (CPC)
clinocephaly
clinodactyly
clinoid
clinoid process
clinometer
Clinoril (sulindac)
clinoscope
clinostatism
clip
clipping, aneurysm
  (basilar)
clipping, aneurysm
  (carotid)
clipping, aneurysm
  (cerebellar)
clipping, aneurysm
  (cerebellopontine)
clipping, aneurysm
  (communicating artery)
clipping, aneurysm
  (vertebral)
clipping, arteriovenous
  fistula
clipping, frenulum
clipping, labia (lips)
clipping, linguae
  (tongue)
clipping, tip of uvula
clipping, vena cava

cliseometer
Clistin (carbinoxamine
  maleate)
clithrophobia
clition
clitoridectomy
clitoriditis
clitoridotomy
clitoris
clitoris crises
clitorism
clitoritis
clitoromegaly
clivogram
clivus
clivus, blumenbachii
clo
cloaca
clobetasol propionate
clock, biological
clofazimine
clofibrate
Clomid (clomiphene
  citrate)
clomiphene citrate
clonal
clonazepam
clonazepam test
clone
clonic
clonic spasm
clonicity
clonicotonic
clonidine hydrochloride
cloning
clonism
clonismus
clonography
Clonopin (clonazepam)
clonorchiasis
Clonorchis sinensis
clonus
Cloquet's canal
Cloquet's node excision
Clorpactin WCS-90 (sodium
  oxychlorosene)
Clos-O-Mat
Clostridium

Clostridium botulinum
Clostridium chauvoei
Clostridium difficile
Clostridium histolyticum
Clostridium novyi
Clostridium perfringens
Clostridium septicum
Clostridium sporogenes
Clostridium tetani
Clostridium welchii
closure
clot
clot, agony
clot, antemortem
clot, chicken fat
clot, currant jelly
clot, distal
clot, external
clot, heart
clot, internal
clot, laminated
clot lysis
clot, muscle
clot, passive
clot, plastic
clot, postmortem
clot, proximal
clot retraction test
clot, stratified
clothes louse
clothing
clotrimazole
clotting
clotting factor
clotting inhibitors
clouding of consciousness
cloudy swelling
clove oil
cloven spine
clownism
cloxacillin sodium
Cloxapen (cloxacillin
  sodium)
clubbing
clubfoot
clubfoot capsulotomy,
  midfoot
clubhand

clue cells
clump
clumping
clunes
Clusivol (vitamin
  supplement with
  minerals)
cluster headache
cluttering
Clutton's joint
clysis
clysma
clyster
cnemial
cnemis
cnemitis
cnemoscoliosis
Co-Gesic (hydrocodone
  bitartrate and
  acetaminophen)
co-twin
coacervate
Coactin (amdinocillin)
coadaptation
coadunation
coagglutination
coagula
coagulability
coagulable
coagulant
coagulase
coagulate
coagulated
coagulated proteins
coagulation
coagulation factors
coagulation time
coagulative
coagulometer
coagulopathy
coagulopathy, consumption
coagulum
coal tar
coal worker's
  pneumoconiosis
coalesce
coalescence
coapt

coaptation
coarctate
coarctation, aorta
coarctotomy
coat
coating, aneurysm of
  brain
Coats' disease
cobalamin
cobalamin concentrate
cobalt (Co)
cobalt-57
cobalt-60 therapy
cobra
cobra venom solution
coca
cocaine hydrochloride
cocaine hydrochloride
  poisoning
cocainism
cocainization
cocainomania
cocarboxylase
cocarcinogen
coccal
cocci
Coccidia
coccidian
Coccidioides
coccidioidin
Coccidioidomycosis
Coccidioidomycosis skin
  test
coccidiosis
coccobacilli
coccobacteria
coccogenous
coccoid
coccus
coccyalgia
coccydynia
coccygeal
coccygeal body
coccygeal nerves
coccygectomy
coccygeus
coccygodynia
coccygotomy

coccyx
cochineal
cochlea
cochlear
cochlear implant
cochlear nerve
cochleare
cochleariform
cochleitis
cochleo-orbicular reflex
cochleopalpebral reflex
cochleovestibular
cochlitis
"cocked hat" procedure
cock-up fifth toe
cock-up splint
cock-up toe
Coco-Quinine (quinine
  sulfate)
Cockett operation
cockroach
cocktail
cocktail, lytic
cocoa butter
coconsciousness
cocontraction
coconut "water"
coctolabile
coctoprecipitin
coctostabile
cod liver oil
Codalan (codeine
  phosphate,
  acetaminophen and
  caffeine)
Code for Nurses
code, genetic
code, triplet
codeine phosphate
codeine poisoning
codeine sulfate
Codiclear DH Syrup
Codimal DH
Codimal DM
Codimal Expectorant
Codimal PH
Codimal-L.A. Capsules
codon

Codroxomin
  (hydroxocobalamin)
Cody tack
coefficient
coefficient, isotonic
coefficient of absorption
Coelenterata
coelom
coelom, extraembryonic
coenocyte
coenzyme
coenzyme A (CoA)
Coenzyme Q10 (essential
  nutrient)
coetaneous
coexcitation
cofactor
coferment
coffee
coffee-ground vomitus
Coffey operation
Cogan's syndrome
Cogentin (benztropine
  mesylate)
cognition
cognitive
cogwheel respiration
cogwheeling
cohension
coherent
cohesive
Cohnheim's theory
Cohnheims's areas
cohort
cohort study
coil
coilonychia
coin counting
coin test
coital
coition
coitophobia
coitus
coitus, à la vache
coitus, interruptus
coitus, reservatus
coitus, Saxonius
col

Cola
Colace (docusate sodium)
colalgia
colation
colauxe
ColBENEMID (probenecid-
  colchicine)
colchicine
cold agglutinin
cold agglutinin disease
cold agglutinins test
cold auto absorption
cold, chest
cold, common
cold cream
cold packs
cold pressor test
cold sore
coldspray
Cole operation
colectomy
coleocystitis
coleoptosis
coleotomy
Colestid (colestipol HCl)
colestipol hydrochloride
colibacillemia
colibacillosis
colibacilluria
colibacillus
colic, biliary
colic, infantile
colic, intestinal
colic, lead
colic, menstrual
colic, renal
colic, uterine
colica
colicin
colicky
colicolitis
colicoplegia
colicystitis
colicystopyelitis
coliform
colilysin
colinephritis
colipase

coliplication
colipuncture
colipyuria
colisepsis
colistimethate sodium
colistin sulfate
colitis, amebic
colitis, mucous
colitis, pseudomembranous
colitis, ulcerative
colitoxemia
colitoxicosis
colitoxin
coliuria
colla
collagen
collagen vascular
  diseases
collagenase
collagenation
collagenic
collagenoblast
collagenolysis
collagenosis
collapse
collapse, circulatory
collapse, lung
collapse of lung
collapsing
collapsing pulse
collapsotherapy
collar
collar of Venus
collarbone
collateral
collateral circulation
collateral eminence
collateral fissure
collateral ganglia
collateral trigone
collaterals
collecting tubules
collection
collection, sperm
Colles' fascia
Colles' fracture
colliculectomy
colliculitis

colliculus
colliculus bulbi
colliculus bulbi
  intermedius
colliculus cervicalis
colliculus inferior
colliculus, seminalis
colliculus superior
colliculus urethralis
collimation
collimator
colliquation
colliquative
Collis-Nissen operation
collodion
collodion, flexible
collodion, salicylic acid
colloid
colloid chemistry
colloid cyst
colloid degeneration
colloid suspension
colloid therapy
colloidal
colloidal dispersion
colloidin
colloidoclasia
colloidopexy
colloma
collonema
collopexia
collum
collyrium
Collyrium Eye Lotion
  (neutral borate
  solution)
coloboma
colocecostomy
colocentesis
colocholecystostomy
coloclysis
coloclyster
colocolostomy
colocutaneous
colocynth
colocystoplasty
coloenteritis
colofixation

colofixation
Cologel (methylcellulose)
coloileotomy
colon
colon, ascending
colon, bacteria of
colon biopsy
colon, descending
colon, irritable
colon, sigmoid
colon, toxic dilatation
   of
colon, transverse
colonalgia
colonic
colonic irrigation
colonitis
colonization
Colonna operation
colonometer
colonopathy
colonopexy
colonorrhagia
colonorrhea
colonoscope
colonoscopy
colonospasm
colony
colony counter
colony-stimulating factor
colopexia
colopexostomy
colopexotomy
colopexy
coloplication
coloproctectomy
coloproctitis
coloproctostomy
coloptosia
coloptosis
colopuncture
color blindness
color deficient
color gustation
color hearing
color index (CI)
color sense
color vision examination

color's, primary
colorectitis
colorectosigmoidostomy
colorectostomy
colorectum
colorimeter
colorrhaphy
coloscopy
colosigmoidostomy
colostomy
colostomy, double barrel
colostomy, terminal
colostomy, wet
colostrorrhea
colostrum
colotomy
colovaginal
colovesical
colpalgia
colpatresia
colpectasia
colpectomy
colpeurynter
colpeurysis
colpitis
colpo-urethrocystopexy
colpocele
colpoceliocentesis
colpoceliotomy
colpocentesis
colpocleisis
colpocystitis
colpocystocele
colpocystoplasty
colpocystosyrinx
colpocystotomy
colpocytology
colpodynia
colpohyperplasia
colpohyperplasia cystica
colpohysterectomy
colpomicroscope
colpomyomectomy
colpomyomotomy
colpoperineoplasty
colpoperineorrhaphy
colpopexy
colpoplasty

colpopoiesis
colpoptosis
colporrhagia
colporrhaphy
colporrhexis
colposcope
colposcopy
colpospasm
colpospasmus
colpostat
colpostenosis
colpostenotomy
colpotherm
colpotomy
colpoureterocystotomy
colpoureterotomy
colpoxerosis
columbium
columella
columella cochleae
columella nasi
column, anal
column, anterior
column, Clarke's
column, fornix
column, gray
column, lateral
column of Burdach
column of Goll
column of Gowers
column of Morgagni
column, posterior
column, rectal
column, renal
column, spinal
column, vertebral
column, vesicular
columna
columna carnea
columna nasi
columna rugarum vaginae
columna vaginalis
columnar layer
columning
Coly-Mycin M Parenteral
(colistimethate sodium)

Coly-Mycin S for Oral
Suspension (colistin
sulfate)
Coly-Mycin S Otic (with
neomycin and
hydrocortisone)
Colyte (polyethylene
glycol and electrolytes
for oral solution)
coma
coma, alcoholic
coma, apoplectic
coma, barbiturate
coma, diabetic
coma, hepatic
coma, hypoglycemic
coma, irreversible
coma, Kussmaul's
coma scale
coma, uremic
coma, vigil
comatose
Combipres (clonidine HCl
and chlorthalidone)
combustion
comedo
comedode
CoMega (natural fish oil
concentrate)
comes
Comfolax (docusate
sodium)
Comhist LA
comma bacillus
comma tract of Schultze
Commando operation
commensal
commensalism
comminute
comminuted
comminuted fracture
comminution
Commission Certified (CC)
commissural
commissura
commissure, anterior
cerebral

commissure, anterior gray
commissure, anterior
  white
commissure, of fornix
commissure, posterior, of
  brain
commissure, posterior, of
  spinal cord
commissurorrhaphy
commissurotomy
commitment
common bile duct
common mode rejection
  ratio (CMRR)
commotio
commotio retinae
commotio spinalis
communicable disease
communicans
communication board
communicator
communis
community medicine
Comolli's sign
compact
compact bone
compaction
comparative anatomy
compartmental syndrome
compatibility
compatible
Compazine
  (prochlorperazine
  maleate)
compensating
compensation
compensation, failure of
competence
competition
complaint
complement
complement (C3) test
complement (C4) test
complement fixation
complement fixation test
  (CFT)
complemental air
complemental colors

complementarity
complementary
complementophil
complete blood count
  (CBC)
complete heart block
  (CHB)
complex
complex, castration
complex, Electra
complex, Ghon
complex, Golgi
complex, inferiority
complex, Oedipus
complex, superiority
complexion
complexus
compliance
complication
component
component blood therapy
compos mentis
composite graft
compound astigmatism
compound, dental
compound fracture
compound, inorganic
compound microscope
compound, organic
compound S test
Compound W (salicylic
  acid)
Comprehensive
  Occupational Assessment
  and Training System
  (COATS)
compress
compress, chest
compress, cold
compress, forehead
compress, hot
compress, wet
compressed spectral array
  (CSA)
compression, cerebral
compression, digital
compression gloves
compression, myelitis

compressor
compulsion
compulsion neurosis
compulsive
compulsive ideas
compulsory
computer
computer interface
computer-assisted design
  (CAD)
computerized assisted
  design (CAD)
computerized axial
  tomography (CAT)
computerized tomography
  (CT)
Comtrex (multi-symptom
  cold reliever)
conarium
conation
conative
concanavalin A
concatenation
Concato's disease
concave
concavity
concavoconcave
concavoconvex
conceive
concentration
concentration, hydrogen
  ion
concentration, minimum
  inhibitory
concentric
concept
conception
Conceptrol (birth control
  cream)
Conceptrol (contraceptive
  gel)
conceptus
concha
conchectomy
conchitis
conchoidal
conchoscope
conchotomy

concoction
concomitant
concordance
concrement
concrescence
concrete
concretio cordis
concretion
concussion
concussion of brain
concussion of labyrinth
concussion, spinal
condensation
condenser
condenser, electrical
condenser, substage
condiment
condition
conditioned reflex (CR)
conditioning
conditioning, operant
condom
Condom Mate Lubricant
conductance
conduction
conduction study, nerve
conduction system,
cardiac
conduction velocity study
conductivity
conductor
conduit
conduit, ileal
conduitogram, ileum
condylar
condylarthrosis
condyle
condylectomy
condylion
condyloid
condyloid process
condyloid tubercle
condyloma
condyloma acuminatum
condyloma latum
condylomata
condylomatous
condylotomy

condylus
cone
cone, ocular
cone of light
cone, retinal
conexus
confabulation
confectio
confection
conference
confidentiality
configuration
confinement
conflict
confluence of sinuses
confluent
conformation
confrontation
confusion
confusion, mental
congelation
congener
congenerous
congenital
congenital anomaly
Congespirin (cough syrup)
Congess Sr & Jr Capsules
  (expectorant/
  decongestant)
congested
congestion, active
congestion, passive
congestion, pulmonary
congestive
congestive heart failure
  (CHF)
congius
conglobate
conglobation
conglomerate
conglutin
conglutinant
conglutinate
conglutination
coniasis
conidia
conidiophore
coniofibrosis

coniology
coniosis
coniosporosis
coniotomy
conization
conjugata
conjugate
conjugate deviation
conjugate, diagonal
conjugate diameter
conjugate, external
conjugate, true
conjugation
conjunctiva
conjunctival reflex
conjunctivitis
conjunctivitis, actinic
conjunctivitis, acute
  contagious
conjunctivitis, angular,
  of Morax-Axenfeld
conjunctivitis, catarrhal
conjunctivitis, epidemic
  hemorrhagic
conjunctivitis,
  follicular
conjunctivitis,
  gonorrheal
conjunctivitis, granular
conjunctivitis, inclusion
conjunctivitis,
  membranous
conjunctivitis of newborn
conjunctivitis,
  phlyctenular
conjunctivitis, purulent
conjunctivitis, vernal
conjunctivo-tarso-levator
conjunctivo-
  cystorhinostomy
conjunctivodacryo-
  cystostomy
conjunctivodacryo-
  cystorhinostomy (CDCR)
conjunctivoma
conjunctivoplasty
conjunctivorhinostomy
Conn's syndrome

connective
connective tissue
connective tissue disease
conoid
conoid ligament
conoid tubercle
consanguinity
conscience
conscious
consciousness
consciousness, clouding
  of
consciousness, cosmic
consciousness,
  disintegration of
consciousness, levels of
consensual
consensual light index
consensual light reflex
consensual reflex
consent
consent, implied
consent, informed
consenting adult
conservative
consolidation
constant
Constant-T (theophylline
  anhydrous)
constellation
constipation
constipation, atonic
constipation, obstructive
constipation, spastic
constitution
constitutional
constitutional disease
constriction
constriction of globe,
  for scleral buckling
constrictor
constructive metabolism
consultant
consultation
consummation
consumption
consumption-coagulopathy
consumptive

contact
contact, complete
contact dermatitis
contact, direct
contact, indirect
contact lens
contact lens, bifocal
contact lens, hard
contact lens, soft
contact, mediate
contact, occlusal
contact, proximal
contact, proximate
contact surface
contactant
contagion
contagious
contagious pustular
  dermatitis
contagium
containers
contaminant
contaminate
contamination
contamination, radiation
content
contiguity
contiguity, amputation in
contiguity, law of
contiguity, solution of
continence
continent
continued
continuity
continuity, amputation in
continuity, solution of
continuous
continuous ambulatory
  peritoneal dialysis
  (CAPD)
continuous arteriovenous
  hemodialysis (CAH)
continuous cycle
  peritoneal dialysis
  (CCPD)
continuous negative
  ventilation pressure
  (CNP)

continuous positive air
  pressure (CPAP)
continuous positive
  airway ventilation
  pressure (CPAP)
continuous positive-
  pressure breathing
  (CPPB)
continuous positive-
  pressure ventilation
  (CPPV)
continuous spectrum
continuous subcutaneous
  insulin infusion (CSII)
contortion
contour, gingival
contour, gingival denture
contoured
contra-aperture
contraception
contraceptive
contract
contractile
contractility
contraction
contraction, Braxton
  Hicks
contraction, carpopedal
contraction, Dupuytren's
contraction, isometric
contraction, isotonic
contraction, postural
contraction stress test
  (CST)
contraction, tetanic
contraction, tonic
contracture
contracture, Dupuytren's
contracture, functional
contracture, ischemic
contracture,
  physiological
contracture, Volkmann's
contrafissura
contraindication
contralateral
contralateral reflexes
contrast

contrast enhancement of
  computed tomographic
  (CECT)
contrast medium
contrast sprays
contravolitional
contrecoup
contrecoup injury
contrectation
control
controlled substance act
contrude
contrusion
contuse
contusion
conus
conus arteriosus
conus medullaris
convalescence
convalescent
convalescent diet
convection
convergence
convergent
conversion
conversion reaction
conversion symptom
convex
convexoconcave
convexoconvex
convolute
convoluted
convoluted tubule
convolution
convolution, angular
convolution, anterior
  choroid
convolution, anterior
  orbital
convolution, Arnold's
convolution, ascending
  frontal
convolution, ascending
  parietal
convolution, Broca's
convolution, callosal
convolution, cuneate
convolution, dentate

convolution, hippocampal
convolution, inferior
  frontal
convolution, inferior
  occipital
convolution, insular
convolution, marginal
convolution, middle
  frontal
convolution, middle
  occipital
convolution, middle
  temporosphenoidal
convolution of the corpus
  callosum
convolution of the
  sylvian fissure
convolution, olfactory
convolution, posterior
  orbital
convolution, second
  frontal
convolution, superior
  frontal
convolution, superior
  occipital
convolution, superior
  temporosphenoidal
convolution,
  supramarginal
convolution, transverse
  orbital
convolution, uncinate
convolutions, annectant
convolutions, cerebral
convolutions, exterior
  olfactory
convolutions, intestinal
convolutions,
  occipitotemporal
convolutions, orbital
convolutions, parietal
convulsant
convulsant poisons
convulsion
convulsion, clonic
convulsion, febrile
convulsion, hysterical

convulsion, mimetic
convulsion, oscillating
convulsion, puerperal
convulsion, salaam
convulsion, tonic
convulsion, toxic
convulsion, uremic
convulsive
convulsive reflex
convulsive tic
cooking
Cooley's anemia
cooling, gastric
Coombs' direct test
Coombs' indirect test
Coombs' test
coordination
cope
coping
copodyskinesia
copolymer
copper (Cu)
copper sulfate
copper sulfate poisoning
copperas
copperhead
Coppertrace (cupric
  chloride injection)
copremesis
coproantibody
coprolagnia
coprolalia
coprolith
coprology
coproma
coprophagy
coprophilia
coprophilic
coprophobia
coproporphyria
coproporphyrin
coproporphyrinuria
coprostanol
coprozoa
coprozoic
copula
copulation
cor pulmonale

coracoacromial
coracoacromial ligament
  release
coracoid
coracoid process
coracoid process transfer
Coramine (nikethamide)
cord
cord bladder
cord, spermatic
cord, spinal
cord, umbilical
cord, vocal
corda willisii
cordal
Cordarone (amiodarone
  HCl)
cordate
cordectomy, vocal
cordiform
corditis
cordopexy
cordopexy, vocal
cordotomy
Cordran (flurandrenolide)
Cordran-N (neomycin
  sulfate with
  flurandrenolide)
core
core temperature
coreclisis
corectasia
corectasis
corectome
corectomy
corectopia
coredialysis
corediastasis
corelysis
coremorphosis
coreometer
coreometry
coreoplasty
corepressor
corestenoma
corestenoma congenitum
coretomedialysis
coretomy

Corgard (nadolol)
Cori cycle
corium
corm
cornea
corneal
corneal contact lens
corneal impression
corneal reflex
corneal section
corneal transplant
corneitis
Cornell Medical Index
corneoblepharon
corneoconjunctivoplasty
corneoiritis
corneomandibular reflex
corneosclera
corneoscleral contact
  lens
corneoscleral section
corneous
corneous layer
corneovitreal adhesions
corneum
corniculate
corniculum
cornification
cornified
cornu
cornu ammonis
cornu anterius
cornu coccygeum
cornu cutaneum
cornu inferius
cornu of the hyoid
cornu of the sacrum
cornu posterius
cornua
cornual
corona
corona capitis
corona ciliaris
corona dentis
corona glandis
corona radiata
corona veneris
coronal

coronal computerized
  tomography (CCT)
coronal plane
coronal suture
coronary
coronary angiography
coronary angioplasty
coronary arteries
coronary artery
coronary artery bypass
  (CAB)
coronary artery bypass
  graft surgery (CABG)
coronary artery disease
  (CAD)
coronary artery spasm
coronary blood flow
coronary bypass
coronary care unit (CCU)
coronary heart disease
  (CHD)
coronary occlusion
coronary plexus
coronary sinus
coronary thrombolysis
coronary thrombosis
coronaviruses
coroner
coronoid
coronoidectomy
coronoid fossa
coronoid process
coroparelcysis
coroscopy
corotomy
corpora
corpora arantii
corpora arenacea
corpora cavernosa
corpora cavernosa-corpus
  spongiosum shunt
corpora cavernosa-glans
  penis fistulization
corpora cavernosa-
  saphenous vein shunt
corpora cavernosography
corpora olivaria
corpora paraaortica

corpora quadrigemina
corporeal
corpse
corpsman
corpulence
corpulent
corpus
corpus albicans
corpus amygdaloideum
corpus amylaceum
corpus annulare
corpus callosum
corpus cavernosum
corpus cavernosum penis
corpus cerebellum
corpus ciliare
corpus dentale
corpus fimbriatum
corpus flavum
corpus fornicis
corpus geniculatum
corpus hemorrhagicum
corpus highmorianum
corpus interpedunculare
corpus luteum
corpus Luysii
corpus mammillare
corpus restiforme
corpus rhomboidale
corpus spongiosum
corpus striatum
corpus subthalamicum
corpus trapezoideum
corpus uteri
corpus vitreum
corpus wolffianum
corpuscle
corpuscle, axile
corpuscle, axis
corpuscle, blood
corpuscle, bone
corpuscle, cancroid
corpuscle, cartilage
corpuscle, chromophil
corpuscle, collid
corpuscle, colostrum
corpuscle, ghost
corpuscle, lymph

corpuscle, malpighian
corpuscle, Meissner's
corpuscle, pacinian
corpuscle, phantom
corpuscle, Purkinje's
corpuscle, red
corpuscle, renal
corpuscle, splenic
corpuscle, tactile
corpuscle, terminal
corpuscle, white
corpuscles, chyle
corpuscles, corneal
corpuscles, Drysdale's
corpuscles, genital
corpuscles, Gierke's
corpuscles, Golgi-Mazzoni
corpuscles, Hassall's
corpuscles, Krause's
corpuscles, Mazzoni's
corpuscles, milk
corpuscles, reticulated
corpuscles, thymic
corpuscular
corpusculum
correction
corrective
correlation
correspondence
correspondence, retinal
corresponding
corresponding points of
  retina
Corrigan's pulse
corrosion
corrosive
corrosive alkalies
corrosive poisoning
corrugator
Cort-Dome
  (hydrocortisone)
Cortaid
Cortef (hydrocortisone)
Cortef Acetate
  (hydrocortisone
  acetate)
Cortenema (hydrocortisone
  retention enema)

cortex
cortex, adrenal
cortex, cerebellar
cortex, cerebral
cortex, interpretive
cortex, renal
cortex, temporal
Corti, Alfonso
Corti, canal of
Corti, organ of
Corti's membrane
cortiadrenal
Corticaine
  (hydrocortisone
  acetate)
cortical
cortical artery
  anastomosis
corticate
corticectomy
cortices
corticifugal
corticipetal
corticoadrenal
corticoafferent
corticobulbar
corticoefferent
corticoid
corticopeduncular
corticopleuritis
corticopontine
corticospinal
corticosteroid
corticosterone
corticothalamic
corticotrophic
corticotrophin
corticotropic
corticotropin
corticotropin-releasing
  factor (CRF)
Cortifoam (hydrocortisone
  acetate)
cortin
cortisol
cortisol test
cortisone

Cortisone administration
test
Cortisporin
(antibacterial)
Cortone (cortisone
acetate)
Cortone Acetate
(cortisone acetate)
Cortril (hydrocortisone)
Cortril Acetate-AS
(hydrocortisone
acetate)
Cortrophin
(corticotropin)
Cortrophin Zinc ACTH
(corticotropin zinc
hydroxide)
Cortrosyn (corticotropin)
coruscation
corybantism
Corynebacterium
Corynebacterium
diphtheriae
Corynebacterium vaginale
coryza
Corzide 40/5 (nadolol and
bendroflumethiazide)
Corzide 80/5 (nadolol and
bendroflumethiazide)
cosensitize
Cosmegen (dactinomycin)
cosmetic
cosmetic surgery
cosmic
costa
costa fluctuans
costa spuria
costa vera
costal
costal cartilage
costal pit
costalgia
costectomy
Costen's syndrome
costive
costiveness
costocervical
costochondral

costochondral cartilage
graft
costochondrectomy
costoclavicular
costocoracoid
costophrenic
costopneumopexy
costosternal
costosternoplasty
costotome
costotomy
costotransverse
costotransversectomy
costovertebral
costoxiphoid
cosyntropin
Cotazym (pancrelipase)
Cotazym-S (enteric
coated-pancrelipase)
cotinine
cotton
cotton, purified
cotton, styptic
cotton-wool spot
cotyledon
CoTYLENOL (cold
medication)
cotyloid
cotyloid cavity
couching
cough
cough, aneurysmal
cough, asthmatic
cough, brassy
cough, bronchial
cough, diphtherial
cough, dry
cough, ear
cough, effective
cough, hacking
cough, harsh
cough, moist
cough, paroxysmal
cough, productive
cough, pulmonary
cough, reflex
cough, uterine
cough, whooping

coulomb (C)
Coumadin (warfarin
  sodium)
counseling
count
counter
counter, Coulter
counter electrophoresis
counter, Geiger
counter, scintillation
counteract
counteraction
countercurrent exchanger
counterextension
counterimmuno-
  electrophoresis
counterincision
counterirritant
counterirritation
counteropening
counterpressure
  instrument
counterpulsation, intra-
  aortic balloon (IABC)
counterpuncture
countershock
counterstain
countertraction
countertransference
counts per minute (c/m)
counts per minute (c/min)
counts per minute (cpm)
coup de soleil
  (sunstroke)
couple
coupling
course
Courvoisier's law
couvade
Couvelaire uterus
covalence
covalent
covariance
covariant
Coventry operation
cover
cover glass
cover slip

Cowden's disease
Cowling's rule
Cowper's glands
cowperitis
cowpox
coxa
coxa plana
coxa valga
coxa vara
coxalgia
coxarthrosis
Coxiella
Coxiella burnetii
coxitis
coxodynia
coxofemoral
coxotuberculosis
coxsackievirus
cozymase
crab louse
"crack"
cracked pot sound
cradle
cradle cap
cramp
cranial
cranial bones
cranial decompression
cranial nerves
craniectomy
cranioacromial
craniocaudal
craniocele
craniocerebral
cranioclasis
cranioclasis, fetal
cranioclast
cranioclasty
craniocleidodysostosis
craniodidymus
craniofacial
craniograph
craniology
craniomalacia
craniometer
craniometric points
craniometry
craniopagus

craniopharyngeal
craniopharyngioma
cranioplasty
craniopuncture
craniorhachischisis
cranioslerosis
cranioscopy
craniospinal
craniostenosis
craniostosis
craniosynostosis
craniotabes
craniotome
craniotomy
craniotonoscopy
craniotrypesis
craniotympanic
cranium
crapulent
crapulous
crater
crateriform
craterization
cravat bandage
Crawford operation
crazing
crazy bone
cream of tartar
crease
crease, gluteofemoral
creatinase
creatine
creatine kinase
creatine phosphokinase
  (CPK)
creatinemia
creatinine (creat)
creatinine clearance test
creatinuria
creation
creatorrhea
Credé maneuver
Credé's method
Cremacoat (throat coating
  cough medicine)
cremains
cremaster
cremasteric

cremasteric fascia
cremasteric reflex
cremate
crematorium
crenate
crenation
crenocyte
Creon (pancreatin)
creosote
crepitant
crepitation
crepitus
crepitus redux
crepuscular
crescent
crescent, articular
crescent bodies
crescent, myopic
crescent of Giannuzzi
crescentic
Crescormon (somatropin)
cresol
cresomania
crest
crest, alveolar
CREST syndrome
cretin
cretinism
cretinoid
cretinous
crevice
crevice, gingival
crevicular
cri du chat syndrome
crib
crib death
cribbing
cribrate
cribration
cribriform
cribriform fascia
cribriform plate
crick
cricoarytenoid
cricoderma
cricoid
cricoid cartilage
cricoidectomy

cricoidynia
cricopharyngeal
cricopharyngeal myotomy
cricothyroid
cricothyroidectomy
cricothyroidostomy
cricothyrotomy
cricotomy
cricotracheotomy
Crigler-Najjar syndrome
criminal
criminology
crinogenic
cripple
crisis
crisis, abdominal
crisis, addisonian
crisis, celiac
crisis, Dietl's
crisis intervention
crisis, salt-losing
crisis, sickle cell
crisis, tabetic
crisis, thyroid
crisis, true
crispation
crista
crista ampullaris
crista galli
crista lacrimalis
  posterior
crista spiralis
criterion
critical
critical care (CC)
critical period
Criticare HN (high
  nitrogen elemental
  diet)
crocodile tears
croesomania
Crohn's disease
cromolyn sodium
Crookes' dark space
Crookes' tube
cross
cross bite
cross education

cross finger pedicle flap
cross lip pedicle flap
cross-bridges
cross-dress
cross-eye
cross-fertilization
crossbirth
crossbreeding
crossed
crossed reflexes
crossing over
crossmatch (XM)
crossmatch, blood
crossmatching
crossover
Crotalus
crotamiton
crotaphion
croton oil
crotonism
croup
croup, catarrhal
croup, diphtheritic
croup, membranous
croup, spasmodic
croupous
Crouzon's disease
crowing
crown
crown, anatomic
crown, clinical
crown, dental
crown-rump (CR)
crowning
crownwork
crucial
cruciate
cruciate ligament
crucible
cruciform
crude
Cruex (antifungal powder,
  spray powder and cream)
crura
crura cerebelli
crura cerebri
crura of diaphragm
crura of the fornix

crural
crural arch
crural hernia
crural nerve
crural palsies
crus
crus cerebri
crush syndrome
crushing
crust
crust cryosurgery
crusta
crutch
crutch paralysis
Crutchfield tongs
Cruveilhier-Baumgarten
  syndrome
cry
cry, cephalic
cry, epileptic
cry, hydrocephalic
cry, night
cry reflex
cryalgesia
cryanesthesia
cryesthesia
crymodynia
crymophilic
crymophylactic
crymotherapy
cryoaerotherapy
cryobank
cryobiology
cryocautery
cryoconization, cervix
cryodestruction
cryoextraction
cryoextraction, lens
cryofibrinogen
cryogen
cryogenic
cryoglobulin
cryoglobulinemia
cryoglobulins test
cryohypophysectomy
cryoleucotomy
cryometer
cryopexy, retinal

cryophilic
cryoprecipitate
cryopreservation
cryoprobe
cryoprotectants
cryoprotective
cryoprotein
cryoretinopexy
cryospray
cryostat
cryosurgery
cryothalamotomy
cryotherapy
cryotolerant
crypt
crypt, anal
crypt, bony
crypt of iris
crypt of Lieberkühn
crypt, synoviparous
crypt, tonsillar
cryptanamnesia
cryptectomy
cryptesthesia
cryptic
cryptitis
cryptocephalus
cryptococcosis
Cryptococcus
cryptodidymus
cryptogenic
cryptogenic infection
cryptolith
cryptomenorrhea
cryptomerorachischisis
cryptomnesia
cryptophthalmus
cryptoplasmic
cryptopodia
cryptopyic
cryptorchid
cryptorchidectomy
cryptorchidism
cryptorchis
cryptorchism
cryptorrhea
cryptorrheic
cryptorrhetic

cryptoscope
cryptosporidiosis
Cryptosporidium
cryptotomy
cryptotoxic
cryptoxanthin
crystal
crystal, apatite
crystals, Charcot-Leyden
crystals, Charcot-Robin
crystals, Charcot-Neumann
crystals of hemin
crystals, spermin
crystallin
crystalline
crystalline deposits
crystalline lens
crystallization
crystallography
crystalloid
crystalloiditis
crystallophobia
crystalluria
Crystodigin (digitoxin)
CS gas
Ctenocephalides
Cu-7 (intrauterine copper
  contraceptive)
cubic centimeter (cc)
cubic measure
cubital
cubital fossa
cubitus
cubitus valgus
cubitus varus
cuboid
cuboid bone
cucurbit
cue
cued speech
cuff
cuff, attached gingival
cuff, gingival
cuffed endotracheal tube
cuffing
cuirass
cul-de-sac
culdocentesis

culdoplasty
culdoscope
culdoscopy
culdotomy
Culex
Culex pipiens
Culex quinquefasciatus
Culicidae
culicide
culicifuge
Cullen's sign
culmen
Culp-Deweerd operation
Culp-Scardino operation
cult
cultivation
cultural
culture
culture and sensitivity
  (C&S)
culture, blood
culture, blood test
culture, cell
culture, contaminated
culture, continuous flow
culture, gelatin
culture, hanging block
culture, hanging drop
culture medium
culture medium, defined
culture, negative
culture, positive
culture, pure
culture shock
culture, slant
culture, sputum test
culture, stab
culture, stock
culture, stool test
culture, streak
culture, throat test
culture, tissue
culture, type
culture, urine test
culture, wound test
cumulative
cumulative drug action
cumulus

cumulus oophorus
cuneate
cuneate fasciculus
cuneate nucleus
cuneiform
cuneiform bones
cuneiform cartilage
cuneocuboid
cuneohysterectomy
cuneus
cuniculus
cunnilinguist
cunnilingus
cunnus
cup
cup arthroplasty of hip
cup, favus
cup, glaucomatous
cup, optic
cup, physiologic
Cupid's bow
cupola
cupping
cupric
cupric sulfate
Cuprid (trientine HCl)
Cuprimine (penicillamine)
cuprous
cuprum
cupruresis
cupula
cupulolithiasis
curare
curarization
curative
curd
cure
curet
curettage
curettage, periapical
curettage, suction
curettage, uterine
curette
curette evacuation, lens
curettement
Curie
curie (Ci)
curiegram

curietherapy
curium (Cm)
curled
Curling's ulcer
currant jelly clot
current
current, alternating (AC)
current, direct (DC)
Curretab
   (medroxyprogesterone
   acetate)
curriculum
Curschmann's spirals
curse
curse, Ondine's
curvature
curvature, angular
curvature of spine
curve
curve, dye-dilution
curve, learning
curve, normal
curve of Carus
curve of Spee
curvilinear
Cushing, Harvey
Cushing's disease
Cushing's syndrome
cushingoid
cushion
cusp
cuspid
cuspidate
cuspidor
custom
cut
cut throat
cutaneolipectomy
cutaneous
cutaneous nerves
cutaneous respiration
cutdown
cutdown, veins
cuticle
cuticle, acquired
cuticle, attachment
cuticle, dental
cuticle, enamel

cuticula
cuticula dentis
cuticularization
cutin
cutireaction
cutireaction, von
  Pirquet's
cutis
cutis anserina
cutis aurantiasis
cutis hyperelastica
cutis laxa
cutis marmorata
cutis pendula
cutis testacea
cutis unctosa
cutis vera
cutis verticis gyrata
cutization
cutting
cuvette
cyanemia
cyanephidrosis
cyanhemoglobin
cyanhidrosis
cyanide
cyanide poisoning
cyanoacrylate adhesives
cyanocobalamin (vitamin
  B_{12})
cyanoderma
cyanogen (CN)
cyanomycosis
cyanopathy
cyanophil
cyanophilous
cyanopia
cyanopsia
cyanosed
cyanosis
cyanosis, congenital
cyanosis, delayed
cyanosis, enterogenous
cyanosis retinae
cyanosis, tardive
cyanotic
cyanuria
cybernetics

cyberphilia
cyberphobia
cycad
cycasin
cyclacillin
cyclamate
cyclandelate
Cyclapen-W (cyclacillin)
cyclarthrosis
cycle
cycle, cardiac
cycle, Cori
cycle, gastric
cycle, genesial
cycle, glycolytic
cycle, Krebs
cycle, life
cycle, menstrual
cyclectomy
cycles per second (CPS)
cyclic
cyclic AMP
cyclic AMP synthetase
cyclic vomiting
cyclicotomy
cyclitis
cyclitis, plastic
cyclitis, purulent
cyclitis, serous
cyclizine hydrochloride
cycloanemization
cyclobenzaprine
  hydrochloride
cycloceratitis
cyclochoroiditis
Cyclocort (amcinonide
  ointment)
cyclocryotherapy
cyclodialysis
cyclodiathermy
cycloelectrolysis
cyclokeratitis
cyclomethycaine sulfate
Cyclopar (tetracycline
  HCl)
cyclopentolate
  hydrochloride
cyclophoria

cyclophosphamide
cyclophotocoagulation
cyclopia
cycloplegia
cycloplegic
cyclopropane
cyclops
cycloserine
cyclosis
cyclosporine
cyclothiazide
cyclothymia
cyclotomy
cyclotron
cyclotropia
cycrimine hydrochloride
cyesis
Cyklokapron (tranexamine acid)
Cylert (pemoline)
cylicotomy
cylinder
cylinders, crossed
cylinders, urinary
cylindroadenoma
cylindroid
cylindroma
cylindruria
cyllosis
cyloid
cymbocephalic
cynamethemoglobin
cynanthropy
cynic spasm
cynophobia
cypridophobia
cypriphobia
cyproheptadine hydrochloride
cyrtometer
cyrtosis
cyst
cyst, adventitious
cyst, alveolar
cyst, apical
cyst, blood
cyst, blue dome
cyst, brachial

cyst, cervical
cyst, chocolate
cyst, colloid
cyst, congenital
cyst, daughter
cyst, dental
cyst, dentigerous
cyst, dermoid
cyst, distention
cyst, echinococcus
cyst, epidermal
cyst, extravasation
cyst, exudation
cyst, follicular
cyst, Gartner's
cyst, hydatid
cyst, implantation
cyst, intraligamentary
cyst, involutional
cyst, keratin
cyst, meibomian
cyst, mucoid
cyst, mucous
cyst, nabothian
cyst, odontogenic
cyst, ovarian
cyst, parasitic
cyst, parovarian
cyst, pilonidal
cyst, porencephalic
cyst, proliferative
cyst, radicular
cyst, retention
cyst, sebaceous
cyst, seminal
cyst, suprasellar
cyst, tubo-ovarian
cyst, unilocular
cyst, vaginal
cyst, vitelline
cystadenocarcinoma
cystadenoma
cystadenoma, pseudomucinous
cystadenoma, serous
cystalgia
cystathionine
cystathioninuria

cystauxe
cystectasy
cystectomy
cysteic acid
cysteine hydrochloride
cystelcosis
cystic
cystic duct
cystic fibrosis (CF)
cystic hygroma
cysticercoid
cysticercosis
cysticercus
cysticotomy
cystiform
cystigerous
cystine
cystinemia
cystinosis
cystinuria
cystistaxia
cystitis
cystitis, interstitial
cystitome
cystitomy
cystiytaxia
cystoadenoma
cystocarcinoma
cystocele
cystocolostomy
cystodiaphanoscopy
cystodynia
cystoelytroplasty
cystoepiplocele
cystoepithelioma
cystofibroma
cystogastrostomy
cystogram
cystography
cystoid
cystojejunostomy
cystolith
cystolithectomy
cystolithiasis
cystolithic
cystolitholapaxy
cystolithotomy
cystolutein

cystoma
cystometaplasia
cystometer
cystometrogram
cystometrography
cystomorphous
cystopexy
cystoplasty
cystoplegia
cystoproctostomy
cystoprostatectomy
cystoptosia
cystoptosis
cystopyelitis
cystopyelography
cystopyelonephritis
cystoradiography
cystorectostomy
cystorrhagia
cystorrhaphy
cystorrhea
cystosarcoma
cystoscope
cystoscopy (cysto)
cystoskeleton
cystospasm
cystostomy
cystotome
cystotomy
cystotrachelotomy
cystoureteritis
cystoureterogram
cystourethritis
cystourethrocele
cystourethrogram
cystourethrography
cystourethrography, chain
cystourethrography,
  voiding
cystourethropexy
cystourethropexy,
  retropubic
cystourethroplasty
cystourethroscopy
cystourethroscope
cystovesiculography
Cytadren
  (aminoglutethimide)

cytarabine
cytase
cytidine
cytoanalyzer
cytoarchitectonic
cytobiology
cytobiotaxis
cytoblast
cytocentrum
cytocerastic
cytochalasin B
cytochemism
cytochemistry
cytochrome
cytochrome oxidase
cytochrome P-450
cytochylema
cytocidal
cytocide
cytoclasis
cytoclastic
cytoclesis
cytodendrite
cytodiagnosis
cytodieresis
cytodistal
cytogenesis
cytogenetic
cytogenetics
cytogenic
cytogenous
cytogeny
cytoglycopenia
cytohistogenesis
cytohyaloplasm
cytoid
cytoinhibition
cytokalipenia
cytokerastic
cytokines
cytologist
cytology
cytolymph
cytolysin
cytolysis
cytomegalic inclusion
  disease
cytomegalovirus (CMV)

Cytomel (liothyronine
  sodium)
cytometer
cytometer, flow
cytometry
cytometry, flow
cytomicrosome
cytomitome
cytomorphology
cytomorphosis
cyton
cytopathic
cytopathogenic effect
cytopathology
cytopenia
cytophagocytosis
cytophagous
cytophagy
cytophilic
cytophotometry
cytophylaxis
cytophyletic
cytophysics
cytophysiology
cytopipette
cytoplasm
cytoplast
cytoproximal
cytoreticulum
cytorrhyctes
Cytosar-U (cytarabine)
cytosine
cytosine arabinoside
cytosol
cytosome
cytospongium
cytost
cytostasis
cytostatic
cytostome
cytotactic
cytotaxia
cytotaxis
cytotherapy
cytothesis
cytotoxic
cytotoxic agents
cytotoxin

cytotrophoblast
cytotropic
cytotropism
Cytoxan
  (cyclophosphamide)
cytozoic
cytozoon
cyturia
Czermak's spaces

D

DHE 45 (dihydroergotamine
  mesylate)
D'Ombrain operation
D-Vert (meclizine HCl)
daboia
daboya
dacarbazine
dacnomania
dacrocystography
dacryadenalgia
dacryadenitis
dacryadenoscirrhus
dacryagogatresia
dacryagogue
dacrycystalgia
dacryelcosis
dacryoadenalgia
dacryoadenectomy
dacryoadenitis
dacryoadenotomy
dacryoblennorrhea
dacryocele
dacryocyst
dacryocystalgia
dacryocystectomy
dacryocystitis
dacryocystoblennorrhea
dacryocystocele
dacryocystogram
dacryocystography
dacryocystoptosis
dacryocystorhinostomy
dacryocystorhinotomy

dacryocystorhinostenosis
dacryocystostomy
dacryocystosyringotomy
dacryocystotome
dacryocystotomy
dacryocyte
dacryogenic
dacryohelcosis
dacryohemorrhea
dacryolin
dacryolite
dacryolith
dacryolithiasis
dacryoma
dacryon
dacryops
dacryopyorrhea
dacryopyosis
dacryorrhea
dacryostenosis
dacryosyrinx
dactinomycin
dactyl
dactyledema
dactylic
dactylion
dactylitis
dactylocampsodynia
dactylogram
dactylography
dactylogryposis
dactylology
dactylolysis
dactylomegaly
dactyloscopy
dactylospasm
dactylus
Dahlman operation
daily living skills
dairy food substitute
Dakin's solution
Dalalone D.P.
  (dexamethasone acetate
  suspension)
Dale reaction
Dalmane (flurazepam HCl)
dalton (Da)
Dalton's law

Dalton-Henry law
dam
Damason-P (hydrocodone bitartrate, aspirin, caffeine)
damp
damp, after
damp, black
damp, cold
damp, fire
damp, white
damping
Dana operation
danazol
dance, Saint Vitus'
dancing disease
dancing mania
dander
dandruff
dandy fever
Dandy-Walker syndrome
Dane particles
Danex (protein enriched dandruff shampoo)
Danforth operation
Danocrine (danazol)
danthron
Dantrium (dantrolene sodium)
dantrolene sodium
Danysz phenomenon
Dapsone
Daranide (dichlorphenamide)
Daraprim (pyrimethamine)
Darbid (isopropamide iodide)
Darier's disease
darkroom
Darling's disease
Darrach operation
dartoid
dartos
dartos muscle reflex
dartrous
Darvocet-N 100 (propoxyphene napsylate and acetaminophen)

Darvon (propoxyphene HCl)
Darvon-N (propoxyphene napsylate)
Darvon-N with A.S.A. (propoxyphene napsylate and aspirin)
darwinian ear
darwinian tubercle
darwinism
dasymeter
date of birth (DOB)
Datril (acetaminophen)
Datura
daughter
daunorubicin hydrochloride
Davidsohn's sign
Davis operation
dawn phenomenon
day blindness
day-care center
Dayalets Filmtab (multivitamin supplement)
daydream
DDD pacing
de Grandmont operation
De Lee maneuver
de Musset's sign
de Pezzer's catheter
de Quervain's disease
de-efferented state
de-lead
deacidification
deactivation
dead
dead on arrival (DOA)
deaf
deaf training
deaf-mute
deafferentation
deafness
deafness, aviator's
deafness, bass
deafness, central
deafness, cerebral
deafness, ceruminous
deafness, conduction

deafness, cortical
deafness, high frequency
deafness, nerve
deafness, occupational
deafness, ototoxic
deafness, perceptive
deafness, psychic
deafness, tone
deafness, word
deamidase
deamidization
deaminase
deamination
deaminization
deaquation
dearterialization
dearticulation
death
death, black
death, brain
death, crib
death, fetal
death, functional
death, local
death, molecular
death rate
death rattle
"death with dignity"
deathbed
deathbed statement
debilitant
debilitate
debility
débouchement
Debove's membrane
debride
debridement
debridement, abdominal
  wall
debridement, arm
debridement, bone
debridement, brain
debridement, canal
debridement, carpal,
  metacarpal
debridement, cerebral
  meninges

debridement, dental
debridement, enzymatic
debridement, epithelial
debridement, femur
debridement, fibula
debridement, flap graft
debridement, foot
debridement, fracture
debridement, hand
debridement, heart valve
debridement, humerus
debridement, infection
debridement, leg
debridement, meninges
debridement, muscle
debridement, nerve
debridement, open
  fracture
debridement, patella
debridement, pedicle
  graft
debridement, phalanges
debridement, radius
debridement, root canal
debridement, skin or
  subcutaneous tissue
debridement, skull
debridement, spinal cord
debridement, tarsal,
  metatarsal
debridement, tibia
debridement, ulna
debridement, wound
debris
Debrisan (wound cleaning
  beads and paste)
debrisoquin
Debrox (carbamide
  peroxide)
debt
debt, oxygen
Deca-Durabolin
  (nandrolone decanoate)
Decaderm (dexamethasone)
  in **Estergel** (isopropyl
  myristate gel)
Decadron (dexamethasone)

Decadron phosphate
   injection
   (dexamethasone sodium
   phosphate)
Decadron phosphate
 Respihaler(dexamethasone
 sodium phosphate)
Decadron phosphate
 Turbinaire(dexamethasone
 sodium phosphate)
Decadron phosphate with
   Xylocaine
Decadron-LA
   (dexamethasone acetate)
decagram (dg)
decalcification
decalcify
decaliter (dl)
decameter (dm)
decannulation
decanormal
decant
decantation
decapitation
decapitation, fetal
decapsulation
decapsulation, kidney
decarboxylase
decarboxylation
decarboxylization
Decaspray (dexamethasone)
decavitamin capsules
decay
decay, radioactive
decayed, extracted, and
   filled teeth (DEF)
decayed, missing, and
   filled teeth (DMF
   Index)
deceleration
decerebrate
decerebrate posture
decerebrate rigidity
decerebration
dechloridation
dechlorination
decholesterolization

Decholin (dehydrocholic
   acid)
decibel (db, dB)
decidophobia
decidua
decidua basalis
decidua capsularis
decidua menstrualis
decidua parietalis
decidua reflexa
decidua serotina
decidua vera
decidual
deciduation
deciduitis
deciduoma
deciduoma, benign
deciduoma, Loeb's
deciduoma, malignant
deciduomatosis
deciduosarcoma
deciduous
deciduous teeth
decigram (dg)
decinormal
decipara
decision analysis
decision making
decision tree
Declaration of Geneva
Declaration of Hawaii
declination
declinator
decline
declivis cerebelli
Declomycin
   (demeclocycline HCl)
declotting
decoction
decollation
décollement
decompensation
decomplementize
decomposition
decomposition, double
decomposition, hydrolytic
decomposition, simple
decompress

decompression
decompression, anus
decompression, auditory
  nerve
decompression, brain
decompression, carpal
  tunnel
decompression, cauda
  equina
decompression, chamber
decompression, common
  bile duct
decompression, cranial
decompression, cranial
  nerve
decompression,
  endolymphatic sac
decompression, explosive
decompression, gastric
decompression, hand
decompression, heart
decompression illness
decompression, intestine
decompression,
  intracranial
decompression, labyrinth
decompression,
  laminectomy
decompression, laminotomy
decompression, median
  nerve
decompression, muscle
decompression, myotomy
decompression, nerve
decompression, orbit
decompression,
  pericardium
decompression, rectum
decompression, skull
  fracture
decompression, tendon
  sheath
decompression, tenotomy
decompression, thoracic
  outlet
decompression, trigeminal
decompression, trigeminal
  nerve

Deconamine
  (chlorpheniramine
  maleate and
  d-pseudoephedrine HCl)
decongestant
Deconsal Sprinkle
  (phenylephrine HCl and
  guaifenesin)
decontamination
decorticate posture
decortication
decortication, arterial
decortication, brain
decortication, cerebral
  meninges
decortication, heart
decortication, kidney
decortication, lung
decortication, nose
decortication, ovary
decortication,
  periarterial
decortication,
  pericardium
decortication, pulmonary
decortication, renal
decortication, ventricle,
  heart
decrement
decrepitate
decrepitation
decrepitude
decrudescence
decubation
decubital
decubitus, acute
decubitus, Andral's
decubitus, dorsal
decubitus, lateral
decubitus projections
decubitus ulcer
decubitus, ventral
decurrent
decussate
decussation
decussation of pyramids
decussation, optic
decussorium

dedifferentiation
dedolation
deduction
deep
deep reflexes
deepening, alveolar ridge
deepening, buccolabial
  sulcus
deepening, lingual sulcus
deer fly fever
defatted
defatting, flap
defatting, pedicle graft
defecalgesiophobia
defecation
defecation syncope
defect
defect, congenital
defect, filling
defect, septal
defective
defeminization
defense
defense mechanism
defense reflex
defensive
defensive medicine
deferens
deferent
deferentectomy
deferential
deferentitis
deferoxamine mesylate
deferred shock
defervescence
defibrillation, electric
defibrillation,
  electrical
defibrillator
defibrination
defibrinization
deficiency
deficiency disease
deficit
defined medium
definition
definitive
deflection

defloration
deflorescence
defluvium
defluvium capillorum
defluxio
defluxio capillorum
defluxio ciliorum
defluxion
deformability
deformation
deformity
deformity, anterior
deformity, gunstock
deformity, Madelung's
deformity, mutilans
deformity, seal fin
deformity, silverfork
deformity, Sprengel's
deformity, Velpeau's
deformity, Volkmann's
defundation
defurfuration
deganglionate
degenerate
degeneration,
  Abercrombie's
degeneration, adipose
degeneration, albuminoid
degeneration, amyloid
degeneration, ascending
degeneration, calcareous
degeneration, caseous
degeneration, cloudy
  swelling
degeneration, colloid
degeneration, congenital
  macular
degeneration, cystic
degeneration, descending
degeneration, fatty
degeneration, fibroid
degeneration, gray
degeneration,
  hepatolenticular
degeneration, hyaline
degeneration, hydropic
degeneration, lardaceous
degeneration, lipoidal

degeneration, macular
degeneration, mucoid
degeneration, mucous
degeneration, myxomatous
degeneration, Nissl
degeneration,
  parenchymatous
degeneration, pigmentary
degeneration, polypoid
degeneration, secondary
degeneration, senile
degeneration, spongy
degeneration, subacute
  combined, of spinal
  cord
degeneration, vitreous
degeneration, wallerian
degeneration, Zenker's
degenerative
degenerative joint
  disease (DJD)
deglutible
deglutition
deglutitive
degradation
degree
degustation
dehiscence
dehumanization
dehumidifier
dehydrate
dehydration
dehydroandrosterone
dehydrocholesterol
dehydrocholic acid
dehydrocorticosterone
dehydroepiandrosterone
dehydrogenase
dehydrogenate
dehydroisoandrosterone
deinstitutionalization
deionization
Deiters' cells
Deiters' nucleus
Deiters' process
déjà entendu
déjà vu
dejecta

dejection
dejecture
Déjérine's disease
Déjérine's syndrome
Déjérine-Sottas atrophy
delacrimation
delactation
delamination
delaying of pedicle graft
Delcid (antacid)
deleterious
deletion
Delfen (contraceptive
  foam)
Delhi boil
deligation
delimitation
delinquent
deliquesce
deliquescence
deliquescent
délire de toucher
deliriant
delirifacient
delirium
delirium, acute
delirium, alcoholic
delirium, chronic
delirium, constantium
delirium, cordis
delirium, epilepticum
delirium, febrile
delirium, lingual
delirium, mussitans
delirium of negation
delirium of persecution
delirium, partial
delirium, toxic
delirium, traumatic
delirium tremens (DTs)
delitescence
deliver
delivery (Del)
delivery, abdominal
delivery, assisted
  spontaneous
delivery, Barton's

delivery, breech
  extraction
delivery, Credé maneuver
delivery, De Lee maneuver
delivery, forceps
delivery, high with
  episiotomy
delivery, instrumental
delivery, key-in-lock
  rotation
delivery, Kielland
  rotation
delivery, low with
  episiotomy
delivery, Malström's
  extraction
delivery, manually
delivery, mid with
  episiotomy
delivery, outlet (low)
  with episiotomy
delivery, postmortem
delivery, precipitate
delivery, premature
delivery, rotation of
  fetal head
delivery, spontaneous
delivery, unassisted
delivery, vacuum
  extraction
delivery, vaginal
dellen
delomorphous
delomorphous cells
Delorme operation
delousing
Delsym (dextromethorphan
  polistirex)
delta
delta fornicis
delta-aminolevulinic acid
  test
deltacortisone
Deltasone (prednisone)
deltoid ligament
deltoid ridge
delusion

delusion, depressive
delusion, expansive
delusion, fixed
delusion, fleeting
delusion, nihilistic
delusion of grandeur
delusion of negation
delusion of persecution
delusion, reference
delusion, systematized
delusion, unsystematized
delusional
demand
demand, biological oxygen
demarcation
demecarium bromide
demeclocycline,
  hydrochloride
dement
demented
dementia
dementia, alcoholic
dementia, apoplectic
dementia, dialysis
dementia, epileptic
dementia, paralytica
dementia, postfebrile
dementia, presenile
dementia, primary
dementia, senile
dementia, syphilitic
dementia, toxic
Demerol Hydrochloride
  (meperidine HCl)
Demi-Regroton
  (chlorthalidone and
  reserpine)
demibain
demic
demilune
demineralization
demise
demodectic
Demodex
Demodex folliculorum
demography
demorphinization
demotivate

Demours' membrane
Demser (metyrosine)
demucosation
demulcent
Demulen 1/35-21
  (ethynodiol diacetate
  with ethinyl estradiol)
Demulen 1/35-28
  (ethynodiol diacetate
  with ethinyl estradiol)
Demulen 1/50-21
  (ethynodiol diacetate
  with ethinyl estradiol)
Demulen 1/50-28
  (ethynodiol diacetate
  with ethinyl estradiol)
demutization
demyelinate
demyelination
denarcotize
denaturation
denatured
denatured protein
dendraxon
dendric
dendriform
dendrite
dendrites, extracapsular
dendrites, intracapsular
dendritic
dendritic calculus
dendroid
dendron
dendrophagocytosis
denervated
denervation
denervation, aortic body
denervation, carotid body
denervation, facet,
  percutaneous
denervation, ovarian
denervation, paracervical
  uterine
denervation, uterosacral
dengue
denial
denial and isolation
denidation

Denis-Browne operation
Denker operation
Dennis-Barco operation
dens
dens bicuspidus
dens caninus
dens deciduus
dens incisivus
dens molaris
dens permanens
dens premolaris
dens sapientiae
dens serotinus
densimeter
densitometer
densitometry
density
dental
dental arch
dental assistant
dental caries
dental chart
dental consonant
dental curve
dental disk
dental dysfunction
dental engine
dental engineering
dental floss
dental formula
dental geriatrics
dental handpiece
dental hygienist
dental index
dental instruments
dental materials
dental plaque
dental prosthesis
dental pulp
dental sealants
dental tape
dentalgia
dentaphone
dentate
dentes
dentia
dentia praecox
dentia tarda

dentibuccal
denticle
denticulate
denticulate body
dentification
dentiform
dentifrice
dentigerous
dentilabial
dentilingual
dentimeter
dentin
dentinal
dentinification
dentinitis
dentinoblast
dentinoclast
dentinogenesis
dentinogenesis imperfecta
dentinoid
dentinoma
dentinosteoid
dentinum
dentiparous
dentist
dentistry
dentistry, esthetic
dentistry for children
dentistry, forensic
dentistry, four-handed
dentistry, geriatric
dentistry, hospital
dentistry, operative
dentistry, prosthodontic
dentistry, public health
dentition
dentition, diphyodont
dentition, heterodont
dentition, homodont
dentition, mixed
dentition, monophyodont
dentition, permanent
dentition, polyphyodont
dentition, primary
dentoalveolar
dentoalveolitis
dentofacial
dentoid

dentoidin
dentulous
denture, full
denture, immediate
denture, partial
denturism
denturist
denucleated
denudation
denutrition
Denver classification
Denver Developmental
  Screening Test (DDST)
deodorant
deodorize
deodorizer
deontology
deorsum
deorsum vergens
deorsumduction
deorsumversion
deossification
deoxidate
deoxidation
deoxidizer
deoxycholic acid
deoxycorticosterone
deoxygenation
deoxyribonuclease (DNase)
deoxyribonucleic acid
  (DNA)
deoxyribonucleoprotein
deoxyribonucleoside
deoxyribose
Depakene (valproic acid)
Depakote (divalproex
  sodium)
depancreatize
Department of Health and
  Human Services (HHS)
Depen (penicillamine)
dependence
depersonalization
  disorder
depersonalize
dephosphorylation
depigmentation
depilate

depilation
depilation, skin
depilatory
depilatory techniques
deplete
depletion
deplumation
Depo-Estradiol
Depo-Provera
  (medroxyprogesterone
  acetate)
Depo-Testosterone
  (testosterone
  cypionate)
depolarization
depolymerization
Deponit (nitroglycerin
  trandermal delivery
  system)
deposit
deposit, calcareous
deposit, tooth
depot
depravation
depressant, cardiac
depressant, cerebral
depressant, motor
depressant, respiratory
depressant, secretory
depressed
depression
depression, bipolar
depression, endogenous
depression, situational
  or reactive
depression, unipolar
depressomotor
depressor
depressor fibers
depressor nerve
depressor reflex
depressor, tongue
deprivation
deprivation, emotional
deprivation, sensory
deprivation, sleep
Deprol (meprobamate +
  benactyzine HCl)

depth
depth dose
depth perception
depth psychology
depulization
depurant
depuration
depurative
depurator
deradelphus
deradenitis
deradenoncus
derangement
Dercum's disease
derealization
dereism
dereistic
derencephalus
Derfil (chlorophyllin
  copper complex)
derivation
derivative
Derlacki operation
derm
derma
dermabrasion
Dermacentor
Dermacentor andersoni
Dermacentor variabilis
dermad
dermadrome
Dermaide Aloe Cream (aloe
  vera jel)
dermal
dermalaxia
dermalgia
dermamyiasis
dermapostasis
dermatalgia
dermatatrophia
dermatauxe
dermatides
dermatitis
dermatitis, actinic
dermatitis, aestivalis
dermatitis, allergic
dermatitis, atopic
dermatitis, berlock

dermatitis, berloque
dermatitis, calorica
dermatitis, cercarial
dermatitis, contact
dermatitis, cosmetic
dermatitis, exfoliative
dermatitis, herpetiformis
dermatitis hiemalis
dermatitis infectiosa
  eczematoides
dermatitis medicamentosa
dermatitis multiformis
dermatitis papillaris
  capillitii
dermatitis, poison ivy
dermatitis, primary
dermatitis, radiation
dermatitis, rhus
dermatitis seborrheica
dermatitis, stasis
dermatitis venenata
dermatitis verrucosa
dermatitis, x-ray
dermatoautoplasty
Dermatobia
Dermatobia hominis
dermatocele
dermatocele lipomatosa
dermatocelidosis
dermatocellulitis
dermatoconiosis
dermatocyst
dermatodynia
dermatofibroma
dermatofibrosarcoma
dermatogen
dermatogenous
dermatoglyphics
dermatographia
dermatography
dermatoheliosis
dermatoheteroplasty
dermatokelidosis
dermatologist
dermatology
dermatolysis
dermatoma
dermatome

dermatomere
dermatomucosomyositis
dermatomycosis
dermatomyoma
dermatomyositis
dermatoneurosis
dermatopathia
dermatopathology
dermatopathy
dermatophiliasis
dermatophilosis
dermatophobia
dermatophylaxis
dermatophyte
dermatophytid
dermatophytosis
dermatoplastic
dermatoplasty
dermatorrhagia
dermatorrhea
dermatosclerosis
dermatoscopy
dermatosis
dermatosis papulosa nigra
dermatosis, progressive
  pigmentary
dermatosome
dermatotherapy
dermatotome
dermatotropic
dermatoxerasia
dermatozoon
dermatozoonosis
dermatrophia
dermic
dermis
dermoblast
dermographia
dermography
dermoid
dermoid cyst
dermoidectomy
dermolipoma
dermomycosis
dermonosology
dermopathy
dermophlebitis
dermophyte

Dermoplast
dermoskeleton
dermosynovitis
dermotropic
dermovascular
derodidymus
DES daughters
DES syndrome
desalination
desaturation
Desault's apparatus
Descement's membrane
descemetitis
descemetocele
descendens
descendens hypoglossi
descensus
descensus testis
descensus uteri
Desenex (antifungal
    powder, spray , cream,
    ointment, liquid)
desensitization
desensitization, allergy
desensitization,
    psychologic
desensitization,
    systematic
desensitize
desert fever
desert rheumatism
desexualize
Desferal (deferoxamine
    mesylate)
desferrioxamine
desiccant
desiccate
desiccation
"designer drug"
desipramine hydrochloride
Desitin (ointment)
deslanoside
desmalgia
desmectasis
desmepithelium
desmitis
desmocranium
desmocyte

desmocytoma
desmodynia
desmoenzyme
desmogenous
desmography
desmoid
desmoid tumor
desmology
desmona
desmoneoplasm
desmopathy
desmoplasia
desmoplastic
desmopressin acetate
desmopyknosis
desmorrhexis
desmosis
desmosome
desmotomy
Desowen (desonide)
desoximetasone
desoxycorticosterone
desoxycorticosterone
    acetate
Desoxyn (methamphetamine
    HCl)
desoxyribonucleic acid
despumation
Desquam-E (benzoyl
    peroxide)
desquamate
desquamation
desquamation,
    furfuraceous
desquamative
desquamative interstitial
    pneumonitis (DIP)
destruction
destructive lesion
desudation
desulfhydrase
desynchronosis
Desyrel (trazodone HCl)
det. (let it be given)
det. in dup (let twice as
    much be given)
detachment
detachment, retinal

detachment, uterosacral
  ligaments
detail
detector
detector, lie
detector, optical
detector, radiation
detergent
deterioration
determinant
determination
determination, mental
  status
determination,
  psychologic
determination, vital
  capacity
determinism
detersive
detonation
detorsion
detorsion, intestine
detorsion, kidney
detorsion, large
detorsion, ovary
detorsion, small
detorsion, spermatic cord
detorsion, testis
detorsion, volvulus
detortion
detoxicate
detoxification
detoxification therapy
detoxify
detrition
detritus
detruncation
detrusor urinae
detumescence
detur
deutencephalon
deuteranomalopia
deuteranopia
deuteranopsia
deuterate
deuterium
deuterium oxide
deuteron (d)

deuteropathia
deuteropathy
deuteroplasm
deutoscolex
devasation
devascularization
devascularization,
  stomach
developer
development, cognitive
development, psychomotor
  and physical, of infant
developmental
developmental milestones
deviance
deviant
deviant behavior
deviant, sex
deviate
deviation
deviation, axis
deviation, conjugate
deviation, minimum
deviation, standard (SD)
device
device, intrauterine
  contraceptive
devil's grip
deviometer
devisceration
devitalization
devolution
dew cure
dew point
dewebbing, esophagus
dewebbing, syndactyly
dexamethasone
dexamethasone suppression
  test
dexbrompheniramine
  maleate
dexchlorpheniramine
  maleate
Dexedrine
  (dextroamphetamine
  sulfate)
dexter
dexterity

dextose
dextrad
dextral
dextrality
dextran
dextrase
dextraural
dextriferron
dextrin
dextrinuria
dextroamphetamine sulfate
dextrocardia
dextrocardiogram
dextrocular
dextrocularity
dextroduction
dextrogastria
dextroglucose
dextrogyre
dextromanual
dextromethorphan
dextropedal
dextrophobia
dextroposition
dextropropoxyphene
dextrorotatory
dextrose
dextrose and sodium
  chloride injection
dextrosinistral
dextrosuria
dextrothyroxine sodium
dextrotropic
dextrotropous
dextroversion
dezymotize
dhobie itch
DHS Conditioning Rinse
DHS Shampoo
DHS Tar Shampoo
DHS Zinc Dandruff Shampoo
DHT (dihydrotachysterol)
Dia-Gesic (hydrocodone
  bitartrate and aspirin)
DiaBeta (glyburide)
diabetes
diabetes, bronze
diabetes insipidus

diabetes mellitus (DM)
diabetes mellitus,
  brittle
diabetes mellitus,
  chemical
diabetes mellitus,
  endocrine
diabetes mellitus,
  iatrogenic
diabetes mellitus,
  insulin-dependent, Type
  I (IDDM)
diabetes mellitus, latent
diabetes mellitus,
  noninsulin-dependent,
  Type II (NIDDM)
diabetes, pancreatic
diabetes, phlorizin
diabetes, renal
diabetes, true
diabetic
diabetic acidosis
diabetic center
diabetic coma
diabetic ear
diabetic neuritis
diabetic tabes
diabetogenic
diabetogenous
Diabinese
  (chlorpropamide)
diabrosis
diabrotic
diacele
diacetate
diacetemia
diacetic acid
diacetonuria
diaceturia
diacetylmorphine
diacid
diaclasia
diacrinous
diacrisis
diacritic
diacritical
diaderm
diadochokinesia

diagnose
diagnosis (diag, Dx)
diagnosis, antenatal
diagnosis by exclusion
diagnosis, clinical
diagnosis, cytological
diagnosis, differential
diagnosis, medical
diagnosis, nursing
diagnosis, oral
diagnosis, pathological
diagnosis, physical
diagnosis, radiographic
diagnosis, serological
diagnosis-related groups
  (DRGs)
diagnostic
Diagnostic and
  Statistical Manual of
  Mental Disorders (DSM
  III-R)
diagnostic ultrasound
diagnostician
diakinesis
dial
dial, astigmatic
dialcast
Dialose
Dialume (aluminum
  hydroxide)
dialysance
dialysate
dialysis
dialysis acidosis
dialysis, continuous
  ambulatory peritoneal
dialysis dementia
dialysis disequilibrium
dialysis,
  hemodiafiltration
dialysis, hemofiltration
dialysis, kidney
  (extracorporeal)
dialysis, peritoneal
dialysis, renal
dialysis, renal
  (extracorporeal)
dialytic

dialyzable
dialyze
diamagnetic
diameter,
  anteroposterior, of
  pelvic cavity
diameter,
  anteroposterior, of
  pelvic inlet
diameter, bigonial
diameter, biparietal
diameter, bitemporal
diameter, bitrochanteric
diameter, bizygomatic
diameter, buccolingual
diameter,
  cervicobregmatic
diameter, diagonal
  conjugate, of pelvis
diameter, external
  conjugate
diameter, frontomental
diameter, interspinous
diameter, labiolingual
diameter, mentobregmatic
diameter, mesiodistal
diameter, obstetric, of
  pelvic inlet
diameter, occipitofrontal
diameter of fetal skull
diameter of pelvis
diamide
diamidine
diamine
diaminuria
Diamox (acetazolamide)
dianoetic
diapason
diapause
diapedesis
diaphane
diaphanography
diaphanometer
diaphanometry
diaphanoscope
diaphanoscopy
diaphemetric
diaphorase

diaphoresis
diaphoretic
diaphragm
diaphragm, Bucky
diaphragm, hernia of
diaphragm, pelvic
diaphragm, urogenital
diaphragmalgia
diaphragmatic
diaphragmatic hernia
diaphragmatocele
diaphragmitis
diaphragmodynia
diaphyseal
diaphysectomy
diaphysis
diaphysitis
Diapid Nasal Spray
  (lypressin)
diaplexus
diapophysis
diarrhea
diarrhea, acute
diarrhea, dysenteric
diarrhea, emotional
diarrhea, epidemic, in
  newborn
diarrhea, fatty
diarrhea, infantile
diarrhea, lienteric
diarrhea, membranous
diarrhea, mucous
diarrhea, purulent
diarrhea, simple
diarrhea, summer
diarrhea, travelers' (TD)
diarthric
diarthrodial
diarthrosis
diarticular
diascope
diastalsis
diastaltic
diastase
diastasis
diastasis recti
diastema
diastematocrania

diastematomyelia
diastematopyelia
diaster
diastole
diastolic
diastolic pressure (DP)
diataxia
diatela
diatele
diaterma
diathermal
diathermanous
diathermia
diathermic
diathermy
diathermy, medical
diathermy, short-wave
diathermy, surgical
diathesis
diathetic
diatolic presssure,
  augmented
diatom
diatomaceous earth
diatomic
diatrizoate meglumine
diatrizoate sodium
diaxon
diaxone
diazepam
diazo reaction
diazotize
diazoxide
dibasic
Dibenzyline
  (phenoxybenzamine HCl)
diblastula
Dibothriocephalus
dibucaine hydrochloride
Dical-D (dibasic calcium
  phosphate with
  vitamin D)
dicalcic
dicalcium
dicalcium phosphate
dicentric
dicephalus
dichloramine-T

dichlorodiphenyl-
  trichloroethane (DDT)
2,4-dichlorophenoxyacetic
  acid (2,4-D)
dichlorphenamide
dichorionic
dichotomization
dichotomy
dichroic
dichroic mirror
dichroism
dichromate
dichromatic
dichromatism
dichromatopsia
dichromic
dichromophil
dichromophilism
Dick method
Dickson operation
Dickson-Diveley operation
dicloxacillin sodium
dicoelus
dicophane
dicoria
dicoumarol
dicrotic
dicrotic notch
dicrotic wave
dicrotism
dictyoma
dictyosome
Dicumarol (coumarin
  anticoagulant)
dicyclomine hydrochloride
dicylic
didactic
didactylism
didelphic
Didronel (etidronate
  disodium)
didymalgia
didymitis
didymodynia
didymus
die
diechoscope
diecious

Dieffenbach operation
dieldrin
dielectric
diembryony
diencephalon
dienestrol
Dientamoeba
Dientamoeba fragilis
dieresis
dieretic
diet
diet, balanced
diet, minimum residue
diet, reduction
dietary
dietary fiber
dietetic
dietetics
diethazine hydrochloride
diethylcarbamazine
  citrate
diethylpropion
  hydrochloride
diethylstilbestrol (DES)
diethyltoluamide
diethyltryptamine (DET)
dietitian
Dietl's crisis
dietotherapy
Dieulafoy's triad
differential
differential blood count
differential diagnosis
differentiation
diffraction
diffraction grating
diffusate
diffuse
diffusible
diffusion
digastric
digenesis
Digenetica
digest
digestant
digestible
digestion
digestion, artificial

digestion, duodenal
digestion, extracellular
digestion, gastric
digestion, intestinal
digestion, intracellular
digestion, oral
digestion, pancreatic
digestion, salivary
digestion, secondary
digestive
digestive juice
Digibind (digoxin)
digit
digital
digital amniotome
digital radiography
digital reflex
digital subtraction
  angiography (DSA)
digitalis
digitalis poisoning
digitalization
digitate
digitation
digiti
digitiform
digitoxin
digitus
diglossia
diglyceride
dignathus
digoxin
digoxin immune FAB
  (ovine) for injection
digoxin toxicology test
dihydric
dihydrocodeinone
  bitartrate
dihydroergotamine
  mesylate (DHE-45)
dihydrosphingosine
dihydrotachysterol
dihydrotheelin
dihydroxyaluminum
  aminoacetate
dihydroxyaluminum sodium
  carbonate
dihydroxycholecalciferol

3,4-
  dihydroxyphenylalanine
dihysteria
diiodohydroxyquin
diisopropyl
  fluorophosphate (DFP)
diisopropyl
  phosphorofluoridate
diktyoma
dilaceration
Dilantin (phenytoin
  sodium)
dilatant
dilatation (dilation) &
  curettage (D&C)
dilatation, digital
dilatation, heart
dilatation, stomach
dilate
dilation
dilation, achalasia
dilation, ampulla of
  Vater
dilation and evacuation
  (D and E)
dilation, anus, anal
  (sphincter)
dilation, bladder
dilation, bronchus
dilation, cervix
dilation, choanae
dilation, colostomy stoma
dilation, endoscopic
dilation, endoscopic
  retrograde
dilation, enterostomy
  stoma
dilation, esophagus
dilation, fallopian tube
dilation, foreskin
dilation, frontonasal
  duct
dilation, heart valve
dilation, ileostomy stoma
dilation, intestinal
  stoma
dilation, lacrimal duct

dilation, lacrimal papilla
dilation, lacrimal punctum
dilation, larynx
dilation, lymphatic structure
dilation, nares
dilation, nasolacrimal duct
dilation, nasopharynx
dilation, pancreatic duct
dilation, pharynx
dilation, rectum
dilation, salivary duct
dilation, sphenoid ostia
dilation, sphincter of Oddi
dilation, sphincter-anal
dilation, sphincter-cardiac
dilation, sphincter-pancreatic
dilation, Stenson's duct
dilation, trachea
dilation, ureter
dilation, ureterovesical orifice
dilation, urethra
dilation, urethrovesical junction
dilation, urinary meatus
dilation, vagina
dilation, vesical neck
dilation, Wharton's duct
dilation, Wirsung's duct
dilator
dilator, Barnes'
dilator, Bossi's
dilator, Goodell's
dilator, gynecologic
dilator, Hegar's
dilator, tent
dilator, vaginal
Dilatrate-SR (isosorbide dinitrate)
Dilaudid (hydromorphone HCl)

dildo
dildoe
Dilor (dyphylline)
Dilor-G (dyphylline, guaifenesin)
diluent
dilution
dim
Dimacol Caplets
Dimacol Liquid
dimenhydrinate
dimension
dimer
dimercaprol
Dimetane (brompheniramine maletate)
Dimetane Decongestant Elixir
Dimetane Decongestant Tablets
Dimetane Extentabs (brompheniramine maleate)
Dimetane-DC Cough Syrup
Dimetane-DX Cough Syrup
Dimetapp Elixir
Dimetapp Extentabs
dimethicone
dimethindene maleate
dimethisterone
dimethyl phthalate
dimethyl sulfoxide (DMSO)
dimethylamine
dimethyltryptamine
dimetria
diminution, ciliary body
dimorphous
dimple sign
dimpling
dineuric
dinical
2,4-dinitrophenol
Dinoflagellata
dinoprost tromethamine
dinucleotide
Dioctophyma
dioctyl calcium sulfosuccinate

dioctyl sodium
  sulfosuccinate
Diogenes syndrome
diopter
dioptometer
dioptometry
dioptral
dioptre
dioptric
dioptrics
diovulatory
dioxide
dioxin
dioxybenzone
dipeptid
dipeptidase
dipeptide
diperodon
Dipetalonema perstans
diphallus
diphasic
diphemanil methylsulfate
diphenhydramine
  hydrochloride
diphenoxylate
  hydrochloride
diphenylhydantoin sodium
diphenylpyraline
  hydrochloride
diphonia
2,3-diphosphoglycerate
  (2,3-DPG)
diphtheria
diphtheria and tetanus
  toxoids and pertussis
  vaccine absorbed
diphtheria antitoxin
diphtheria, cutaneous
diphtheria, laryngeal
diphtheria, surgical
diphtherial
diphtheriaphor
diphtheric
diphtherin
diphtheritic
diphtheroid
diphtherotoxin
diphthongia

Diphyllobothrium
Diphyllobothrium cordatum
Diphyllobothrium erinacei
Diphyllobothrium latum
diphyodont
diplacusis
diplegia
diplegia, infantile
diplegia, spastic
diplegic
diploalbuminuria
diplobacillus
diplobacterium
diploblastic
diplocardia
diplocephaly
diplococcemia
diplococci
Diplococcus
Diplococcus pneumoniae
diplocoria
diploë
diploetic
diplogenesis
diploic
diploid
diplokaryon
diplomellituria
diplomyelia
diploneural
diplopagus
diplophonia
diplopia
diplopia, binocular
diplopia, crossed
diplopia, direct
diplopia, heteronymous
diplopia, monocular
diplopia, uncrossed
diplopia, unocular
diplopia, vertical
diplopiometer
diploscope
diplosomatia
diplosomia
diplotene
dipole
dipping

Diprolene (betamethasone
  dipropionate)
Diprosone (betamethasone
  dipropionate)
diprosopus
dipsesis
dipsogen
dipsomania
dipsophobia
dipsosis
dipsotherapy
dipstick
Diptera
dipterous
dipygus
dipylidiasis
Dipylidium
Dipylidium caninum
direct
direct current (DC)
direct light reflex
direct reflex
directionality
director
dirigomotor
Dirofilaria
Dirofilaria immitis
disability
disability, developmental
disaccharidase
disaccharide
Disalcid (salsalate)
disarticulation
disassimilation
disaster
discharge (DC)
discharge abstract
discharge,
  cerebrocortical
discharge, convective
discharge, disruptive
discharge, lochial
discharging
discharging lesion
dischronation
discission
discitis
disclosing agent

discoblastic
discoblastula
discogenic
discogram
discography
discoid
disconnection syndromes
discontinue (DC)
discoplacenta
discordance
discrete
discrimination
discrimination, one-point
discrimination, tonal
discrimination, two-point
discus
discus articularis
discus proligerus
disdiaclast
disdiadochokinesia
disease
disease, acute
disease, anticipated
disease, autoimmune
disease, chronic
disease, chronic
  granulomatous (CGD)
disease, collagen
disease, communicable
disease, complicating
disease, congenital
disease, constitutional
disease, contagious
disease, cystine storage
disease, deficiency
disease, degenerative
disease, degenerative
  joint
disease, demyelinating
disease, endemic
disease, epidemic
disease, epizootic
disease, extrapyramidal
disease, familial
disease, focal
disease, functional
disease, glycogen storage
disease, heavy chain

disease, hemolytic, of the newborn
disease, hemorrhagic, of the newborn
disease, hereditary
disease, hookworm
disease, hypokinetic
disease, iatrogenic
disease, idiopathic
disease, infectious
disease, intercurrent
disease, iron storage
disease, malignant
disease, Mediterranean
disease, metabolic
disease, motor neuron
disease, occupational
disease, organic
disease, pandemic
disease, parasitic
disease, periodontal
disease, psychosomatic
disease, secondary
disease, self-limited
disease, sporadic
disease, storage
disease, subacute
disease, systemic
disease, thyrotoxic heart
disease, veneral (VD)
disengagement
disequilibrium
dish, Petri
disinfect
disinfectant
disinfection
disinfection, concurrent
disinfection of blankets and woolens
disinfection of excreta
disinfection of field of operation
disinfection, terminal
disinfestation
disinhibition
disinsected
disinsertion
disintegration

Disipal (orphenadrine HCl)
disjoint
disjunction
disk, anisotropic
disk, articular
disk, Bowman's
disk, choked
disk, dental
disk, embryonic
disk, epiphyseal
disk, germinal
disk, herniated intervertebral
disk, intervertebral
disk, M.
disk, Merkel's
disk, optic
disk, proligerous
disk, Q.
disk, slipped
disk, tactile
disk, Z.
diskectomy
diskiform
diskitis
diskogram
diskography
dislocation
dislocation, closed
dislocation, complete
dislocation, complicated
dislocation, compound
dislocation, congenital
dislocation, consecutive
dislocation, divergent
dislocation, habitual
dislocation, incomplete
dislocation, metacarpophalangeal joint
dislocation, Monteggia's
dislocation, Nelation's
dislocation, old
dislocation, partial
dislocation, pathologic
dislocation, primitive
dislocation, recent

dislocation, simple
dislocation, slipped
dislocation,
 subastragalar
dislocation, traumatic
dismember
dismutase
dismutase, superoxide
disocclude
disodium edetate
disomus
Disonate (dioctyl sodium
 sulfosuccinate)
disopyramide phosphate
disorder
disorder, character
disorganization
disorientation
disparate points
dispensary
dispensatory
dispense
dispensing
dispersate
disperse
dispersion
dispersion, coarse
dispersion, colloidal
dispersion, medium
dispersion, molecular
dispersoid
dispersonalization
dispireme
displacement
disposition
disproportion
disproportion,
 cephalopelvic
dissect
dissection
disseminated
disseminated
 intravascular
 coagulation (DIC)
dissipation
dissociation
dissociation,
 atrioventricular

dissociation, microbic
dissociation of
 personality
dissociation,
 psychological
dissolution
dissolve
dissolvent
dissolving
dissonance
dissonance, cognitive
distad
distal
distance
distance, focal
distance, focal-film
distance, interocclusal
distance, interocular
distance, source-skin
distance, source-to-image
 receptor
distance, target-skin
distance visual acuity
 (DVA)
distemper
distend
distensibility
distention
distichiasis
distill
distillate
distillation
distillation, destructive
distillation, dry
distillation, fractional
disto-occlusal
distobuccal
distoclusion
distogingival
distolabial
distolingual
Distoma
distome
distomia
distomiasis
Distomum
distortion
distractibility

distraction
distraught
distress
distress, fetal
distribution
districhiasis
distrix
disturbance
disturbance, emotional
disulfate
disulfiram
disulfiram poisoning
dithiazanine iodide
Ditropan (oxybutynin
  chloride)
Dittrich's plugs
Diucardin
  (hydroflumethiazide)
Diulo (metolazone)
Diupres (reserpine-
  chlorothiazide)
diurese
diuresis
diuretic
Diuril (chlorothiazide)
diurnal
Diutensen (cryptenamine
  and methyclothiazide)
Diutensen-R
  (methyclothiazide and
  reserpine)
divagation
divalent
diver's paralysis
divergence
divergent
diversion
diversion, urinary
diversional therapy
diverticula
diverticulectomy
diverticulitis
diverticulitis, acute
diverticulitis, chronic
diverticulosis
diverticulum
diverticulum, false
diverticulum, Meckel's

diverticulum of colon
diverticulum of duodenum
diverticulum of jejunum
diverticulum of stomach
diverticulum, true
diverticulum, Zenker's
diving reflex
division
divulsion
divulsor
divulsor, pterygium
divulsor, tendon
Dix, Dorothea Lynde
dizygotic twins
dizziness
DML Moisturizing Lotion
DNA probe
do not resuscitate (DNR)
Dobell's solution
Dobie's globule
Dobutrex (dobutamine HCl)
doctor of podiatric
  medicine (DPM)
doctor (DR,Dr)
doctor, barefoot
doctor of chiropractic
  (DC)
doctor of dental medicine
  (DMD)
doctor of dental surgery
  (DDS)
doctor of divinity (DD)
doctor of medicine (MD)
doctor of osteopathy (DO)
doctor of pharmacy (DP)
doctor of philosophy
  (PhD)
doctor of science (D.Sc.)
doctor of science in
  nursing (DSN)
doctor of veterinary
  medicine (DVM)
doctrine
docusate calcium
docusate sodium
dog bite
Döhle's bodies
dol

Dolacet (hydrocodone
  bitartrate and
  acetaminophen)
Doleris operation
dolichocephalic
dolichocolon
dolichofacial
dolichohieric
dolichomorphic
dolichopellic
dolichopelvic
dolichosigmoid
dolichuranic
Dolobid (diflunisal)
Dolophine Hydrochloride
  (methadone HCl)
dolor
dolorific
dolorimeter
dolorogenic
domatophobia
Dome-Paste (medicated
  bandage for leg or arm,
  Unna's boot)
Domeboro (astringent wet
  dressing)
domestic task therapy
domiciliary
dominance
dominance, ocular
dominant
Domol (di-isopropyl
  sebacate, isopropyl
  myristate)
Don Juan
Donath-Landsteiner
  phenomenon
donee
Donnagel-PG
Donnan's equilibrium
Donnatal Capsules
Donnatal Elixir
Donnatal Extentabs
Donnatal Tablets
Donnazyme Tablets
donor
donor card
donor, universal

Donovan body
Donovania granulomatis
dopa
dopa-oxidase
dopamine
dopamine hydrochloride
dopaminergic
doping
doping, blood
Doppler effect
Doppler flow mapping
Doppler ultrasound
Dopplergram
Dopram (doxapram HCl)
doraphobia
Dorcol
Dorello's canal
Dorendorf's sign
Doriden (glutethimide)
dornase
dornase, pancreatic
Dorrance operation
dorsa
dorsabdominal
dorsad
dorsal
dorsal cavity
dorsal cord stimulation
dorsal elevated position
dorsal ganglia
dorsal inertia posture
dorsal nerves
dorsal recumbent position
dorsal reflex
dorsal rigid posture
dorsal slit
dorsalgia
dorsalis
dorsiduct
dorsiduction
dorsiflect
dorsiflexion
dorsimesal
dorsimeson
dorsispinal
dorsocephalad
dorsodynia
dorsolateral

dorsoplantar
dorsosacral
dorsosacral position
dorsoventral
dorsum
Doryx (doxycycline
  hyclate pellets)
dosage
dose
dose, absorbed
dose, air
dose, bolus
dose, booster
dose, cumulative
dose, curative
dose, divided
dose, erythema
dose, fatal
dose, infective
dose, maintenance
dose, maximum
dose, maximum permissible
dose, median curative
dose, median infective
dose, median lethal
dose, minimum
dose, primary
dose response curve
dose, skin
dose, therapeutic
dose, threshold
dose, tissue tolerance
dose, toxic
dosimeter
dosimetric
dosimetry
dot
dot, Trantas
dotage
Dotter operation
double
double personality
double touch
double uterus
double-blind technique
double-contrast
  examination
double-valve replacement

douche
douche, air
douche, alternating
douche, astringent
douche, circular
douche, cleansing
douche, deodorizing
douche, high
douche, jet
douche, low
douche, medicated
douche, neutral
douche, perineal
douche, Scotch
douche, vaginal
Douglas operation
Douglas' cul-de-sac
Douglas' fold
Douglas' pouch
Douglas' space
dowel
down
Down syndrome (DS)
doxapram hydrochloride
doxorubicin hydrochloride
doxycycline
doxycycline hyclate
doxylamine succinate
Doyère's eminence
Doyle operation
drachm (dr)
dracontiasis
dracunculiasis
dracunculosis
Dracunculus
Dracunculus medinensis
draft
drag
drain
drain, capillary
drain, cigarette
drain, Mikulicz's
drain, nonabsorbable
drain, Penrose
drainage
drainage, capillary
drainage, closed
drainage, closed sterile

drainage, funnel
drainage, negative
  pressure
drainage, open
drainage, postural
drainage, suction
drainage, tidal
drainage tube
drained weight
dram (dr)
Dramamine
  (dimenhydrinate)
dramatism
drapetomania
drastic
draught
draw sheet
Draw-a-Person Test
drawer sign
drawing test
dream
drench
drepanocyte
drepanocytemia
drepanocytic
dressing
dressing, absorbent
dressing, antiseptic
dressing, clear
  transparent covering
dressing, dry
dressing, fixed
dressing, hot moist
dressing, nonadherent
dressing, occlusive
dressing, pressure
dressing, protective
dressing stick
dressing, transparent
  synthetic
dressing, universal
dressing, water
drift
drift, genetic
drift, mesial
drill
drilling, bone
Drinker respirator

drip
drip, intravenous
drip, Murphy
drip, nasal
drip, postnasal (PND)
Dristan (phenylephride
  HCl and pheniramine
  maleate)
Dritho-Scalp (anthralin)
Drithocreme (anthralin)
drive
drive controls
Drixoral Plus
Drize (chlorpheniramine
  maleate and
  phenylpropanolamine
  HCl)
dromomania
dromostanolone propionate
dromotropic
dronabinol
drop
drop, culture
drop, foot
drop, hanging
drop, wrist
drops, ear
drops, eye
drops, nose
droperidol
droplet
droplet infection
dropper
dropper, medicine
dropsy
Drosophila
Drosophila melanogaster
drowning
drownproofing
drowsiness
drowsiness, day-time
drug
drug action
drug addiction
drug administration
drug dependence
drug eruption
drug fever

drug interaction
drug overdose
drug rashes
drug reaction
drug receptors
drug-fast
druggist
drum
drunkenness
drusen
dry eye
dry ice
dry measure
dry mouth
Drysdale's corpuscles
Drysol
DTIC-Dome (dacarbazine)
dual personality
dualism
duazomycin
Dubin-Johnson syndrome
Dubini's disease
duboisine
Dubowitz score
Dubowitz tool
Duchenne, Guillaume
Duchenne's disease
Duchenne's muscular
  dystrophy
Duchenne's paralysis
Duchenne-Aran disease
Duchenne-Erb paralysis
Ducrey's bacillus
duct
duct, accessory
  pancreatic
duct, alveolar
duct, Bartholin's
duct, cochlear
duct, common bile
duct, cystic
duct, efferent
duct, ejaculatory
duct, endolymphatic
duct, excretory
duct, Gartner's
duct, interlobular
duct, lacrimal

duct, Leydig's
duct, lymphatics
duct, mesonephric
duct, metanephric
duct, nasolacrimal
duct of Santorini
duct of the epoophoron
duct of Wirsung
duct, omphalomesenteric
duct, pancreatic
duct, paramesonephric
duct, parotid
duct, segmental
duct, spermatic
duct, Stensen's
duct, striated
duct, submandibular
duct, testicular
duct, thoracic
duct, umbilical
duct, utriculosaccular
duct, vitelline
duct, Wharton's
duct, wolffian
ducts, biliary
ducts, hepatic
ducts, lactiferous
ducts, mammary
ducts, milk
ducts, mullerian
ducts of Rivinus
ducts, papillary
ducts, paraurethral
ducts, prostatic
ducts, salivary
ducts, secretory
ducts, semicircular
ducts, seminal
ducts, Skene's
ducts, sublingual
ducts, tear
ductile
ductless
ductless glands
ductogram, mammary
ductule
ductule, aberrant
ductulus

ductus arteriosus
ductus arteriosus, patent
ductus choledochus
ductus cochlearis
ductus deferens
ductus epoophori
  longitudinalis
ductus hemithoracicus
ductus hepaticus
ductus hepaticus dexter
ductus hepaticus sinister
ductus prostatici
ductus reuniens
ductus utriculosaccularis
ductus venosus
Duffy system
Duhamel operation
Duhrssen's incisions
Duhrssen's operation
duipara
Duke method
dulcite
Dulcolax (bisacodyl)
dull
dullness
dumb
dumbness
dumping
dumping syndrome
Dunn operation
Duo-Medihaler
  (isoproterenol HCl and
  phenylephrine
  bitartrate)
Duocet (hydrocodone and
  acetaminophen)
duodenal
duodenal bulb
duodenal delay
duodenal ulcer
duodenectasis
duodenectomy
duodenitis
duodenocholecystostomy
duodenocholedochotomy
duodenocystostomy
duodenoduodenostomy
duodenoenterostomy

duodenogram
duodenography
duodenohepatic
duodenoileostomy
duodenojejunostomy
duodenorrhaphy
duodenoscopy
duodenostomy
duodenotomy
duodenum
Duotrate (pentaerythritol
  tetranitrate)
duplication
duplicature
duplicitas
dupp
Dupuytren, Baron G.
Dupuytren operation
Dupuytren's contracture
Dupuytren's fracture
dura
dura mater
Dura-Gest
Dura-Vent
  (phenylpropanolamine
  HCl and
  chlorpheniramine
  maleate)
Dura-Vent/DA
dural
duramatral
Duramorph (morphine
  sulfate)
Durand-Nicolas-Favre
  disease
Duranest (etidocaine HCl)
Duraphyl (anhydrous
  theophylline)
duraplasty
duration
durematoma
Durham operation
Duricef (cefadroxil)
duritis
duroarachnitis
Durofilm
Duroziez' murmur
dust

dust, blood
dust cells
dust, ear
dust, house
dusting powder
DuToit and Roux operation
Duverney's fracture
Duverney's gland
DuVries operation
DV (dienestrol)
dwarf
dwarf, achondroplastic
dwarf, asexual
dwarf, hypophyseal
dwarf, infantile
dwarf, Levi-Lorain
dwarf, micromelic
dwarf, ovarian
dwarf, phocomelic
dwarf, physiologic
dwarf, pituitary
dwarf, primordial
dwarf, rachitic
dwarf, renal
dwarf, thanatophoric
dwarfism
Dwyer operation
dyad
dyadic
Dyazide
   (hydrochlorothiazide
   and triamterene)
Dyclone (dyclonine HCl)
dyclonine hydrochloride
dye
dying
dynamia
dynamic
dynamic splint
dynamics, group
dynamics, population
dynamogenesis
dynamogenic
dynamograph
dynamometer
dynamoneure
dynamoscope
dynamoscopy

dyne
dyphylline
Dyrenium (triamterene)
dysacousia
dysacousma
dysacusis
dysadrenalism
dysantigraphia
dysaphia
dysarthria
dysarthroisis
dysautonomia
dysbarism
dysbasia
dysboulia
dyscalculia
dyscephaly
dyschezia
dyschiria
dyschondroplasia
dyschroa
dyschroia
dyschromatopsia
dyschromia
dyschronism
dyscinesia
dyscoria
dyscrasia
dyscrasic
dyscrinism
dysdiadochokinesia
dysembryoplasia
dysemia
dysenteric
dysentery
dysentery, amebic
dysentery, bacillary
dysentery, balantidial
dyserethesia
dysergasia
dysergastic
dysergia
dysesthesia
dysesthesia, auditory
dysesthesia, pedis
dysfunction
dysfunctional uterine
   bleeding (DUB)

dysgalactia
dysgammaglobulinemia
dysgenesis
dysgenesis, gonadal
dysgenic
dysgenitalism
dysgerminoma
dysgeusia
dysglandular
dysglobulinemia
dysgnathia
dysgonesis
dysgonic
dysgonsia
dysgraphia
dyshematopoiesia
dyshidria
dyshidrosis
dysidrosis
dyskaryosis
dyskeratosis
dyskinesia
dyskinesia, algera
dyskinesia, biliary
dyskinesia, intermittens
dyskinesia, tardive
dyskinesia, uterine
dyskinetic
dyslalia
dyslexia
dyslochia
dyslogia
dysmasesis
dysmaturity
dysmegalopsia
dysmelia
dysmenorrhea
dysmenorrhea, congestive
dysmenorrhea,
   inflammatory
dysmenorrhea, membranous
dysmenorrhea, primary
dysmenorrhea, secondary
dysmenorrhea, spasmodic
dysmetria
dysmetropsia
dysmimia
dysmnesia

dysmorphophobia
dysmorphosis
dysmyotonia
dysodontiasis
dysomnias
dysontogenesis
dysontogenetic
dysopia
dysopsia
dysorexia
dysosmia
dysostosis
dysostosis, cleidocranial
dysostosis,
   craniocerebral
dysostosis,
   mandibulofacial
dysoxia
dysoxidizable
dyspancreatism
dyspareunia
dyspepsia
dyspepsia, acid
dyspepsia, alcoholic
dyspepsia, biliary
dyspepsia, cardiac
dyspepsia, gastric
dyspepsia,
   gastrointestinal
dyspepsia, hepatic
dyspepsia, hysterical
dyspeptic
dyspermasia
dyspermatism
dyspermia
dysphagia
dysphagia, constricta
dysphagia, lusoria
dysphagia, paralytica
dysphagia, spastica
dysphagy
dysphasia
dysphemia
dysphonia
dysphonia clericorum
dysphonia puberum
dysphonia, spasmodic
dysphoria

dysphrasia
dysphylaxia
dyspigmentation
dyspituitarism
dysplasia, anhidrotic
dysplasia, cervical
dysplasia,
  chondroectodermal
dysplasia, hereditary
  ectodermal
dysplasia, monostotic
  fibrous
dysplasia, polyostotic
  fibrous
dyspnea
dyspnea, cardiac
dyspnea, expiratory
dyspnea, inspiratory
dyspneic
dyspraxia
dysprosium (Dy)
dysprosody
dysraphia
dysraphism
dysrhythmia
dysstasia
dysstatic
dyssynergia
dystaxia
dystectia
dysteleology
dystenery, malignant
dystenery, viral
dysthymia
dysthyreosis
dysthyroidism
dystocia
dystonia
dystonia musculum
  deformans
dystonic
dystopia
dystopia canthorum
dystopic
dystopy
dystrophia
dystrophic
dystrophoneurosis

dystrophy
dystrophy, adiposogenital
dystrophy, Landouzy-
  Déjérine
dystrophy, progressive
  muscular
dystrophy,
  pseudohypertrophic
  muscular
dystrypsia
dysuria
dysuriac
dyszooamylia
dyszoospermia

E

E.E.S. (erythromycin
  ethylsuccinate)
E-Mycin (erythromycin)
E-Mycin E (erythromycin
  ethylsuccinate)
each (ea)
Eagleton operation
Eales' disease
ear
ear, Blainville's
ear bones
ear, Cagot
ear, cauliflower
ear dust
ear, external
ear, foreign bodies
ear, internal
ear, middle
ear oximeter
ear, pierced
ear plug
earache
eardrops
eardrum
earth
earth, alkaline
earth, diatomaceous
earth eating

earth, fuller's
earwax
Easprin (aspirin)
eastern equine
encephalitis
eat
Eaton agent
Eberthella
Ebner's glands
Ebola-Marburg virus
disease
ebonation
Ebstein's anomaly
ebullism
eburnation
eburneous
ecaudate
ecbolic
eccentric
eccentro-
osteochondrodysplasia
eccentropiesis
ecchondroma
ecchondrotome
ecchymoma
ecchymosis
ecchymotic
eccrine
eccrine sweat glands
eccritic
eccyclomastopathy
eccyesis
ecdemomania
ecderon
ecdysis
echeosis
echidnase
echidnin
Echidnophaga
Echidnophaga gallinacea
echinate
echinococcosis
echinococcotomy
Echinococcus
Echinococcus granulosus
Echinococcus
hydatidosus
echinocyte

echinosis
Echinostoma
echinulate
echo
echo, amphoric
echo sign
echoacousia
echocardiogram (ECHO)
echocardiography
echoencephalography
echoencephalogram
echogram
echography
echogynography
echokinesia
echolalia
echolocation
echomimia
echomotism
echopathy
echophotony
echophrasia
echoplacentogram
echopraxia
echothiophate iodide
Eck's fistula
eclabium
eclampsia
eclamptic
eclamptogenic
eclectic
eclecticism
ecmnesia
ecology
Economo's disease
écorché
ecosphere
ecostate
ecosystem
Ecotrin (aspirin)
écouvillonage
ecphoria
écrasement
écraseur
ecstasy
ecstrophy
ectad
ectal

ectasia
ectasia, hypostatic
ectasia iridis
ectasia ventriculi
  paradoxa
ectasis
ectatic
ectental
ectental line
ectethmoid
ecthyma
ectiris
ectoantigen
ectoblast
ectocardia
ectocervical
ectocervix
ectochoroidea
ectocinerea
ectocolostomy
ectocondyle
ectocornea
ectocuneiform
ectocytic
ectodactylism
ectoderm
ectodermal
ectodermatosis
ectodermatosis, erosiva
  pluriorificialis
ectodermic
ectodermoidal
ectodermosis
ectoentad
ectoenzyme
ectogenous
ectoglia
ectoglobular
ectogony
ectolecithal
ectomere
ectomesoblast
ectomorph
ectonuclear
ectopagus
ectoparasite
ectoperitonitis
ectophyte

ectopia cordis
ectopia lentis
ectopia pupillae
  congenita
ectopia renis
ectopia testis
ectopia vesicae
ectopia, visceral
ectopic
ectopic beat, complex
ectopic pregnancy
ectopic rhythm
ectopic secretion
ectoplasm
ectoplasmic
ectoplast
ectoplastic
ectopotomy
ectopterygoid
ectopy
ectoretina
ectostosis
ectothrix
Ectotrichophyton
ectozoon
ectrodactylism
ectrogeny
ectromelia
ectromelus
ectropic
ectropion
ectropionize
ectrosyndactyly
eczema
eczema, erythematous
eczema fissum
eczema herpeticum
eczema, hypertrophicum
eczema, lichenoid
eczema marginatum
eczema, nummular
eczema, pustular
eczema, seborrheic
eczema vaccinatum
eczematous
Edecrin (ethacrynic acid)
edema

edema, acute
  circumscribed
edema, angioneurotic
edema, blue
edema, brain
edema bullosum vesicae
edema, cardiac
edema, cerebral
edema, dependent
edema, high-altitude
edema, inflammatory
edema, laryngeal
edema, malignant
edema neonatorum
edema of glottis
edema, pitting
edema, pulmonary
edema, purulent
edema, salt
edematogenic
edematous
Eden-Hybinette operation
edentia
edentulous
edetate calcium disodium
edge
edge, bevel
edge, chamber
edge, cutting
edge, denture
edge, incisal
edible
edrophonium chloride
edrophonium test
eduction
edulcorant
edulcorate
EFA plus (omega 3,6, and
  essential fatty acids)
Efed II (Black)
  (theionized caffeine)
Efed II (Yellow)
  (theionized
  phenylpropanolamine)
effacement
effect
effect, additive
effect, Bainbridge

effect, cumulative
effective dose (ED)
effectiveness
effector
effector organ
effeminate
effemination
Effer-Syllium
efferent
efferent nerves
effervesce
effervescence
effervescent
Effler operation
effleurage
efflorescence
efflorescent
effluent
effluvium
efforts syndrome
effuse
effusion, pericardial
effusion, pleural
Efudex (fluorouracil)
egersis
egesta
egg
eglandulous
ego
ego strength
ego-dystonic
ego-syntonic
egocentric
egoism
egomania
egophony
egotism
egotropic
Ehlers-Danlos syndrome
Ehrenritter's ganglion
Ehrlich's side-chain
  theory
eicosanoids
eidetic
eidoptometry
eighth cranial nerve
Eikenella corrodens
eikonometry

eiloid
Eimeria
Eimeria hominis
einsteinium (Es)
Eisenmenger's complex
eisodic
ejaculatio
ejaculatio praecox
ejaculation
ejaculation, retrograde
ejaculatory
ejaculatory duct
ejecta
ejection
ejection fraction
ejection, ventricular
ekphorize
elaboration
elaiopathy
Elase (fibrinolysin and desoxyribonuclease, combined [bovine])
Elase-Chloromycetin
elastase
elastic
elastic bandage
elastic cartilage
elastic hosiery
elastic, intermaxillary
elastic, intramaxillary
elastic skin
elastic stocking
elastic tissue
elastic, vertical
elasticity
elastin
elastinase
elastofibroma
elastoid
elastoma
elastomer
elastometer
elastometry
elastorrhexis
elastose
elastosis
elation

Elavil (amitriptyline HCl)
elbow
elbow conformer
elbow jerk
elbow joint
elbow reflex
elbow, tennis
elbow unit
Eldercaps (vitamins and minerals)
Eldertonic (vitamins and minerals)
Eldopaque Forte (hydroquinone)
elective therapy
Electra complex
electric
electric light baker
electric shock
electrical
electrical stimulation
electricity
electricity, frictional
electricity, galvanic
electricity, induced
electricity, magnetic
electricity, negative
electricity, positive
electricity, static
electrify
electrization
electro-oculogram (EOG)
electroaffinity
electroanalgesia
electroanalysis
electroanesthesia
electrobiology
electrobioscopy
electrocardiography
electrocardiograph
electrocardiogram (ECG,EKG)
electrocardiographic stress testing
electrocardiophonograph
electrocatalysis
electrocautery

electrochemistry
electrochemy
electrocision
electrocoagulation
electrocochleography
electroconization, cervix
electrocontractility
electroconvulsive therapy
  (ECT)
electrocorticography
electrocryptectomy
electrocution
electrode
electrode, active
electrode, calomel
electrode, depolarizing
electrode, dispersive
electrode, gas-sending
electrode, glass
electrode, hydrogen
electrode,immmobilized
  enzyme
electrode, indifferent
electrode, internal
  reference
electrode, ion-selective
electrode, multiple point
electrode, negative
electrode, point
electrode, positive
electrode, spark-ball
electrode, subcutaneous
electrode, surface
electrode, therapeutic
electrodermal
electrodermal audiometry
electrodesiccation
electrodiagnosis
electrodialysis
electrodynamometer
electroejaculation
electroencephalograph
electroencephalogram
  (EEG)
electroencephalography
  (EEG)
electrogastrogram
electrogoniometer

electrograph
electrohemostasis
electrohydraulic
  fragmentation
electrohysterography
electrokardiogram (EKG)
electrology
electrolysis
electrolysis, ciliary
  body
electrolysis epilation
electrolysis, hair
  follicle
electrolysis, retina
electrolysis, skin
electrolysis,
  subcutaneous tissue
electrolyte, amphoteric
electrolyte profile
electrolytes test
electrolytic
electrolytic conduction
electromagnet
electromagnetic
electromagnetic induction
electromagnetic spectrum
electromagnetism
electromassage
electrometer
electromotive
electromotive force (EMF)
electromyogram (EMG)
electromyography (EMG)
electron
electron microscope
electron microscopy
electron paramagnetic
  resonance (EPR)
electron spin resonance
  (ESR)
electron volt (EV)
electron-dense
electronarcosis
electronegative
electroneurography
electroneurolysis
electronic
electronic gaiter

electronic musical
  instrument (EMI)
  scanning
electronic voice
electronics
electronization
electronystagmography
electronystagmogram (ENG)
electropathology
electrophoresis
electrophoresis, serum
  protein test
electrophorus
electrophrenic
electrophrenic
  respiration
electrophysiology
electropositive
electropuncture
electroradiometer
electroresection
electroresection, bladder
  neck
electroresection,
  esophagus
electroresection,
  prostate
electroresection, stomach
electroretinogram (ERG)
electroscission
electroscope
electroshock
electroshock therapy
  (EST)
electrosleep
electrostatic
electrostatic generator
electrostatic unit
electrostimulation
electrosurgery
electrosynthesis
electrotaxis
electrothanasia
electrotherapeutics
electrotherapist
electrotherapy
electrothermotherapy

electrothrombosis,
  intracranial
electrotome
electrotonic
electrotonus
electrotropism
electrovalence
electroversion
electuary
eleidin
element
element's, trace
eleoma
eleopathy
eleoptene
eleosaccharum
eleotherapy
elephantiasis
elephantiasis, scrotal
elevation
elevation, bone fragments
elevation, orbit
elevation, pedicle graft
elevation, sinus
elevation, skull
elevation, spinal
elevation's, tactile
elevator
elevator, periosteal
eleventh cranial nerve
elileptogenous
eliminant
eliminate
elimination
elimination diet
elinguation
elixir
Elixophyllin
  (theophylline
  anhydrous)
Elixophyllin-GG
  (theophylline
  anhydrous-guaifenesin)
Elixophyllin-KI
  (theophylline anhydrous
  and potassium iodide)
Elliot operation
ellipsis

ellipsoid
elliptocyte
elliptocytosis
elliptocytosis,
  hereditary
Ellis Jones operation
Ellis-van Creveld
  syndrome
Elmslie-Cholmeley
  operation
Elocon (mometasone
  furoate)
Eloesser operation
elongation
elope
Elspar (asparaginase)
eluate
eluent
elution
elutriation
emaciate
emaciated
emaciation
emaculation
emailloid
emanation
emanation, actinium
emanation, radium
emanation, thorium
emasculation
embalming
embarrass
Embden-Meyerhof pathway
embedding
embolalia
embole
embolectomy
embolectomy, abdominal
embolectomy, aorta
embolectomy, head and
  neck
embolectomy, intracranial
embolectomy, lower limb
embolectomy, thoracic
embolectomy, upper limb
embolectomy with
  endarterectomy
Embolex

embolic
emboliform
embolism
embolism, air
embolism, fat
embolism, pulmonary
embolism, pyemic
embolization
embololalia
embolophrasia
embolus
embolus, air
embolus, amniotic fluid
embolus, coronary
embolus, pulmonary
emboly
embolysis
embrace reflex
embrasure
embrasure, buccal
embrasure, labial
embrasure, lingual
embrasure, occlusal
embrocation
embryectomy
embryo
embryo transfer
embryocardia
embryocidal
embryoctony
embryogenetic
embryogenic
embryogeny
embryography
embryology
embryoma
embryonal
embryonic
embryonization
embryonoid
embryopathy
embryoplastic
embryoscopy
embryotocia
embryotome
embryotomy
embryotoxon
embryotroph

embryotrophy
embryulcia
embryulcus
Emcyt (estramustine
  phosphate sodium)
emedullate
emergency
emergency cardiac care
  (ECC)
emergency medical service
  (EMS)
emergency medical
  technician (EMT)
emergency readiness
emergency room (ER)
emergent
emesis
emesis basin
emesis, gastric
emesis gravidarum
emesis, irritation
emesis, nervous
emesis, reflex
Emete-Con (benzquinamide
  HCl)
emetic
emetic, direct
emetic, indirect
emetine
emetine bismuth iodide
emetine hydrochloride
emetism
emetocathartic
emetology
emigration
eminence
eminence, arcuate
eminence, articular, of
  the temporal bone
eminence, bicipital
eminence, blastodermic
eminence, canine
eminence, collateral
eminence, frontal
eminence, germinal
eminence, hypothenar
eminence, iliopectineal
eminence, intercondyloid

eminence, mamillary
eminence, median
eminence, nasal
eminence, occipital
eminence of Doyère
eminence, olivary
eminence, parietal
eminence, pyramidal
eminence, thenar
eminences, portal
eminentia
emiocytosis
emissary
emissary veins
emissio
emission
emission, nocturnal
emission, thermionic
emmenagogue
emmenagogue, direct
emmenagogue, indirect
emmenia
emmenic
emmeniopathy
emmenology
Emmet operation
emmetrope
emmetropia (E)
emollient
emotion
emotional
emotional need
emotivity
empasm
empasma
empathic
empathy
emperipolesis
emperor of pruritus
emphractic
emphraxis
emphysatherapy
emphysema
emphysematous
empiric
empirical
empiricism

Empirin with codeine
  (aspirin and codeine
  phosphate)
emplastic
emplastrum
Empracet with codeine
  (acetaminophen and
  codeine phosphate)
emprosthotonos
empty follicle syndrome
empty nest syndrome
empty-sella syndrome
emptysis
empyema
empyema, interlobular
empyema, necessitatis
empyema, pulsating
empyemectomy
empyesis
empyocele
empyreuma
emulsification
emulsifier
emulsify
emulsion
emulsoid
Emulsoil (self-emulsifyin
  castor oil)
emunctory
en bloc
enamel
enamel, aprismatic
enamel, cervical
enamel, gnarled
enamel hypoplasia
enamel, mottled
enamel organ
enamelum
enanthem
enanthema
enanthematous
enanthesis
enanthrope
enantiobiosis
enantiomorph
enantiopathy
enarthritis
enarthrosis

encanthis
encapsulated
encapsulation
encatarrhaphy
enceinte
encepahlomyelitis, benign
  myalgic
encephalalgia
encephalatrophy
encephalic
encephalitis
encephalitis, acute
  disseminated
encephalitis, cortical
encephalitis, epidemic
encephalitis, equine
encephalitis, equine,
  eastern
encephalitis, equine,
  western
encephalitis, hemorrhagic
encephalitis, herpes
encephalitis
  hyperplastica
encephalitis, infantile
encephalitis, Japanese (B
  type)
encephalitis, lead
encephalitis, lethargica
encephalitis, meningo
encephalitis neonatorum
encephalitis periaxialis
encephalitis,
  postinfection
encephalitis,
  postvaccinal
encephalitis, purulent
encephalitis, Russian
  spring-summer
encephalitis, St. Louis
encephalitis, toxic
encephalocele
encephalocentesis
encephalocystocele
encephalogram
encephalography
encephaloid
encephalolith

encephaloma
encephalomalacia
encephalomeningitis
encephalomeningocele
encephalomere
encephalometer
encephalomyelitis
encephalomyelitis, acute
  disseminated
encephalomyelitis, equine
encephalomyelitis,
  postinfectious
encephalomyelitis,
  postvaccinal
encephalomyeloneuropathy
encephalomyelopathy
encephalomyeloradiculitis
encephalomyocarditis
encephalon
encephalopathy
encephalopathy, hepatic
encephalopuncture
encephalopyosis
encephalorrhagia
encephalosclerosis
encephalosis
encephalospinal
encephalotome
encephalotomy
encephalpathy
enchondroma
enchondrosarcoma
enchondrosis
encircling procedure
enclave
enclitic
encolpitis
encopresis
encranial
encyesis
encysted
end artery
end organ
end organ, neuromuscular
end organ, neurotendinous
end organ, sensory
end product
end result

end-bud
end-bulb of Krause
end-feet
endadelphos
Endamoeba
endangeitis
endangiitis
endangium
endaortitis
endarterectomy
endarterectomy, abdominal
endarterectomy, aorta
endarterectomy, coronary
  artery
endarterectomy, head and
  neck
endarterectomy,
  intracranial
endarterectomy, lower
  limb
endarterectomy, thoracic
endarterectomy, upper
  limb
endarterial
endarteritis
endarteritis, acute
endarteritis, chronic
endarteritis deformans
endarteritis obliterans
endarteritis, syphilitic
endaural
endbrain
endemic
endemoepidemic
Endep (amitriptyline HCl)
endergonic
endermatic
endermic
endermosis
ending
endoaneurysmorrhaphy
endoangiitis
endoantitoxin
endoappendicitis
endoarteritis
endoauscultation
endobiotic
endoblast

endobronchitis
endocardiac
endocardial
endocardial cushion
  defect
endocardial resection
endocarditis
endocarditis, acute
  bacterial
endocarditis, atypical
  verrucous
endocarditis, bacterial
endocarditis, chronic
endocarditis, infective
endocarditis, Libman-
  Sacks
endocarditis, malignant
endocarditis, mural
endocarditis, rheumatic
endocarditis, subacute
  bacterial
endocarditis, syphilitic
endocarditis, tuberculous
endocarditis, ulcerative
endocarditis, valvular
endocarditis, vegetative
endocarditis, verrucous
endocarditis, viridans
endocardium
endocervical
endocervicitis
endocervix
endochondral
endochondral ossification
endochorion
endocolitis
endocolpitis
endocorpuscular
endocranial
endocranitis
endocranium
endocrinasthenia
endocrine
endocrinologist
endocrinology
endocrinopathic
endocrinopathy
endocrinotherapy

endocyst
endocystitis
endocytosis
endoderm
endodermal
Endodermophyton
endodiascope
endodiascopy
endodontia
endodontics
endodontist
endodontitis
endodontium
endodontologist
endodontology
endoectothrix
endoenteritis
endoenzyme
endogamy
endogastric
endogastritis
endogenic
endogenous
endogenous opiate-like
  substance
endogeny
endoglobar
endoglobular
endognathion
endointoxication
endolabyrinthitis
endolaryngeal
Endolimax nana
endolumbar
endolymph
endolymphatic
endolymphatic duct
endolysin
endolysis
endomastoiditis
endometer
endometrectomy
endometrial
endometrial biopsy
endometrial cyst
endometrial dating
endometrial jet washing
endometrioma

endometriosis
endometriosis, direct
endometriosis,
  implantation
endometriosis, internal
endometriosis, metastatic
endometriosis, peritoneal
endometriosis, primary
endometriosis,
  transplantation
endometritis
endometritis, cervical
endometritis, decidual
endometritis, dissecans
endometritis, puerperal
endometrium
endometry
endomorph
endomyocardial biopsy
endomyocarditis
endomysium
endoneuritis
endoneurium
endonuclease
endoparasite
endopathy
endopelvic
endopelvic fasciae
endopeptidase
endopericarditis
endoperimyocarditis
endoperitonitis
endophasia
endophlebitis
endophlebitis obliterans
endophlebitis portalis
endophthalmitis
endoplasm
endoplasmic reticulum
  (ER)
endorhinitis
Endorphan (D-
  phenylalanine, D-
  leucine, L-tryptophan)
endorphins
endorrhachis
endosalpingitis
endosalpingoma

endosalpinx
endoscope
endoscopic retrograde
  cannulation of
  pancreatic duct (ERCP)
endoscopic retrograde
  cholangio-
  pancreatography (ERCP)
endoscopy
endoscopy, anus
endoscopy, biliary tract
endoscopy, bladder
endoscopy, bronchus
endoscopy, colon
endoscopy, cul-de-sac
endoscopy, ear
endoscopy, esophagus
endoscopy, fiberoptic
endoscopy, ileum
endoscopy, jejunum
endoscopy, kidney
endoscopy, large
  intestine
endoscopy, larynx
endoscopy, mediastinum
endoscopy, nose
endoscopy, pelvis
endoscopy, peritoneum
endoscopy, pharynx
endoscopy, rectum
endoscopy, small
  intestine
endoscopy, stomach
endoscopy, thorax
endoscopy, through stoma
endoscopy, trachea
endoscopy, transabdominal
endoscopy, transpleural
endoscopy, ureter
endoscopy, urethra
endoscopy, uterus
endoscopy, vagina
endoscopy, with biopsy
endosepsis
endoskeleton
endosmometer
endosmosis
endosome

endospore
endosteitis
endosteoma
endosteum
endostitis
endostoma
endostosis
endotendineum
endothelial
endotheliocyte
endotheliocytosis
endotheliolysin
endotheliolytic
endothelioma
endotheliomyoma
endotheliomyxoma
endotheliosis
endotheliotoxin
endothelium
endothermal
endothermic
endothermy
endothrix
endothyropexy
endotoscope
endotoxemia
endotoxicosis
endotoxin
endotoxin, bacterial
endotoxin shock
endotracheal
endotracheal tube, cuffed
endotracheitis
endotrachelitis
endovasculitis
endovenous
endplate
endplate, motor
Enduron
  (methyclothiazide)
Enduronyl
  (methyclothiazide and
  deserpidine)
endyma
enema
enema, antispasmodic
enema, barium
enema, carminative

enema, cleansing
enema, double-contrast
enema, emollient
enema, high
enema, lubricating
enema, medicinal
enema, nutrient
enema, one-two-three
enema, physiological salt
  solution
enema, retention
enema, saline
enema, soapsuds
Ener-B (intra-nasal
  vitamin B_{12} Gel)
energetics
energy (E)
energy, conservation of
energy expenditure, basal
  (BEE)
energy, kinetic
energy, latent
energy, potential
energy, radiant
enervation
Enfamil (low iron infant
  formula)
Enfamil Nursette (low
  iron and iron
  fortified)
Enfamil with iron (infant
  formula with iron)
enflagellation
enflurane
engagement
Engelmann's disk
engine
engine, dental
engine, high-speed
engine, ultraspeed
englobe
engorged
engorgement
engram
enhancement
enissophobia
Enkaid (encainide HCl)
enkatarrhaphy

enkephalins
enlargement
enlargement, aortic lumen
enlargement, atrial
 septal defect
enlargement, eye socket
enlargement, foramen
 ovale
enlargement, intestinal
 stoma
enlargement, introitus
enlargement, palpebral
 fissure
enlargement, punctum
enlargement, sinus tract
Enlon (edrophonium
 chloride)
enol
enolase
enology
enomania
enophthalmos
enosimania
enostosis
Enovid 5 mg
 (norethynodrel with
 mestranol)
Enovid 10 mg
 (norethynodrel with
 mestranol)
Enovid-E 21
 (norethynodrel with
 mestranol)
Enrich (liquid nutrition
 with fiber)
enriched
ensiform
ensisternum
enstrophe
Ensure (liquid nutrition)
Ensure HN (high nitrogen
 liquid nutrition)
Ensure Plus (high calorie
 liquid nutrition)
Ensure Plus HN (high
 calorie, high nitrogen
 liquid nutrition)
Ensure Pudding

entad
ental
entamebiasis
Entamoeba
Entamoeba buccalis
Entamoeba coli
Entamoeba gingivalis
Entamoeba histolytica
Entamoeba kartulisi
Entamoeba tetragena
Entamoeba undulans
enteogastritis
enteradenitis
enteral
enteral tube feeding
enteralgia
enterectasia
enterectomy
enterelcosis
enteric
Enteric Cytopathogenic
 Human Orphan (ECHO)
 virus
enteric fever
enteric-coated
enteritis
enteroanastomosis
enteroantigen
enteroapokleisis
Enterobacter
Enterobacter aerogenes
Enterobacteriaceae
enterobacteriotherapy
enterobiasis
enterobiliary
Enterobius
Enterobius vermicularis
enterocele
enterocele repair
enterocelectomy
enterocentesis
enterocholecystotomy
enterocholecystostomy
enterocinesia
enterocinetic
enteroclysis
enterococcus
enterocoelic fistula

enterocolectomy
enterocolitis
enterocolitis, neonatal
  necrotizing
enterocolostomy
enterocrinin
enterocutaneous
enterocyst
enterocystoma
enterocystoplasty
enterodynia
enteroentectropy
enteroenteric fistula
enteroenterostomy
enteroepiplocele
enterogastrone
enterogastrostomy
enterogenous
enterogram
enterography
enterohepatic
enterohepatitis
enterohydrocele
enteroidea
enteroitomy, transverse
  colon
enterokinase
enterokinesia
enterolith
enterolithiasis
enterolithotomy
enterology
enterolysis
enteromegalia
enteromegaly
Enteromonas hominis
enteromycosis
enteromyiasis
enteron
enteroneuritis
enteroparesis
enteropathogen
enteropathy
enteropeptidase
enteropexy
enteroplasty
enteroplegia
enteroplex

enteroplexy
enteroproctia
enteroptosis
enterorrhaphy
enterorrhexis
enteroscope
enteroscopy
enterosepsis
enterospasm
enterostasis
enterostenosis
enterostomal therapist
enterostomy
enterostomy, cecum
enterostomy, delayed
  opening
enterostomy, duodenum
enterostomy, feeding
enterostomy, ileum
enterostomy, jejunum
enterostomy, loop
enterostomy, sigmoid
  colon
enterotome
enterotomy
enterotoxemia
enterotoxigenic
enterotoxin
enterotoxism
enterotropic
enterovesical fistula
enterovirus
enterozoic
enterozoon
Entex (phenylephrine HCl,
  phenylpropanolamine
  HCl, guaifenesin)
enthalsis
entheomania
enthesis
enthetic
enthlasis
entity
entoblast
entocele
entochondrostosis
entochoroidea
entocineria

entocone
entocornea
entocyte
entoderm
entoectad
Entolase (pancrelipase)
Entolase-HP
  (pancrelipase)
entome
entomion
entomology
entomology, medical
entophyte
entopic
entoptic
entoptic phenomena
entoretina
entotic
entozoon
Entozyme
entrain
entrocystocele
entropion
entropion, cicatricial
entropion, spastic
entropionize
entropy
Entuss (hydrocodone
  bitartrate and
  guaifenesin)
enucleate
enucleation
enucleator
enuresis, diurnal
enuresis, nocturnal
enuresis, primary
enuresis, secondary
envelope
envelope, nuclear
envenomation
environment
environmental control
  unit
envy
Enzactin (triacetin)
enzootic
enzygotic

enzygotic twins
enzyme
enzyme, activating
enzyme, amylolytic
enzyme, autolytic
enzyme, bacterial
enzyme, coagulating
enzyme, deamidizing
enzyme, debranching
enzyme, decarboxylating
enzyme, digestive
enzyme, extracellular
enzyme, fermenting
enzyme, glycolytic
enzyme, hydrolytic
enzyme induction
enzyme, inhibitory
enzyme, inorganic
enzyme, intracellular
enzyme, inverting
enzyme, lipolytic
enzyme, mucolytic
enzyme, oxidizing
enzyme, proteolytic
enzyme, redox
enzyme, reducing
enzyme, respiratory
enzyme, splitting
enzyme, steatolytic
enzyme, transferring
enzyme, uricolytic
enzyme, yellow
enzyme's, allosteric
enzyme's, branching
enzyme-linked
  immunosorbent assay
  (ELISA)
enzymology
enzymolysis
enzymopathy
enzymopenia
enzymuria
eonism
eosin
eosinoblast
eosinopenia
eosinophil

eosinophile
eosinophilia
eosinophilia, urinary
eosinophilic
eosinophilic leukocytes
eosinophilous
eosinotactic
epactal
eparterial
epaxial
epencephalon
ependyma
ependymal cells
ependymal layer
ependymitis
ependymoblast
ependymocyte
ependymoma
ephebiatrics
ephebic
ephebology
ephedrine
ephedrine hydrochloride
ephedrine sulfate
ephelis
ephemeral
ephidrosis
ephidrosis cruenta
ephidrosis tincta
epiandrosterone
epiblast
epiblastic
epiblepharon
epibole
epiboly
epibulbar
epicanthus
epicardia
epicardiectomy
epichordal
epichorion
epicomus
epicondylalgia
epicondyle
epicondylitis, lateral
  humeral
epicranium
epicranius

epicrisis
epicritic
epicystitis
epicystotomy
epicyte
epidemic
epidemic viral
  gastroenteropathy
epidemiologic
epidemiologist
epidemiology
epidermal
epidermatoplasty
epidermic
epidermis
epidermitis
epidermization
epidermodysplasia
epidermoid
epidermolysis
epidermolysis bullosa
epidermoma
epidermomycosis
Epidermophyton
Epidermophyton floccosum
epidermophytosis
epidermosis
epididymectomy
epididymis
epididymitis
epididymodeferential
epididymodeferentectomy
epididymogram
epididymography
epididymoorchitis
epididymoplasty
epididymorrhaphy
epididymotomy
epididymovasostomy
epididymovesiculography
epidural
epidural space
epifascial
Epifoam (hydrocortisone
  acetate and pramoxine
  HCl)
epifolliculitis
epigaster

epigastralgia
epigastric
epigastric reflex
epigastrium
epigastrocele
epigastrorrhaphy
epigenesis
epiglottidean
epiglottidectomy
epiglottis
epiglottitis
epihyal
epikeratophakia
epilate
epilating
epilation
epilation, cryosurgical
epilation,
    electrosurgical
epilation, eyebrow
epilation, eyelid
epilation, skin
epilemma
epilepsy
epilepsy, television
epilepsy, traumatic
epileptic
epileptiform
epileptogenic
epileptoid
epileptology
epiloia
epimandibular
epimer
epimere
epimerite
epimorphosis
epimysium
epinephrine
epinephrine bitartrate
epinephrinemia
epinephritis
epinephroma
epineural
epineurium
epiotic
epiotic center
epipastic

Epipen (epinephrine auto
    injector)
epipharynx
epiphenomenon
epiphora
epiphylaxis
epiphyseal
epiphyseal separation
epiphyseolysis
epiphyseopathy
epiphysial
epiphysiodesis
epiphysiolysis
epiphysis
epiphysitis
epipial
epiplocele
epiploectomy
epiploenterocele
epiploic
epiploic foramen
epiploitis
epiplomerocele
epiplomphalocele
epiploon
epiplopexy
epiplorrhaphy
epiplosarcomphalocele
epiploscheocele
epipygus
episclera
episcleral
episcleritis
episioelytrorrhaphy
episioperineoplasty
episioperineorrhaphy
episioplasty
episioproctotomy
episiorrhaphy
episiostenosis
episiotomy
episome
epispadias
episplenitis
epistasis
epistaxis
episternal
episternum

epistropheus
epitaxy
epitendineum
epitenon
epithalamus
epithalaxia
epithélia
epithelial cancer
epithelial casts
epithelial cells
epithelial tissue
epithelialization
epitheliitis
epithelioblastoma
epitheliogenetic
epitheliogenic
epithelioglandular
epithelioid
epitheliolysin
epitheliolysis
epithelioma
epithelioma adamantinum
epithelioma adenoides
   cysticum
epithelioma, basal cell
epithelioma, deep-seated
epitheliomatous
epitheliosis
epithelium, attachment
epithelium, ciliated
epithelium, columnar
epithelium, cuboidal
epithelium, germinal
epithelium, glandular
epithelium, laminated
epithelium, mesenchymal
epithelium, pavement
epithelium, pigmented
epithelium,
   pseudostratified
epithelium, reduced
   enamel
epithelium, squamous
epithelium, stratified
epithelium, sulcular
epithelium, transitional
epitope
epitrichial layer

epitrichium
epitrochlea
epitrochlear
epiturbinate
epitympanum
epizoic
epizoicide
epizoon
epizootic
eponychium
eponym
epoophorectomy
epoxide
epoxy
epsilon-aminocaproic acid
Epstein's pearls
Epstein-Barr virus (EBV)
epulis
epuloid
epulosis
epulotic
Equagesic (meprobamate
   with aspirin)
equalization, by bone
   fusion
equalization, by
   epiphyseal stapling
equalization, leg
Equanil (meprobamate)
equation
equator
equator oculi
equator of cell
equator of crystalline
   lens
equatorial
equatorial plate
equilibrating
equilibration
equilibrium
equilibrium, nitrogenous
equilibrium,
   physiological
equilin
equiloudness balance
equine
equine infectious anemia
   (EIA)

equinovarus
equipotential
equivalence
equivalent
equivalent weight
eradication
erasion
Erb's palsy
Erb's paralysis
Erb's point
Erben's reflex
erbium (Er)
erectile
erectile tissue
erection
erector
erector spinae reflex
eremophobia
erepsin
erethism
erethism mercurialis
erethismic
erethisophrenia
erethistic
erethitic
ereuthrophobia
ergasiomania
ergasiophobia
ergasthenia
ergastic
ergastoplasm
ergocalciferol
ergogenic
ergograph
ergometer
ergometer, bicycle
ergonomics
ergonovine maleate
ergophobia
ergophore
ergostat
Ergostat (ergotamine
  tartrate)
ergosterol
ergot
ergot poisoning
ergotamine
ergotamine tartrate

ergotherapy
ergotism
ergotrate
ergotropic
ergotropy
Eristalis
erode
erogenous
erogenous zone
erosion
erosion, dental
erosion of cervix uteri
erosive
erotic
eroticism
eroticism, allo
eroticism, anal
eroticism, auto
eroticism, oral
erotism
erotogenic
erotology
erotomania
erotopathia
erotophobia
erratic
errhine
error
error, type I
error, type II
erubescence
eructation
eruption
eruption, active
eruption, creeping
eruption, delayed
eruption, drug
eruption, passive
eruption, serum
eruption, tooth
eruptive
eruptive stage
Ery-Tab (erythromycin)
ERYC (erythromycin)
Erycette (erythromycin)
Eryderm (erythromycin)
Erymax (erythromycin)

Eryped (erythromycin
  ethylsuccinate)
erysipelas
erysipelatous
erysipeloid
*Erysipelothrix
  rhusiopathiae*
erysipelotoxin
erysiphake
erythema ab igne
erythema annulare
erythema congestivum
erythema, diffuse
erythema dose (ED)
erythema induratum
erythema infectiosum
erythema intertrigo
erythema marginatum
erythema migrans (EM)
erythema multiforme
erythema neonatorum
erythema nodosum
erythema, punctate
erythema toxicum
  neonatorum
erythema, venenatum
erythematic
erythematous
erythemogenic
erythralgia
erythrasma
erythredema
erythremia
erythrism
erythristic
erythrityl tetranitrate
erythroblast
erythroblastemia
erythroblastic
erythroblastoma
erythroblastosis
erythroblastosis fetalis
erythrochloropia
erythrochromia
**Erythrocin Lactobionate
  I.V.** (erythromycin
  lactobionate)

Erythrocin Piggyback
  (erythromycin
  lactobionate)
Erythrocin Stearate
  (erythromycin stearate)
erythroclasis
erythroclastic
erythrocyanosis
erythrocyte
erythrocyte, achromatic
erythrocyte, basophilic
erythrocyte, crenated
erythrocyte, immature
erythrocyte maturation
  factor (EMF)
erythrocyte,
  orthochromatic
erythrocyte,
  polychromatic
erythrocyte sedimentation
  rate
erythrocythemia
erythrocytolysin
erythrocytolysis
erythrocytometer
erythrocytoopsonin
erythrocytopenia
erythrocytopoiesis
erythrocytorrhexis
erythrocytoschisis
erythrocytosis
erythroderma
erythroderma
  desquamativum
erythroderma
  ichthyosiforme
  congenitum
erythrodermia
erythrodextrin
erythrodontia
erythrogenesis
erythroid
erythrokeratodermia
erythrokinetics
erythroleukemia
erythroleukosis
erythrolysin
erythrolysis

erythromania
erythromelalgia
erythromelia
Erythromycin Base Filmtab
   (erythromycin)
erythromycin stearate
erythron
erythroneocytosis
erythronoclastic
erythroparasite
erythropathy
erythropenia
erythrophage
erythrophagia
erythrophile
erythrophilous
erythrophobia
erythrophose
erythrophthisis
erythropia
erythroplasia
erythroplasia of Queyrat
erythropoiesis
erythropoietic
erythropoietic
   stimulating factor
   (ESF)
erythropoietin
erythroprosopalgia
erythropsia
erythropsin
erythrorrhexis
erythrosine sodium
erythrosis
erythrostasis
erythrotoxin
erythruria
Esbach method
escape
escape beat
escape phenomenon
escape, vagal
escape, ventricular
escharectomy
escharotic
escharotomy
Escherich's reflex
Escherichia (E.)

Escherichia coli (E.coli)
eschrolalia
escorcin
esculent
escutcheon
eserine
Esgic (butalbital,
   acetaminophen and
   caffeine)
Esgic with Codeine
Esimil (guanethidine
   monosulfate and
   hydrochlorothiazide)
Eskalith (lithium
   carbonate)
Esmarch's bandage
esodic
esoethmoiditis
esogastritis
esophagalgia
esophageal
esophageal acidity test
esophageal manometry
esophageal voice training
esophageal web
esophagectasia
esophagectomy
esophagismus
esophagitis
esophagobronchial
esophagocele
esophagocolostomy
esophagoduodenostomy
esophagodynia
esophagoenterostomy
esophagoesophagostomy
esophagogastrectomy
esophagogastric
   fundoplasty
esophagogastric manometry
esophagogastroanastomosis
esophagogastro-
   duodenoscopy
esophagogastromyotomy
esophagogastropexy
esophagogastroplasty
esophagogastroscopy
esophagogastrostomy

esophagoileostomy
esophagojejunostomy
esophagomalacia
esophagomycosis
esophagomyotomy
esophagoplasty
esophagoplication
esophagoptosia
esophagoptosis
esophagorrhaphy
esophagoscope
esophagoscopy
esophagospasm
esophagostenosis
esophagostomy
esophagotome
esophagotomy
esophagotracheal
esophagus
esophagus, foreign bodies
  in
esophoria
esosphenoiditis
Esoterica (medicated fade
  cream)
esotropia (ST)
essence
essential
essential fatty acids
  (EFA)
Estar (therapeutic tar
  gel)
ester
esterase
esterification
esterize
Estes operation
esthematology
esthesia
esthesiology
esthesiomania
esthesiometer
esthesioneurosis
esthesiophysiology
esthesioscopy
estheticokinetic
esthetics
esthiomene

estimated blood loss
  (EBL)
Estinyl (ethinyl
  estradiol)
estival
estivoautumnal
Estlander operation
Estrace (estradiol)
Estraderm (estradiol
  transdermal system)
estradiol (E2)
estradiol dipropionate
Estradurin (polyestradiol
  phosphate)
Estratab (exterified
  estrogen)
Estratest (androgen-
  estrogen therapy)
estrin
estrinization
estriol
estriol (E3)
estrogen's conjugated
estrogenic
estrone (E1)
estropipate
Estrovis (quinestrol)
estrual
estruation
estrus
estrus cycle
estuarium
état criblé
état mamelonné
etching
etching, acid
ethacrynic acid
ethambutol hydrochloride
ethamivan
ethanol
Ethatab (ethaverine HCl)
ethaverine hydrochloride
ethchlorvynol
ethene
ether
ether anesthesia
ether asphyxia
ether bed

ethereal
etherization
etherize
etheromania
ethics
ethinamate
ethinyl estradiol
Ethiodol (ethiodized oil
  injection)
ethionamide
ethionine
ethmocarditis
ethmoid
ethmoid bone
ethmoid sinus
ethmoidal
ethmoidectomy
ethmoiditis
ethmoidotomy
ethnic
ethnobiology
ethnography
ethnology
ethology
ethopropazine
  hydrochloride
ethosuximide
ethotoin
ethoxzolamide
Ethrane (enflurane)
Ethril '250'
  (erythromycin
  stearate)
Ethril '500'
  (erythromycin
  stearate)
ethyl acetate
ethyl alcohol
ethyl aminobenzoate
ethyl biscoumacetate
ethyl chaulmoograte
ethyl chloride
ethyl, vanillin
ethylamine
ethylcellulose
ethylene(C_2H_4)
ethylene anesthesia
ethylene glycol

ethylene oxide
ethylenediamine
ethylenediaminetetra-
  acetic acid (EDTA)
ethylmorphine
ethylnorepinephrine
  hydrochloride
ethynodiol diacetate
ethynyl
etiocholanolone
etiologic
etiological
etiotropic
Etrafon (perphenazine,
  amitriptyline HCl)
etretinate
ETS-2% (erythromycin)
etymology
Eubacteriales
Eubacterium
eubiotics
eubolism
eucalyptol
eucalyptus
eucapnia
eucatropine hydrochloride
Eucerin (unscented
  moisturizing formula)
euchlorhydria
eucholia
euchromatin
euchylia
eucrasia
eudiaphoresis
eudiometer
euesthesia
eugenics
eugenol
euglobulin
euglobulin lysis
eugonic
eukaryon
eukaryote
eukinesia
Eulenburg's disease
Eumycetes
eunoia
eunuch

eunuchism
eunuchism, pituitary
eunuchoid
eunuchoidism
eupancreatism
eupepsia
eupeptic
euphonia
euphoria
euplastic
euploidy
eupnea
eupraxia
eupraxic
Eurax (crotamiton)
europium (Eu)
Eurotium
eurycephalic
eustachian catheter
eustachian tube
eustachian valve
eustachianography
eustachitis
eusystole
eutectic
eutectic mixture
euthanasia
euthenics
Eutheria
Euthroid (liotrix)
euthyroid
eutocia
Eutonyl Filmtab
  (pargyline HCl)
Eutrombicula
eutrophication
Evac-Q-Kit (bowel
  evacuant)
Evac-Q-Kwik (bowel
  evacuant)
evacuant
evacuate
evacuation
evacuation, abscess
evacuation, anterior
  chamber (eye)
evacuation, breast
evacuation, cyst

evacuation, hematoma
evacuation, hemorrhoids
evacuation, incisional
evacuation, kidney
evacuation, liver
evacuation, obstetrical
evacuation, pelvic blood
  clot
evacuation, retained
  placenta
evacuation, streptothrix
  from lacrimal duct
evacuator
evaginate
evagination
evaluation
evanescent
Evans blue
Evans operation
Evans syndrome
evaporation
evenomation
eventration
eversion
every other hour
  (alt. hor.)
evidement
evidence
evil
eviration
evisceration
evisceration, eyeball
evisceration, ocular
  contents
evisceration, orbit
evisceration, pelvic
evisceroneurotomy
evocation
evoked potentials
evoked response
evolution
evolution, theory of
evulsion
evulsion, nail
evulsion, skin
evulsion, subcutaneous
  tissue
Ewing's sarcoma

Ewing's tumor
Ex-Lax
exacerbation
exaltation
examination
examination (exam)
exangia
exanthem
exanthem subitum
exanthema
exanthematous
exanthrope
exarticulation
excavation
excavation, atrophic
excavation, dental
excavation of optic nerve
excavation, rectouterine
excavator
Excedrin
excerebration
exchange transfusion
excipient
excise
excision (ex)
excision of esophageal
  diverticulum
excisional biopsy
excitability
excitability, independent
excitability, muscle
excitability, nerve
excitability, reflex
excitant
excitation
excitation, direct
excitation, indirect
excitation wave
exciting
excitoglandular
excitometabolic
excitomotor
excitomuscular
excitor
excitosecretory
excitovascular
exclave
exclusion

exclusion, pyloric
excochleation
excoriation
excrement
excrementitious
excrescence
excrete
excretion
excretory
excursion
excurvation
excystation
exencephalia
exenteration
exenteration, ethmoid air
  cells
exenteration, orbit
exenteration, pelvic
exercise
exercise, active
exercise, assistive
exercise, blowing
exercise bone
exercise, Buerger's
  postural
exercise, Codman's
exercise, corrective
exercise, crawling
exercise,
  electrocardiogram
exercise, free
exercise, isokinetic
exercise, isometric
exercise, isotonic
exercise, muscle-setting
exercise, passive
exercise prescription
exercise, range of motion
exercise, resistive
exercise, static
exercise stress testing
exercise, therapeutic
exercise tolerance test
  (ETT)
exercises, Kegel
exercise-induced asthma
exeresis
exergonic

exfetation
exflagellation
exfoliation
exfoliation, skin
exhalation
exhaustion
exhaustion, heat
exhibit
exhibitionism
exhibitionist
exhilarant
exhumation
exitus
Exna (benzthiazide)
Exner's nerve
Exner's plexus
exobiology
exocardia
exocardial
exocataphoria
exocolitis
exocrine
exocytosis
exodeviation
exodic
exodontia
exodontology
exoenzyme
exoerythrocytic
exogamy
exogastritis
exogenous
exohysteropexy
exometritis
exomphalos
exons
exopathic
exophoria
exophthalmia cachectica
exophthalmia fungosa
exophthalmic
exophthalmic goiter
exophthalmometer
exophthalmos
exophthalmus
exoplasm
exoserosis
exoskeleton

exosmosis
exosplenopexy
exostectomy
exostosis
exostosis bursata
exostosis cartilaginea
exostosis, dental
exostosis, multiple
    osteocartilaginous
exoteric
exothermal
exothermic
exothyropexy
exotic
exotoxin
exotropia (XT)
expander
expansion
expansive delusion
expectant
expectation
expected date of
    confinement (EDC)
expectorant
expectoration
expel
experiment
expiration (exp)
expiration, active
expiration, passive
expiratory
expiratory center
expiratory flow rate
expire
explant
explode
exploration
exploratory
explorer
explosive speech
exponent
expose
exposure
express
expression
expression, trachoma
    follicles
expressivity

expulsion rate
expulsive
exsanguinate
exsanguination
exsanguination
  transfusion
exsanguine
exsection
Exsel (selenium sulfide)
exsiccant
exsiccation
exsiccative
exsomatize
exsorption
exstrophy
exsufflation
extemporaneous
extend
extended care facility
extended family
extender
Extendryl (antihistamine-
  decongestant)
extension
extension, buccolabial
  sulcus
extension, Buck's
extension, limb, forced
extension, lingual sulcus
extension, mandibular
  ridge
extensor
exterior
exteriorization
exteriorize
extern
external
external cardiac
  compression (ECC)
external fixation
external fixator
external occipital
  protuberance (EOP)
external resistance (ER)
externalia
externalize
externe
exteroceptive

exteroceptor
exterofective
extima
extinction
extinguish
extirpation
extorsion
extra beats
extra-articular
extracapsular
extracellular
extracellular fluid (ECF)
extracorporeal
extracorporeal
  circulation
extracorporeal membrane
  oxygenator (ECMO)
extracorporeal shock-wave
  lithotripsy (ESWL)
extracorporeal shock-wave
  lithotriptor
extracorticospinal
extracranial
extracranial nerves
extract
extract, alcoholic
extract, aqueous
extract, aromatic fluid
extract, compound
extract, ethereal
extract, fluid
extract, powdered
extract, soft
extract, solid
extractable nuclear
  antigen (ENA)
extraction
extractive
extractor
extractor, tissue
extractor, tube
extractum (ext.)
extracystic
extradural
extraembryonic
extragenital
extrahepatic

extrahepatic biliary
  ducts
extraligamentous
extramalleolus
extramarginal
extramarital
extramastoiditis
extramedullary
extramural
extraneous
extranuclear
extraocular
extraocular eye muscles
extraocular movement
  (EOM)
extrapetrosal drainage
extrapolar
extrapyramidal
extrapyramidal symptoms
  (EPS)
extrapyramidal syndrome
extrapyramidal system
extrasensory
extrasensory perception
  (ESP)
extrasystole
extrasystole, atrial
extrasystole, junctional
extrasystole, nodal
extrasystole, ventricular
extratubal
extrauterine
extravaginal
extravasate
extravasation
extravascular
extraventricular
extremital
extremity, lower
extremity, upper
extrinsic
extrinsic muscles (e.m.)
extrospection
extroversion
extrovert
extrude
extrusion

extubation
exuberant
exudate
exudation
exudative
exude
exumbilication
exuviae
eye (E)
eye, aphakic
eye bank
eye, black
eye contact
eye, crossed
eye, dark-adapted
eye deviation
eye, dominant
eye, dry
eye, exciting
eye, fixating
eye, foreign body in
eye, light-adapted
eye muscle imbalance
eye, pink-
eye, squinting
eye stones
eye, sympathizing
eye-gaze communicator
eyeball
eyebrow
eyecup
eyedrops
eyeglass
eyeground
eyelash
eyelashes
eyelid
eyelid closure reflex
eyelid, drooping
eyelid, fused
eyelids
eyepiece
eyes, ears, nose, and
  throat (EENT)
eyestrain
eyewash

F

F response
F wave
F-E-P Creme
  (hydrocortisone acetate
  and pramoxine HCl)
fabella
fabism
fabrication
Fabry's disease
face
face lift
face, moon
facet
facetectomy
facetectomy, vertebra
facette
facial
facial bones
facial center
facial nerve
facial paralysis
facial reflex
facial spasm
facial-hypoglossal
  anastomosis
facial-phrenic
  anastomosis
facial-spinal accessory
  anastomosis
facies
facies abdominalis
facies, adenoid
facies aortica
facies hepatica
facies hippocratica
facies leontina
facies, masklike
facies mitralis
facies, myopathic
facies, parkinsonian
facies, typhoid
facilitation

facilitation, intraoculae
  circulation
facing
faciobrachial
faciocephalalgia
faciocervical
faciolingual
facioplasty
facioplegia
facioscapulohumeral
factitious
factitious disorders
factor
factor, accessory food
factor, antianemic
factor, antihemophilic
factor, lethal
factor, milk
factor, proliferation
  inhibiting
factor, Rh
factor assay
Factor I (fibrinogen)
Factor II (prothrombin)
Factor III (tissue
  factor)
Factor IV (calcium ions)
Factor V (unstable
  protein)
Factor VII (proconvertin)
Factor VIII
  (antihemophilic factor)
Factor IX (plasma
  thromboplastin-
  Christmas factor)
Factor X (Stuart factor
  or Prower factor)
Factor XI (plasma
  thrombloplastin
  antecedent)
Factor XII (Hageman or
  glass factor)
Factor XIII (fibrin
  stabilizing factor)
factor's coagulation
Factrel (gonadorelin HCl)
facultative
faculty

fagopyrism
Fahrenheit (F)
failure
failure, heart
failure, kidney
failure, renal
failure, respiratory
failure to thrive
faint
faintness
faith healing
falcate
falces
falcial
falciform
falciform ligament
falciform ligament of
  liver
falciform process
falcular
fallectomy
falling drop
fallopian canal
fallopian ligament
fallopian tube
fallopian tubes
Fallot, tetralogy of
fallotomy
fallout
false
false ribs
false-negative
false-positive
falsification
falx
falx cerebelli
falx cerebri
falx inguinalis
falx ligmentosa
fames
familial
familial Mediterranean
  fever
familial periodic
  paralysis
family
family history (FH)
family planning

family practice (FP)
family therapy (FT)
Fanconi's syndrome
fang
fango
Fannia
Fansidar (sulfadoxine and
  pyrimethamine)
fantast
fantasy
Farabeuf operation
farad
faraday
faradic
faradism
faradization
faradotherapy
farcy
farcy, button
farina
farinaceous
farmer's lung
farpoint
Farre's tubercles
farsighted
farsightedness
fart
fascia
fascia, Abernethy's
fascia, anal
fascia, aponeurotic
fascia, Buck's
fascia, cervical, deep
fascia, cervical,
  superficial
fascia, Cloquet's
fascia, Colles'
fascia, cremasteric
fascia, cribriform
fascia, crural
fascia, deep
fascia, dentate
fascia, endothoracic
fascia, extrapleural
fascia, intercolumnar
fascia, lata femoris
fascia, lumbodorsal
fascia, pectineal

fascia, pelvic
fascia, pharyngobasilar
fascia, plantar
fascia, Scarpa's
fascia sling operation
fascia, superficial
fascia, thyrolaryngeal
fascia, transversalis
fasciae
fascial
fascial reflex
fasciaplasty
fascicle
fascicular
fasciculation
fasciculus
fasciculus cuneatus
fasciculus, dorsolateral
fasciculus, fundamental
fasciculus gracillis
fasciculus, longitudinal,
  inferior
fasciculus, longitudinal,
  medial
fasciculus, longitudinal,
  posterior
fasciculus, unciform
fasciectomy
fasciitis
fasciodesis
fasciola
fasciola cinerea
Fasciola
Fasciola hepatica
fasciolar
fasciolopsiasis
Fasciolopsis buski
fascioplasty
fasciorrhaphy
fasciotomy
fascitis
fast
fast, acid
fastidium
fastigium
Fastin (phentermine HCl)
fasting
fasting blood sugar (FBS)

fat
fat emulsion
fat, neutral
fatal
fatal dose (FD)
fatigability
fatigue
fatigue, acute
fatigue, chronic
fatigue, muscular
fats
fatty
fatty acid (FA)
fatty acid, essential
fatty acid, free (FFA)
fatty acids
fatty acids, omega 3
fatty casts
fatty change
fatty degeneration
fauces
faucial
faucial reflex
faucitis
fauna
faveolate
faveolus
favism
favus
fear
febricide
febrifacient
febrific
febrifugal
febrifuge
febrile
febrile agglutinins test
febrile convulsions
febrile state
febriphobia
febris
febris, enterica
febris, falva
febris, undulans
fecal
fecal fat test
fecal impaction
fecal vomit

fecalith
fecaloid
fecaloma
fecaluria
feces
Fechner's law
fecula
feculent
fecundate
fecundation
fecundation, artificial
fecundity
Fedahist (pseudoephedrine HCl and chlorpheniramine maleate)
Fedrazil
feedback
feeder
feeding
feeding, artificial
feeding, breast
feeding, forcible
feeding, intravenous
feeding, rectal
feeding, tube
feeling
Feer's disease
feet
Fehling's solution
Feingold diet
Feldene (piroxicam)
feline
fellatio
felon
feltwork
Felty's syndrome
female
feminine
feminism
feminization
feminization, testicular
femoral
femoral arteriography
femoral artery
femoral hernia repair
femoral reflex
femoral vein

femoral-anterior bypass graft
femorocele
femoropopliteal artery
femorotibial
Femstat (butoconazole nitrate)
Femstat Prefill (butoconazole nitrate)
femur
fenestra
fenestra cochleae
fenestra rotunda
fenestra vestibuli
fenestrated
fenestration
fenfluramine hydrochloride
fenoprofen calcium
fentanyl citrate
Feosol (ferrous sulfate)
Feosol Elixir (ferrous sulfate)
Feostat (ferrous fumarate)
Fer-In-Sol (iron supplement)
feral
Ferancee (chewable hematinic)
Ferancee-HP (high potency hematinic)
Fergon (ferrous gluconate)
Ferguson operation
ferment
fermentation
fermentation, acetic
fermentation, alcoholic
fermentation, amylolytic
fermentation, autolytic
fermentation, butyric
fermentation, citric acid
fermentation, invertin
fermentation, lactic
fermentation, oxalic acid
fermentation, propionic acid

fermentation, viscous
fermentum
fermium (Fm)
fern
fern pattern, ferning
Fern test
Fero-Folic-500 Filmtab
  (iron with folic acid
  and vitamin C)
Ferralet (ferrous
  gluconate)
ferrated
ferric
ferric chloride
ferrin
ferritin
ferrokinetics
ferropexia
ferroprotein
Ferro-Sequels (iron)
ferrotherapy
ferrous
ferrous fumarate
ferrous gluconate
ferrous sulfate
ferruginous
ferrule
ferrum
fertile
fertility
fertilization
fertilization, in vitro
fertilizin
fervescence
Festalan (lipase,
  amylase, protease,
  atropine methyl
  nitrate)
fester
festinant
festination
festoon
fetal
fetal alcohol syndrome
  (FAS)
fetal biophysical profile
fetal circulation
fetal distress

fetal echocardiography
fetal echography
fetal heart rate (FHR)
fetal heart sound (FHS)
fetal hemoglobin
fetal membranes
fetal monitoring
fetal non-stress test
fetal oxytocin stress
  test
fetal scalp, blood
  sampling
fetal study
fetal transfusion,
  intrauterine
fetalism
feticide
fetid
fetish
fetishism
feto protein, alpha-1
fetochorionic
fetoglobulin
fetography
fetology
fetometry
fetoplacental
fetoprotein
fetor
fetor ex ore
fetor hepaticus
fetor oris
fetoscope
fetoscopy
fetotoxic
fetus
fetus amorphus
fetus, calcified
fetus in fetu
fetus, mummified
fetus papyraceus
fetus, parasitic
fever
fever blister
fever, childbed
fever, continuous
fever, drug
fever, induced

fever, intermittent
fever of unknown origin
  (FUO)
fever, periodic
fever, relapsing
fever, remittent
fever, septic
fiat
fiat mistura (f.m.)
fiber
fiber, accelerator
fiber, afferent
fiber, dietary
fiber, efferent
Fiber Guard (high fiber
  supplement)
fiber, inhibitory
fiber, medullated
fiber, nerve
fiber, nonmedullated
fiber, unmyelinated
fiber's, Purkinje
fiber-illuminated
Fiberall
fibercolonoscope
Fibercon (bulk-forming
  fiber laxative)
fibergastroscope
fiberglass
Fibermed (high-fiber
  supplement)
fiberoptic
fiberoscopy
fiberscope
fibra
fibralbumin
fibremia
fibril
fibril, muscle
fibril, nerve
fibrilla
fibrillar
fibrillary
fibrillated
fibrillation
fibrillation, atrial
fibrillation, ventricular
fibrillogenesis

fibrillolysis
fibrillolytic
fibrin
fibrin degradation
  product test
fibrin foam
fibrinocellular
fibrinogen
fibrinogenic
fibrinogenolysis
fibrinogenopenia
fibrinogenous
fibrinoid
fibrinoid change
fibrinoid material
fibrinokinase
fibrinolysin
fibrinolysin tests
fibrinolysis
fibrinolytic
fibrinopenia
fibrinopeptide
fibrinoplastic
fibrinopurulent
fibrinoscopy
fibrinosis
fibrinous
fibrinuria
fibro-osteoma
fibroadenia
fibroadenoma
fibroadipose
fibroangioma
fibroareolar
fibroblast
fibroblastoma
fibrobronchitis
fibrocalcific
fibrocarcinoma
fibrocartilage
fibrocellular
fibrochondritis
fibrochondroma
fibrocutaneous
fibrocyst
fibrocystic
fibrocystic disease of
  pancreas

fibrocystic disease of
  the breast
fibrocystoma
fibrocyte
fibrodysplasia
fibroelastic
fibroelastosis
fibroelastosis,
  endocardial
fibroenchondroma
fibroepithelioma
fibroglia
fibroglioma
fibroid
fibroid, interstitial
fibroid tumor
fibroid, uterine
fibroidectomy
fibrolipoma
fibroma
fibroma, intramural
fibroma of breast
fibroma, submucous
fibroma, subserous
fibroma, uterine
fibromatosis
fibromatosis gingivae
fibromatosis, palmar
fibromatous
fibromectomy
fibromembranous
fibromuscular
fibromyalgia
fibromyitis
fibromyoma
fibromyomectomy
fibromyositis
fibromyotomy
fibromyxoma
fibromyxosarcoma
fibroneuroma
fibropapilloma
fibroplasia
fibroplasia, retrolental
fibroplastic
fibropurulent
fibrosarcoma
fibrose

fibroserous
fibrosis
fibrosis,
  arteriocapillary
fibrosis, diffuse
  interstitial pulmonary
fibrosis of lungs
fibrosis, postfibrinosis
fibrosis, proliferative
fibrosis, pulmonary
fibrosis, retroperitoneal
fibrosis uteri
fibrositis
fibrothorax
fibrotic
fibrous
fibula
fibular
fibulocalcaneal
ficin
Fick method
Fick operation
field
field, auditory
field, high-power
field, low-power
field of vision
fifth cranial nerve
Fifth disease
fifth ventricle
FIGLU excretion test
figurate
figure
figure-ground
  discrimination
fila
filaceous
filament
filamentous
filar
filaria
Filaria
Filaria bancrofti
Filaria loa
Filaria medinensis
Filaria sanguinis
  hominis
filarial

filariasis
filaricidal
Filarioidea
file
filial generation
Filibon (prenatal
  vitamins and minerals)
Filibon Forte (prenatal
  vitamins and minerals)
filiform
filipuncture
fillet
filleting
filling
filling, tooth
film
film badge
film, bite-wing
film, spot
film, x-ray
filopressure
filovaricosis
filter
filter bed
filter, Berkefeld
filter, infrared
filter, Kitasato's
filter, membrane
filter, Millipore
filter, optical
filter, Pasteur-
  Chamberland
filter, umbrella
filter, Wood's
filterable
filterable agent (FA)
filtrate
filtrate, glomerular
filtration
filtration of roentgen
  rays
filtrum
filum
filum coronaria
filum terminale
fimbria ovarica
fimbria tubae
fimbriae

fimbriate
fimbriated
fimbriectomy
fimbriocele
fimbrioplasty
fine motor skills
fine needle aspiration
finer, webbed
finger
finger, clubbed
finger cot
finger, dislocation
finger, hammer
finger ladder
finger, mallet
finger, seal
finger spelling
finger spreader
finger spring
finger-stall
fingerprint
finite
Finney operation
Fiogesic
Fioricet
Fiorinal
Fiorinal with Codeine
fire, St. Anthony's
first aid (FA)
first intention healing
first-degree A-V block
fish poisoning
Fishberg concentration
  test
fishskin disease
fission
fissiparous
fissural
fissure
fissure, anal
fissure, auricular
fissure, branchial
fissure, Broca's
fissure, Burdach's
fissure, calcarine
fissure, callosomarginal
fissure, central
fissure, Clevenger's

fissure, collateral
fissure, hippocampal
fissure, inferior orbital
fissure, interparietal
fissure, longitudinal
fissure, occipitoparietal
fissure of Bichat
fissure of Sylvius
fissure, palpebral
fissure, portal
fissure, Rolando's
fissure, sphenoidal
fissure, transverse
fissure, umbilical
fissure, Wernicke's
fissure, zygal
fissure's, Henle's
fissurectomy
fistula
fistula, anal
fistula, arteriovenous
fistula, biliary
fistula, blind
fistula, branchial
fistula, cervical
fistula, complete
fistula, craniosinus
fistula, enterovaginal
fistula, fecal
fistula, gastric
fistula, horseshoe
fistula, incomplete
fistula, metroperitoneal
fistula, parotid
fistula, perineovaginal
fistula, pulmonary
  arteriovenous,
  congenital
fistula, rectovaginal
fistula, thyroglossal
fistula, umbilical
fistula, ureterovaginal
fistula, vesicouterine
fistula, vesicovaginal
fistulatome
fistulectomy
fistulization
fistuloenterostomy

fistulogram
fistulotomy
fistulotomy, anus
fistulous
fit
fitness, biologic
fitting
Fitzgerald factor assay
five-in-one repair, knee
fix
fixation
fixation, complement
fixation, field of
fixation of eyes
fixation point
fixative
fixed eruption
fixed partial denture
fixing
flaccid
flaccid paralysis
flagella
flagellant
flagellate
flagellation
flagelliform
flagellum
Flagyl I.V.
  (metronidazole HCl)
flail chest
flail joint
flame ionization detector
  (FID)
flames, inhalation of
flange
flank
flap
flap, amputation
flap, extraction
flap, island
flap, jump
flap, pedicle
flap, periodontal
flap, skin
flap, sliding
flap, tube
flare
flash

flash method
flash point
flashbacks
flask
flatfoot
flatfoot, spasmodic
flatness
flatplate
flatulence
flatulent
flatus
flatus tube
flatworm
flavedo
flavescent
flavin
flavin adenine
    dinucleotide (FAD)
flavism
flavivirus
Flavobacterium
flavone
flavoprotein
flavor
Flaxedil (gallamine
    triethiodide)
flaxseed
flea
flea bites
flea infestation
fleam
flecainide acetate
Flechsig's areas
fleece of Stilling
Fleet Enema (sodium
    biphosphate and sodium
    phosphate)
**Fleet Flavored Castor Oil
    Emulsion** (stimulant
    laxative)
Fleet Mineral Oil Enema
    (mineral oil)
Fleet Phospho-Soda
    (buffered laxative)
Fleet Prep Kits (bowel
    cleansing system)
Fleet Relief (anesthetic
    hemorrhoidal ointment)

Fleming, Sir Alexander
flesh
Fletcher factor
fletcherism
flex
Flexeril (cyclobenzaprine
    HCl)
flexibilitas cerea
flexibility
flexible
**Flexiflo Enteral Delivery
    System**
flexile
flexion
flexor
flexor tendon
flexura
flexure
flexure, colic, left
flexure, colic, right
flexure, dorsal
flexure, duodenojejunal
flexure, hepatic
flexure, sigmoid
flexure, splenic
flicker
flicker phenomenon
flight of ideas
flint disease
Flint SSD (1% silver
    sulfadiazine cream)
flip-flop
floaters
floating
floating kidney
floating ribs
floats
floccillation
floccitation
floccose
floccular
flocculation
flocculation reaction
flocculence
flocculent
flocculus
Flood's ligament
flooding

floor
floppy-valve syndrome
flora
florid
Florone (diflorasone diacetate)
Floropryl (isoflurophate)
floss
floss, dental
flour
flow
flow cytometry
flow state
flower
flowmeter
flowmetry, Doppler
floxuridine
flucticuli
fluctuant
fluctuation
flucytosine
flucytosine test
fludrocortisone
fludrocortisone acetate
fluid (Fl)
fluid, allantoic
fluid, amniotic
fluid balance
fluid, cerebrospinal
fluid diet
fluid, extracellular
fluid, extravascular
fluid, interstitial
fluid, intracellular
fluid, intraocular
fluid, repair
fluid retention
fluid, seminal
fluid, serous
fluid, spinal
fluid, synovial
fluidextract
fluidextract, aromatic cascara
fluidextract, glycyrrhiza
fluidextract, ipecac
fluidextractum
fluke

fluke, blood
fluke, intestinal
fluke, liver
fluke, lung
flumethasone pivalate
flumina pilorum
fluocinolone acetonide
Fluogen (influenza virus vaccine)
Fluonid (fluocinolone acetonide)
fluor albus
fluorescein angiography
fluorescein blood flow test
fluorescein sodium
fluorescein-sting test
fluorescence
fluorescent
fluorescent antibody (FA)
fluorescent culture typing
fluorescent screen
fluorescent stain
fluorescent treponemal antibody absorption test (FTA-ABS)
fluoridation
fluoride
fluoride dental treatment
fluoride poisoning
fluoride, stannous
fluorine (F)
Fluoritab (sodium fluoride)
fluoroacetate
fluorocarbon
fluorometer
fluorometholone
Fluoroplex (fluorouracil)
fluoroscope
fluoroscopy
fluorosis
Fluorouracil
Fluothane (halothane)
fluoxymesterone
fluphenazine enanthate
fluprednisolone

flurandrenolide
flurazepam hydrochloride
fluroapatite
flurogestone acetate
flurothyl
fluroxene
flush
flush aortogram
flush, hectic
flush, hot
flush, malar
flutter
flutter, atrial
flutter, diaphragmatic
flutter, mediastinal
flutter, ventricular
flutter-fibrillation
flux
fly
fly, black
fly, blow
fly, bot
fly, flesh
fly, house
fly, sand
fly, screwworm
fly, Spanish
fly, tsetse
fly, warble
foam
foam stability test
focal
focal distance (FD)
focal film distance (FFD)
focal infection
focal lesion
focal spot
foci
focus
focus, real
focus, virtual
focus-object distance
  (FOD)
fog
fog therapy
fogging
foil
Folate test

fold
fold, amniotic
fold, aryepiglottic
fold, circular
fold, costocolic
fold, Douglas'
fold, genital
fold, gluteal
fold, lacrimal
fold, mesouterine
fold, mucosal
fold, nail
fold, palmate
fold, semilunar, of
  conjunctiva
fold, transverse, of
  rectum
fold, ventricular
fold, vestibular
fold, vocal
folds, gastric
folding, eye muscle
Folex (methotrexate
  sodium)
Foley catheterization
Foley operation
Foley Y-pyeloplasty
folia
foliaceous
folic acid
folie
folie à deux
folie du doute
folie du pourquoi
folie gemellaire
folinic acid
folium
folium vermis
follicle
follicle, aggregated
follicle, atretic
follicle, dental
follicle, gastric
follicle, graafian
follicle, growing
follicle, hair
follicle, lymphatic
follicle, nabothian

follicle, ovarian
follicle, primordial
follicle, sebaceous
follicle, solitary
follicle, thyroid
follicle, vesicular
follicle-stimulating
  hormone (FSH)
follicular
follicular tonsillitis
follicular tumor
folliculitis
folliculitis barbae
folliculitis decalvans
folliculitis, keloidal
folliculoma
folliculose
folliculosis
folliculus
follow-up
Folvite (folic acid)
fomentation
fomes
fomites
Fontana's spaces
fontanel
fontanel, anterior
fontanel, posterior
fontanelle
fonticulus
food (cib)
food additives
food adulterant
food allergies
Food and Drug
  Administration (FDA)
food ball
food chain
food, contamination of
food, convenience
food, dietetic
food, enriched
food exchange
food, nutrient substances
  of
food poisoning
food requirements
food, textured

foot
foot and mouth disease
foot, arches of
foot, athlete's
foot board
foot, cleft
foot, contracted
foot, flat
foot, immersion
foot, Madura
foot, march
foot pound
foot, splay
foot, trench
foot, weak
foot-candle
footdrop
footling presentation
footplate
footprint
forage
foramen
foramen, apical
foramen, condyloid,
  anterior
foramen, condyloid,
  posterior
foramen, epiploic
foramen, ethmoidal
foramen, external
  auditory
foramen, incisive
foramen, infraorbital
foramen, internal
  auditory
foramen, interventricular
foramen, intervertebral
foramen, jugular
foramen, Magendie's
foramen, magnum
foramen, mandibular
foramen, mastoid
foramen, mental
foramen, obturator
foramen of Monro
foramen of Vesalius
foramen of Winslow
foramen, olfactory

foramen, optic
foramen ovale
foramen, palatine
foramen, rotundum
foramen, sacral, anterior
foramen, sacral, posterior
foramen, Scarpa's
foramen, sciatic, greater
foramen, sciatic, lesser
foramen, sphenopalatine
foramen, spinous
foramen, supraorbital
foramen, thebesian
foramen, transverse
foramen, vena caval
foramen, vertebral
foramen, Weitbrecht's
foramen, zygomatic-orbital
foramina
foraminotomy
Forane (isoflurane)
Forbes' disease
force
force, catabolic
force, electromotive (EMF)
force, G.
force, reserve
force, unit of
forced expiratory volume (FEV)
forceps
forceps, ACMI
forceps, Adair's
forceps, Adson's
forceps, alligator
forceps, Allis'
forceps, Allis-Ochsner
forceps, Andrews-Hartmann
forceps, Arruga's
forceps, artery
forceps, Asch's
forceps, Babcock's
forceps, Backhaus'
forceps, Bacon's

forceps, Bailey-Williamson
forceps, Bainbridge's
forceps, Ballenger's
forceps, Bane's
forceps, Barlow's
forceps, Barraquer's
forceps, Barraya's
forceps, Barrett-Allen
forceps, Barrett's
forceps, Barton's
forceps, bayonet
forceps, Beaupre's
forceps, Beebe's
forceps, Benaron's
forceps, Bengolea's
forceps, Bennett's
forceps, Berens'
forceps, Berke's
forceps, Berne's
forceps, Berry's
forceps, Bevan's
forceps, Beyer's
forceps, Billroth's
forceps, Bishop-Harmon
forceps, Blake's
forceps, Blakesley's
forceps, Blanchard's
forceps, Boettcher's
forceps, Boies'
forceps, Bonaccolto's
forceps, Bond's
forceps, bone
forceps, Bonn's
forceps, Boys-Allis
forceps, Bozeman's
forceps, Braasch's
forceps, Bracken's
forceps, Bradford's
forceps, Brophy's
forceps, Brown-Adson
forceps, Brown's
forceps, Broyles'
forceps, Bruening's
forceps, Brunner's
forceps, Buerger-McCarthy
forceps, Buie's
forceps, Bumpus'

forceps, Bunim's
forceps, Cairns'
forceps, Campbell's
forceps, capsule
forceps, Carmalt's
forceps, Carmody's
forceps, Cassidy-Brophy
forceps, Castroviejo-
  Arruga
forceps, Castroviejo's
forceps, chalazion
forceps, Chamberlen's
forceps, Chandler's
forceps, Cherry-Kerrison
forceps, Cicherelli's
forceps, clamp
forceps, Coakley's
forceps, Cohen's
forceps, Colibri's
forceps, Collin's
forceps, Colver's
forceps, Cooley's
forceps, Coppridge's
forceps, Corbett's
forceps, Cordes'
forceps, Cordes-New
forceps, Corey's
forceps, Cottle-Arruga
forceps, Cottle-Jansen
forceps, Cottle-Kazanjian
forceps, Cottle's
forceps, Crafoord's
forceps, Craig's
forceps, Crenshaw's
forceps, Crile's
forceps, Curtis
forceps, Cushing's
forceps, Davis'
forceps, De Alvarez's
forceps, Dean's
forceps, DeBakey-Bahnson
forceps, DeBakey-
  Bainbridge
forceps, DeBakey-Cooley
forceps, DeBakey's
forceps, D'Errico's
forceps, DeLee's
forceps, delivery

forceps, Dennis'
forceps, dental
forceps, Desjardin's
forceps, Desmarres'
forceps, DeVilbiss'
forceps, Dewey's
forceps, Dingman's
forceps, Doyen's
forceps, dressing
forceps, Dufourmentel's
forceps, Duval-Crile
forceps, Eber's
forceps, Eder's
forceps, Ehrhardt's
forceps, Elliott's
forceps, Elschnig-O'Brien
forceps, Elschnig's
forceps, Erich's
forceps, Evan's
forceps, Farabeuf-
  Lambotte
forceps, Farabeuf's
forceps, Farrington's
forceps, Farris'
forceps, Fauvel's
forceps, Feilchenfeld's
forceps, Ferguson's
forceps, Ferris-Smith
forceps, Ferris-Smith-
  Kerrison
forceps, Ferris'
forceps, Finochietto's
forceps, Fish's
forceps, Fitzgerald's
forceps, fixation
forceps, Fletcher-Van
  Doren
forceps, Foerster's
forceps, Foley
forceps, Foss'
forceps, Fraenkel's
forceps, Frankfeldt's
forceps, Fuchs'
forceps, Fulpit's
forceps, Garrigue's
forceps, Gaylor's
forceps, Gellhorn's
forceps, Gelpi-Lowrie

forceps, Gerald's
forceps, Gifford's
forceps, Glassman-Allis
forceps, Glassman's
forceps, Glenner's
forceps, Glover's
forceps, Goldman-Kazanjian
forceps, Goodhill's
forceps, Gordon's
forceps, Gray's
forceps, Green's
forceps, Gruenwald-Bryant
forceps, Gruenwald's
forceps, Guggenheim's
forceps, Gutglass'
forceps, Hajek-Koffler
forceps, Hale's
forceps, Halsted's
forceps, Harken's
forceps, Harrington-Mayo
forceps, Harrington's
forceps, Harris
forceps, Hartmann-Citelli
forceps, Hartmann-Gruenwald
forceps, Hartmann's
forceps, Hartman's
forceps, Hawkins'
forceps, Hawks-Dennen
forceps, Healy's
forceps, Heaney-Ballantine
forceps, Heaney-Kanter
forceps, Heaney-Rezek
forceps, Heaney's
forceps, Heath's
forceps, Heise's
forceps, Hendren's
forceps, Henrotin's
forceps, Hess'
forceps, Hess-Barraquer
forceps, Hess-Horwitz
forceps, Hibbs'
forceps, Hirschman's
forceps, Henrotin's
forceps, Hirst-Emmett
forceps, Hodge's

forceps, Hoffmann's
forceps, Holinger's
forceps, Holth's
forceps, Horsley's
forceps, House's
forceps, Howard's
forceps, Hoxworth's
forceps, Hudson's
forceps, Hunt's
forceps, Hurd's
forceps, Imperatori's
forceps, Iowa
forceps, Jackson's
forceps, Jacobs'
forceps, Jacobson's
forceps, Jameson's
forceps, Jansen-Middleton
forceps, Jansen's
forceps, Jansen-Struycken
forceps, Jarcho's
forceps, Johns Hopkins
forceps, Johnson's
forceps, Jones'
forceps, Judd-Allis
forceps, Judd-DeMartel
forceps, Judd's
forceps, Juers-Lempert
forceps, Julian's
forceps, Jurasz's
forceps, Kahler's
forceps, Kalt's
forceps, Kazanjian's
forceps, Katzin-Barraquer
forceps, Kelly's
forceps, Kelman's
forceps, Kennedy's
forceps, Kern's
forceps, Kerrison's
forceps, Kielland-Luikart
forceps, Kielland's (Kjelland's)
forceps, Kiffler's
forceps, Killian's
forceps, Kirby's
forceps, Kittner's
forceps, Knapp's
forceps, Knight's
forceps, Knight-Sluder

forceps, Kocher's
forceps, Koffler-Lillie
forceps, Kiffler's
forceps, Kolb's
forceps, Krause's
forceps, Kronfeld's
forceps, Kuhnt's
forceps, Kulvin-Kalt
forceps, Lahey-Pean
forceps, Lahey's
forceps, Lambert's
forceps, Lambotte's
forceps, Lane's
forceps, Laufe-Barton-
  Kielland
forceps, Laufe-Piper
forceps, Laufe's
forceps, Lebsche's
forceps, Leksell's
forceps, Leland-Jones
forceps, Lempert's
forceps, Leriche's
forceps, Levret's
forceps, Lewin's
forceps, Lewis'
forceps, Lewkowitz's
forceps, Leyro-Diaz
forceps, Lillie's
forceps, Lister's
forceps, Liston-Stille
forceps, Littauer-Liston
forceps, Littauer's
forceps, Lockwood's
forceps, Long Island
forceps, Long's
forceps, Love-Gruenwald
forceps, Love-Kerrison
forceps, Lovelace's
forceps, Lower's
forceps, Lowsley's
forceps, Lucae's
forceps, Luc's
forceps, Luer's
forceps, Luikart's
forceps, Luikart-Simpson
forceps, Lutz's
forceps, Lynch's
forceps, Maier's

forceps, Mann's
forceps, Marshik's
forceps, Martin's
forceps, Maryan's
forceps, Mathieu's
forceps, Mayo-Blake
forceps, Mayo-Ochsner
forceps, Mayo-Robson
forceps, Mayo-Russian
forceps, Mayo's
forceps, McCarthy-Alcock
forceps, McCarthy's
forceps, McCullough's
forceps, McHenry's
forceps, McKay's
forceps, McKenzie's
forceps, McLane's
forceps, McLane-Tucker
forceps, McLane-Tucker-
  Luikart
forceps, McNealy-
  Glassman-Babcock
forceps, McNealy-
  Glassman-Mixter
forceps, McPherson's
forceps, Metzenbaum's
forceps, Millin's
forceps, Mitchell-Diamond
forceps, Mixter's
forceps, Moersch's
forceps, Moritz-Schmidt
forceps, mosquito
forceps, Mount-Mayfield
forceps, mouse-tooth
forceps, Moynihan's
forceps, Mundie's
forceps, Museholdt's
forceps, Myerson's
forceps, Myles'
forceps, Nelson's
forceps, New's
forceps, Newman's
forceps, needle
forceps, Noble's
forceps, Noyes'
forceps, Nugent's
forceps, O'Brien's
forceps, obstetric

forceps, Ochsner-Dixon
forceps, Ochsner's
forceps, O'Hanlon's
forceps, Oldberg's
forceps, O'Shaughnessy's
forceps, Overstreet's
forceps, ovum
forceps, Palmer's
forceps, Pang's
forceps, Parker-Kerr
forceps, Paterson's
forceps, Patterson's
forceps, Pean's
forceps, Pennington's
forceps, Percy's
forceps, Perritt's
forceps, Phaneuf's
forceps, Piper's
forceps, Pitha's
forceps, placental
forceps, Pley's
forceps, polyp
forceps, Porter's
forceps, Potts-Smith
forceps, Poutasse's
forceps, Pratt-Smith
forceps, Price-Thomas
forceps, Prince's
forceps, Providence
forceps, Quevedo's
forceps, Randall's
forceps, Randall's stone
forceps, Raney's
forceps, Rankin's
forceps, Ratliff-Blake
forceps, Ray's
forceps, Reese's
forceps, Reiner-Knight
forceps, Rienhoff's
forceps, ring
forceps, Robb's
forceps, Roberts'
forceps, Robertson's
forceps, Rochester-
  Carmalt
forceps, Rochester-Ewald
forceps, Rochester-Mixter

forceps, Rochester-
  Ochsner
forceps, Rochester-Pean
forceps, Rochester-Rankin
forceps, Rochester's
forceps, Rockey's
forceps, Roeder's
forceps, Rolf's
forceps, rongeur
forceps, Rowland's
forceps, Rumel's
forceps, Ruskin's
forceps, Russell's
forceps, Russian
forceps, Sam Roberts
forceps, Sarot's
forceps, Satinsky's
forceps, Sauerbruch's
forceps, Sauer's
forceps, Sawtell's
forceps, Scheinmann's
forceps, Schlesinger's
forceps, Schoenberg's
forceps, Schroeder's
forceps, Schubert's
forceps, Schutz's
forceps, Schwartz's
forceps, Schweigger's
forceps, Schweizer's
forceps, Scoville's
forceps, Scudder's
forceps, Segond's
forceps, Seiffert's
forceps, Selman's
forceps, Semb's
forceps, Semken's
forceps, Senn
forceps, Sewall's
forceps, Shaaf's
forceps, Shallcross'
forceps, Shearer's
forceps, Simpson-Luikart
forceps, Simpson's
forceps, Singley's
forceps, Skene's
forceps, Skillern's
forceps, Smart's
forceps, Smith's

forceps, Smithwick's
forceps, Somers'
forceps, Spence-Adson
forceps, Spencer Wells
forceps, Spence's
forceps, Spero's
forceps, sponge
forceps, Spurling's
forceps, Staude-Moore
forceps, Staude's
forceps, Stevens'
forceps, Stevenson's
forceps, Stille-Liston
forceps, Stille-Luer
forceps, Stille's
forceps, stone
forceps, Stone's
forceps, Struempel's
forceps, Struyken's
forceps, Sweet's
forceps, Takahashi's
forceps, Tarnier's
forceps, Teale's
forceps, Thoms'
forceps, Thoms-Allis
forceps, Thoms-Gaylor
forceps, Thorek-Mixter
forceps, Thorpe's
forceps, Tischler's
forceps, tissue
forceps, Tivnen's
forceps, Tobold-Fauvel
forceps, Tobold's
forceps, towel
forceps, Tucker-McLean
forceps, Tuttle's
forceps, Tydings'
forceps, Tydings-Lakeside
forceps, Van Buren's
forceps, Van Doren
forceps, Van Struycken
forceps, Vanderbilt's
forceps, Verhoeff's
forceps, Virtus'
forceps, von Graefe's
forceps, von Mondak's
forceps, vulsellum
forceps, Waldeau's

forceps, Walsham's
forceps, Walter's
forceps, Walther's
forceps, Walton's
forceps, Walton-Schubert
forceps, Wangensteen's
forceps, Watson-Williams
forceps, Weil's
forceps, Weingartner's
forceps, Weisenbach's
forceps, Weisman's
forceps, Welch-Allyn
forceps, Wertheim-Cullen
forceps, Wertheim's
forceps, White-Lillie
forceps, White-Oslay
forceps, White's
forceps, Wilde's
forceps, Willett's
forceps, Williams'
forceps, Wittner's
forceps, Wullstein-House
forceps, Wullstein's
forceps, Yankauer-Little
forceps, Yankauer's
forceps, Yeomans'
forceps, Young's
forceps, Ziegler's
forcipate
forcipressure
Fordyce's disease
Fordyce's spots
Fordyce-Fox disease
forearm
forebrain
forefinger
forefoot
foregut
forehead
foreign body
foreign bodies
forelock
forensic
forensic dentistry
forensic medicine
foreplay
forepleasure
foreskin

forewaters
forgetting
fork, tuning
form
form sense
formaldehyde (HCOH)
formaldehyde poisoning
formalin
formate
formatio
formatio reticularis
formation
formation, reticular
forme fruste
formic
formic acid (HCOOH)
formic aldehyde
formic ether
formication
formiciasis
formilase
formiminoglutamic acid
  (FIGLU)
formol
formula (F)
formula, Arneth's
formula, chemical
formula, dental
formula, empirical
formula, molecular
formula, official
formula, spatial
formula, stereochemical
formula, structural
formulary
formulary, National (NF)
formyl
fornicate
fornication
fornices
fornicolumn
fornicommissure
fornix
fornix conjunctivae
fornix uteri
fornix vaginae
Fort Bragg fever
Fortaz (ceftazidime)

fortification spectrum
Fosfree (calcium-
  vitamins-iron)
Foshay's test
fossa
fossa, amygdaloid
fossa, articular, of
  mandible
fossa, articular, of
  temporal bone
fossa, axillary
fossa, canine
fossa, cerebral
fossa, Claudius'
fossa, condylar
fossa, coronoid
fossa, cranial
fossa, digastric
fossa, epigastric
fossa, ethmoid
fossa, glenoid
fossa, hyaloid
fossa, hypophyseal
fossa, iliac
fossa, incisive
fossa, infratemporal
fossa, intercondyloid
fossa, interpeduncular
fossa, ischiorectal
fossa, lacrimal
fossa, mandibular
fossa, mastoid
fossa, nasal
fossa, navicular
fossa, olecranon
fossa ovalis
fossa ovalis cordis
fossa, ovarian
fossa, pituitary
fossa, Rosenmüller's
fossa, sphenomaxillary
fossa, sublingual
fossa, submandibular
fossa, subpyramidal
fossa, supraspinous
fossa supratonsillaris
fossa, temporal
fossae

fossette
fossula
Fothergill operation
Fothergill's disease
Fototar (coal tar)
foulage
fourchet
fourchette
fourth cranial nerve
fovea
fovea capitus
fovea centralis
fovea centralis retinae
foveate
foveation
foveola
Fowler operation
Fowler's position
Fowler's solution
Fox operation
Fox-Fordyce disease
foxglove
fraction
fraction of inspired
  oxygen (FiO_2)
fractional
fractional test meal
fractionation
fracture (Fx)
fracture, avulsion
fracture, blow-out
fracture, closed
fracture, Colles'
fracture, comminuted
fracture, complete
fracture, complicated
fracture, compound
fracture, compression
fracture, depressed
fracture, direct
fracture, dislocation
fracture, double
fracture, Duverney's
fracture, epiphyseal
fracture, fatigue
fracture, fissured
fracture, greenstick
fracture, hairline

fracture, hangman's
fracture, impacted
fracture, incomplete
fracture, indirect
fracture, intrauterine
fracture, lead pipe
fracture, LeFort
fracture, march
fracture, oblique
fracture, open
fracture, overriding
fracture, pathologic
fracture, ping-pong
fracture, Pott's
fracture, pretrochanteric
fracture, simple
fracture, Smith's
fracture, spiral
fracture, spontaneous
fracture, stellate
fracture, stress
fracture, surgical
fracture, transcervical
fracture, transverse
fragile X syndrome
fragile-X, chromosome
  analysis
fragilitas
fragilitas crinium
fragilitas ossium
fragilitas unguium
fragility
fragility, capillary
fragility, erythrocyte
fragility of blood
fragment
fragment antigen binding
  (FAB)
fragmentation
frambesia
frambesioma
frame
frame, Balkan
frame, Bradford
frame, quadriplegic
  standing
frame, Stryker
frame, trial

framework
Franceschetti's syndrome
Franciscella tularensis
francium (Fr)
Franco operation
frank
Frank's operation
Frankenhaüser's ganglion
Frankfort horizontal
  plane
Franklin glasses
fraternal twins
fratricide
Fraunhofer's lines
Frazier operation
freckle
freckle, Hutchinson's
Fredet-Ramstedt operation
free association
free base
free radical
free thyroxine index
  (FTI)
freebasing
freeing
freeze-drying
freezing
freezing, gastric
freezing mixtures
freezing point
Freiberg's infraction
fremitus
fremitus, tactile
fremitus, tussive
fremitus, vocal
frenal
French scale
Frenckner operation
frenectomy
frenoplasty
frenosecretory
frenotomy
frenulectomy
frenuloplasty
frenulum
frenulum clitoridis
frenulum labiorum pudendi
frenulum linguae

frenulum of ileocecal
  valve
frenulum of the lips,
  labialis oris
frenulum of tongue
frenulum preputii
frenulumectomy
frenum
frenumectomy
frenzy
frequency
fresh frozen plasma (FFP)
fretum
Freud, Sigmund
freudian
Freund's adjuvant
friable
Frickman operation
friction
friction, dry
friction, moist
friction rub
friction rub, pericardial
frictional electricity
Friedländer's bacillus
Friedländer's disease
Friedman's test
Friedreich's ataxia
Friedreich's sign
fright
fright neuroses
fright, precordial
frigid
frigidity
frigolabile
frigorific
frigorism
frigostabile
frigotherapy
frit
frog belly
frog face
Fröhlich's syndrome
Froin's syndrome
frolement
Froment's sign
Frommann's lines
Frommel operation

frons
front-tap reflex
frontad
frontal
frontal bone
frontal lobe
frontal plane
frontal sinuses
frontomalar
frontomaxillary
frontoparietal
frontotemporal
frost
frost, uremic
frostbite
frost-itch
frottage
frotteur
frozen blood
frozen plasma
frozen section
fructofuranose
fructokinase
fructose
fructose intolerance
fructosemia
fructoside
fructosuria
fruit
frumentaceous
frustration
Fryns syndrome
fuchsin
fucose
fucosidosis
FUDR (floxuridine)
fugitive
fugue
fugue, psychogenic
fulgurant
fulgurating
fulguration
full mouth extraction
   (FME)
full range of motion
   (FROM)
full term
full weight bearing (FWB)

fulling
fulminant
fulminating
Fulvicin P/G
   (griseofulvin
   ultramicrosize)
Fulvicin-U/F
   (griseofulvin microsize)
fumarase
fumaric acid
fumes
fumes, nitric acid
fumigant
fumigation
fuming
function (F)
functional
functional disease
functional overlay
functional psychosis
functioning tumor
funda
fundal
fundament
fundectomy
fundectomy, uterine
fundic
fundiform
fundoplasty
fundoplication
fundoscopy
fundus
fundus oculi
fundus of bladder
fundus of gallbladder
fundus of stomach
fundus tympani
fundus uteri
funduscope
fundusectomy
fundusectomy, gastric
fungal
fungal septicemia
fungate
fungating
fungemia
fungi
Fungi

Fungi-Nail
fungicide
fungiform
fungiform papillae
fungistasis
fungistat
fungistatic
Fungizone (amphotericin B)
fungoid
Fungoid Creme and Solution
Fungoid Tincture
fungosity
fungous
fungus
funic
funic souffle
funicle
funicular
funicular process
funiculitis
funiculopexy
funiculus
funiform
funis
funnel
funnel breast
funnel chest
funny bone
Furacin (nitrofurazone)
Furadantin (nitrofurantoin)
furcal
furcation
furcula
furfur
furfuraceous
furibund
Furonatal FA
furor
furor femininus
furosemide
furred
furrow
furrow, atrioventricular
furrow, digital
furrow, gluteal

furuncle
furuncular
furunculoid
furunculosis
furunculous
furunculus
Fusarium
fuscin
fuse
fusible
fusiform
fusimotor
fusion
fusion, diaphyseal-epiphyseal
fusion, nuclear
fusion, spinal
Fusobacterium
fusocellular
fusospirochetal
fusospirochetosis
fustigation
fututrix

G

G-1 (acetaminophen, butalbital, caffeine)
G-Myticin Creme and Ointment (gentamicin sulfate)
G-suit
gadfly
gadolinium (Gd)
gag
gag reflex
gage
gain
gain, secondary
Gaisböck's syndrome
gait
gait, ataxic
gait, cerebellar
gait, double step
gait, drag-to

gait, equine
gait, festinating
gait, gluteal
gait, helicopod
gait, hemiplegic
gait, scissor
gait, spastic
gait, steppage
gait, swing-through
gait, swing-to
gait, tabetic
gait, three-point
gait, two-point
gait, waddling
galactacrasia
galactagogue
galactan
galactase
galactemia
galactic
galactidrosis
galactischia
galactoblast
galactocele
galactogram
galactoid
galactokinase
galactolipin
galactoma
galactometer
galactopexic
galactopexy
galactophagous
galactophore
galactophoritis
galactophorous
galactophthisis
galactophygous
galactophylsis
galactoplania
galactopoietic
galactopyra
galactorrhea
galactosamine
galactose
galactose-1-phosphate
  uridyl transferase test
galactosemia

galactosidase
galactosis
galactostasis
galactosuria
galactotherapy
galactotoxin
galactotoxism
galactotrophy
galactozymase
galacturia
galea
galea aponeurotica
galeanthropy
galeaplasty
Galeazzi's sign
Galen, Claudius
Galen's veins
galena
galenic
galenicals
galenics
galeophilia
galeophobia
galeropia
galeropsia
gall
gall duct
gallamine triethiodide
gallate
gallbladder (GB)
gallium (Ga)
gallium scan
gallon
gallop rhythm
gallstone
Galton's whistle
galvanic
galvanic battery
galvanic cell
galvanic current
galvanic skin response
  (GSR)
galvanism
galvanization
galvanocautery
galvanocontractility
galvanofaradization
galvanoionization

galvanometer
galvanopalpation
galvanopuncture
galvanoscope
galvanosurgery
galvanotaxis
galvanotherapeutics
galvanotherapy
galvanothermy
galvanotonus
galvanotropism
Gamastan (immune globulin
[human])
gamete
gamete intrafallopian
transfer (GIFT)
gametic
gametocide
gametocyte
gametogenesis
gametogony
gametophyte
gamic
gamma
gamma benzene
hexachloride
gamma globulin (GG)
gamma ray
gamma-aminobutyric acid
(GABA)
gamma-glutamyl
transferase (GGT) test
gammacism
GAMMAGARD (immune
globulin [human])
Gammar (immune globulin,
[human])
gammopathy
Gamna nodules
Gamna's disease
gamogenesis
gamont
gamophobia
gampsodactylia
Gamulin Rh (Rh$_o$(D) immune
globulin, [human])
ganglia
ganglial

gangliated
gangliectomy
gangliform
ganglioblast
gangliocyte
gangliocytoma
ganglioglioma
ganglioglioneuroma
ganglioma
ganglion
ganglion, abdominal
ganglion, anterior
cerebral
ganglion, aorticorenal
ganglion, Arnold's
auricular
ganglion, auricular
ganglion, autonomic
ganglion, basal
ganglion, basal optic
ganglion, cardiac
ganglion, carotid
ganglion, celiac
ganglion, cephalic
ganglion, cerebral
ganglion, cervical
ganglion, cervicothoracic
ganglion, cervicouterine
ganglion, ciliary
ganglion, coccygeal
ganglion, collateral
ganglion, Corti's
ganglion, dorsal root
ganglion, false
ganglion, Frankenhäuser's
ganglion, gasserian
ganglion, geniculate
ganglion, inferior
mesenteric
ganglion, intervertebral
ganglion, jugular
ganglion, lateral
ganglion, lenticular
ganglion, lumbar
ganglion, lymphatic
ganglion, nodose
ganglion, ophthalmic
ganglion, otic

ganglion, parasympathetic
ganglion, petrous
ganglion, pharyngeal
ganglion, phrenic
ganglion, pterygopalatine
ganglion, renal
ganglion, sacral
ganglion, Scarpa's
ganglion, semilunar
ganglion, sensory
ganglion, simple
ganglion, sphenopalatine
ganglion, spinal
ganglion, spiral
ganglion, stellate
ganglion, submandibular
ganglion, superior mesenteric
ganglion, suprarenal
ganglion, sympathetic
ganglion, temporal
ganglion, terminal
ganglion, thoracic
ganglion, trigeminal
ganglion, tympanic
ganglion, vestibular
ganglion, Wrisberg's
ganglion, wrist
ganglionated
ganglionectomy
ganglioneuroma
ganglionic
ganglionic blockade
ganglionitis
ganglionostomy
ganglioplegia
ganglioside
gangliosidosis
ganglitis
gangosa
gangrene
gangrene, angioneurotic
gangrene, diabetic
gangrene, dry
gangrene, embolic
gangrene, gas
gangrene, humid
gangrene, idiopathic

gangrene, inflammatory
gangrene, moist
gangrene, primary
gangrene, secondary
gangrene, symmetric
gangrene, traumatic
gangrenous
ganoblast
Ganser's syndrome
Gant operation
Gantanol (sulfamethoxazole)
Gantrisin Ophthalmic Ointment (sulfisoxazole diolamine)
Gantrisin Ophthalmic Solution (sulfisoxazole diolamine)
Gantrisin Pediatric Suspension (acetyl sulfisoxazole)
Gantrisin Pediatric Syrup (acetyl sulfisoxazole)
Gantrisin Tablets (sulfisoxazole)
gantry
gap
gap, auscultatory
Garamycin (gentamicin sulfate)
Garceau operation
Gardner operation
Gardner's syndrome
Gardnerella vaginalis
Gardnerella vaginalis vaginitis
gargarism
gargle
gargoylism
garlic
garment, front-opening
Garré's disease
Garren gastric bubble
Gartner's duct
gas
gas bacillus
gas, binary
gas, Clayton

gas, coal
gas distention
gas endarterectomy
gas gangrene
gas, illuminating
gas, inert
gas, laughing
gas, lewisite
gas, lung irritant
gas, marsh
gas, mustard
gas, nerve
gas, nose irritant
gas pains
gas, sewer
gas, suffocating
gas, tear
gas, toxic
gas, vesicant
gas, vomiting
gases, blood
gases, digestive tract
gases, war
gas-liquid chromatography
  (GLC)
gaseous
gasoline
gasoline poisoning
gasometric
gasometry
gasp
gasserectomy
gasserian ganglion
gasteralgia
Gasterophilus
Gasterophilus
  hemorrhoidalis
Gasterophilus
  intestinalis
Gasterophilus nasalis
gastorrhagia
gastralgia
gastratrophia
gastrectasia
gastrectasis
gastrectomy
gastric
gastric analysis (GA)

gastric bypass
gastric cytology
gastric digestion
gastric glands
gastric inhibitory
  polypeptide (GIP)
gastric intubation
gastric juice
gastric lavage
gastric ulcer
gastricism
gastrin
gastrinoma
gastritis, acute
gastritis, atrophic
gastritis, chronic
gastritis, giant
  hypertrophic
gastritis, toxic
gastroanastomosis
gastrocamera
gastrocardiac
gastrocele
gastrocnemius
gastrocnemius neurectomy
gastrocolic
gastrocolic fistula
gastrocolic omentum
gastrocolic reflex
gastrocolitis
gastrocoloptosis
gastrocolostomy
gastrocolotomy
gastrocolpotomy
gastrocutaneous
gastrodialysis
gastrodidymus
gastrodisciasis
Gastrodiscoides
Gastrodiscoides hominis
gastroduodenal
gastroduodenectomy
gastroduodenitis
gastroduodenoscopy
gastroduodenostomy
gastrodynia
gastroenteralgia
gastroenteric

gastroenteritis
gastroenteroanastomosis
gastroenterocolitis
gastroenterocolostomy
gastroenterologist
gastroenterology
gastroenteropathy
gastroenteroptosis
gastroenterostomy
gastroenterotomy
gastroepiploic
gastroesophageal
gastroesophageal reflux
gastroesophagitis
gastroesophagostomy
gastrofiberscope
gastrogastrostomy
gastrogavage
gastrogenic
gastrohelcosis
gastrohepatic
gastrohepatitis
gastroileac
gastroileal reflex
gastroileitis
gastroileostomy
gastrointestinal (GI)
gartrointestinal (GI)
  series
gastrointestinal bleeding
gastrointestinal
  decompression
gastrointestinal
  scintigraphy
gastrojejunoscopy
gastrojejunostomy
gastrolienal
gastrolith
gastrolithiasis
gastrology
gastrolysis
gastromalacia
gastromegaly
gastromycosis
gastromyotomy
gastromyxorrhea
gastropancreatitis
gastroparalysis

gastropathy
gastropexis
gastropexy
gastropharyngostomy
gastrophrenic
gastroplasty
gastroplegia
gastroplication
gastroptosis
gastropulmonary
gastropylorectomy
gastropyloric
gastroradiculitis
gastrorrhagia
gastrorrhaphy
gastrorrhea
gastroschisis
gastroscope
gastroscopy
gastrospasm
gastrosplenic
gastrostaxis
gastrostenosis
gastrostenosis cardiaca
gastrostenosis pylorica
gastrostogavage
gastrostolavage
gastrostoma
gastrostomy
gastrosuccorrhea
gastrotherapy
gastrothoracopagus
gastrotome
gastrotomy
gastrotonometer
gastrotropic
gastrotympanites
gastrula
gastrulation
Gatch bed
gate
gate theory
gatism
Gaucher, Philippe C.E.
Gaucher's cells
Gaucher's disease
gauge
Gault's reflex

gauntlet
gauss
Gauss' sign
gauze
gauze, absorbent
gauze, antiseptic
gauze, aseptic
gauze, petrolatum
gavage
Gavard's muscle
Gaviscon (aluminum hydroxide and magnesium carbonate)
gay
Gay's glands
Gay-Lussac's law
gaze
Gee, Samuel J.
Gee's disease
Gee-Thaysen disease
gegenhalten
Geigel's reflex
Geiger counter
gel
gel, aluminum hydroxide
gelasmus
gelate
gelatin
gelatin culture
gelatin, nutrient
gelatin sponge, absorbable
gelatinase
gelatiniferous
gelatinize
gelatinoid
gelatinolytic
gelatinous
gelation
Gellé's test
Gelman operation
gelose
gelosis
gelotherapy
gelotripsy
Gelpirin (acetaminophen, aspirin, caffeine)

Gelpirin-CCF (cold, cough and fever tablets)
gemellipara
gemellology
gemellus
gemfibrozil
geminate
gemination
gemistocyte
gemma
gemmation
gemmule
Gemnisyn
Gemonil (metharbital)
gena
genal
Genapax (gentian violet)
gender (g)
gender identity
gender role
gender testing
gene
gene amplification
gene, dominant
gene, histocompatibility
gene, holandric
gene, inhibiting
gene, lethal
gene map
gene, modifying
gene, mutant
gene, operator
gene, pleiotropic
gene, recessive
gene, regulator
gene, sex-linked
gene splicing
gene, structural
gene therapy
gene transfer
gene, X-linked
genes, allelic
genes, complementary
general
general adaptation syndrome (GAS)
general practice (GP)
general practitioner (GP)

general surgery (GS)
generalize
generally recognized as safe GRAS List (food additives)
generation
generation, alternate
generation, asexual
generation, filial
generation, parental
generation, sexual
generative
generator
generator, electric
generator, pulse
generator, x-ray
generic
generic drugs
genesiology
genesis
genetic
genetic code
genetic counseling
genetic engineering
geneticist
genetics
genetics, biochemical
genetics, clinical
genetics, molecular
genetotrophic
genetous
Geneva Convention
genial
genic
genicular
geniculate
geniculate otalgia
geniculocalcarine tract
geniculum
genion
genioplasty
genital
genital herpes
genital warts
genitalia
genitalia, ambiguous
genitalia, female
genitalia, male

genitals
genitocrural
genitofemoral
genitoplasty
genitourinary (GU)
genitourinary system
genius
genocide
genodermatosis
genome
genotoxic
genotoxic damage
genotype
gentamicin
gentamicin sulfate
gentian
gentian violet
gentianophil
gentianophile
gentianophobic
genu
genu extrorsum
genu introrsum
genu recurvatum
genu valgum
genu varum
genua
genuclast
genucubital
genucubital position
genupectoral
genupectoral position
genus
genyplasty
geobiology
Geocillin (carbenicillin indanyl sodium)
geode
geographic tongue
geomedicine
Geopen (carbenicillin disodium)
geophagia
geophagism
geophagy
geotaxis
geotragia
geotrichosis

Geotrichum
geotropism
gephyrophobia
Gerdy's fibers
geriatrician
geriatrics
Geritonic (elixir with
  vitamin B complex and
  iron)
Gerlach's valve
germ
germ cell
germ, dental
germ epithelium
germ, hair
germ layers
germ plasm
germ theory
germ, wheat
German measles
German measles antibody
  test
germanium (Ge)
germicidal
germinal
germinal center
germinal disk
germinal epithelium
germinal vesicle
germination
germinoma
Gerobion (geriatric
  elixir)
geroderma
gerodermia
gerodontology
geromarasmus
geromorphism
gerontal
gerontology
gerontophilia
gerontopia
gerontotherapeutics
gerontoxon
Gerota's capsule
gestagen
gestalt
gestalt, therapy

gestation
gestation, abdominal
gestation, cornual
gestation, ectopic
gestation, interstitial
gestation, ovarian
gestation, plural
gestation, prolonged
gestation sac
gestation, secondary
gestation, secondary
  abdominal
gestation time
gestation, tubal
gestation, tuboabdominal
gestation, tubo-ovarian
gestation, uterotubal
gestational assessment
gestosis
gesture
geumaphobia
Gevrabon (vitamin-mineral
  supplement)
Gevral (multivitamin and
  multimineral
  supplement)
Ghon's primary lesion,
  tubercle
Ghormley operation
ghost corpuscle
Giannuzzi's cells
giant
giant cell
giant cell tumor
Giardia
Giardia lamblia
giardiasis
Gibbon's hydrocele
gibbosity
gibbous
gibbus
Gibney's boot, bandage
Gibson's murmur
giddiness
Giemsa's stain
Gifford operation
Gifford's reflex
giga (G)

gigantism
gigantism, acromegalic
gigantism, eunuchoid
gigantism, normal
gigantoblast
gigantocyte
gigantosoma
Gigli's saw
Gilbert's syndrome
Gilchrist's disease
Gill operation
Gill-Stein operation
Gilles de la Tourette's
  syndrome
Gilliam operation
Gimbernat's ligament
gingiva
gingiva, alveolar
gingiva, attached
gingiva, free
gingiva, labial
gingiva, lingual
gingiva, marginal
gingival (g)
gingivalgia
gingivally
gingivectomy
gingivitis
gingivitis, acute
  necrotizing
gingivitis, expulsive
gingivitis, gravidum
gingivitis, hyperplastic
gingivitis, interstitial
gingivitis, phagedenic
gingivitis, Vincent's
gingivoglossitis
gingivolabial
gingivosis
gingivostomatitis
gingivostomatitis, acute
  necrotizing ulcerative
gingivostomatitis,
  herpetic
ginglyform
ginglymoarthrodial
ginglymoid
ginglymus

ginseng
ginvivoplasty
Giraldés' organ
girdle
girdle pain
girdle, pelvic
girdle, shoulder
girdle symptom
Girdlestone operation
Girdlestone-Taylor
  operation
gitalin
gitter cell
giving-up
gizzard
glabella
glabellomeatal line (GML)
glabrate
glabrous
glacial
gladiate
gladiolus
glairy
gland, absorbent
gland, accessory
gland, acinotubular
gland, acinous
gland, adrenal
gland, apocrine
gland, bulbourethral
gland, carotid
gland, coccygeal
gland, compound
gland, compound tubular
gland, conglobate
gland, Cowper's
gland, cytogenic
gland, ductless
gland, eccrine
gland, endocrine
gland, gastric
gland, genal
gland, holocrine
gland, interscapular
gland, interstitial
gland, lacrimal
gland, Luschka's
gland, lymph

gland, lymphatic
gland, mammary
gland, merocrine
gland, Méry's
gland, mixed
gland, parotid
gland, peptic
gland, pineal
gland, pituitary
gland, prostate
gland, racemose
gland, Rivinus
gland, saccular
gland, salivary
gland, sebaceous
gland, sentinel
gland, seromucous
gland, sex
gland, sublingual
gland, submandibular
gland, suprarenal
gland, target
gland, thymus
gland, thyroid
gland, tubular
gland, unicellular
gland, Zuckerkandl's
glands, aggregate
glands, albuminous
glands, anal
glands, areolar
glands, auricular
glands, axillary
glands, Bartholin's
glands, Blandin's
glands, Bowman's
glands, brachial
glands, bronchial
glands, Bruch's
glands, Brunner's
glands, buccal
glands, cardiac
glands, celiac
glands, ceruminous
glands, cervical
glands, ciliary
glands, circumanal
glands, Cobelli's

glands, cutaneous
glands, duodenal
glands, Ebner's
glands, female
glands, Fraenkel's
glands, fundic
glands, Gay's
glands, genital
glands, hair
glands, haversian
glands, hematopoietic
glands, hemolymph
glands, hepatic
glands, inguinal
glands, intestinal
glands, jugular
glands, Krause's
glands, labial
glands, lactiferous
glands, Lieberkühn's
glands, lingual
glands, Littré's
glands, lumbar
glands, meibomian
glands, Moll's
glands, Montgomery's
glands, Morgagni's
glands, muciparous
glands, nabothian
glands, odoriferous
glands of Zies
glands, olfactory
glands, oxyntic
glands, palatine
glands, palpebral
glands, parathyroid
glands, paraurethral
glands, Peyer's
glands, preputial
glands, pyloric
glands, serous
glands, Skene's
glands, solitary
glands, sudoriferous
glands, sweat
glands, synovial
glands, tarsal
glands, tracheal

glands, Tyson's
glands, urethral
glands, vaginal
glands, vestibular
glands, vulvovaginal
glands, Waldeyer's
glands, Weber's
glanders
glandilemma
glandula
glandular
glandular therapy
glandule
glans
glans, clitoridis
glans penis
Glanzmann's
  thrombasthenia
glare
glaserian artery
glaserian fissure
Glasgow Coma Scale
glass
glass, leaded
glass, photochromic
glass, polarized
glass, safety
glass, tempered
glass, ultraviolet
  transmitting
glass, watch
glasses
glasses, bifocal
glasses, safety
glasses, sun
glasses, trifocal
glassy
Glauber's salt
glaucoma
glaucoma, absolutum
glaucoma, chronic
glaucoma, congenital
glaucoma, infantile
glaucoma, narrow angle
glaucoma, open angle
glaucoma, simplex
glaucomatous
gleet

Glénard's disease
Glenn operation
glenohumeral
glenohumeral joint
  arthrotomy
glenohumeral ligaments
glenoid
glenoid bone block
glenoid cavity
glenoid fossa
glenoid lip
glenoplasty
glia
glia cells
gliacyte
gliadin
glial
gliarase
glide
glide, mandibular
glioblastoma
glioblastoma multiforme
gliocyte
gliocytoma
gliogenous
glioma
glioma retinae
gliomatosis
gliomatous
gliomyoma
glioneuroma
gliosarcoma
gliosis
gliosome
gliotoxin
Glisson, Francis
Glisson's capsule
Glisson's disease
glissonian cirrhosis
glissonitis
globi
globin
globoid
globular
globule
globulin
globulin, Ac
globulin, antihemophilic

globulin, gamma
globulin, immune
globulin, Rh$_o$(D) immune
globulin, serum
globulin, varicella-
  zoster immune
globulinuria
globulose
globus
globus hystericus
globus major
globus minor
globus pallidus
glomangioma
glomectomy
glomerate
glomerular
glomerular disease
glomerular filtration
  rate (GFR)
glomeruli
glomerulitis
glomerulonephritis
glomerulopathy
glomerulosclerosis
glomerulosclerosis,
  diabetic
glomerulosclerosis,
  intercapillary
glomerulus
glomerulus, olfactory
glomoid
glomus
glomus caroticum
glomus choroideum
glomus coccygeum
glomus tumor
glossa
glossal
glossalgia
glossectomy
Glossina
glossitis
glossitis, acute
glossitis areata
  exfoliativa
glossitis desiccans

glossitis, median
  rhomboid
glossitis, Moeller's
glossitis parasitica
glossocele
glossodynamometer
glossodynia
glossodynia exfoliativa
glossoepiglottic
glossoepiglottidean
glossoepiglottidean folds
glossoepiglottidean
  ligament
glossograph
glossohyal
glossokinesthetic
glossolabial
glossolalia
glossology
glossolysis
glossopalatine
glossopathy
glossopexy
glossopharyngeal
glossopharyngeal nerve
glossophytia
glossoplasty
glossoplegia
glossoptosis
glossopyrosis
glossorrhaphy
glossoscopy
glossospasm
glossotomy
glossotrichia
glossy
glossy skin
glottis
glottis, edema of
glottitis
glottology
glucagon
glucagonoma
gluciphore
glucocerebroside
glucocorticoid
glucofuranose
glucogenesis

glucohemia
glucokinase
glucokinetic
Glucometer
gluconeogenesis
glucopenia
glucophore
glucoprotein
glucopyranose
glucosamine
glucose
glucose, blood level of
glucose, liquid
glucose polymer
glucose tolerance test
  (GTT)
glucose-6-phospahte
  dehydrogenase (G-6-PD)
glucosidase
glucosidase, beta
glucoside
glucosin
glucosulfone sodium
glucosuria
Glucotrol (glipizide)
glucuronic acid
glucuronide
glue ear
glue-sniffing
Gluge's corpuscles
glutamate
glutamate dehydrogenase
glutamic acid
glutamic acid amide
glutamic oxaloacetic
  transaminase (GOT)
glutamic pyruvic
  transaminase (GPT)
glutaminase
glutamine
glutamyl transpeptidase,
  gamma (GGT)
glutaral
glutaraldehyde
glutathione
gluteal
gluteal fold
gluteal reflex

gluteal-iliotibial
  fasciotomy
glutelin
gluten
gluten-free diet
gluten-induced
  enteropathy
glutethimide
glutin
glutinous
glutitis
Glutose (dextrose gel)
Gly-Oxide (carbamide
  peroxide)
glycase
glyceride
glycerin
glycerite
glycerol
glyceryl
glyceryl monostearate
glyceryl triacetate
glyceryl trinitrate
glycine
glycobiarsol
glycocalyx
glycocholate
glycocholic acid
glycocin
glycoclastic
glycocoll
glycogen
glycogen storage disease
glycogen storage disease,
  phosphorylase b kinase
  deficiency
glycogen storage disease
  type Ia
glycogen storage disease
  type Ib
glycogen storage disease
  type II
glycogen storage disease
  type III
glycogen storage disease
  type IV
glycogen storage disease
  type V

glycogen storage disease
  type VI
glycogen storage disease
  type VII
glycogenase
glycogenesis
glycogenetic
glycogenic
glycogenolysis
glycogenolytic
glycogenosis
glycogeusia
glycohemia
glycohemoglobin test
glycol
glycolipid
glycolipide
glycolysis
glycolytic
glycolytic enzyme
glycometabolic
glycometabolism
glyconeogenesis
glyconucleoprotein
glycopenia
glycopexic
glycopexis
glycophorin
glycopolyuria
glycoprival
glycoprivous
glycoprotein
glycoptyalism
glycopyrrolate
glycorrhea
glycosecretory
glycosemia
glycosialia
glycosialorrhea
glycoside
glycosphingolipids
glycostatic
glycosuria
glycosuria, alimentary
glycosuria, diabetic
glycosuria, emotional
glycosuria, phloridzin
glycosuria, pituitary

glycosuria, renal
glycosyl
glycosylated hemoglobin
glycosylated hemoglobin
  test
glycotropic
glycuresis
glycuronuria
glycylglycine
glycyltryptophan
glycyrrhiza
glyoxalase
glyoxylic acid
gnashing
gnat
gnat, buffalo
gnathalgia
gnathic
gnathion
gnathitis
gnathocephalus
gnathodynamometer
gnathodynia
gnathoplasty
gnathoschisis
Gnathostoma
gnathostomiasis
gnosia
gnotobiotics
goat's milk
goblet cell
Goebel-Frangenheim-
  Stoeckel operation
goggle-eyed
goiter
goiter, aberrant
goiter, acute
goiter, adenomatous
goiter, colloid
goiter, congenital
goiter, cystic
goiter, diffuse
goiter, diver
goiter, endemic
goiter, exophthalmic
goiter, fibrous
goiter, follicular
goiter, hyperplastic

goiter, intrathoracic
goiter, lingual
goiter, nodular
goiter, parenchymatous
goiter, perivascular
goiter, retrovascular
goiter, simple
goiter, substernal
goiter, suffocative
goiter, toxic
goiter, vascular
goitrogens
goldbeater's skin
gold (Au)
gold alloy
gold alloy, dental
  casting
gold sodium thiomalate
gold standard
Gold Au 198 injection
Goldblatt kidney
Goldmann exam
Goldner operation
Goldthwaite operation
Golgi apparatus
Golgi's cells
Golgi's corpuscle
Goll's tract
GoLYTELY (polyethylene
  glycol 3350 and
  electrolytes)
gomphosis
gonad
gonadal
gonadal dysgenesis
gonadectomy
gonadial
gonadopathy
gonadotherapy
gonadotrope
gonadotrophic
gonadotrophic hormones
gonadotropin, chorionic
gonadotropin releasing-
  hormone (GnRH)
gonadotropin's, anterior
  pituitary
gonaduct

gonalgia
gonangiectomy
gonarthritis
gonarthromeningitis
gonarthrotomy
gonatocele
gonecyst
gonecystis
gonecystitis
gonecystolith
Gongylonema
goniometer
goniometer, finger
gonion
goniopuncture
gonioscope
gonioscopy
goniospasis
goniosynechia
goniosynechiae
goniotomy
gonocide
gonococcal
gonococcemia
gonococci
gonococcic
gonococcic smears
gonococcide
gonococcus
gonocyte
gonohemia
gonophore
gonorrhea (GC)
gonorrhea culture
gonorrheal
gonorrheal arthritis
Gonyaulax catanella
gonycampsis
gonycrotesis
gonyectyposis
gonyocele
gonyoncus
Good Samaritan Law
Goodal-Power operation
Goodell's sign
Goodpasture's syndrome
goose flesh
Gordon's reflex

Gordon-Taylor operation
gorget
Gossypium
gossypol
gouge
goundou
gout
gout, abarticular
gout, chronic
gout, tophaceous
gouty
gouty diathesis
Gowers' sign
Gowers' tract
graafian follicle
graafian follicles
Graber-Duvernay operation
gracile
gracile nucleus
gracilis
gradatim
graded exercise test
  (GxT)
Gradenigo's syndrome
gradient
gradient, axial
graduate
graduated
graduated tenotomy
Graefe's sign
graft, allogeneic
graft, allograft
graft, arteriovenous
  fistula
graft, arteriovenous
  shunt
graft, artery
graft, autodermic
graft, autogenous
graft, autologous
graft, avascular
graft, blood vessel
graft, bone
graft, bronchus
graft, cable
graft, cadaver
graft, cartilage
graft, conjunctiva

graft, delayed
graft, dermal
graft, fascia
graft, fascicular
graft, free
graft, full-thickness
graft, hair transplant
graft, heterodermic
graft, heteroplastic
graft, homologous
graft, isologous
graft, lamellar
graft, lid margin
graft, mucosa
graft, muscle
graft, myocutaneous
graft, nerve
graft, nipple
graft, Ollier-Thiersch
graft, omental
graft, ovarian
graft, pedicle
graft, periosteum
graft, pinch
graft, postmortem
graft, pterygium
graft, rectal
graft, renal
graft, rope
graft, sclera
graft, sieve
graft, skin
graft, sponge
graft, tendon
graft, thick-split
graft, Thiersch's
graft, vein
graft versus host disease
  (GVH)
graft, zooplastic
grafts, split-skin
grafts, Wolfe's
graft-verus-host reaction
grafting
Graham's law
gram (g, Gm)
gram molecule
Gram's method

gram-equivalent
gramicidin
grammeter
gram-negative
gram-positive
Grancher's disease
Grancher's sign
grand mal
grandiose
grandiosity
granular
granular cast
granulatio
granulation
granulation, arachnoidal
granulation, exuberant
granule
granule, agminated
granule, albuminous
granule, Altmann's
granule, amphophil
granule, azurophil
granule, basal
granule, beta
granule, chromophil
granule, epsilon
granule, glycogen
granule, Kölliker's
  interstitial
granule, Nissl
granule, Plehn's
granule, protein
granule, rod
granule, Schüffner's
granule, seminal
granules, acidophil
granules, basophil
granules, chromatic
granules, cone
granules, delta
granules, eosinophil
granules, hyperchromatin
granules, iodophil
granules, juxtaglomerular
granules, metachromatic
granules, Much's
granules, neutrophil
granules, pigment

granules, secretory
granules, thread
granules, zymogen
granulitis
granuloadipose
granuloblast
granulocyte
granulocyte-macrophage
  colony stimulating
  factor (GM-CSF)
granulocytopenia
granulocytopoiesis
granulocytosis
granuloma
granuloma annulare
granuloma, benign, of
  thyroid
granuloma, coccidioidal
granuloma, dental
granuloma, eosinophilic
granuloma fissuratum
granuloma, foreign body
granuloma fungoides
granuloma, infectious
granuloma inguinale
granuloma iridis
granuloma, lipoid
granuloma, lipophagic
granuloma, Majocchi's
granuloma, malignant
granuloma,
  paracoccidioidal
granuloma pyogenicum
granuloma, swimming pool
granuloma,
  telangiectaticum
granulomas, trichophytic
granulomatosis
granulomatosis siderotica
granulomatosis, Wegener's
granulomatous
granulopenia
granuloplasm
granuloplastic
granulopoiesis
granulopotent
granulosa
granulosa cell tumor

granulosa-theca cell
  tumor
granulose
granulosis
granulosis rubra nasi
granum
grape
grape sugar
graph
graphesthesia
graphite
graphology
graphomotor
graphophobia
graphorrhea
graphospasm
grasp
grass
grating
grattage
grattage, conjunctiva
grave
grave wax
gravel
Graves' disease
gravid
gravida
gravidism
graviditas
gravidity
gravidocardiac
gravimetric
gravistatic
gravitation
gravity
gravity, specific
Gravlee jet washer
gray
gray matter
gray syndrome of the
  newborn
greater trochanter
greater tuberosity
  fracture
green
green blindness
green, brilliant
green, indocyanine

green, malachite
Green operation
green soap
green soap tincture
green vitriol
Greenfield's disease
greffotome
grenz rays
Grice operation
grid
grid, Fixott-Everett
grief reaction
griffe des orteils
Grifulvin V (griseofulvin
  microsize)
grinder
grinders' disease
grinding
grinding, selective
grip
grip, strength
gripes
griping
grippe
Gris-PEG (griseofulvin
  ultramicrosize)
Grisactin (griseofulvin
  microsize)
Grisactin Ultra
  (griseofulvin
  ultramicrosize)
griseofulvin
gristle
grits
Gritti-Stokes operation
grocers' itch
groin
grommet
groove
groove, bicipital
groove, branchial
groove, carotid
groove, costal
groove, costovertebral
groove, Harrison's
groove, infraorbital
groove, intertubercular
groove, labial

groove, lacrimal
groove, laryngotracheal
groove, malleolar
groove, medullary
groove, musculospiral
groove, mylohyoid
groove, nasolacrimal
groove, nasopalatine
groove, neural
groove, obturator
groove, olfactory
groove, palatine
groove, peroneal
groove, pharyngeal
groove, primitive
groove, pterygopalatine
groove, radial
groove, rhombic
groove, sagittal
groove, sigmoid
groove, subcostal
groove, tympanic
groove, urethral
groove, vertebral
groove, visceral
grooves, meningeal
gross anatomy
gross lesion
gross motor skills
Gross operation
ground
ground bundle
ground itch
ground substance
group
group, alcohol
group, azo
group, coli-aerogenes
group, colon-typhoid-
  dysentery
group dynamics
group, peptide
group, prosthetic
group, saccharide
group therapy
group transfer
grouping
grouping serum

growing pains
growth
growth hormone (GH)
gruel
grumose
grumous
Grünfelder's reflex
Gruntzig balloon
  arterioplasty
gryposis
guaiac
guaiacol
Guaifed (pseudoephedrine
  HCl and guaifenesin)
guaifenesin
guanase
guanethidine
guanethidine, sulfate
guanidine
guanidinemia
guanidoacetic acid
guanine
guanosine
gubernaculum
gubernaculum dentis
gubernaculum testis
Gubler's line
Gubler's paralysis
Gubler's tumor
Gudden's inferior
  commissure
Gudden's law
guidance
guide
guide dog
guidewire
Guillain-Barré syndrome
  (GBS)
guillotine
guilt
guinea pig
guinea worm
Gull's disease
gullet
Gullstrand's slit lamp
gum
gumboil
gumma

gummatous
gummose
gummy
Gunderson conjunctival
  flap
Gunn's dots
gunshot wound
gunstock deformity
Günther's disease
gurney
Gustase (gastrointestinal
  enzyme)
Gustase Plus
  (gastrointestinal
  enzyme with
  phenobarbital)
gustation
gustatory
gustatory sweating
gustometry
gut
Guthrie test
gutta
gutta-percha
guttate
guttatim
guttering
guttering, bone
guttur
guttural
gutturotetany
Guyon operation
Guyon's sign
Gwathmey's method
gymnastics
gymnastics, ocular
gymnastics, Swedish
gymnophobia
gynander
gynandrism
gynandroid
gynatresia
gynecic
gynecogenic
gynecoid
gynecologic
gynecologic operative
  procedures

gynecologist
gynecology (gyn)
gynecomania
gynecomastia
gynecopathy
gynecophonus
Gyne-Lotrimin
  (clotrimazole)
gynephobia
gynesic
gyniatrics
Gynol II (contraceptive
  jelly)
gynopathic
gynoplastics
gynoplasty
gypsum
gyrate
gyration
gyre
gyrectomy
gyrencephalic
gyri
gyri breves insulae
gyrochrome
gyroma
gyrometer
gyrose
gyrospasm
gyrous
gyrus
gyrus, angular
gyrus, annectent
gyrus, anterior central
gyrus, Broca's
gyrus, callosal
gyrus, cerebelli
gyrus, cingulate
gyrus, dentate
gyrus, fornicatus
gyrus, frontal, inferior
gyrus, frontal, middle
gyrus, frontal, superior
gyrus, fusiform
gyrus, Heschl's
gyrus, hippocampal
gyrus, infracalcarine
gyrus, lingual

gyrus, longus insulae
gyrus, marginal
gyrus, middle temporal
gyrus, occipital
gyrus, occipitotemporal
gyrus, orbital
gyrus, paracentral
gyrus, parahippocampal
gyrus, paraterminal
gyrus, parietal
gyrus, postcentral
gyrus, precentral
gyrus, profundi cerebri
gyrus, rectus
gyrus, Retzius
gyrus, subcallosal
gyrus, subcollateral
gyrus, supracallosus
gyrus, supramarginal
gyrus, temporal
gyrus transitivus
gyrus, uncinate

H

H reflex
H.P. Acthar Gel
  (repository
  corticotropin)
H.T. Factorate
  (antihemophilic factor,
  [human])
**H.T. Factorate Generation
  II** (antihemophilic
  factor, [human])
H-Big (hepatitis B immune
  globulin [human])
H-substance
Haab's reflex
habena
habenal
habenar
habenula
habenular
habenular commissure

habenular trigone
habilitation
habit
habit, chorea
habit, masticatory
habit, spasm
habit training
habituation
habitus
hachement
hacking cough
Haemadipsa
Haemadipsa ceylonica
Haemagogus
Haemaphysalis
Haemophilus
Haemosporidia
hafnium (Hf)
Hagedorn needle
Hageman clotting factor
Hageman factor (HF)
Hagner operation
Hailey-Hailey disease
hair
hair analysis
hair, auditory
hair, bamboo
hair, beaded
hair bulb
hair, burrowing
hair cell
hair follicle
hair, gustatory
hair, ingrown
hair, kinky
hair, lanugo
hair, moniliform
hair papilla
hair, pubic
hair, sensory
hair, tactile
hair, taste
hair, terminal
hair transplantation
hair, twisted
hairball
hairy tongue
halation

halazone
halcinonide
Halcion (triazolam)
Haldol (haloperidol)
Haldol decanoate
  (haloperidol decanoate)
Haleys's M-O (magnesium
  hydroxide and mineral
  oil)
half-life
half-value layer
half-value thickness
halfway house
halibut liver oil
halide
halisteresis
halisteretic
halitosis
halitus
Haller's anastomotic
  circle
Hallervorden-Spatz
  disease
Hallervorden-Spatz
  syndrome
hallex
hallucination, auditory
hallucination,
  extracampine
hallucination, gustatory
hallucination, haptic
hallucination, hypnagogic
hallucination, kinetic
hallucination, microptic
hallucination, motor
hallucination, olfactory
hallucination, somatic
hallucination, tactile
hallucination, visual
hallucinogen
hallucinogenesis
hallucinosis
hallucinosis, acute
  alcoholic
hallus
hallux
hallux dolorosus
hallux flexus

hallux malleus
hallux rigidus
hallux valgus
hallux valgus (bunion)
hallux varus
halo
halo appliance
halo, Fick's
halo, glaucomatous
halo, senile
  peripapillary
halo symptom
halodermia
Halog (halcinonide)
halogen
haloid
haloid salt
halometer
haloperidol
halophilic
halosteresis
Halotestin
  (fluoxymesterone)
Halotex (haloprogin)
halothane
Halsted's operation
Halsted's suture
ham
Ham test
hamartia
hamartoma
hamartomatosis
hamate
hamate bone
hamatum
Hamman, Louis
Hamman's disease
Hamman-Rich syndrome
hammer
hammer, dental
hammer finger
hammer, percussion
hammer, reflex
hammertoe
hammertoe operation
Hampton operation
hamster

Hamster penetration test
hamstring
hamstring recession
hamstring tendon
hamstrings
hamular
hamulus
hamulus cochleae
hamulus lacrimalis
hamulus pterygoideus
hand
hand, ape
hand, claw
hand, cleft
hand, drop
hand, functional position
  of
hand, lobster-claw
hand, obstetrician's
hand, opera-glass
hand, resting position of
hand, writing
handedness
hand-foot-and-mouth
  disease
handicap
handpiece
handpiece, air-bearing
  turbine
handpiece, contra-angle
handpiece, high-speed
handsock
hanging drop culture
hanging hip operation
hangman's fracture
hangnail
hangover
Hanot's disease
Hansen's bacillus
Hansen's disease
hapalonychia
haphalgesia
haphephobia
haplodont
haploid
haploidy
haplopia

hapten
haptene
haptic
haptics
haptin
haptoglobin (Hp)
haptoglobin (Hp) test
haptometer
haptophil
haptophile
haptophore
haptophoric
haptophorous
hardening
hardening of the arteries
hardness
hardness number
harelip
harelip operation
harelip suture
harlequin fetus
harmony
harmony, functional
  occlusal
harmony, occlusal
harness
harpoon
Harrington rod technique
Harris-Benedict equations
Harrison's groove
Harrison-Richardson
  operation
Hartmann operation
Hartmann's solution
Hartnup disease
  (H disease)
harvest
Harvey, William
Hashimoto's disease
Hashimoto's struma
hashish
Hasner's fold
Hasner's valve
Hassall's corpuscles
Hatchcock's sign
haunch
Hauser operation

haustra
haustra coli
haustral
haustration
haustrum
haustus (H)
Haverhill fever
haversian canal
haversian canaliculi
haversian gland
haversian system
hay fever
Hayflick limit
Haygarth's deformities
hazardous material
   (hazmat)
head
Head & Chest
head, after-coming
Head and Shoulders
head, articular
head injury
head, nerve
head trauma
headache
headache, cluster
headache, exertional
headache, histamine
headache, postlumbar
   puncture
headache, tension
headache, thundering
headgut
heal
healer
healing
health
health, bill of
health, board of
health care worker (HCW)
health certificate
health, department of
health hazard
health, industrial
Health Maintenance
   Organization (HMO)

health, public
health risk appraisal
healthful
healthy
Heaney operation
hearing
hearing aid
hearing distance (HD)
hearing hallucinations
heart
heart, abdominal
heart and lungs (H&L)
heart, armored
heart, artificial
heart attack
heart, beriberi
heart block (HB)
heart block,
   atrioventricular
heart block, bundle
   branch
heart block, complete or
   third-degree
heart block, congenital
heart block, first-degree
heart block,
   interventricular
heart block, partial or
   second-degree
heart block, sinoatrial
heart, boatshaped
heart, bony
heart, cervical
heart, conduction system
   of
heart, dilatation of
heart disease, ischemic
heart disease, risk
   factors
heart failure
heart failure, backward
heart failure, congestive
heart failure, forward
heart failure, high
   output

heart failure, left
  ventricular
heart failure, left-sided
heart failure, low output
heart failure, right
  ventricular
heart failure, right-
  sided
heart, fatty degeneration
  of
heart, fatty infiltration
  of
heart, fibroid
heart, hypertrophy of
heart, irritable
heart, left
heart murmur
heart, palpitation of
heart pump, nuclear-
  powered
heart rate
heart reflex
heart, right
heart sounds
heart test
heart transplant
heart valve, prosthetic
heart-lung machine
heart-lung transplant
heartbeat
heartburn
heat, acclimatization to
heat, application of
heat, conductive
heat, convective
heat, conversive
heat cramps
heat, diathermy
heat, dry
heat exhaustion
heat gun
heat, initial
heat labile
heat, latent
heat, latent, of fusion
heat, latent, of
  vaporization

heat, luminous
heat, mechanical
  equivalent of
heat, moist
heat, molecular
heat, prickly
heat, radiant
heat, sensible
heat, specific
heat unit
heatstroke
heaves
heavy chain disease
heavy metal screen
hebephrenia
hebephrenic
Heberden's disease
Heberden's nodes
hebetic
hebosteotomy
hebotomy
hecateromeric
hecatomeric
hectogram (hg)
hectoliter (hl)
hectometer (hm)
hedonism
hedrocele
heel
heel bone
heel bone, calcaneus
heel pressure ulcer
heel puncture
heel, Thomas
Heerfordt's disease
Hegar operation
Hegar's sign
Heidenhain's demilunes
height (H, Ht)
heimdysesthesia
Heimlich maneuver
Heimlich sign
Heine operation
Heineke-Mikulicz
  operation
Heineke-Mikulicz
  pyloroplasty

Heinz bodies
Heinz body anemia
Heister, spiral valve of
HeLa cells
helcoid
helcology
helcoma
helcoplasty
helcosis
helianthine
helical
helicine
helicine arteries
helicoid
helicopodia
helicotrema
heliophobia
heliosis
heliotaxis
heliotaxis, negative
heliotaxis, positive
heliotherapy
heliotropism
helium (He)
helix
helix, Watson-Crick
Heller operation
Heller's test
Hellin's law
Hellstom operation
helminth
helminthagogue
helminthemesis
helminthiasis
helminthic
helminthicide
helminthoid
helminthology
helminthoma
helminthophobia
heloma
helotomy
helplessness
Helweg's bundle
hemachrosis
hemacytometer
hemacytozoon

hemad
hemadostenosis
hemadsorption
hemafecia
hemagglutination
hemagglutination
    inhibition
hemagglutinin
hemagglutinin, cold
hemagglutinin, warm
hemagogue
hemal
hemal arch
hemal gland
hemal node
hemanalysis
hemangiectasis
hemangioblast
hemangioblastoma
hemangioendo-
    thelioblastoma
hemangioendothelioma
hemangiofibroma
hemangioma
hemangiomatosis
hemangiopericytoma
hemangiosarcoma
hemaphein
hemapoiesis
hemapoietic
hemapophysis
hemarthros
hemarthrosis
hematapostema
hematein
hematemesis
hematencephalon
hematherapy
hemathermal
hemathermous
hemathidrosis
hematic
hematidrosis
hematimeter
hematin
hematinemia
hematinic

hematinuria
hematobilia
hematoblast
hematocele
hematocele, parametric
hematocele, pudendal
hematocelia
hematocephalus
hematochezia
hematochromatosis
hematochyluria
hematocolpometra
hematocolpos
hematocrit (HCT)
hematocyst
hematocytoblast
hematocytolysis
hematocytometer
hematocytozoon
hematocyturia
hematogenesis
hematogenic
hematogenous
hematohidrosis
hematoid
hematoidin
hematokolpos
hematologist
hematology
hematolymphangioma
hematolysis
hematolytic
hematoma
hematoma auris
hematoma, epidural
hematoma, intracerebral
hematoma, pelvic
hematoma, subarachnoid
hematoma, subdural
hematoma, vulvar
hematomediastinum
hematometra
hematometry
hematomphalocele
hematomyelia
hematomyelitis
hematomyelopore
hematopathology

hematopericardium
hematoperitoneum
hematopexin
hematophage
hematophagia
hematophagous
hematophilia
hematophobia
hematophyte
hematoplastic
hematopoiesis,
   extramedullary
hematopoietic
hematopoietic system
hematoporphyrin
hematoporphyrinuria
hematorrhachis
hematorrhea
hematosalpinx
hematoscheocele
hematoscope
hematoscopy
hematose
hematosepsis
hematospectroscopy
hematospectroscope
hematospermatocele
hematospermia
hematospermia spuria
hematospermia vera
hematostatic
hematosteon
hematothermal
hematothorax
hematotrachelos
hematotropic
hematotympanum
hematoxylin
hematoxylin and eosin (H
   and E)
hematozoon
hematozymosis
hematuria
hematuria, renal
hematuria, urethral
hematuria, vesical
heme

hemeralopia
hemiacephalus
hemiachromatopsis
hemiageusia
hemialbumin
hemialbumose
hemialbumosuria
hemialgia
hemiamaurosis
hemiamblyopia
hemianacusia
hemianalgesia
hemianencephaly
hemianesthesia
hemianopia
hemianopsia
hemianopsia, altitudinal
hemianopsia, binasal
hemianopsia, bitemporal
hemianopsia, complete
hemianopsia, crossed
hemianopsia, heteronymous
hemianopsia, homonymous
hemianopsia, incomplete
hemianopsia, quadrant
hemianopsia, unilateral
hemianosmia
hemiaparaxia
hemiarthroplasty of the
  hip
hemiarthrosis
hemiasynergia
hemiataxia
hemiathetosis
hemiatrophy
hemiballism
hemiblock
hemic
hemicanities
hemicardia
hemicastration
hemicellulose
hemicentrum
hemicephalia
hemicephalus
hemicerebrum
hemichorea
hemichromatopsia

hemicolectomy
hemicorporectomy
hemicrania
hemicraniectomy
hemicraniosis
hemicystectomy
hemidesmosome
hemidiaphoresis
hemidiaphragm
hemidrosis
hemidysergia
hemidystrophy
hemiectromelia
hemiepilepsy
hemifacial
hemigastrectomy
hemigeusia
hemiglossal
hemiglossectomy
hemiglossitis
hemignathia
hemihepatectomy
hemihidrosis
hemihypalgesia
hemihyperesthesia
hemihyperidrosis
hemihyperplasia
hemihypertonia
hemihypertrophy
hemihypesthesia
hemihypoesthesia
hemihypoplasia
hemihypotonia
hemikaryon
hemilaminectomy
hemilaryngectomy
hemilateral
hemilesion
hemilingual
hemimacroglossia
hemimandibulectomy
hemimastectomy
hemimaxillectomy
hemimelus
hemin
heminephrectomy
hemineurasthenia
hemiopalgia

hemiopia
hemiopic
hemipagus
hemiparalysis
hemiparaplegia
hemiparesis
hemiparesthesia
hemipatellectomy
hemipelvectomy
hemiphalangectomy
hemiplegia
hemiplegia, capsular
hemiplegia, cerebral
hemiplegia, facial
hemiplegia, spastic
hemiplegia, spinal
hemiplegic
Hemiptera
hemipyocyanin
hemirachischisis
hemisacralization
hemisection
hemisomus
hemispasm
hemisphere
hemisphere, dominant
hemispherectomy
hemispheric
  specialization
hemistrumectomy
hemisyndrome
hemithermoanesthesia
hemithorax
hemithyroidectomy
hemitomias
hemitremor
hemivertebra
hemizygosity
hemlock
hemlock poisoning
hemoagglutination
hemoagglutinin
hemobilinuria
hemoblast
hemoccult
hemochorial
hemochromatosis

hemochromatosis,
  exogenous
hemochrome
hemochromogen
hemochromometer
hemochromoprotein
hemoclasia
hemoclasis
hemoclastic
hemoconcentration
hemoconia
hemoconiosis
hemocryoscopy
hemocrystallin
hemocuprein
hemocyanin
hemocyte
Hemocyte (ferrous
  fumarate)
Hemocyte-F (ferrous
  fumarate and folic
  acid)
Hemocyte Plus (iron-
  vitamin-mineral
  complex)
hemocytoblast
hemocytoblastoma
hemocytogenesis
hemocytology
hemocytolysis
hemocytometer
hemocytophagia
hemocytopoiesis
hemocytotripsis
hemocytozoon
hemodiagnosis
hemodialysis
hemodialyzer
hemodiastase
hemodilution
hemodynamic
hemodynamics
hemodynamometer
hemoendothelial
Hemofil CT
  (antihemophilic factor
  [human], factor VIII)
hemofiltration

hemoflagellate
hemofuscin
hemogenesis
hemoglobin (Hb, Hbg, Hgb)
hemoglobin, fetal
hemoglobin, glycosylated
hemoglobinemia
hemoglobinocholia
hemoglobinolysis
hemoglobinometer
hemoglobinopathies
hemoglobinopepsia
hemoglobinophilic
hemoglobinous
hemoglobinuria
hemoglobinuria, cold
hemoglobinuria, epidemic
hemoglobinuria, intermittent
hemoglobinuria, malarial
hemoglobinuria, march
hemoglobinuria, paroxysmal
hemoglobinuria, toxic
hemoglobinuric
hemogram
hemoid
hemokinesis
hemokonia
hemolith
hemolymph
hemolymphangioma
hemolysate
hemolysin
hemolysis
hemolytic
hemolytic anemia
hemolytic disease of the newborn
hemolytic jaundice
hemolytic uremic syndrome
hemolytopoietic
hemolyze
hemomediastinum
hemometra
hemonephrosis
Hemopad (absorable collagen hemostat)

hemopathic
hemopathology
hemopathy
hemoperfusion
hemopericardium
hemoperitoneum
hemopexin
hemophagocyte
hemophagocytosis
hemophil
hemophilia
hemophilia A
hemophilia B
hemophilia, vascular
hemophiliac
hemophilic
Hemophilus
Hemophilus aegyptius
Hemophilus ducreyi
Hemophilus influenza B
Hemophilus influenzae
Hemophilus pertussis
Hemophilus vaginalis
hemophobia
hemophoric
hemophthalmia
hemophthalmus
hemopleura
hemopneumopericardium
hemopneumothroax
hemopoiesis
hemoprecipitin
hemoprotein
hemopsonin
hemoptysis
hemorrhage
hemorrhage, accidental
hemorrhage, antepartum
hemorrhage, arterial
hemorrhage, capillary
hemorrhage, carotid artery
hemorrhage cerebral
hemorrhage, concealed
hemorrhage, fibrinolytic
hemorrhage, internal
hemorrhage, intracranial
hemorrhage, lung

hemorrhage of knee
hemorrhage, petechial
hemorrhage,
  postmenopausal
hemorrhage, postpartum
hemorrhage, primary
hemorrhage, secondary
hemorrhage, stomach
hemorrhage, typhoid
hemorrhage, unavoidable
hemorrhage, uterine
hemorrhage, venous
hemorrhage, vicarious
hemorrhagenic
hemorrhagic
hemorrhagic disease of
  the newborn
hemorrhagic fevers
hemorrhagic
  nephrosonephritis
hemorrhagiparous
hemorrhoid
hemorrhoid, external
hemorrhoid, internal
hemorrhoid, prolapsed
hemorrhoid, strangulated
hemorrhoidal
hemorrhoidectomy
hemosalpinx
hemosiderin
hemosiderosis
hemospasia
hemospermia
Hemosporida
hemostasia
hemostasis
hemostat
hemostatic
hemostatic agent
hemostyptic
hemotherapeutics
hemotherapy
hemothorax
hemothymia
hemotoxin
hemotrophe
hemotrophic
hemotrophic nutrition

hemotropic
hemotympanum
hemozoin
hemozoon
Henderson-Hasselbalch
  equation
Henle, Friedrich G. J.
Henle's ampulla
Henle's fissure
Henle's layer
Henle's ligament
Henle's loop
Henle's membrane
Henle's sheath
Henle's tubules
Henley operation
Henoch-Schönlein purpura
henry (H)
Henry hernia repair
Henry's law
Hensen's cells
Hensen's disk
Hensen's stripe
Hep-B-Gammagee (hepatitis
  B immune globulin
  [human])
Hep-Forte (protein, B
  factors and other
  nutritional factors)
hepar
heparin assay
heparin lock flush
  solution
heparin sodium
heparin-protamine
  tolerance test
heparinize
hepatalgia
hepatalgic
hepatatrophia
hepatectomize
hepatectomy
hepatic
hepatic amebiasis
hepatic antigen (HAA,
  HBsAG) test
hepatic artery
hepatic coma

hepatic duct
hepatic encephalopathy
hepatic flexure
hepatic function panel
hepatic lobes
hepatic sequestration
hepatic veins
hepatic zones
hepaticochol-
  angiojejunostomy
hepaticocystoduodenostomy
hepaticodochotomy
hepaticoduodenostomy
hepaticoenterostomy
hepaticogastrostomy
hepaticojejunostomy
hepaticolithectomy
hepaticolithotomy
hepaticolithotripsy
hepaticostomy
hepaticotomy
hepatitis
hepatitis, A
hepatitis A antibody, RIA
hepatitis A antigen
  (HaAg)
hepatitis A virus (HAV)
hepatitis, acute
  anicteric
hepatitis, acute viral
hepatitis associated
  agent (HAA)
hepatitis B (HB)
hepatitis B antigen (HB
  Ag)
hepatitis B core antibody
hepatitis B core antigen
hepatitis B immune
  globulin
hepatitis B immunization
hepatitis B surface
  antibody
hepatitis B surface
  antigen (HBsAg)
hepatitis B virus (HBV)
hepatitis B virus vaccine
  inactivated
hepatitis Be antibody

hepatitis Be antigen
hepatitis, chronic
hepatitis, delta agent
hepatitis, drug-induced
hepatitis, fulminant
hepatitis, infectious
hepatitis, non-A
hepatitis, non-B
hepatitis panel
hepatitis, serum
hepatitis, toxic
hepatitis, viral
hepatitis-associated
  antigen
hepatitis-associated
  antigen (HAA) test
hepatization
hepatobiliary ductal
  system imaging
hepatobiliary imaging
hepatoblastoma
hepatocarcinogen
hepatocarcinoma
hepatocele
hepatocellular
hepatocholangio-
  cystoduodenostomy
hepatocholangio-
  enterostomy
hepatocholangio-
  gastrostomy
hepatocholangiostomy
hepatocholangitis
hepatocholedochostomy
hepatocirrhosis
hepatocolic
hepatocuprein
hepatocystic
hepatocyte
hepatoduodenostomy
hepatodynia
hepatoenteric
hepatogastric
hepatogastrostomy
hepatogenic
hepatogenous
hepatogram
hepatography

hepatohemia
hepatoid
hepatojejunostomy
hepatojugular reflex
hepatolenticular
hepatolenticular
  degeneration
hepatolienography
hepatolienomegaly
hepatolith
hepatolithectomy
hepatolithiasis
hepatolithotomy
hepatologist
hepatology
hepatolysin
hepatolysis
hepatolytic
hepatoma
hepatomalacia
hepatomegaly
hepatomelanosis
hepatomphalocele
hepatonecrosis
hepatonephric
hepatonephritis
hepatonephromegaly
hepatonephromegaly
  glycogenica
hepatopathy
hepatoperitonitis
hepatopexy
hepatophage
hepatopleural
hepatopneumonic
hepatoportogram
hepatoptosia
hepatoptosis
hepatopulmonary
hepatorenal
hepatorrhaphy
hepatorrhexis
hepatoscan
hepatoscopy
hepatosis
hepatosplenitis
hepatosplenography
hepatosplenomegaly

hepatosplenopathy
hepatostomy
hepatotherapy
hepatotomy
hepatotoxemia
hepatotoxic
hepatotoxin
heptachromic
heptapeptide
heptaploidy
Heptavax-B (hepatitis B
  vaccine)
heptose
heptosuria
Heptuna Plus
  (hematopoietic
  formulation)
herb
herbivorous
herd
hereditary
heredity
heredoataxia
heredodegeneration
heredofamilial
heredoimmunity
Hering, Karl Ewald K.
Hering-Breuer reflex
Hering's nerves
Hering's theory
heritable
heritage
hermaphrodism
hermaphrodite
hermaphroditism
hermaphroditism,
  bilateral
hermaphroditism, complex
hermaphroditism,
  dimidiate
hermaphroditism, false
hermaphroditism, lateral
hermaphroditism, spurious
hermaphroditism,
  transverse
hermaphroditism, true
hermaphroditism,
  unilateral

hermetic
hernia
hernia, abdominal
hernia, acquired
hernia, bladder
hernia, cerebral
hernia, Cloquet's
hernia, complete
hernia, concealed
hernia, congenital
hernia, crural
hernia, cystic
hernia, diaphragmatic
hernia, direct
hernia, diverticular
hernia, encysted
hernia, epigastric
hernia, fascial
hernia, femoral
hernia, funicular
hernia, hiatal
hernia, Holthouse's
hernia, incarcerated
hernia, incisional
hernia, incomplete
hernia, indirect
hernia, inguinal
hernia, inguinocrural
hernia, internal
hernia, interstitial
hernia, intervertebral
  disk
hernia, irreducible
hernia, labial
hernia, lumbar
hernia, lung
hernia, medial
hernia, mesocolic
hernia, nuckian
hernia, oblique
hernia, obturator
hernia of diaphragm
hernia, omental
hernia, ovarian
hernia, phrenic
hernia, posterior vaginal
hernia, properitoneal
hernia, reducible

hernia repair
hernia, retroperitoneal
hernia, Richter's
hernia, scrotal
hernia, sliding
hernia, spigelia
hernia, strangulated
hernia, umbilical
hernia, uterine
hernia, vaginal
hernia, vaginolabial
hernia, ventral
hernial
hernial sac
herniated
herniated disk
herniated disk syndrome
  (HDS)
herniation
herniation of nucleus
  pulposus
herniation, tonsillar
herniation,
  transtentorial
hernioenterotomy
herniography
hernioid
herniolaparotomy
herniology
hernioplasty
herniopuncture
herniorrhaphy
herniotomy
heroin
heroin toxicity
heroinism
herpangina
Herpecin-L
herpes corneae
herpes facialis
herpes febrilis
herpes, genitalia
herpes genitalis
herpes labialis
herpes menstrualis
herpes, ocular
herpes praeputialis
herpes progenitalis

herpes simplex (HS)
herpes simplex virus
  (HSV)
herpes test
herpes, traumatic
herpes zoster
herpes zoster
  ophthalmicus
herpes zoster virus (HZV)
herpesvirus simiae
  encephalomyelitis
herpesviruses
herpetic
herpetic neuralgia
herpetic sore throat
herpetiform
herpetism
Herring bodies
Herring track
hersage
Herter's infantilism
Hertig-Rock embryos
Hertig-Rock ovum
Hertwig's root sheath
hertz (Hz)
Hespan (hetastarch in
  sodium chloride)
hesperidin
Hesselbach's hernia
Hesselbach's triangle
hetacillin
heteradelphia
heteradenia
heteradenic
heteradenoma
heterecious
heterecism
heteresthesia
heteroagglutination
heteroagglutinin
heteroalbumose
heteroantibody
heteroantigen
heteroautoplasty
heteroblastic
heterocellular
heterocephalus
heterochiral

heterochromatin
heterochromatosis
heterochromia
heterochromia, iridis
heterochromosome
heterochromous
heterochronia
heterochronic
heterochthonous
heterocinesia
heterocladic
heterocrisis
heterocyclic
heterodermic
heterodont
heterodromus
heteroecious
heteroecism
heteroerotism
heterogametic
heterogamy
heterogeneity
heterogeneous
heterogeneous vaccine
heterogenesis
heterogenetic
heterogeusia
heterograft
heterograft, skin
heterography
heterohemagglutination
heterohemagglutinin
heterohemolysin
heteroimmunity
heteroinfection
heteroinoculation
heterokeratoplasty
heterolalia
heterolateral
heterologous
heterology
heterolysin
heterolysis
heteromeric
heterometaplasia
heterometropia
heteromorphosis
heteromorphous

heteronomous
heteronymous
hetero-osteoplasty
heterophany
heterophasia
heterophemia
heterophemy
heterophil
heterophile
heterophile antibodies
heterophilic
heterophonia
heterophoralgia
heterophoria
heterophthalmos
Heterophyes
Heterophyes heterophyes
heterophyiasis
Heterophyidae
heteroplasia
heteroplastic
heteroploid
heteroprosopus
heteropsia
heteroptics
heteropyknosis
heteroscopy
heteroserotherapy
heterosexual
heterosexuality
heterosis
heterosmia
heterotaxia
heterothermy
heterotopia
heterotopic
heterotopy
heterotoxin
heterotransplantation
heterotransplant
heterotrichosis
heterotroph
heterotropia
heterotypic
heterovaccine
heteroxanthine
heteroxenous
heterozygosis

heterozygote
heterozygous
hettocyrtosis
Heubner, Johann Otto L.
Heubner-Herter disease
Heubner's disease
heuristic
heurteloup
hex
hexabasic
hexachlorophene
hexachromic
hexad
hexadactylism
hexadecimal
Hexadrol (dexamethasone)
Hexadrol Strip Packs
  (dexamethasone)
hexafluorenium bromide
hexaploidy
Hexapoda
hexatomic
hexavaccine
hexavalent
hexavitamin capsules
hexavitamin tables
hexestrol
hexing
hexobarbital
hexokinase
hexone
hexonic
hexosamine
hexose
hexosephosphate
hexylcaine hydrochloride
hexylresorcinol
Hey operation
Hey's ligament
Hey-Groves operation
Heyman operation
Heyman-Herndon operation
hiatal hernia
hiatus
hiatus aorticus
hiatus canalis facialis
hiatus esophageus
hiatus fallopii

hiatus maxillaris
hiatus, sacral
hiatus semilunaris
Hibbs operation
hibernation
hibernoma
Hibiclens (chlorhexidine
  gluconate)
Hibistat (germicide hand
  rinse)
HibVAX (Haemophilus b
  polysaccharide vaccine)
hiccough
hiccup
Hick's sign
hidebound disease
hidradenitis
hidradenoma
hidrocystoma
hidropoiesis
hidropoietic
hidrorrhea
hidrosadenitis
hidroschesis
hidrosis
hidrotic
hieralgia
hierarchy
hierolisthesis
hierophobia
Higgins operation
high blood pressure (HBP)
high forceps delivery
high frequency (HF)
high performance liquid
  chromatography (HPLC)
high pressure liquid
  chromatography (HPLC)
high, runners'
high-calorie diet
high-cellulose diet
high-density lipoprotein
  (HDL)
high-residue diet
Highmore, antrum of
Highmore's body
hila
hilar

hilitis
Hill sign
Hill-Allison operation
hillock
hillock, anal
hillock, axon
hillock, seminal
Hilton's law
Hilton's line
Hilton's muscle
Hilton's sac
hilum
hilus
himantosis
hind-kidney
hindbrain
hindfoot
hindgut
Hines and Brown test
hinge joint
Hinton's test
hip
hip, congenital
  dislocation of
hip, dislocation of
hip joint
hip, snapping
hip, total replacement
hip-joint disease
Hippel's disease
hippocampal
hippocampal commissure
hippocampal fissure
hippocampal formation
hippocampal major
hippocampus major,
  digitations of
hippocampus minor
Hippocrates
hippocratic facies
Hippocratic oath
hippurase
hippuria
hippuric acid
hippuricase
hippus
hippus, respiratory

Hiprex (methanamine
  hippurate)
hirci
hircismus
hircus
Hirschberg's reflex
Hirschsprung's disease
hirsute
hirsuties
hirsutism
hirudicide
hirudin
Hirudinea
hirudiniasis
Hirudo
His, bundle of
His, bundle recording
His, Jr., Wilhelm
His-Werner disease
Hispanic
Hispril (diphenylpyraline
  HCl)
Hispril Spansule
  (diphenylpyraline HCl)
Histafed LA
  (pseudoephedrine HCl,
  chlorpheniramine
  maleate)
Histalet DM Syrup
Histalet Forte
Histalet S Tablets
Histalet Syrup
Histalet X Syrup
Histamic
histaminase
histamine
histamine blocking agents
histamine headache
histamine phosphate
histaminemia
histaminia
histase
Histaspan-D
Histaspan-Plus
histenzyme
histidase
histidine
histidinemia

histidinuria
histioblast
histiocyte
histiocytoma
histiocytosis
histiocytosis, lipid
histiocytosis X
histiogenic
histioid
histioirritative
histioma
histionic
histoblast
histochemical staining
  with frozen section
histochemistry
histochromatosis
histoclastic
histocompatibility
histocompatibility
  antigens
histocompatibility genes
histocyte
histodiagnosis
histodialysis
histodifferentiation
histogenesis
histogenetic
histogram
histography
histohematin
histohematogenous
histoid
histokinesis
histological
histologist
histology
histolysis
histolytic
histoma
histone
histonomy
histonuria
histopathology
histophysiology
Histoplasma
Histoplasma capsulatum
histoplasmin

histoplasmosis
histoplasmosis skin test
historetention
history (Hx)
history and physical
  (H&P)
history, dental
history, family
history, medical
histotherapy
histothrombin
histotome
histotomy
histotoxic
histotribe
histotroph
histotrophic
histotropic
histozoic
histozyme
histrionic
histrionic mania
histrionic personality
  disorder
Hitchcock operation
hives
hoarseness
hobnail liver
Hochsinger's sign
Hodara's disease
Hodgkin's disease
Hodgson's disease
hodoneuromere
hof
Hofbauer cell
Hoffmann's reflex
Hoffmann's sign
Hofmeister operation
Hoke operation
holandric
holarthritis
Holden's line
holergastric
holism
holistic
holistic medicine
Hollenhorst plaques
Hollerhorst bodies

hollow
hollow, Sebileau's
hollow-back
Holmgren's test
holmium (Ho)
holoacardius
holoblastic ova
holocrine
holodiastolic
holoendemic
holoenzyme
holography
hologynic
holomastigote
holophytic
holoprosencephaly
holosystolic
holotetanus
holotonia
holotonic
holotrichous
holozoic
Holter monitor
Holth operation
Holthouse's hernia
homalocephalus
Homan operation
Homans' sign
homatropine hydrobromide
homatropine methylbromide
homaxial
home assessment
home health care
homeo-osteoplasty
homeomorphous
homeopathic
homeopathist
homeopathy
homeoplasia
homeoplastic
homeostasis
homeostatic
homeotherapy
homeothermal
homeotransplantation
homeotypical
homesickness
homicide

hominid
Homo sapiens
homoblastic
homocentric
homochronous
homocladic
homocysteine
homocystine
homocystinuria
homocytotropic
homodromous
homoerotic
homogametic
homogenate
homogeneous
homogenesis
homogenize
homogentisic acid
homogentisuria
homoglandular
homograft
homoiopodal
homoiotherm
homokeratoplasty
homolateral
homologous
homologous organs
homologous series
homologous tissues
homologous vaccine
homologue
homology
homolysin
homonomous
homonymous
homonymous diplopia
homophil
homophile
homoplastic
homoplasty
homosexual
homosexuality
homostimulant
homothallic
homotherm
homothermal
homotonic
homotopic

homotransplant
homotransplantation
homotransplantation,
  renal
homotype
homozygosis
homozygote
homozygous
homunculus
honey
hook
hookworm
hopelessness
hora (H)
hora decubitus (hd)
hordeolum internum
horseshoe fistula
horizontal (H)
horizontal position
hormesis
hormion
hormonagogue
hormonal
hormone
hormone, adaptive
hormone, adrenocortical
hormone,
  adrenocorticotropic
  (ACTH)
hormone, androgenic
hormone, antidiuretic
  (ADH)
hormone, calcitonin
hormone, corpus luteum
hormone, cortical
hormone, ectopic
hormone, estrogenic
hormone, follicle
hormone, follicle-
  stimulating (FSH)
hormone, follicle-
  stimulating releasing
hormone, gastric
hormone, gonadotropic
hormone, gonadotropin-
  releasing
hormone, growth

hormone, human placental
  lactogen
hormone, inhibitory
hormone, interstitial
  cell-stimulating
hormone, lipolytic
hormone, luteal
hormone, luteinizing
hormone, luteinizing,
  releasing
hormone, luteotropic
hormone, melanocyte-
  stimulating
hormone, ovarian
hormone, pancreatic
hormone, parathyroid
hormone, posterior
  pituitary
hormone, progestational
hormone, progesterone
hormone, prolactin
hormone, releasing
hormone replacement
  therapy (HRT)
hormone, somatotrophic
hormone, somatrophin
  releasing
hormone, testicular
hormone, thyroid
hormone, thyrotropic
hormones, adrenomedullary
hormones, anterior
  pituitary
hormones, placental
hormones, sex
hormonic
hormonogenesis
hormonogenic
hormonology
hormonopoiesis
hormonopoietic
hormonotherapy
hormonotropic
horn
horn, anterior, of spinal
  cord
horn, cicatricial
horn, cutaneous

horn, dorsal
horn of Ammon
horn, posterior
horn, sebaceous
horn, ventral
horn, warty
Horner's syndrome
hornet sting
horny
horopter
horripilation
horsepower
horseshoe kidney
hospice
hospital
hospital, base
hospital, camp
hospital, evacuation
hospital, field
hospital visit (HV)
hospitalism
hospitalization
host
host, accidental
host, alternate
host, definitive
host, final
host, immunocompromised
host, intermediate
host of predilection
host, primary
host, reservoir
host, secondary
host, transfer
hostility
hot
hot flashes
hot packs
hot water bag
hotline
Hottentot apron
hottentotism
hour (H)
hour of going to bed (hd)
hourglass contraction
hourglass stomach
house physician
house staff

house surgeon (HS)
housefly
housemaid's knee
Houston's muscle
Howell-Jolly bodies
Howship's lacunae
Howship's symptom
HT Profilate
  (antihemophilic factor
  [human], factor VIII)
Hubbard tank
Huguier's canal
Huhner test
Huhner-Sims test
hum
human
human bite
human chorionic
  gonadotropin hormone
  test
  (HCG)
human diploid cell
  vaccine (HDCV)
human growth factor (HGF)
human growth hormone
  antibody
human immunodeficiency
  virus (HIV)
human leukocyte antigen
  (HLA)
human menopausal
  gonadotropin (HMG)
human pituitary
  gonadotropin (HPG)
human placental lactogen
  (HPL)
human rabies immune
  globulin (HRIG)
Humate-P (antihemophilic
  factor [human])
Humatin (paromomycin
  sulfate)
Humatrope (somatropin
  [rDNA origin])
humectant
humeral
humeroradial
humeroscapular

humeroulnar
humerus
Humibid (guaifenesin)
humid
humid gangrene
humidifier
humidity
humor
humor, aqueous
humor, crystalline
humor, vitreous
humoral
Humorsol (demecarium
  bromide)
humpback
Humulin BR (buffered
  regular insulin
  [rDNA origin])
Humulin L (Lente human
  insulin [rDNA origin])
Humulin N (NPH human
  insulin [rDNA origin])
Humulin R (human insulin
  [rDNA origin])
Humulin U Ultralente
  (human insulin [rDNA
  origin])
hunchback
hunger
hunger, air
hunger contractions
hunger cure
Hunner's ulcer
Hunt's neuralgia
Hunter's canal
Hunter's disease
hunterian chancre
Huntington chorea
Huntington's disease (HD)
Hurler's syndrome
Hurricaine (benzocaine)
Hürthle cell tumor
Hürthle cells
Huschke's auditory teeth
Huschke's canal
Huschke's foramen
Huschke's valve
Hutch operation

Hutchinson, Sir Jonathan
Hutchinson-Gilford
  disease
Hutchinson's patch
Hutchinson's pupil
Hutchinson's teeth
Hutchinson's triad
Huxley's layer
Hy-Phen (hydrocodone
  bitartrate and
  acetaminophen)
hyalin
hyaline
hyaline bodies
hyaline cartilage
hyaline casts
hyaline membrane disease
  (HMD)
hyalinization
hyalinosis
hyalinuria
hyalitis
hyalitis, asteroid
hyalitis, punctata
hyalitis, suppurativa
hyaloenchondroma
hyalogen
hyaloid
hyaloid artery
hyaloid canal
hyaloid membrane
hyaloiditis
hyalomere
hyalomucoid
hyalonyxis
hyalophagia
hyalophagy
hyalophobia
hyaloplasm
hyaloserositis
hyaloserositis,
  progressive multiple
hyalosis
hyalosis, asteroid
hyalosome
hyalotome
hyaluronic acid
hyaluronidase

Hybinette-Eden operation
hybrid
hybridization
hybridoma
Hycodan (hydrocodone
  bitartrate/homatropine
  methylbromide)
Hycomine (hydrocodone
  bitartrate)
Hycomine Compound
Hycotuss (hydrocodone
  bitartrate and
  guaifenesin)
hydantoin
hydatid
hydatid disease
hydatid fremitus
hydatid mole
hydatid of Morgagni
hydatid, sessile
hydatid, stalked
hydatidiform
hydatidiform mole
hydatidocele
hydatidoma
hydatidosis
hydatidostomy
hydatiform
hydatism
Hydeltra-T.B.A.
  (prednisolone tebutate)
Hydeltrasol (prednisolone
  sodium phosphate)
Hydergine (ergoloid
  mesylates)
Hydergine LC (ergoloid
  mesylates)
hydradenitis
hydradenoma
hydraeroperitoneum
hydragogue
hydralazine hydrochloride
hydramnion
hydramnios
hydranencephaly
hydrargyria
hydrarthrosis

hydrarthrosis,
  intermittent
hydrase
hydrate
hydrated
hydration
hydraulics
hydrazine
Hydrea (hydroxyurea)
hydremia
hydrencephalocele
hydrencephalomeningocele
hydrencephalus
hydrepigastrium
hydriatric
hydriatrist
hydride
Hydrisalic Gel
Hydrisinol Creme and
  Lotion
hydroappendix
hydrobilirubin
hydrobromate
hydrocalycosis
hydrocarbon
hydrocarbon, alicyclic
hydrocarbon, aliphatic
hydrocarbon, aromatic
hydrocarbon, cyclic
hydrocarbon, saturated
hydrocarbon, unsaturated
hydrocele
hydrocele, acute
hydrocele, cervical
hydrocele, congenital
hydrocele, encysted
hydrocele feminae
hydrocele hernialis
hydrocele, infantile
hydrocele muliebris
hydrocele, spermatic
hydrocele spinalis
hydrocelectomy
hydrocephalic
hydrocephalocele
hydrocephaloid
hydrocephaloid disease

hydrocephalus
hydrocephalus,
  communicating
hydrocephalus, congenital
hydrocephalus, external
hydrocephalus, internal
hydrocephalus,
  noncommunicating
hydrocephalus, normal
  pressure
hydrocephalus, secondary
hydrochlorate
hydrochloric acid (HCl)
hydrochlorothiazide
hydrocholecystis
hydrocholeresis
hydrocholeretic
Hydrocil Instant
hydrocirsocele
hydrocodone bitartrate
hydrocolloid
hydrocolpos
hydroconion
hydrocortisone
hydrocortisone acetate
Hydrocortone
  (hydrocortisone)
hydrocyanic acid
hydrocyst
hydrocystoma
hydrodiascope
hydrodictiotomy
HydroDIURIL
  (hydrochlorothiazide)
hydroencephalocele
hydroflumethiazide
hydrogel
hydrogen (H)
hydrogen acceptor
hydrogen breath test
hydrogen cyanide
hydrogen dioxide
hydrogen donor
hydrogen iodide
hydrogen ion (H^+)
hydrogen ion
  concentration (pH)

hydrogen ion scale
hydrogen peroxide
hydrogen sulfide
hydrogenase
hydrogenate
hydrogenation
hydroglossa
hydrogymnasium
hydrogymnastics
hydrohematonephrosis
hydrohymenitis
hydrokinetics
hydrolabile
hydrolase
hydrology
hydrolysate
hydrolysis
hydrolytic
hydrolyze
hydroma
hydromeiosis
hydromeningitis
hydromeningocele
hydrometer
hydrometra
hydrometrocolpos
hydromicrocephaly
hydromorphone
   hydrochloride
Hydromox (quinethazone)
Hyrdromox R
   (quinethazone-
   reserpine)
hydromphalus
hydromyelia
hydromyelocele
hydromyelomeningocele
hydromyoma
hydronephrosis
hydroparasalpinx
hydroparotitis
hydropathic
hydropathy
hydropenia
hydropericarditis
hydropericardium
hydroperinephrosis
hydroperion

hydroperitoneum
hydropexis
hydrophilia
hydrophilic lyophilic
   colloid
hydrophilic ointment
hydrophilism
hydrophilous
hydrophobia
hydrophobophobia
hydrophthalmos
hydrophysometra
hydropic
hydropneumatosis
hydropneumopericardium
hydropneumoperitoneum
hydropneumothorax
Hydropres (reserpine-
   hydrochlorothiazide)
hydrops
hydropsy
hydropyonephrosis
hydroquinone
hydrorheostat
hydrorrhachis
hydrorrhachitis
hydrorrhea
hydrorrhea gravidarum
hydrosalpinx
hydrosarcocele
hydroscheocele
hydrosis
hydrosol
hydrosphygmograph
hydrostat
hydrostatic
hydrostatic densitometry
hydrostatic test
hydrostatic weighing
hydrostatics
hydrosudotherapy
hydrosulfuric acid
hydrosyringomyelia
hydrotaxis
hydrotherapeutics
hydrotherapist
hydrotherapy
hydrothermic

hydrothionammonemia
hydrothionemia
hydrothionuria
hydrothorax
hydrotis
hydrotomy
hydrotropism
hydrotympanum
hydroureter
hydrous
hydrovarium
hydroxide
hydroxocobalamin
hydroxy acids
hydroxyamphetamine
  hydrobromide
hydroxyapatite
hydroxybenzene
hydroxybutyric acid
hydroxybutyric
  dehydrogenase
hydroxybutyric
  dehydrogenase, alpha
hydroxychloroquine
  sulfate
hydroxycorticosteroids
17-hydroxycorticosteroids
  (17-OHCS) test
hydroxydione sodium
  succinate
hydroxyindolacetic acid
5-hydroxyindolacetic acid
  (5-HIAA) test
hydroxyl
hydroxylase
hydroxylysine
hydroxyprogesterone
hydroxyprogesterone
  caproate
hydroxyproline
hydroxypropyl
  methycellulose
hydroxystilbamidine
  isethionate
hydroxyurea
hydroxyzine hydrochloride
hydruria
hygiene

hygiene, community
hygiene, dental
hygiene, industrial
hygiene, mental
hygiene, oral
hygienic
hygienics
hygienist
hygienist, dental
hygienization
hygric
hygroblepharic
hygroma
hygroma, cystic
hygrometer
hygroscopic
hygroscopy
hygrostomia
Hygroton (chlorthalidone)
hyla
hyloma
Hylorel (quanadrel
  sulfate)
hymen
hymen, annular
hymen, biforis
hymen, cribriform
hymen, denticulatus
hymen, fenestrated
hymen, imperforate
hymen, lunar
hymen, ruptured
hymen, septate
hymen, unruptured
hymenal
hymenectomy
hymenitis
Hymenolepis
Hymenolepis nana
hymenology
hymenoplasty
Hymenoptera
hymenorrhyphy
hymenotome
hymenotomy
hyobasioglossus
hyoepiglottic
hyoepiglottidean

hyoglossal
hyoglossus
hyoid
hyoid arch
hyoid bone
hyopharyngeus
hyoscine hydrobromide
hyoscyamus
hyoscyamus poisoning
hypacousia
hypacusia
hypacusis
hypalbuminosis
hypalgesia
hypalgia
hypamnios
hypaphrodisia
hypaxial
Hyper-Tet (tetanus immune globulin [human])
Hyperab (rabies immune globulin [human])
hyperacid
hyperacidaminuria
hyperacidity
hyperactive child syndrome
hyperactivity
hyperacuity
hyperacusis
hyperacute
hyperadenosis
hyperadiposis
hyperadiposity
hyperadrenalism
hyperadrenocorticalism
hyperalbuminemia
hyperaldosteronism
hyperalgesia
hyperalgia
hyperalimentation
hyperalkalinity
hyperaminoacidemia
hyperammonemia
hyperamylasemia
hyperanacinesia
hyperanacinesis
hyperanakinesis

hyperaphia
hyperaphic
hyperazotemia
hyperbaric chamber
hyperbaric oxygen
hyperbaric oxygen therapy (HBOT)
hyperbaric oxygenation
hyperbarism
hyperbetalipoproteinemia
hyperbilirubinemia
hyperbrachycephaly
hyperbulia
hypercalcemia
hypercalciuria
hypercapnia
hypercarbia
hypercatharsis
hypercellularity
hypercementosis
hyperchloremia
hyperchlorhydria
hyperchloridation
hypercholesterolemia
hypercholesterolia
hypercholia
hyperchromasia
hyperchromatic
hyperchromatic cell
hyperchromatism
hyperchromatopsia
hyperchromatosis
hyperchromia
hyperchromic
hyperchylia
hyperchylomicronemia
hypercoagulability
hypercorticism
hypercrinism
hypercryalgesia
hypercryesthesia
hypercupremia
hypercyanosis
hypercyanotic
hypercyesis
hypercythemia
hypercytosis
hyperdactylia

hyperdicrotic
hyperdistention
hyperdontia
hyperdynamia
hypereccrisia
hypereccrisis
hypereccritic
hyperemesis
hyperemesis gravidarum
hyperemesis lactentium
hyperemia
hyperemia, active
hyperemia, arterial
hyperemia, Bier's
hyperemia, constriction
hyperemia, leptomeningeal
hyperemia, passive
hyperemia, reactive
hyperemia, venous
hyperemization
hyperemotivity
hypereosinophilia
hypereosinophilic
  syndrome
hyperepinephrinemia
hyperequilibrium
hypererethism
hyperergia
hyperergy
hyperesophoria
hyperesthesia
hyperesthesia, acoustic
hyperesthesia, cerebral
hyperesthesia, gustatory
hyperesthesia, muscular
hyperesthesia, optic
hyperesthesia, sexualis
hyperesthesia, tactile
hyperesthetic
hyperexophoria
hyperexplexia
hyperextension
hyperferremia
hyperfibrinogenemia
hyperflexion
hyperfunction
hypergalactia
hypergammaglobulinemia

hypergamy
hypergasia
hypergenesis
hypergenitalism
hypergeusesthesia
hypergeusia
hypergia
hyperglandular
hyperglobulinemia
hyperglycemia
hyperglycemic-
  glycogenolytic factor
  (HGF)
hyperglyceridemia
hyperglycinemia
hyperglycogenolysis
hyperglycoplasmia
hyperglycorrhachia
hyperglycosemia
hyperglycosuria
hypergnasia
hypergonadism
hyperguanidinemia
hyperhedonia
hyperhedonism
Hyper-Hep (hepatitis B
  immune globulin
  [human])
hyperhidrosis
hyperhydration
hyperimmune
hyperinflation
hyperinosemia
hyperinosis
hyperinsulinism
hyperinvolution
hyperinvolution uteri
hyperirritability
hyperisotonic
hyperkalemia
hyperkaliemia
hyperkeratinization
hyperkeratomycosis
hyperkeratosis
hyperkeratosis
  congenitalis
hyperkeratosis,
  epidermolytic

hyperketonemia
hyperketonuria
hyperketosis
hyperkinesia
hyperkinesis
hyperlactation
hyperlipemia
hyperlipoproteinemia
hyperliposis
hyperlithuria
hypermastia
hypermature
hypermature cataract
hypermegasoma
hypermelanosis
hypermenorrhea
hypermetabolic state
hypermetabolism
hypermetaplasia
hypermetria
hypermetrope
hypermetropia (Ht)
hypermetropic
hypermimia
hypermnesia
hypermobility
hypermorph
hypermotility
hypermyatrophy
hypermyesthesia
hypermyotonia
hypermyotrophy
hypernatremia
hyperneocytosis
hypernephroma
hyperneurotization
hypernitremia
hypernormal
hypernormocytosis
hypernutrition
hyperonychia
hyperope
hyperopia
hyperopia, absolute
hyperopia, axial
hyperopia, facultative
hyperopia, latent
hyperopia, manifest

hyperopia, relative
hyperopia, total
hyperorchidism
hyperorexia
hyperorthocytosis
hyperosmia
hyperosmolar
  hyperglycemic
  nonketotic coma (HHNC)
hyperosmolarity
hyperostosis
hyperostosis, frontal
  internal
hyperostosis, infantile
  cortical
hyperostosis, Morgagni's
hyperovaria
hyperoxaluria
hyperoxaluria, enteric
hyperoxaluria, primary
hyperoxemia
hyperoxia
hyperpancreatism
hyperparasitism
hyperparathyroidism
hyperpathia
hyperpepsia
hyperpepsinia
hyperperistalsis
hyperphalangism
hyperphasia
hyperphenylalaninemia
hyperphonia
hyperphoria
hyperphosphatasemia
hyperphosphatemia
hyperphosphaturia
hyperphospheremia
hyperphrenia
hyperpiesia
hyperpiesis
hyperpietic
hyperpigmentation
hyperpituitarism
hyperplasia
hyperplasia, fibrous
hyperplasia, lipoid
hyperplastic

hyperploidy
hyperpnea
hyperpotassemia
hyperpragic
hyperpraxia
hyperprolactinemia
hyperprolinemia
hyperproteinemia
hyperproteinuria
hyperptyalism
hyperpyretic
hyperpyrexia
hyperpyrexial
hyperreactive
hyperreflexia
hyperresonance
hypersalemia
hypersalivation
hypersecretion
hypersensibility
hypersensitiveness
hypersensitivity
hypersensitization
hypersialosis
hypersomnia
hypersplenism
Hyperstat I.V.
  (diazoxide)
hypersthenia
hypersthenic
hypersthenuria
hypersusceptibility
hypersystole
hypersystolic
hypertelorism
hypertelorism correction
hypertensinogen
hypertension
hypertension, benign
hypertension, essential
hypertension, Goldblatt
hypertension, malignant
hypertension, portal
hypertension, primary
hypertension, renal
hypertensive

hypertensive
  arteriosclerotic heart
  disease (HASHD)
hyperthecosis
hyperthelia
hyperthermalgesia
hyperthermia
hyperthermoesthesia
hyperthrombinemia
hyperthymia
hyperthyroidism
hyperthyrosis
hyperthyroxinemia
hypertonia
hypertonic
hypertonicity
hypertonus
hypertoxicity
hypertrichiasis
hypertrichophobia
hypertrichophrydia
hypertrichosis
hypertriglyceridemia
hypertrophia
hypertrophic
hypertrophy, adaptive
hypertrophy, benign
  prostatic
hypertrophy, cardiac
hypertrophy, compensatory
hypertrophy, concentric
hypertrophy, eccentric
hypertrophy, false
hypertrophy, Marie's
hypertrophy, numerical
hypertrophy,
  physiological
hypertrophy,
  pseudomuscular
hypertrophy, simple
hypertrophy, true
hypertrophy, ventricular
hypertrophy, vicarious
hypertropia
hyperuricemia
hyperuricuria
hypervalinemia
hypervascular

hyperventilation
hyperviscosity
hypervitaminosis
hypervolemia
hypesthesia
hyphedonia
hyphema
hyphidrosis
Hyphomycetes
hypinosis
hypnagogic
hypnagogic state
hypnagogue
hypnalgia
hypnic
hypnoanalysis
hypnoanesthesia
hypnodontics
hypnodrama
hypnogenetic
hypnoidal
hypnoidization
hypnolepsy
hypnology
hypnonarcoanalysis
hypnonarcosis
hypnophobia
hypnopompic
hypnosis
hypnosophy
hypnotherapy
hypnotic
hypnotics
hypnotism
hypnotist
hypnotize
hypnotoxin
hypoacidity
hypoacusis
hypoadenia
hypoadrenalism
hypoadrenocorticism
hypoaffectivity
hypoalbuminemia
hypoaldosteronism
hypoalimentation
hypoallergenic
hypoazoturia

hypobaric
hypobaropathy
hypoblast
hypoblastic
hypobulia
hypocalcemia
hypocalciuria
hypocapnia
hypocarbia
hypocellularity
hypochloremia
hypochlorhydria
hypochlorite salts
hypochlorite salts
  poisoning
hypochlorization
hypochlorous acid (HClO)
hypochloruria
hypocholesteremia
hypochondria
hypochondriac
hypochondriac region
hypochondriacal
hypochondrial reflex
hypochondriasis
hypochondrium
hypochromasia
hypochromatism
hypochromatosis
hypochromia
hypochromic
hypochylia
hypocinesia
hypocomplementemia
hypocondylar
hypocone
hypoconid
hypocorticism
hypocrinism
hypocupremia
hypocyclosis
hypocyclosis, ciliary
hypocyclosis, lenticular
hypocystotomy
hypocythemia
hypodactylia
Hypoderma
hypodermatoclysis

hypodermatomy
hypodermiasis
hypodermic
hypodermic,
  intracutaneous
hypodermic, intramuscular
hypodermic, intraspinal
hypodermic, intravenous
hypodermic, subcutaneous
hypodermoclysis
hypodipsia
hypodontia
hypodynamia
hypoeccrisia
hypoeccritic
hypoendocrinism
hypoendocrisia
hypoeosinophilia
hypoepinephria
hypoergasia
hypoergia
hypoergic
hypoergy
hypoesophoria
hypoesthesia
hypoexophoria
hypoferremia
hypofibrinogenemia
hypofunction
hypogalactia
hypogammaglobulinemia
hypogammaglobulinemia,
  acquired
hypogammaglobulinemia,
  congenital
hypogastric
hypogastric artery
hypogastric artery repair
hypogastric plexus
hypogastrium
hypogenesis
hypogenitalism
hypogeusia
hypoglossal
hypoglossal alternating
  hemiplegia
hypoglossal nerve (XII)
hypoglottis

hypoglycemia
hypoglycemic
hypoglycemic agents, oral
hypoglycemic shock
hypoglycogenolysis
hypoglycorrhachia
hypognathous
hypogonadism
hypogonadotropic
hypohepatia
hypohidrosis
hypohyloma
hypoinsulinism
hypoisotonic
hypokalemia
hypokalemic
hypokinesia
hypokinetic
hypolemmal
hypoleydigism
hypolipidemic
hypoliposis
hypologia
hypolymphemia
hypomagnesemia
hypomania
hypomastia
hypomazia
hypomelanoses
hypomenorrhea
hypomere
hypometabolism
hypometria
hypometropia
hypomnesia
hypomnesis
hypomorph
hypomotility
hypomyotonia
hypomyxia
hyponanosoma
hyponatremia
hyponeocytosis
hyponoia
hyponychium
hyponychon
hypo-orthocytosis
hypopallesthesia

hypopancreatism
hypoparathyreosis
hypoparathyroidism
hypopepsia
hypopepsinia
hypoperistalsis
hypophalangism
hypopharynx
hypophonesis
hypophonia
hypophoria
hypophosphatasia
hypophosphatemia
hypophosphaturia
hypophrenia
hypophrenic
hypophysectomy
hypophyseoportal
hypophyseoprivic
hypophysis
hypophysis cerebri
hypophysis sicca
hypophysitis
hypopiesis
hypopigmentation
hypopinealism
hypopituitarism
hypoplasia
hypopnea
hypoporosis
hypoposia
hypopotassemia
hypopraxia
hypoproteinemia
hypoproteinosis
hypoprothrombinemia
hypopselaphesia
hypoptyalism
hypopyon
hyporeactive
hyporeflexia
hyposalemia
hyposalivation
hyposarca
hyposcleral
hyposecretion
hyposensitive
hyposensitization

hyposialadenitis
hyposmia
hyposmolarity
hyposomnia
hypospadia
hypospadias
hyposphresia
hypostasis
hypostatic
hypostatic pneumonia
hyposteatolysis
hyposthenia
hypostheniant
hyposthenic
hyposthenuria
hyposthenuria, tubular
hypostomia
hypostosis
hypostypsis
hypostyptic
hyposynergia
hypotaxia
hypotelorism
hypotension
hypotension, orthostatic
hypotensive
hypothalamus
hypothenar
hypothenar eminence
hypothermal
hypothermia
hypothermia blanket
hypothesis
hypothrombinemia
hypothymia
hypothymism
hypothyroid
hypothyroidism
hypotonia
hypotonic
hypotoxicity
hypotrichosis
hypotrophy
hypotropia
hypotympanotomy
hypotympanum
hypouricuria
hypourocrinia

hypovaria
hypovenosity
hypoventilation
hypovitaminosis
hypovolemia
hypovolia
hypoxanthine
hypoxemia
hypoxia
hypoxic lap swimming
HypRho-D (Rh$_o$(D) immune
  globulin [human])
HypRho-D Mini-Dose
  (Rh$_o$(D) immune globulin
  [human])
hypsarrhythmia
hypsibrachycephalic
hypsicephalic
hypsicephaly
hypsiconchous
hypsiloid
hypsiloid ligament
hypsistenocephalic
hypsokinesis
hypsophobia
hypurgia
Hyskon Hysteroscopy Fluid
  (dextran-70 in
  dextrose)
hysocephalous
hysteralgia
hysteratresia
hysterectomy
hysterectomy, abdominal
hysterectomy, cesarean
hysterectomy, Porro
hysterectomy, radical
hysterectomy, subtotal
hysterectomy,
  supracervical
hysterectomy,
  supravaginal
hysterectomy, total
hysterectomy, vaginal
hysteresis
hystereurynter
hysteria
hysteria, anxiety

hysteria, major
hysteria, mass
hysteria, minor
hysteriac
hysteric
hysteric ataxia
hysteric chorea
hysterical
hystericoneuralgic
hysteritis
hysterobubonocele
hysterocele
hysterocleisis
hysterocolpectomy
hysterocystocleisis
hysterodynia
hysterogastrorrhaphy
hysterogenic
hysterogram
hysterography
hysteroid
hysterolaparotomy
hysterolith
hysterology
hysterolysis
hysteromania
hysterometer
hysterometry
hysteromyoma
hysteromyomectomy
hysteromyotomy
hystero-oophorectomy
hysteropathy
hysteropexy
hysteropia
hysteroplasty
hysteropsychosis
hysteroptosia
hysteroptosis
hysterorrhaphy
hysterorrhexis
hysterosalpingectomy
hysterosalpingography
hysterosalpingogram (HSG)
hysterosalpingo-
  oophorectomy
hysterosalpingostomy
hysteroscope

hysteroscopy
hysterospasm
hysterostomatocleisis
hysterostomatomy
hysterotome
hysterotomy
hysterotrachelectomy
hysterotracheloplasty
hysterotrachelorrhaphy
hysterotrachelotomy
hysterotraumatic
hysterotubography
hysterovagino-enterocele
Hytone (hydrocortisone)
Hytrin (terazosin HCl)

I

I band
I.V. push
ianthinopsia
iatraliptics
iatric
iatrochemistry
iatrogenic disorder
iatrogeny
iatrology
iatrotechniques
Iberet-Folic-500 Filmtab
   (iron with folic acid,
   sodium ascorbate)
ibuprofen
ice
ice bag
ice, dry
ice treatment
iceberg phenomenon
Iceland disease
Iceland moss
ichnogram
ichor
ichoremia
ichorous
ichthammol
ichthyism

ichthyismus
ichthyoacanthotoxism
ichthyohemotoxin
ichthyoid
ichthyology
ichthyootoxin
ichthyophagous
ichthyophobia
ichthyosarcotoxin
ichthyosis
ichthyosis congenita
ichthyosis fetalis
ichthyosis hystrix
ichthyosis, lamellar, of
   newborn
ichthyosis vulgaris
ichthyotic
ichthyotoxicology
ichthyotoxin
icing
iconolagny
ictal
icteric
icteritious
icteroanemia
icterogenic
icterogenous
icterohematuric
icterohemoglobinuria
icterohepatitis
icteroid
icterus gravis neonatorum
icterus, hemolytic
icterus index (ict ind)
icterus, neonatorum
icterus, nonobstructive
icterus, obstructive
ictus
ictus cordis
ictus epilepticus
ictus sanguinis
ictus solis
id
idea
idea, autochthonous
idea, compulsive
idea, dominant
idea, fixed

idea of reference
ideas, flight of
ideal
ideal body weight (IBW)
ideation
idée fixe
identical
identification (ID)
identification, dental
identification, palm and
  sole system
identity
identity, ego
identity, gender
ideogenetic
ideogenous
ideology
ideomotion
ideomotor
ideomuscular
ideophrenic
ideoplastia
ideovascular
idiochromosome
idiocrasy
idiocratic
idiocy
idiocy, complete
idiocy, cretinoid
idiocy, epileptic
idiocy, genetous
idiocy, hemiplegic
idiocy, hydrocephalic
idiocy, intrasocial
idiocy, microcephalic
idiocy, paralytic
idiocy, paraplegic
idiocy, sensorial
idiocy, traumatic
idiogamist
idiogenesis
idioglossia
idiogram
idioisolysin
idiolalia
idiolysin
idiometritis
idiomiasma

idiomuscular
idiomuscular contraction
idiopathic
idiopathic pulmonary
  fibrosis
idiopathic
  thrombocytopenia
  purpura (ITP)
idiopathy
idiophrenic
idiopsychologic
idioreflex
idiospasm
idiosyncrasy
idiosyncrasy of effect
idiosyncrasy to a drug
idiosyncratic
idiot
idiot-savant
idiotic
idiotrophic
idiotropic
idiotropic type
idiotype
idiotypic
idiovariation
idioventricular
idoxuridine
IgA immunodiffusion
IgE radioallergosorbent
  test (RAST)
IgE radioimmunosorbent
  test (RIST)
ignatia
igniextirpation
ignioperation
ignipuncture
ignis
ignis infernalis
ignis sacer
ignis Sancti Antonii
ilea
ileac
ileal
ileal bladder,
  ureteroileal conduit
ileal bypass
ileal conduit

ileectomy
ileitis
ileocecal
ileocecal orifice
ileocecal valve
ileocecostomy
ileocecum
ileocolectomy
ileocolic
ileocolitis
ileocolostomy
ileocolotomy
ileocystoplasty
ileocystostomy
ileoduodenotomy
ileoectomy
ileoentectropy
ileoesophagostomy
ileoileostomy
ileoloopogram
ileopancreatostomy
ileopexy
ileoproctostomy
ileorectal
ileorectostomy
ileorrhaphy
ileoscopy
ileoscopy, fiberoptic
ileosigmoidostomy
ileostomy
ileostomy, urinary
ileotomy
ileotransversostomy
ileoureterostomy
Iletin (regular and
  modified insulin)
ileum
ileum, duplex
ileus
ileus, adynamic
ileus, dynamic
ileus, mechanical
ileus, meconium
ileus, paralyticus
ileus, postoperative
ileus, spastic
ileus, subparta
ilia

iliac
iliac artery
iliac fascia
iliac fossa
iliac region
iliac roll
iliac spine
iliac
  thromboendarterectomy
iliac vein
iliococcygeal
iliocolotomy
iliocostal
iliofemoral
iliofemoral bypass graft
iliohypogastric
iliohypogastric nerve
  injection
ilioiliac bypass graft
ilioinguinal
ilioinguinal nerve
  injection
iliolumbar
iliopagus
iliopectineal
iliopelvic
iliopsoas
iliopsoas abscess
iliopsoas, transfer
iliosacral
iliosciatic
iliospinal
iliothoracopagus
iliotibial
iliotibial band
ilioxiphopagus
ilium
ill
illaqueation
illegitimate
illinition
illness
illness, catastrophic
illuminating gas
illumination
illumination, axial
illumination, central
illumination, dark-field

illumination, direct
illumination, focal
illumination, oblique
illumination, transmitted
  light
illuminism
illusion
illusion, optical
illusional
Ilopan (dexpanthenol)
Ilosone (erythromycin
  estolate)
Ilotycin (erythromycin)
Ilotycin Gluceptate
  (erythromycin
  gluceptate)
ima
image
image, body
image, direct
image, double
image, false
image intensifier
image, inverted
image, latent
image, mirror
image, radiographic
image, real
image, true
image, virtual
imagery
imagery, auditory
imagery, smell
imagery, tactile
imagery, taste
imagery, visual
imagination
imaging
imago
imbalance
imbalance, autonomic
imbalance, sympathetic
imbalance, vasomotor
imbecile
imbecility
imbed
imbibition
imbricate

imbricated
imbrication
Imferon (iron dextran)
imidazole
imide
imipramine hydrochloride
immature
immediate
immediate postoperative
  prosthesis (IPOP)
immediately (stat)
immedicable
immersion
immersion foot
immersion, homogeneous
immersion lens, oil
immiscible
immobilization
immune
immune body
immune globulin
  crossmatch, Rh
Immune Globulin
  Intravenous (Human)
immune reaction
immune response
Immune-Aid (natural fatty
  acid)
immunifacient
immunity, acquired
immunity, active
immunity, cell-mediated
immunity, congenital
immunity deficiency state
  (IDS)
immunity, herd
immunity, local
immunity, natural
immunity, passive
immunization
immunization, deliberate
immunization, natural
immunizing unit (IU)
immunoassay
immunobiology
immunochemistry
immunochemotherapy

immunocompetence
immunocompromised
immunoconglutinin
immunocytochemistry
  stains
immunodeficiency
immunodiagnosis
immunodiffusion
immunoelectrophoresis
immunofluorescence
immunofluorescent method
immunofluorescent study
immunogen
immunogenetics
immunogenic
immunogenicity
immunoglobulin
immunoglobulin assay
immunoglobulin gamma A
  (IgA)
immunoglobulin gamma D
  (IgD)
immunoglobulin gamma E
  (IgE)
immunoglobulin gamma G
  (IgG)
immunoglobulin gamma M
  (IgM)
immunoglobulin test
immunohematology
immunologic
immunologic disease
immunologist
immunology
immunopathology
immunoperioxidase
  histochemistry stains
immunoprecipitation
immunoproliferative
immunoprotein
immunoreactant
immunoreaction
immunoselection
immunostimulant
immunosuppression
immunosuppressive
immunosuppressive agent
immunosurgery

immunosurveillance
immunotherapy
immunotoxin
immunotransfusion
immunoassay
Imodium (loperamide HCl)
Imogam Rabies (rabies
  immune globulin
  [human])
Imovax Rabies (rabies
  vaccine human diploid
  cell)
impacted
impaction
impaction, fecal removal
impairment
impalpable
impar
imparidigitate
impatent
impedance
impedance plethysmography
  (IPG)
impedance testing
imperative
imperception
imperforate
imperforate hymen
imperforation
imperious acts
impermeable
impervious
impetiginous
impetigo
impetigo contagiosa
impetigo herpetiformis
implant
implant, brain
implant, dental
implant, tooth
implantation
implantation, hypodermic
implantation, teratic
implosion
implosion flooding
imponderable
impostors, medical
impotence

impotence, anatomic
impotence, atonic
impotence, functional
impotence, organic
impotence, psychic
impotence, symptomatic
impotence, vasculogenic
impotency
impotent
impotentia
impregnate
impregnated
impregnated carbon
impregnation
impregnation, artificial
impressio
impressio cardiaca
  hepatis
impressio colica
impressio duodenalis
impressio gastrica
impressio renalis
impression
impression, digitate
impression, final
impression materials
impression tray
impressiones digitatae
imprinting
impulse
impulse, cardiac
impulse, ectopic
impulse, enteroceptive
impulse, excitatory
impulse, exteroceptive
impulse, inhibitory
impulse, nervous
impulse, proprioceptive
impulsion
Imuran (azathioprine)
in articulo mortis
in extremis
in situ
in utero
in vacuo
in vitro
in vitro fertilization
  (IVF)

in vivo
inaction
inactivate
inactivation
inactivation of
  complement
inadequacy
inanimate
inanition
inapparent
inappetence
Inapsine (droperidol)
inarticulate
inassimilable
inborn
inbreeding
incandescent
incaparina
incarcerated
incarceration
incarial bone
incarnatio
incarnatio unguis
incasement
incentive spirometry
inception
incest
incidence
incident
incineration
incipient
incisal
incise
incised
incision
incision and drainage
  (I&D)
incisive
incisive bone
incisor
incisor, prostatic
incisors, central
incisura
incisura angularis
  gastrica
incisure
incisure of Rivinus

incisures of Schmidt-
  Lanterman
incitant
inclination
inclinometer
inclusion
inclusion blennorrhea
inclusion bodies
inclusion bodies smear
inclusion, cell
inclusion conjunctivitis
inclusion, dental
inclusion, fetal
incoagulability
incoercible
incoherence
incoherent
incombustible
incompatibility
incompatibility,
  physiological
incompatible
incompetence
incompetence, aortic
incompetence, ileocecal
incompetence, mental
incompetence, muscular
incompetence, pyloric
incompetence, relative
incompetence, valvular
incompetency
incompetent
incompetent palatal
  syndrome
incompressible
incontinence
incontinence, active
incontinence, anal
incontinence, giggle
incontinence,
  intermittent
incontinence of milk
incontinence of urine
incontinence, overflow
incontinence, paralytic
incontinence, passive
incontinence, urinary
  stress

incoordinate
incoordination
incorporation
increment
Incremin with Iron
  (vitamins B_1, B_6, B_{12}-
  lysine-iron)
incretogenous
incrustation
incubation
incubator
incubus
incudal
incudectomy
incudiform
incudomalleal
incudostapedial
incurable
incurvation
incus
incus, lenticular process
  of
incyclophoria
incyclotropia
indagation
indecision
indentation
independent living
independent living skills
Inderal (propranolol HCl)
Inderide (propranolol HCl
  and
  hydrochlorothiazide)
index
index, alveolar
index, cardiac
index case
index, cephalic
index, cerebral
index, leukopenic
index of dental health
  and caries
index, opsonic
index, oral hygiene
index, pelvic
index, periodontal
  (Ramfjord)
index, phagocytic

index, refractive
index, therapeutic
index, thoracic
index, vital
indican
indicanemia
indicant
indicanuria
indication
indication, causal
indication, symptomatic
indicator
indicator dilution
  studies
indices, blood
indifferent
indigenous
indigestible
indigestion
indigitation
indigo
indigotindisulfonate
  sodium
indigouria
indirect Coombs' test
  (ICT)
indisposition
indium (In)
indium chlorides in 113m
  injection
individuation
Indocin (indomethacin)
Indocin I.V.
  (indomethacin sodium
  trihydrate)
indocyanine green
indolaceturia
indole
indolent
indolent ulcer
indologenous
indoluria
indomethacin
indoxyl
indoxylemia
indoxyluria
induced
inducer

inductance
induction
inductor
inductorium
inductotherm
inductothermy
indulin
indulinophil
indulinophile
indurate
indurated
induration
induration, black
induration, brown
induration, cyanotic
induration, granular
induration, gray
induration, red
indurative
indusium
indusium griseum
Industrial Medical
  Association (IMA)
inebriant
inebriate
inebriation
inelastic
inert
inertia
inertia, uterine
infant
infant, development of
infant, post-term
infant, preterm
infant, respiration of
infant, temperature of
infant, term
infanticide
infantile
infantilism
infantilism, angioplastic
infantilism, Brissaud's
infantilism, cachectic
infantilism, celiac
infantilism, dysthyroidal
infantilism, hepatic
infantilism, hypophyseal
infantilism, idiopathic

infantilism, intestinal
infantilism, myxedematous
infantilism, pituitary
infantilism, renal
infantilism, sex
infantilism, symptomatic
infantilism, universal
infarct
infarct, anemic
infarct, bland
infarct, calcareous
infarct, cicatrized
infarct, hemorrhagic
infarct, infected
infarct, pale
infarct, red
infarct, septic
infarct, uric acid
infarct, white
infarction
infarction, cardiac
infarction, cerebral
infarction, evolution of
infarction, extension of
infarction, myocardial
infarction, pulmonary
infect
infection
infection, acute
infection, airborne
infection, apical
infection, chronic
infection, concurrent
infection, contagious
infection, cross
infection, droplet
infection, dustborne
infection, endogenous
infection, exogenous
infection, fungus
infection, local
infection, low-grade
infection, metastatic
infection, mixed
infection, opportunistic
infection, protozoal
infection, pyogenic
infection, secondary

infection, simple
infection, subacute
infection, subclinical
infection, systemic
infection, terminal
infection, waterborne
infectious
infectious disease
infectious hepatitis (IH)
infectious mononucleosis
infective dose (ID)
infecundity
inferior (inf)
inferior alveolar nerve
    transection
inferior vena cava
inferior vena cava
    pressure (IVCP)
inferiority complex
infertility
infest
infestation
infibulation
infiltrate
infiltration
infiltration, adipose
infiltration, amyloid
infiltration, anesthesia
infiltration, calcareous
infiltration, cellular
infiltration, fatty
infiltration, glycogenic
infiltration, lymphocytic
infiltration, pigmentary
infiltration, purulent
infiltration, serous
infiltration, urinous
infiltration, waxy
infinite distance
infinity
infirm
infirmary
infirmity
inflammation, acute
inflammation, adhesive
inflammation, bacterial
inflammation, catarrhal
inflammation, chronic

inflammation, exudative
inflammation, fibrinous
inflammation,
  granulomatous
inflammation, hemorrhagic
inflammation,
  hyperplastic
inflammation,
  interstitial
inflammation,
  parenchymatous
inflammation, productive
inflammation,
  proliferative
inflammation,
  pseudomembranous
inflammation, purulent
inflammation, reactive
inflammation, serous
inflammation, specific
inflammation, subacute
inflammation, suppurative
inflammation, toxic
inflammation, traumatic
inflammation, ulcerative
inflammatory
inflammatory response
inflation
inflator
inflection
influenza
influenza, Asian
influenza virus vaccine
influenzal
infolding
informed consent
infra-axillary
infrabulge
infraclavicular
infracortical
infracostal
infracotyloid
infraction
infradentale
infradiaphragmatic
infraglenoid
infraglottic
infrahyoid

inframammary
inframandibular
inframarginal
inframaxillary
infranuclear
infraocclusion
infraorbital
infraorbital nerve
  transection
infraorbitomeatal line
  (IOML)
infrapatellar
infrapatellar tendon,
  suture
infrapsychic
infrapubic
infrared (IR)
infrared physiotherapy
infrared rays
infrared spectroscopy
infrascapular
infrasonic
infraspinous
infrasternal
infratemporal
infratentorial
infratentorial burr holes
  or trephine
infratentorial
  craniectomy
infratonsillar
infratrochlear
infraumbilical
infraversion
infriction
infundibular resection
infundibulectomy
infundibuliform
infundibulopelvic
infundibulum
infundibulum, ethmoidal
infundibulum of
  hypothalamus
infundibulum of the
  uterine tube
infusible
infusion (inf)
infusion, continuous

infusion, direct
  intracoronary artery
infusion, intra-arterial
  (percutaneous
  transluminal
  angioplasty)
infusion, intra-arterial
  thrombolytic agent
  (streptokinase)
infusion, intravenous
infusion pump
infusion, subcutaneous
infusion therapy
infusion urography
infusodecoction
Infusoria
infusum
ingesta
ingestant
ingestion challenge test
Ingrassia's apophyses
ingravescent
ingredient
ingrowing
ingrown nail
inguen
inguinal
inguinal canal
inguinal glands
inguinal hernia
inguinal hernia repair
inguinal ligament
inguinal lymph node
  needle biopsy
inguinal reflex
inguinal region
inguinal ring
inguinocrural
inguinodynia
inguinofemoral
  lymphadenectomy
inguinolabial
inguinoscrotal
INH (isoniazid)
Inhal-Aid
inhalant
inhalation

inhalation bronchial
  challenge tests
inhalation therapy
inhalations, aerosol or
  vapor
inhale
inhaler
inherent
inherent cauterization
inheritance
inherited
inhibin
inhibited sexual desire
  (ISD)
inhibited sexual
  excitement
inhibition
inhibition, competitive
inhibition, contact
inhibition,
  noncompetitive
inhibition, psychic
inhibition, selective
inhibitor
inhibitory
inhibitory nerve
inhibitory postsynaptic
  potential (IPSP)
inhibitrope
inhomogeneity
iniac
inial
iniencephalus
inion
iniopagus
iniops
initial
initis
inject
injected
injection, epidural
injection, fractional
injection, hypodermic
injection, intra-alveolar
injection, intracardial
injection, intracutaneous
injection, intralingual
injection, intramuscular

injection, intraosseous
injection, intraperitoneal
injection, intravenous
injection, jet
injection, rectal
injection, sclerosing
injection, spinal
injection, subcutaneous
injection, vaginal
injection, Z-track
injectors
injury
injury, egg-white
injury, internal
injury, steering wheel
ink poisoning
inlay
inlet
innate
innervate
innervation
innervation, collateral
innervation, double
innervation, reciprocal
innidiation
innocent
innocuous
innominate
innominate artery
innominate bone
innominate veins
Innovar (fentanyl citrate/droperidol)
innoxious
inochondritis
inochondroma
Inocor Lactate Injection (amrinone lactate)
inoculability
inoculable
inoculate
inoculation
inoculum
inocyst
inocyte
inogenesis
inogenous

inoglia
inohymenitis
inolith
inomyositis
inomyxoma
inoneuroma
inoperable
inopexia
inophose
inorganic
inorganic acid
inorganic chemistry
inorganic compound
inosclerosis
inoscopy
inosculating
inosculation
inose
inosemia
inosinic acid
inosite
inositis
inositol
inosituria
inosuria
inotropic
inpatient
inquest
insalivation
insalubrious
insane
insanitary
insanity
insatiable
inscriptio
inscriptio tendinea
inscription
insect
insect bites and stings
insect repellents
Insecta
insecticide
insectifuge
insectivora
insectivore
insecurity
insemination, artificial (AI)

insemination,
  heterologous artificial
insemination, homologous
  artificial
insenescence
insensible
insertion
insertion, velamentous
insheathed
inside diameter (ID)
insidious
insight
insipid
insolation
insoluble
insomnia
insomniac
insorption
inspect
inspection
inspectionism
inspersion
inspiration
inspiration, crowing
inspiration, external
inspiration, forcible
inspiration, full
inspiration, internal
inspirator
inspiratory
inspiratory capacity (IC)
inspiratory-expiratory
  ratio (I/E)
inspirometer
inspissate
inspissated
inspissation
Instat (collagen
  absorable hemostat)
instep
instillation
instinct
instinct, death
instinct, herd
instinctive
institutional review
  board (IRB)
instruction

instrument
instrument, dental
instrumental
instrumental activities
  of daily living (IADL)
instrumentarium
instrumentation
insufficiency
insufficiency, adrenal
insufficiency, aortic
insufficiency, cardiac
insufficiency, coronary
insufficiency, gastric
insufficiency, hepatic
insufficiency, ileocecal
insufficiency, mitral
insufficiency, muscular
insufficiency of ocular
  muscles
insufficiency, pulmonary
  valvular
insufficiency, renal
insufficiency,
  respiratory
insufficiency, thyroid
insufficiency, valvular
insufficiency, venous
insufflate
insufflation
insufflation, perirenal
insufflation, tubal
insufflator
insula
insular
Insulatard NPH Human (U-
  100 purified pork
  insulin isophane)
insulation
insulator
insulin
insulin assay
insulin, human
insulin lipodystrophy
insulin, monocomponent
insulin, NPH
insulin pump
insulin shock

insulin, suspension,
 isophane
insulin, suspension,
 protamine zinc
insulin, synthetic
insulin zinc suspension,
 extended
insulin zinc suspension,
 prompt
insulin-dependent
 diabetes mellitus
 (IDDM)
insulinase
insulinemia
insulinogenesis
insulinogenic
insulinoid
insulinoma
insulitis
insuloma
insulopathic
insultus
insusceptibility
intake
intake and output (I&O)
Intal (cromolyn sodium)
integrated electromyogram
 (IEMG)
integration
integrator
integument
integumentary
intellect
intellectual
intellectualization
intelligence
intelligence quotient
 (IQ)
intemperance
intensifying
intensifying screen
intensimeter
intensity
intensive
intensive care unit (ICU)
intensive coronary care
 unit (ICCU)
intention

intention, first
intention, second
intention, third
intention tremor
interacinar
interalveolar
interarticular
interarytenoid
interatrial
interatrial septal defect
 (IASD)
interauricular
interbrain
intercadence
intercalary
intercalated
intercalated ducts
intercanalicular
intercapillary
intercarotic
intercarpal
intercarpal joint
intercartilaginous
intercavernous
intercellular
intercerebral
interchange
interchondral
intercilium
interclavicular
intercoccygeal
intercolumnar
intercolumnar fascia
intercolumnar fibers
intercostal
intercostal muscles,
 external
intercostal muscles,
 internal
intercostal nerve
intercostal space (ICS)
intercostobrachial
intercostohumeral
intercourse
intercricothyrotomy
intercristal
intercrural
intercurrent

intercusping
interdent
interdental
interdental fixation
interdentium
interdigitation
interface
interfascicular
interfemoral
interference
interference of impulses
interferometer
interferon
interfibrillar
interfibrillary
interfilamentous
interfilar
interfilar mass
interganglionic
intergemmal
interglobular
interglobular dentin
interglobular spaces
intergluteal
intergonial
intergyral
interhemicerebral
interictal
interischiadic
interkinesis
interlabial
interlamellar
interleukin (IL)
interleukin-1 (IL-1)
interleukin-2 (IL-2)
interlobar
interlobitis
interlobular
interlobular emphysema
intermalleolar
intermamillary
intermammary
intermarginal adhesions
intermarriage
intermaxillary
intermediary
intermediary metabolism
intermediate

intermedin
intermediolateral
intermedius
intermembranous
intermeningeal
intermenstrual
intermetacarpal
intermission
intermittence
intermittent
intermittent fever
intermittent mandatory
    ventilation (IMV)
intermittent positive-
    pressure breathing
    (IPPB)
intermittent pulse
intermuscular
intern
internal
internal bleeding
internal ear
internal fixation
internal injury
internal, medicine
internal, os
internal resistance (IR)
internal secretion
internalization
internarial
internasal
internatal
International
    Classification of
    Diseases (ICD)
International College of
    Surgeons (ICS)
International Council of
    Nurses (ICN)
International
    Nonproprietary Names
    (INN)
International Standards
    Organization (ISO)
International Symbol of
    Access
International System of
    Units (SI)

international unit (IU)
interneuron
internist
internode
internship
internuclear
internuncial
internuncial neuron
internus
interocclusal
interoceptive
interoceptor
interofective
interoinferior
interolivary
interorbital
interosseous
interpalpebral
interparietal bone
interparietal suture
interparoxysmal
interpeduncular
interpelviabdominal
  amputation
interpersonal
interphalangeal
interphalangeal
  arthroplasty
interphalangeal
  arthrotomy
interphalangeal articular
  fracture
interphalangeal joint
interphalangeal
  synovectomy
interphalangeal tenodesis
interphase
interpolar
interpolar path
interpolation
interposed
interposition
interpretation
interproximal
interproximal space
interpubic
interpupillary

interpupillary distance
interpupillary line (IPL)
interradicular
interradicular bone
interradicular fibers
interrenal
interruption
interscapilium
interscapular
interscapular reflex
interscapulum
intersection
intersegmental
intersex
intersex surgery
intersexuality
interspace
interspinal
interstice
interstitial
interstitial cell
  stimulating hormone
  (ICSH)
interstitial cells of
  testes
interstitial cystitis
interstitial fluid
interstitial fluid
  pressure monitoring
interstitial lung
  disorders (ILD)
interstitial radioactive
  colloid therapy
interstitial radioelement
  application
interstitial tissue
interstitium
intersystole
intertarsal
intertarsal arthrotomy
intertarsal synovectomy
interthoracoscapular
  amputation
intertransverse
intertriginous
intertrigo
intertrochanteric

intertrochanteric bone
  graft
intertrochanteric line
intertrochanteric
  osteotomy
intertubular
interureteral
interureteric
intervaginal
interval, A-V
interval, atriocarotid
interval, cardioarterial
interval, focal
interval, isometric
interval, lucid
interval, P-R
interval, passive
interval, postsphygmic
interval, presphygmic
interval, Q-R
interval, Q-T
interval, QRS
interval, QRST
intervalvular
intervascular
intervention
intervention, crisis
intervention, nursing
interventricular
interventricular septal
  defect (IVSD)
intervertebral
intervertebral disk (IVD)
intervillous
intestinal
intestinal adhesion
intestinal anastomosis
intestinal bypass
intestinal bypass surgery
intestinal cutaneous
  fistula
intestinal endoscopy
intestinal feeding tube
intestinal flora
intestinal gases
intestinal juice
intestinal perforation
intestinal plication

intestinal putrefaction
intestinal reflex
intestinal transplant
intestinal tubes
intestine
intestine, large
intestine, small
intestinum
intestinum crassum
intestinum rectum
intestinum tenue
intima
intimal
intimitis
intolerance
intorsion
intoxicant
intoxication
intra vitam
intra-abdominal
intra-abdominal A-V
  fistula repair
intra-acinous
intra-amniotic injection
  (saline)
intra-amniotic injection,
  abortion
intra-aortic balloon
intra-aortic balloon
  catheter
intra-aortic balloon
  counterpulsation (IABC)
intra-aortic balloon pump
  (IABP)
intra-arterial
intra-arterial
  embolization
intra-articular
intra-atrial
intra-atrial pacing
intrabronchial
intrabuccal
intracanalicular
intracapsular
intracapsular cataract
  extraction (ICCE)
intracapsular fracture
intracapsular lens

intracardiac
intracardiac
  phonocardiogram
intracarpal
intracartilaginous
intracavitary
intracellular
intracerebellar
intracerebral
intracervical
intracisternal
intracostal
intracranial
intracranial abscess
intracranial
  electrothrombosis
intracranial hematoma
intracranial
  microdissection
intractable
intracutaneous
intracutaneous injection
intracutaneous test
intracystic
intrad
intradermal (ID)
intradermal reaction
intraduct
intraduodenal
intradural
intraepidermal
intraepithelial
intrafebrile
intrafilar
intragastric
intragastric balloon
intragemmal
intraglandular
intragyral
intrahepatic
intraintestinal
intralaryngeal
intralesional
intraligamentary
intraligamentous
intralingual
intralobar
intralobular

intralocular
intralumbar
intraluminal
intramastoiditis
intramedullary
intramedullary cyst
intramural
intramuscular
intranasal
intranasal biopsy
intranasal choanal
  atresia repair
intranasal ethmoidectomy
intranasal reconstruction
intranasal sinusotomy
intranasal synechia lysis
intraocular
intraocular foreign body
  removal
intraocular lens
  prosthesis
intraocular pressure
  (IOP)
intraoperative
intraoperative echography
intraoral
intraoral abscess
intraoral abscess, cyst
intraoral drainage
intraoral
  sialolithotomy
intraorbital
intraosseous
intraosseous venography
intraovarian
intraovular amnioscopy
intraparietal
intrapartum
intrapelvic
intrapelvic hip joint
  denervation
intrapelvic transection
intraperitoneal (IP)
intraperitoneal cannula
intraplacental
intrapleural
intrapontine
intrapsychic

intrapsychical
intrapulmonary
intrapyretic
intrarectal
intrarenal
intraretinal
intrascrotal
intraspinal
intratemporal facial
  nerve
intratendinous calcareous
  deposits
intrathecal
intrathecal
  chemotherapeutic agent
  injection
intrathoracic
intrathoracic A-V fistula
  repair
intrathoracic
  tracheoplasty
intratracheal
intratracheal anesthesia
intratubal
intratympanic
intrauterine
intrauterine device (IUD)
intrauterine transfusion
intravasation
intravascular
intravascular device
intravascular occlusion
intravascular
  radionuclide therapy
intravenous
intravenous feeding
intravenous gamma
  globulin (IGIV)
intravenous infusion
intravenous infusion pump
intravenous medication
intravenous pyelogram
  (IVP)
intravenous pyelography
  (IVP)
intravenous therapy
intravenous treatment
intravenous urogram (IVU)

intravenous urography
  (IVU)
intraventricular
intraventricular pacing
intravesical
intravesical lesion
intravital
intravital stain
intravitelline
intravitreous
intrinsic
intrinsic factor
intrinsic muscles
introducer
introflexion
introitus
introitus canalis
  sacralis
introitus laryngis
introitus vaginae
introjection
intromission
intromittent
Intron A (interferon
  alfa-2b [recombinant])
introns
Intropin (dopamine HCl)
introspection
introsusception
introversion
introvert
intubate
intubated ureterotomy
intubation
intubator
intuition
intumesce
intumescence
intumescent
intussusception
intussusceptum
intussuscipiens
Inuit
inulase
inulin
inunction
inustion
invaginate

invaginated
invagination
invalid
invasion
invasive
invasive procedure
invermination
inverse-square law
Inversine (mecamylamine HCl)
inversion
inversion, uterine
invert
invert sugar
invertase
invertebrate
invertin
invertor
investing
investment
inveterate
inviscation
involucre
involucrum
involuntary
involution
involution of uterus
involution, senile
involution, sexual
involutional
involutional melancholia
iocetamic acid
Iodamoeba
Iodamoeba bütschlii
iodate sodium
iodide
iodide, cesium
iodinate
iodine (I)
iodine poisoning
iodine, protein-bound
iodine, radioactive
iodine, tincture of
iodinophilous
iodipamide meglumine injection
iodism
iodize

iodized
iodized salt
iododerma
iodoform
iodoformism
iodoglobulin
iodophilia
iodophor
iodopyracet
iodoquinol
iodotherapy
ion
ion, dipolar
ion, hydrogen
ion-exchange resins
Ionamin (phentermine resin)
ionic
ionic medication
Ionil (antiseborrheic treatment shampoo)
Ionil Plus
Ionil T (antiseborrheic tar shampoo)
Ionil T Plus
ionium (Io)
ionization
ionization chamber
ionize
ionizing radiation
ionogen
ionometer
ionotherapy
iontophoresis
iontophoretic sweat test
iontoquantimeter
iontoradiometer
iontotherapy
iopanoic acid
iophendylate
iophobia
iotacism
iothalamate meglumine injection
ipecac
ipecac syrup
ipodate calcium
ipratropium bromide

iproniazid
ipsilateral
iralgia
irascible
Ircon-FA (folic acid and
  ferrous fumarate)
iridadenosis
iridal
iridalgia
iridauxesis
iridectome
iridectomesodialysis
iridectomize
iridectomy
iridectomy, optical
iridectropium
iridemia
iridencleisis
iridentropium
irideremia
irides
iridescence
iridesis
iridic
iridis, rubeosis
iridium (Ir)
iridium-192
iridoavulsion
iridocapsulitis
iridocapsulotomy
iridocele
iridochorioiditis
iridochoroiditis
iridocoloboma
iridoconstrictor
iridocyclectomy
iridocyclitis
iridocyclitis,
  heterochromic
iridocyclochoroiditis
iridocystectomy
iridodesis
iridodiagnosis
iridodialysis
iridodilator
iridodonesis
iridokeratitis
iridokinesis

iridoleptynsis
iridology
iridomalacia
iridomedialysis
iridomesodialysis
iridomotor
iridoncus
iridoparalysis
iridoparelkysis
iridopathy
iridoperiphacitis
iridoperiphakitis
iridoplegia
iridoplegia,
  accommodative
iridoplegia, complete
iridoplegia, reflex
iridoptosis
iridopupillary
iridorrhexis
iridoschisis
iridosclerotomy
iridosteresis
iridotasis
iridotomy
iris
iris bombe
iris, chromatic asymmetry
  of
iris, piebald
Irish moss
irisopsia
iritic
iritis
iritis, plastic
iritis, primary
iritis, purulent
iritis, secondary
iritis, serous
iritoectomy
iritomy
Iromin-G (hematinic
  supplement)
iron (Fe)
iron dextran injection
iron poisoning
iron sorbitex injection
iron storage disease

iron-binding capacity
  (IBC)
iron-deficiency anemia
irotomy
irradiate
irradiating
irradiation
irrational
irreducible
irrelevance
irrespirable
irreversible
irrigate
irrigation
irrigation, bladder
irrigation, colonic
irrigator
irritability
irritability, muscular
irritability, nervous
irritable
irritable bowel syndrome
  (IBS)
irritant
irritant poisons
irritation
irritative
ischemia
ischemia, intestinal
ischemia, myocardial
ischemic heart disease
  (IHD)
ischemic limb exercise
  test
ischesis
ischia
ischiac
ischiadic
ischial
ischial bursa
ischial fracture
ischial pressure ulcer
ischial ramus
ischial tuberosity
ischialgia
ischiatic
ischiatitis
ischidrosis

ischiectomy
ischioanal
ischiobulbar
ischiocapsular
ischiocavernosus
ischiocele
ischiococcygeus
ischiodynia
ischiofemoral
ischiofibular
ischiohebotomy
ischioneuralgia
ischionitis
ischiopubic
ischiopubiotomy
ischiorectal
ischiorectal abscess
ischiosacral
ischiovaginal
ischium
ischogalactic
ischuretic
ischuria
iseikonia
ishihara
  pseudoisochromatic
  plates
isinglass
island, blood
island of Reil
island, pancreatic
islands of Calleja
islands of Langerhans
islet
islets of Calleja
islets of Langerhans
islets, Walthard's
Ismelin (guanethidine
  monosulfate)
Iso-B (B-complex)
Iso-Bid (isosorbide
  dinitrate)
isoagglutination
isoagglutinin
isoagglutinogen
isoanaphylaxis
isoantibody

isoantigen
isobar
isobaric
isobucaine hydrochloride
Isocal (complete liquid
diet tube-feeding
formulation)
isocarboxazid
isocellular
isochromatic
isochromatophil
isochromatophile
isochromosome
isochronal
isochronia
isochronous
isochroous
isocitrate dehydrogenase
(IDH)
Isoclor (chlorpheniramine
maleate and
pseudoephedrine HCl)
isocolloid
Isocom
isocomplement
isocoria
isocortex
isocytosis
isocytotoxin
isodactylism
isodiametric
isodontic
isodose
isodose calculation
isodose plan
isodynamic
isoelectric
isoelectric period
isoelectric point (IP)
isoenergetic
isoenzyme
isoetharine hydrochloride
isogamete
isogamy
isogeneic
isogeneric
isogenesis
isogenic

isograft
isohemagglutination
isohemagglutinin
isohemolysin
isohemolysis
isohypercytosis
isohypocytosis
isoiconia
isoiconic
isoimmunization
isokinetic exercise
isolate
isolation
isolation, infectious
isolation, protective
isolation, reverse
isoleucine
isologous
isolophobia
isolysin
isolysis
isolytic
isomer
isomerase
isomerase, phosphohexose
isomeric
isomerism
isomerization
isometric
isometric contraction
isometric exercise
isometric muscle
isometropia
Isomil (soy protein
formula with iron)
Isomil SF (sucrose-free
soy protein formula
with iron)
isomorphism
isomorphous
isoniazid (INH)
isonicotinoylhydrazine
isonormocytosis
isopathy
isophoria
isopia
isoplastic

isoprecipitin
isopropamide iodide
isopropanol
isopropyl alcohol
isoproterenol
  hydrochloride
isopters
Isoptin (verapamil HCl)
isopyknosis
Isordil (isosorbide
  dinitrate)
isoserotherapy
isoserum
isosexual
isosmotic
isosorbide dinitrate
Isospora
Isospora hominis
isospore
isosthenuria
isostimulation
isotherapy
isothermal
isothermognosis
isotherms
isotones
isotonia
isotonic
isotonic exercise
isotonic solution
isotonicity
isotope
isotope cisternography
Isotrate Timecelles
  (isosorbide dinitrate)
isotretinoin
isotropic
isotropy
isotypes
isotypical
isovalericacidemia
Isovex (ethaverine HCl)
isoxsuprine hydrochloride
isozyme
issue
isthmectomy
isthmian
isthmitis

isthmoparalysis
isthmoplegia
isthmus
isthmus, aortic
isthmus faucium
isthmus glandulae
  thyroideae
isthmus of eustachian
  tube
isthmus of thyroid
isthmus of uterine tube
isthmus, pharyngeal
isthmus pharyngonasalis
isthmus, thyroid
isthmus tubae auditivae
isthmus tubae uterinae
isthmus, uteri
Isuprel (isoproterenol
  HCl)
isuria
itch
itch, baker's
itch, barber's
itch, dhobie
itch, grain
itch, grocer's
itch, ground
itch, jock
itch mite
itch, seven-year
itch, swimmer's
itch, winter
itching
iteral
iteroparity
ithycyphosis
ithylordosis
ithyokyphosis
ivermectin
Ivy method
ivy poisoning
Ixodes
ixodiasis
ixodic
Ixodidae
Ixodides
Ixodoidea
ixomyelitis

J

Jaboulay's amputation
Jaboulay's button
Jaboulay's operation
jacket, porcelain
jacket, Risser
  application
jacket, Sayre's
jacket, strait
jacket, turnbuckle
  application
jackknife position
jackscrew
jacksonian epilepsy
Jacob, Arthur
Jacob's membrane
Jacob's ulcer
Jacobson, Ludwig
Jacobson's cartilage
Jacobson's nerve
Jacobson's organ
Jacobson's sulcus
Jacquemier's sign
jactatio
jactitation
Jaeger's test types
jamais vu
James fibers
Janeway lesions
Janeway operation
janiceps
Jansky-Bielschowsky
  syndrome
jar, bell
jar, heel
jargon
Jarvis' snare
Jatene operation
jaundice
jaundice, acholuric
jaundice, cholestatic
jaundice, congenital
jaundice, hematogenous

jaundice, hemolytic
jaundice, hemorrhagic
jaundice,
  hepatocanalicular
jaundice, hepatocellular
jaundice, hepatogenous
jaundice, infectious
jaundice, leptospiral
jaundice, malignant
jaundice, nonhemolytic
jaundice, obstructive
jaundice of newborn
jaundice, parenchymatous
jaundice, physiologic
jaundice, posthepatic
jaundice, regurgitation
jaundice, retention
jaundice, spirochetal
jaundice, toxic
Javelle water
jaw
jaw, cleft
jaw, crackling
jaw, dislocation of
jaw, lumpy
jaw, swelling of
jaw winking
jejunal
jejunectomy
jejunitis
jejunocecostomy
jejunocholecystostomy
jejunocolostomy
jejunoileal
jejunoileitis
jejunoileostomy
jejunojejunostomy
jejunopexy
jejunorrhaphy
jejunostomy
jejunotomy
jejunum
jelly
jelly, contraceptive
jelly, mineral
jelly, petroleum
jelly, vaginal
jelly, Wharton's

Jendrassik's maneuver
Jenner, Edward
Jenner's stain
jerk
jerk, Achilles
jerk, ankle
jerk, biceps
jerk, elbow
jerk, jaw
jerk, knee
jerk, tendon
jerk, triceps surae
jet lag
jigger
jimson weed
jitters
jiujitsu
Jobst pressure garment
Jocasta complex
Joffroy's reflex
Joffroy's sign
jogger's heel
jogging
Johannsen urethroplasty
Johanson operation
joint (jt)
joint, amphidiarthrodial
joint approximation
joint, arthrodial
joint, ball-and-socket
joint, biaxial
joint, bilocular
joint, bleeders'
joint, Brodie's
joint, Budin's
joint capsule
joint, cartilaginous
joint cavity
joint, Charcot's
joint, Chopart's
joint, cochlear
joint, compound
joint, condyloid
joint, diarthrodial
joint, dry
joint, ellipsoid
joint, enarthrodial
joint, false

joint, flail
joint fluid
joint, ginglymoid
joint, gliding
joint, hemophilic
joint, hinge
joint, hip
joint imaging
joint, immovable
joint, irritable
joint, knee
joint mice
joint, midcarpal
joint, mixed
joint, movable
joint, multiaxial
joint, pivot
joint, plane
joint, polyaxial
joint protection
joint, receptive
joint, rotary
joint, saddle
joint, simple
joint, spheroid
joint, spiral
joint, sternoclavicular
joint survey
joint, synarthrodial
joint, synovial
joint, trochoid
joint, uniaxial
joint, unilocular
joint's craniomandibular
joint's fibrous
joint's intercarpal
joint's subtalar
joint's tarsometatarsal
joint's temporomandibular
Jones criteria
Jones operation
Jones procedure
Joplin exostectomy
Joplin operation
joule (J)
jugal
jugal bone
jugal process

jugale
jugate
jugomaxillary
jugular
jugular catheterization
jugular foramen
jugular fossa
jugular ganglion
jugular node dissection
jugular phonocardiogram
jugular process
jugular vein ligation
jugular veins
jugular venipuncture
jugular venography
jugular venous pulse
  (JVP)
jugulate
jugulation
jugulum
jugum
jugum penis
jugum petrosum
juice, alimentary
juice, gastric
juice, intestinal
juice, pancreatic
jujitsu
jumentous
Jumping Frenchmen of
  Maine
junction
junction, amelodentinal
junction, cementodentinal
junction, cementoenamel
junction, dentinocemental
junction, dentinoenamel
junction, dentogingival
junction, interneuronal
junction, mucocutaneous
junction, mucogingival
junction, myoneural
junction, sclerocorneal
junction, squamocolumnar
junction, tight
junctional epithelium
junctura
juniper tar

junket
jurisprudence
jury-mast
jusculum
Juster's reflex
justo major
justo minor
jute
juvenile
juvenile cell
juvenile rheumatoid
  arthritis (JRA)
juvenile warts
juxta-articular
juxtaglomerular
juxtaglomerular apparatus
juxtaglomerular cells
juxtangina
juxtaposition
juxtapyloric
juxtaspinal

K

K^+ 10 (potassium
  chloride)
K^+ Care (potassium
  chloride)
K^+ Care ET (potassium
  bicarbonate)
K-Dur (potassium
  chloride)
K-Lor (potassium
  chloride)
K-Lyte (potassium as
  bicarbonate and
  citrate)
K-Norm (potassium
  chloride)
K-Phos M.F. (potassium
  and sodium acid
  phosphates, anhydrous)
K-Phos Neutral
  (phosphorus, sodium,
  potassium)

K-Tab (potassium
  chloride)
Kabikinase
  (streptokinase)
Kader's operation
kaif
kainophobia
kaiserling
kakidrosis
kakke
kakosmia
kakotrophy
kala-azar
kaliemia
kaligenous
kalimeter
kaliopenia
kalium (K)
kaliuresis
kallidin
kallikrein
kallikreinogen
kanamycin
kanamycin sulfate
Kantrex (kanamycin
  sulfate)
Kanulase
Kaochlor (potassium
  chloride)
kaolin
kaolinosis
Kaon Cl-10 (potassium
  chloride)
Kaon Elixir (potassium
  gluconate)
Kaopectate (anti-diarrhea
  medicine)
Kaopectate Concentrate
  (anti-diarrhea
  medicine)
Kaposi, Moritz K.
Kaposi's disease
Kaposi's sarcoma
Kaposi's varicelliform
  eruption
kappa (K)

Kapseals/Capsules
  Chloromycetin
  (chloramphenicol)
karaya gum
Karman catheter
Karnofsky Index
Karnofsky Scale
Kartagener's syndrome
karyochromatophil
karyochrome
karyoclasis
karyocyte
karyogamy
karyogenesis
karyokinetic
karyoklasis
karyolobism
karyolymph
karyolysis
karyolytic
karyomegaly
karyomere
karyomicrosome
karyomitome
karyomitosis
karyomorphism
karyophage
karyoplasm
karyopyknosis
karyorrhexis
karyosome
karyostasis
karyotheca
karyotype
karyotyping chromosome
  analysis
karyozoic
Kasabach-Merritt syndrome
Kasai procedure
Kashin-Beck disease
Kasof (stool softener)
katabolism
kataplasia
katathermometer
katatonia
kathisophobia

kation
KATO (potassium chloride)
katophoria
katotropia
katzenjammer
Kaufman operation
kava
Kawasaki disease
Kay Ciel (potassium
  chloride)
Kayser-Fleischer ring
Kazanjiian operation
keel insertion,
  laryngoplasty
kefir
Keflex (cephalexin)
Kefurox (cefuroxime
  sodium)
kefyr
Kefzol (cefazolin sodium)
Kegel exercises
Keith's bundle, node
Keith-Flack node
Keith-Wagener-Barker
  classification
Kelikian webbing
  operation
kelis
Kell blood group
Keller operation
Kelly operation
Kelly urethral plication
Kelly's pad
Kelly-Stoeckel operation
keloid
keloid, acne
keloidosis
kelotomy
kelp
Kelvin scale
Kemadrin (procyclidine
  HCl)
Kempner rice-fuit diet
Kenalog (triamcinolone
  acetonide)
Kenalog in Orabase
  (triamcinolone
  acetonide dental paste)

Kenny treatment
kenophobia
kenotoxin
Kent's bundles
keoplastic
Keralyt Gel (salicylic
  acid)
kerasin
keratalgia
keratectasia
keratectomy
keratiasis
keratic
keratin
keratin, hard
keratin, soft
keratinase
keratinization
keratinize
keratinocyte
keratinous
keratitic precipitates
keratitis
keratitis, band-shaped
keratitis bullosa
keratitis, deep
keratitis, dendritic
keratitis disciformis
keratitis, fascicular
keratitis, herpetic
keratitis, hypopyon
keratitis, interstitial
keratitis, lagophthalmic
keratitis, mycotic
keratitis, neuroparalytic
keratitis, parenchymatous
keratitis, phlyctenular
keratitis, punctate
keratitis, purulent
keratitis, sclerosing
keratitis, superficial
  punctate
keratitis, trachomatous
keratitis, traumatic
keratitis, xerotic
keratoacanthoma
keratocele
keratocentesis

keratoconjunctivitis
keratoconjunctivitis,
   epidemic
keratoconjunctivitis,
   flash
keratoconjunctivitis,
   phlyctenular
keratoconjunctivitis
   sicca
keratoconjunctivitis,
   virus
keratoconus
keratocyte
keratoderma
keratoderma
   blennorrhagica
keratoderma climactericum
keratodermatitis
keratodermia
keratogenous
keratoglobus
keratohelcosis
keratohemia
keratohyalin
keratoid
keratoiditis
keratoiritis
keratoleptynsis
keratoleukoma
keratolysis
keratolytic
keratoma
keratomalacia
keratome
keratometer
keratometry
keratomileusis
keratomycosis
keratonosis
keratonyxis
keratopathy, band
keratophakia
keratoplasty
keratoplasty (corneal
   transplant)
keratoplasty, optic
keratoplasty, refractive
keratoplasty, tectonic

keratoprosthesis
keratoprotein
keratorrhexis
keratoscope
keratoscopy
keratose
keratosis
keratosis, actinic
keratosis climactericum
keratosis follicularis
keratosis nigrican
keratosis, oral
keratosis palmaris et
   plantaris
keratosis pharyngis
keratosis pilaris
keratosis punctata
keratosis, seborrheic
keratosis senilis
keratotome
keratotomy
keratotomy, radical
keraunoneurosis
keraunophobia
Kerckring's folds
kerectomy
kerion
Kerley lines
kernicterus
Kernig's sign
Kerodex (skin barrier
   cream)
kerosene
Kerr operation
Kessler operation
Ketalar (ketamine HCl)
ketamine hydrochloride
keto acid
ketoacidosis
ketoaciduria
ketogenesis
ketogenic diet
ketogenic steroids
ketohexose
ketolysis
ketolytic
ketone

ketone bodies (acetone, urine) test
ketone bodies (KB)
ketone threshold
ketonemia
ketonuria
ketoplasia
ketose
ketosis
ketosteroids
17-ketosteroids (17-KS) test
ketosuria
ketotic
Key-Retzius foramina
kibe
Kidner operation
Kidnet advancement
kidney
kidney, amyloid
kidney, artificial
kidney, cake
kidney, contracted
kidney, cystic
kidney, embolic contracted
kidney failure
kidney, fatty
kidney, flea-bitten
kidney, floating
kidney function study
kidney, fused
kidney, Goldblatt
kidney, granular
kidney heterophile antibodies
kidney, horseshoe
kidney, hypermobile
kidney imaging
kidney, lardaceous
kidney, lump
kidney, movable
kidney, polycystic
kidney, red contracted
kidney, sacculated
kidney, sponge
kidney stone
kidney, syphilitic

kidney, ureter, and bladder (KUB)
kidney vascular flow
kidney, wandering
kidney, waxy
Kienböck's disease
Kiernan's spaces
Kiesselbach's plexus
Kilian's pelvis
Killian operation
kilocalorie (C;kcal)
kilocycle (kc)
kiloelectron volts (keV)
kilogram (kg)
kilogram-meter (kg-m)
kilohertz (kHz)
kilojoule (kJ)
kilomegacycle (kMc)
kilomegacycles
kilometer (km)
kilopascal (kPa)
kilounit
kilovolt (kV)
kilovoltage peak
kilowatt (kW)
Kimmelstiel-Wilson syndrome
kinanesthesia
kinase
kinase, pyruvic
kinematics
kinematograph
kineplastic
kineplasty
kinesalgia
kinescope
Kinesed (belladonna alkaloids and phenobarbital)
kinesia
kinesialgia
kinesiatrics
kinesics
kinesimeter
kinesiodic
kinesiology
kinesioneurosis
kinesiotherapy

kinesis
kinesitherapy
kinesodic
kinesthesia
kinesthesiometer
kinesthetic
kinetic
kinetic energy (KE)
kinetic perimetry
kinetics
kinetocardiogram (KCG)
kinetocardiography
kinetosis
kinetotherapy
King-Steelquist operation
kingdom
kinin
kininases, plasma
kininogen
kink
kinky hair disease
kinocilium
kinomometer
kinship
kiotome
kiotomy
Kirk operation
Kirschner's wire
Kisch's reflex
kitasamycin
Kite apparatus
Klebs-Loeffler bacillus
Klebsiella
Klebsiella ozaenae
Klebsiella pneumoniae
Klebsiella rhinoscleromatis
Kleihauer hemoglobin
kleptolagnia
kleptomania
kleptomaniac
kleptophobia
Klieg eye
Klinefelter's syndrome
Klippel's disease
Klippel-Feil syndrome
Klonopin (clonazepam)

Klor-Con (potassium chloride)
Klorvess 10% Liquid (potassium chloride)
Klorvess Effervescent Granules (potassium chloride)
Klotrix (potassium chloride)
Klumpke's paralysis
Klüver-Bucy syndrome
Knapp's forceps
kneading
knee
knee, Brodie's
knee, dislocation of
knee, game
knee, housemaid's
knee of internal capsule
knee jerk (KJ)
knee joint
knee kick (KK)
knee, knock-
knee, locked
knee-chest position
knee-jerk reflex
kneecap
Kneipp cure
kneippism
knemometry
knife
knife, electric
knife, gold
knife, interdental
knife, periodontal
knife, plaster
knismogenic
knitting
knob
knock-knee
knock-knee osteotomy
knot
knot, false
knot, granny
knot, Hensen's
knot, primitive
knot, square

knot, surgical
knot, syncytial
knot, true
knuckle
knuckle pads
Koate-HS (factor VIII, AHF, AHG)
Koate-HT (factor VIII, AHF, AHG)
Koch, Robert
Koch, Walter
Koch's bacillus
Koch's law
Koch's node
Koch's phenomenon
Koch's postulates
Kocher's reflex
kocherization
Koebner phenomenon
Köhler's disease
Kohlrausch's fold
Kohnstamm's phenomenon
koilocyte
koilocytotic atypia
koilonychia
koilorrhachic
Kolantyl (wafers and gel)
kolpitis
kolypeptic
Komed Acne Lotion (sodium thiosulfate, salicylic acid, alcohol)
Komex (scrub for oily skin and make-up removal)
Konakion (phytonadione)
Kondoleon's operation
koniocortex
koniology
koniometer
koniosis
Konsyl (psyllium hydrophilic mucilloid)
Konsyl-D (psyllium hydrophilic mucilloid with dextrose)
Konyne-HT (factor IX)
kopf-tetanus

kophemia
Koplik's spots
kopophobia
Korányi's sign
koro
Koro-Flex (arcing spring diaphragm)
Koromex (coil spring diaphragm)
koronion
Korotkoff's sounds
Korotkoff's syndrome
kosher
koumiss
Krabbe's disease
Kraepelin's classification
krait
Kraske proctectomy
kraurosis
kraurosis penis
kraurosis vulvae
Krause, Karl
Krause operation
Krause, Wilhelm
Krause's bulbs
Krause's end bulbs
Krause's glands
Krause's membrane
Krause's valve
Krebs cycle
Kristeller maneuver
Kroener operation
Kroenlein operation
Kroenlein orbitotomy
Krönig operation
Krönig's area
Krukenberg operation
Krukenberg's chopsticks
Krukenberg's tumor
krypton (Kr)
Ku-Zyme (amylase, protease, lipase, cellulase)
Ku-Zyme HP (pancrelipase [lipase, protease, amylase])
kubisagari

Kudrox
Kufs' disease
Kugelberg-Welander
  disease
Kuhnt-Szymanowski
  blepharoplasty
Kuhnt-Szymanowski
  operation
kumiss
Kümmell's disease
Kümmell's spondylitis
kumyss
Kupffer's cells
kuru
Kussmaul, Adolph
Kussmaul's breathing
Kussmaul's disease
Kutrase (digestive
  enzymes)
kwashiorkor
Kwelcof (hydrocodone
  bitartrate and
  guaifenesin)
Kwell (lindane)
Kyasanur Forest disease
kyestein
kyllosis
kymatism
kymogram
kymograph
kymography
kymoscope
kynocephalus
kynurenic acid
kynurenine
kyogenic
kyphorachitis
kyphos
kyphoscoliosis
kyphosis
kyphotic
kyrtorrhachic
kysthitis
kysthoptosis

L

L-Carnitine (crystalline
  L-carnitine)
L-forms
L-phase variants
la belle indifference
la grippe
La Leche League
lab
Labbé operation
Labbé's vein
labeling
labia
labia majora
labia minora
labial
labial frenum
labial glands
labial graft
labialism
labieotomy
labile
lability, emotional
labile, heat
labioalveolar
labiocervical
labiochorea
labioclination
labiodental
labiogingival
labioglossolaryngeal
labioglossopharyngeal
labiograph
labiomental
labiomycosis
labionasal
labiopalatine
labioplasty

labiotenaculum
labioversion
labium
labium cerebri
labium inferius oris
labium majus
labium minus
labium minus pudendi
labium oris
labium superius oris
labium tympanicum
labium urethrae
labium uteri
labium vestibulare
labor
labor, active
labor and delivery (L&D)
labor, arrested
labor, artificial
labor, complicated
labor, dry
labor, false
labor, induction of
labor, instrumental
labor, missed
labor, normal
labor, precipitate
labor, premature
labor, spontaneous
labor, trial of
laboratory (lab)
Laborde's method
labret
labrocyte
labrum
labyrinth
labyrinth, bony
labyrinth, ethmoidal
labyrinth, membranous
labyrinth, olfactory
labyrinth, osseous
labyrinthectomy
labyrinthine
labyrinthitis
labyrinthotomy
labyrinthus
lac

Lac-hydrin (ammonium
  lactate)
lacerable
lacerate
lacerated
laceration
laceration of cervix
laceration of perineum
laceration repair
lacertus
lacertus cordis
lacertus fibrosus
laciniate
lacrima
lacrimal
lacrimal apparatus
lacrimal bone
lacrimal canaliculi
lacrimal duct
lacrimal fistula
lacrimal flow study
lacrimal gland
lacrimal punctum
lacrimal reflex
lacrimal sac
lacrimation
lacrimator
lacrimatory
lacrimonasal
lacrimotome
lacrimotomy
Lacrisert (hydroxypropyl
  cellulose ophthalmic
  insert)
lactacid
lactacidemia
lactaciduria
lactagogue
Lactaid (lactase enzyme)
lactalbumin
lactam
lactase
lactase deficiency
  syndrome
lactase deficiency test
lactate
lactate dehydrogenase

lactation
lacteal
lactenin
lactescence
lactic
lactic acid
lactic acid fermentation
lactic acidosis (LA)
lactic dehydrogenase
  (LDH)
Lacticare-HC Lotion
  (hydrocortisone)
lacticemia
lactiferous
lactiferous ducts
lactiferous glands
lactification
lactifuge
lactigenous
lactigerous
lactinated
Lactisol-C&M
lactivorous
Lactobacillus
Lactobacillus acidophilus
Lactobacillus bulgaricus
Lactobacillus casei
Lactobacillus helveticus
lactobutyrometer
Lactocal-F (multivitamin)
lactocele
lactochrome
lactocrit
lactodensimeter
lactoflavin
lactogen
lactogenic
lactogenic hormone (LTH)
lactoglobulin
lactoglobulins, immune
lactometer
lacto-ovovegetarian
lactophosphate
lactoprotein
lactorrhea
lactose
lactose intolerance
lactose tolerance test

lactoserum
lactosuria
lactotherapy
lactotoxin
lactovegetarin
Lactrase (lactase enzyme)
lactulose
lacuna
lacuna, absorption
lacuna, blood
lacuna, bone
lacuna, Howship's
lacuna, intervillous
lacuna laterales
lacuna magna
lacuna of the urethra
lacuna pharyngis
lacuna, trophoblastic
lacuna vasorum
lacuna, venous
lacunae
lacunar
lacunar disease
lacunes
lacunula
lacunule
lacus
lacus lacrimalis
Ladd operation
Laënnec's cirrhosis
Laënnec's pearls
Laënnec's thrombus
Lafora, Gonzalo R.
Lafora's bodies
lag
lag phase
lageniform
lagophthalmos
lagophthalmus
Lagrange operation
laity
lake
laked
laking
laliatry
lallation
lalognosis
lalopathology

lalopathy
lalophobia
laloplegia
lalorrhea
Lamarck's theory
Lamaze technique
lambda
lambdacism
lambdoid
lambdoid suture
lambdoidal
lambert
Lamblia intestinalis
lambliasis
Lambrinudi operation
lame
lamella
lamella, bone
lamella, circumferential
lamella, concentric
lamella, enamel
lamella, ground
lamella, haversian
lamella, interstitial
lamella, medullary
lamella, periosteal
lamella, triangular
lamella, vitreous
lamellar
lamellar excision
lamellar keratoplasty
lameness
lamina
lamina, alar
lamina, anterior elastic
lamina, basal
lamina basalis choroideae
lamina, Bowman's
lamina cartilaginis
  cricoideae
lamina chorioidcapillaris
lamina cribrosa
lamina cribrosa sclerae
lamina, dental
lamina dura
lamina, epithelial
lamina fusca sclerae

lamina, interpubic
  fibrocartilaginous
lamina, labial
lamina, medullary,
  internal
lamina multiformis
lamina of vertebral arch
lamina papyracea
lamina perpendicular
lamina propria mucosae
lamina pterygoid
lamina, rostral
lamina suprachoroidea
lamina, terminal
lamina, vestibular
lamina vitrea
lamina zonalis
laminae
laminagram
laminagraph
laminagraphy
laminar air flow
Laminaria digitata
laminaria insertion
laminarin
laminated
lamination
laminectomy
laminitis
laminograph
laminography
laminotomy
lamp, Gullstrand's
lamp, infrared
lamp, slit
lamp, sun
lamp, ultraviolet
Lamprene (clofazimine)
lamprophonia
lamprophonic
lana
lanatoside C
lance
Lancefield classification
lancet
lancinating
landmark
landmark, bony

landmark, cephalometric
landmark, craniometric
landmark, orbital
landmark, radiographic
landmark, soft tissue
Landouzy-Déjérine atrophy
Landry's paralysis
Landsteiner's
  classification
Lane's kinks
Lange's test
Langenbeck operation
Langer's lines
Langer's muscle
Langerhans' islands
Langhans' layer
languor
laniary
Laniazid Syrup (isoniazid
  syrup)
lanolin
lanolin, anhydrous
Lanoxicaps (digoxin)
Lanoxin (digoxin)
lanthanum (La)
lanuginous
lanugo
Laora's disease
lap board
laparectomy
laparoamnioscopy
laparocele
laparocholecystotomy
laparocolectomy
laparocolostomy
laparocolotomy
laparocystectomy
laparocystidotomy
laparocystotomy
laparoenterostomy
laparoenterotomy
laparogastroscopy
laparogastrostomy
laparogastrotomy
laparohepatotomy
laparohysterectomy
laparohystero-
  oophorectomy

laparohysteropexy
laparohysterosalpingo-
  oophorectomy
laparohysterotomy
laparoileotomy
laparomyitis
laparomyomectomy
laparonephrectomy
laparorrhaphy
laparosalpingectomy
laparosalpingo-
  oophorectomy
laparosalpingotomy
laparoscope
laparoscopy
laparosplenectomy
laparosplenotomy
laparotomy
laparotrachelotomy
laparotyphlotomy
Lapidus bunion correction
Lapidus operation
lapinization
lapis
lard
lard, benzoinated
lardaceous
large (lg)
Larobec (multivitamin)
Larodopa (levodopa)
Larry operation
larva
larva currens
larva migrans, cutaneous
larva migrans, visceral
larval
larvate
larvicide
larviphagic
larygnotomy, subhyoid or
  superior
larygoplegia
Larylgan Throat Spray
  (analgesic-like)
laryngalgia
laryngeal
laryngeal fracture

laryngeal function
  studies
laryngeal reflex
laryngeal reinnervation
laryngeal vertigo
laryngeal web
laryngectomee
laryngectomy
laryngemphraxis
laryngismal
laryngismus
laryngitic
laryngitis
laryngitis, acute
  catarrhal
laryngitis, chronic
laryngitis, croupous
laryngitis, diphtheritic
laryngitis, membranous
laryngitis, syphilitic
laryngitis, tuberculous
laryngocele
laryngocentesis
laryngoedema
laryngoesophagectomy
laryngofissure
laryngogram
laryngograph
laryngography
laryngologist
laryngology
laryngomalacia
laryngometry
laryngoparalysis
laryngopathy
laryngophantom
laryngopharyngeal
laryngopharyngectomy
laryngopharyngeus
laryngopharyngitis
laryngopharyngo-
  esophagectomy
laryngopharyngography
laryngopharynx
laryngophony
laryngophthisis
laryngoplasty
laryngoptosis

laryngorhinology
laryngorrhagia
laryngorrhaphy
laryngorrhea
laryngoscleroma
laryngoscope
laryngoscopic
laryngoscopist
laryngoscopy
laryngospasm
laryngostenosis
laryngostomy
laryngostroboscope
laryngotomy
laryngotomy, inferior
laryngotomy, median
laryngotracheal
laryngotracheitis
laryngotracheo-
  bronchoscopy
laryngotracheobronchitis
laryngotracheoscopy
laryngotracheostomy
laryngotracheotomy
laryngoxerosis
larynx
Lasan (anthralin)
lascivia
Lasègue's sign
laser
laser angioplasty
laser cane
laser surgery
Lash operation
Lasix (furosemide)
Lassa fever
lassitude
last menstrual period,
  (LMP)
last sacraments
latah
latency
latency period
latent
latent content
latent heat
latent hyperopia (Hl)
latent image

latent period
laterad
lateral (lat)
lateral sinus
lateralis
laterality
laterality, crossed
laterality, dominant
latericeous
lateritious
lateroabdominal
laterodeviation
lateroduction
lateroflexion
lateroposition
lateropulsion
laterosemiprone position
laterotorsion
lateroversion
latex
latex bead rapid test
lathyrism
lathyrogen
Latin (L)
Latino
latissimus
latitude
latrine
latrodectism
Latrodectus
Latrodectus mactans
lattice
latum
latus
Latzko operation
laudable
laudanum
laugh, sardonic
laughing gas
laughter, compulsive
laughter reflex
Laurence-Moon-Biedl
  syndrome
lavage
lavage, gastric
law, all-or-none
law, Avogadro's
law, Bell's

law, biogenetic
law, Boyle's
law, Charles'
law, Courvoisier's
law, Fechner's
law, Gay-Lussac's
law, Graham's
law, Haeckel's
law, Hilton's
law, Hooke's
law, Koch's
law, Marey's
law, Mariotte's
law, Murphy's
law, Nysten's
law of definite
  proportions
law of Magendie
law of mass action
law of multiple
  proportions
law of reciprocal
  proportions
law of the heart
law of the intestine
law, periodic
law, Sutton's
law, Waller's, of
  degeneration
law, Weber's
law, Wolff's
laws, Mendel's
laws, Rubner's
lawrencium (Lr)
lax
laxation
laxative
laxator
laxator tympani
layer
layer, ameloblastic
layer, bacillary
layer, basal
layer, blastodermic
layer, claustral
layer, clear
layer, columnar
layer, compact

layer, cuticular, of
  epithelium
layer, enamel
layer, ependymal
layer, ganglionic
layer, germ
layer, germinative
layer, granular exterior
layer, granular interior
layer, half-value
layer, Henle's
layer, horny
layer, Huxley's
layer, Langhans'
layer, malpighian
layer, mantle
layer, molecular
layer, nervous
layer, odontoblastic
layer, Ollier's
layer, osteogenetic
layer, outer nuclear
layer, papillary
layer, pigment
layer, prickle cell
layer, Purkinje
layer of pyramidal cells
layer of rods and cones
layer, reticular
layer, somatic
layer, spinous
layer, splanchnic
layer, spongy
layer, subendocardial
layer, subendothelial
layer, Tome's granular
layer, Weil's basal
layer, zonal, of
  hypothalamus
lazaretto
Lazerformalyde Solution
Lazersporin-C Solution
LDH isoenzyme test
LE cell prep
Le Fort operation
leachate
leaching
lead (Pb)

lead acetate
lead apron
lead, bipolar
lead colic
lead encephalopathy
lead, esophageal
lead level test
lead, limb
lead line
lead monoxide
lead pipe contraction
lead poisoning, acute
lead poisoning, chronic
lead, precordial
lead, unipolar
Leadbetter operation
Leadbetter-Politano
  operation
leads
leaf
leak, dural/CSF
lean
lean body mass
learning curve
learning disability
learning, latent
learning theory
Leber's disease
Leber's plexus
Leboyer method
Lecat's gulf
lechery
lecithal
lecithin
lecithin/sphingomyelin
  ratio (L/S)
lecithinase
lecithinase, cobra
lecithoprotein
lectin
lectual
Lee and White coagulation
  time
Lee's ganglion
leech
leech, artificial
lees
Leeuwenhoek's disease

Lefort I operation
Lefort II operation
Lefort III operation
left (L)
left anterior descending
  (LAD)
left atrium (LA)
left bundle branch block
  (LBBB)
left ear (AS)
left eye (OS)
left frontoanterior (LFA)
left frontoposterior
  (LFP)
left frontotransverse
  (LFT)
left lateral recumbent
  position
left lower extremity
  (LLE)
left lower lobe (LLL)
left lower quadrant (LLQ)
left lower sternal border
  (LLSB)
left mentoanterior (LMA)
left mentoposterior (LMP)
left mentotransverse
  (LMT)
left occipitoanterior
  (LOA)
left occipitoposterior
  (LOP)
left occipitotransverse
  (LOT)
left sacroanterior (LSA)
left sacroposterior (LSP)
left sacrotransverse
  (LST)
left scapuloanterior
  (LScA)
left scapuloposterior
  (LScP)
left upper extremity
  (LUE)
left upper quadrant (LUQ)
left ventricle (LV)
left-handedness
leg

leg, badger
leg, baker
leg, bandy
leg, Barbadoes
leg, bayonet
leg, bird
leg, boomerang
leg, bow
leg, milk
leg, restless
leg, scissor
leg, white
Legg's disease
Legg-Calvé-Perthes
  disease
leggings
Legionnaires' disease
legitimacy
legume
legumelin
legumin
Leiner's disease
leiodermia
leiomyofibroma
leiomyoma
leiomyoma, epithelioid
leiomyoma, uteri
leiomyosarcoma
leiotrichous
Leishman-Donovan bodies
Leishmania
Leishmania braziliensis
Leishmania donovani
Leishmania tropica
leishmaniasis
leishmaniasis, American
leishmaniasis, cutaneous
leishmaniasis, visceral
lema
LeMesurier operation
lemmocyte
lemniscus
lemon
lemoparalysis
lemostenosis
length (L)
length, basialveolar
length, basinasal

length, crown-heel
length, crown-rump
length, focal
length, wave
lengthening
lenitive
lens
lens, achromatic
lens, aplanatic
lens, apochromatic
lens, biconcave
lens, biconvex
lens, bifocal
lens, concave spherical
lens, contact
lens, convex spherical
lens, convexoconcave
lens, corneal contact
lens, crystalline
lens, cylindrical
lens, implanted
lens, omnifocal
lens, orthoscopic
lens, soft contact
lens, spherical
lens, trial
lens, trifocal
Lente Iletin I (insulin
  zinc suspension)
Lente Insulin (insulin
  zinc suspension)
lentectomy
lenticonus
lenticular
lenticular fossa
lenticular glands
lenticular nucleus
lenticulostriate
lenticulothalamic
lentiform
lentiginosis
lentiginous
lentiglobus
lentigo
lentitis
leontiasis
leontiasis ossea
leotropic

leper
lepidic
Lepidoptera
lepidosis
lepothrix
lepra
lepra Arabum
lepra maculosa
leprid
leprology
leproma
lepromatous
lepromin
lepromin skin test
leprosarium
leprostatic
leprosy
leprotic
leprous
leptocephalia
leptocephalus
leptochromatic
leptocyte
leptocytosis
leptodactyly
leptomeninges
leptomeningitis
leptomeningopathy
leptomeninx
leptonema
leptopellic
leptophonia
leptoprosopia
leptorhine
leptorrhine
leptoscope
leptosome
Leptospira
Leptospira
  icterohaemorrhagiae
leptospire
leptospirosis
leptospiruria
leptotene
leptothricosis
Leptus autumnalis
leresis
Leri's plenonosteosis

Leriche operation
Leriche's syndrome
lesbian
lesbianism
Lesch-Nyhan disease
lesion
lesion, degenerative
lesion, diffuse
lesion, discharging
lesion, focal
lesion, indiscriminate
lesion, initial, of
  syphilis
lesion, irritative
lesion, local
lesion, peripheral
lesion, primary
lesion, structural
lesion, systemic
lesion, toxic
lethal (L)
lethal dose (LD)
lethargic
lethargy, African
lethargy, hysteric
lethargy, induced
lethargy, lucid
lethe
lethologica
Letterer-Siwe disease
leucine (Leu)
leucine aminopeptidase
  (LAP)
leucine tolerance test
leucinosis
leucinuria
leucism
leucismus
leucitis
leucotomy
leucovorin calcium
leukapheresis
leukemia
leukemia, acute
  granulocytic
leukemia, acute
  lymphocytic (ALL)

leukemia, acute
  myelogenous (AML)
leukemia, chronic
  lymphocytic (CLL)
leukemia, chronic
  myelogenous (CML)
leukemia, hairy cell
leukemic
leukemid
leukemogenesis
leukemoid
Leukeran (chlorambucil)
leukin
leukoagglutinin
leukoblast
leukoblastosis
leukocidin
leukocytal
leukocyte
leukocyte, acidophilic
leukocyte, agranular
leukocyte alkaline
  phosphatase
leukocyte antibody
leukocyte, basophil
leukocyte, eosinophilic
leukocyte, granular
leukocyte, heterophilic
leukocyte histamine
  release test (LHR)
leukocyte, lymphoid
leukocyte, neutrophilic
leukocyte, nongranular
leukocyte phagocytosis
leukocyte,
  polymorphonuclear
leukocyte transfusion
leukocythemia
leukocytic
leukocytoblast
leukocytogenesis
leukocytoid
leukocytoma
leukocytopenia
leukocytoplania
leukocytopoiesis
leukocytosis, basophilic
leukocytosis, mononuclear

leukocytosis, pathologic
leukocytotaxis
leukocytotoxin
leukocyturia
leukoderma
leukoderma, syphilitic
leukodiagnosis
leukodystrophy
leukodystrophy,
  metachromatic
leukoedema
leukoencephalitis
leukoerythroblastosis
leukokeratosis
leukokoria
leukokraurosis
leukolymphosarcoma
leukolysis
leukoma
leukoma adherens
leukomaine
leukomainemia
leukomatous
leukomyelitis
leukomyelopathy
leukonecrosis
leukonychia
leukopathia
leukopathia unguium
leukopedesis
leukopenia
leukoplakia
leukoplakia buccalis
leukoplakia lingualis
leukoplakia vulvae
leukoplasia
leukopoiesis
leukopoietic
leukopsin
leukorrhagia
leukorrhea
leukosarcoma
leukosis
leukotactic
leukotaxine
leukotaxis
leukotomy
leukotoxic

leukotoxin
leukotrichia
leukotrienes
leukous
levallorphan tartrate
levarterenol bitartrate
levator
levator ani
levator palpebrae
  superioris
levator resection
LeVeen shunt
level of activities
lever
levigation
Levin's tube
levitation
Levlen 21 (levonorgestrel
  and ethinyl estradiol)
Levlen 28 (levonorgestrel
  and ethinyl estradiol)
Levo-Dromoran
  (levorphanol tartrate)
levocardia
levoclination
levocycloduction
levodopa
levoduction
levography
levogyration
levogyrous
levonordefrin
Levophed Bitartrate
  (norepinephrine
  bitartrate)
levophobia
levopropoxyphene
  napsylate
levorotation
levorotatory
levorphanol tartrate
Levothroid (levothyroxine
  sodium)
levothyroxine sodium
Levsin (hyoscyamine
  sulfate)
levulinic acid
levulose

levulosmia
levulosuria
lewisite
Lewy bodies
Leyden jar
Leydig cells
libidinous
libido
Libman-Sacks disease
Librax (chlordiazepoxide
  HCl and clidinium
  bromide)
Librax (Librium and
  Quarzan)
Libritabs
  (chlordiazepoxide)
Librium (chlordiazepoxide
  HCl)
lice
licensed practical nurse
  (LPN)
licensed vocational nurse
  (LVN)
licensure
licentiate
licentiate of the Royal
  College of Physicians
  (LRCP)
licentiate of the Royal
  College of Surgeons
  (LRCS)
lichen
lichen, myxedematous
lichen nitidus
lichen pilaris
lichen planopilaris
lichen planus
lichen ruber moniliformis
lichen ruber planus
lichen sclerosus et
  atrophicus
lichen scrofulosus
lichen simplex chronicus
lichen spinulosus
lichen striatus
lichen tropicus
lichenification
lichenin

lichenoid
Lichtheim's syndrome
licorice
lid
lid reflex
lid suture operation
Lidex (fluocinonide)
Lidex-E (fluocinonide)
lidocaine
lidocaine HCL toxicology
  test
lidocaine hydrochloride
lie detector
lie, transverse
Lieberkühn crypts
lien
lien accessorius
lien mobilis
lienal
lienitis
lienocele
lienography
lienomalacia
lienomedullary
lienomyelogenous
lienomyelomalacia
lienopancreatic
lienorenal
lienotoxin
lientery
lienunculus
life
life expectancy
life extension
life sciences
life span
life support
lifestyle
ligament (lig)
ligament, accessory
ligament,
  acromioclavicular
ligament, alar
ligament, annular
ligament, apical
ligament, arterial
ligament, broad, of liver

ligament, broad, of
uterus
ligament, caudal
ligament, check
ligament, conoid
ligament, coracoacromial
ligament, coracohumeral
ligament, coronary, of
liver
ligament, costocolic
ligament,
costotransverse, middle
ligament, cricopharyngeal
ligament, cricotracheal
ligament, cruciate
ligament, cruciform
ligament, crural
ligament, deltoid
ligament, dentate
ligament, dentoalveolar
ligament, falciform, of
liver
ligament, fundiform, of
penis
ligament, gastrophrenic
ligament, Gimbernat's
ligament, gingivodental
ligament, glenoid
ligament, Henle's
ligament,
hepaticoduodenal
ligament, iliofemoral
ligament, iliolumbar
ligament, iliopectineal
ligament,
infundibulopelvic
ligament, interclavicular
ligament, interspinal
ligament, ischiocapsular
ligament, lacunar
ligament, lateral
occipitoatlantal
ligament, Lockwood's
ligament, medial
ligament, nuchal
ligament, patellar
ligament, pectineal
ligament, periodontal

ligament, Petit's
ligament, phrenocolic
ligament, popliteal
arcuate
ligament, Poupart's
ligament,
pterygomandibular
ligament, pulmonary
ligament, rhomboid, of
clavicle
ligament, round, of femur
ligament, round, of liver
ligament, round, of
uterus
ligament, sacrospinous
ligament, sacrotuberous
ligament,
sphenomandibular
ligament, spiral, of
cochlea
ligament, stylohyoid
ligament, stylomandibular
ligament, suprascapular
ligament, supraspinal
ligament, suspensory
ligament, suspensory, of
axilla
ligament, suspensory, of
lens
ligament, suspensory, of
ovary
ligament, suspensory, of
penis
ligament,
temporomandibular
ligament,
tendinotrochanteric
ligament, transverse
crural
ligament, transverse
humeral
ligament, transverse, of
atlas
ligament, transverse, of
hip joint
ligament, transverse, of
knee joint
ligament, trapezoid

ligament, umbilical,
  lateral
ligament, umbilical,
  median
ligament,
  uterorectosacral
ligament, uterosacral
ligament, venous, of
  liver
ligament, ventricular, of
  larynx
ligament, vesicouterine
ligament, vestibular
ligament, vocal
ligament, Weitbrecht's
ligaments, arcuate
ligaments, auricular
ligaments, capsular
ligaments,
  costotransverse
ligaments, costovertebral
ligaments, cricothyroid
ligaments, glenohumeral
ligaments, lateral
  odontoid
ligaments, lateral, of
  liver
ligaments, Lisfranc's
ligaments, meniscofemoral
ligaments, nephrocolic
ligaments, palpebral
ligaments, pubic arcuate
ligaments, sacroiliac
ligaments, suspensory, of
  uterus
ligaments, sutural
ligaments, triangular, of
  liver
ligaments, yellow
ligamenta
ligamentopexis
ligamentous
ligamentum
ligand
ligase
ligate
ligation
ligature

light
light adaptation
light amplification by
  stimulated emission of
  radiations (LASER)
light and accommodation
  (L&A)
light, axial
light coagulation
light, cold
light diet
light difference
light, diffused
light, idioretinal
light, intrinsic
light, oblique
light perception (PL)
light, polarized
light, reflected
light reflex
light, refracted
light sense
light therarpy
light, transmitted
light unit
light, white
light, Wood's
light-dark discrimination
  (LDD)
light-emitting diode
  (LED)
lightening
light-headed
lightning safety rules
lightning streaks,
  Moore's
Lignac-Fanconi disease
lignin
lignocaine
lignoceric acid
limb
limb, anacrotic
limb, anterior, of
  internal capsule
limb, ascending, of renal
  tubule
limb, catacrotic

limb, descending, of
  renal tubule
limb, pectoral
limb, pelvic
limb, phantom
limb, thoracic
limbic
limbic system
Limbitrol
  (chlordiazepoxide and
  amitriptyline HCl)
limbus
limbus alveolaris
limbus conjunctivae
limbus corneae
limbus, corneoscleral
limbus fossa ovalis
limbus lamina spiralis
  ossae
limbus palpebrales,
  anteriores
limbus palpebralis,
  posterior
limbus sphenoidalis
lime
lime, chlorinated
lime, slaked
lime, soda
lime, sulfurated
lime, water
limen
limen nasi
limen of insula
limes nul
limes tod
liminal
limit
limit, assimilation
limit, audibility
limit, elastic
limit, Hayflick's
limit of flocculation
limit of perception
limit, quantum
limitans
limitation
limitation of motion
  (LOM)

limotherapy
limulus amebocyte lysate
  (LAL)
limulus amebocyte lysate
  test (LAL)
limulus lysate assay
Lincocin (lincomycin HCl)
lincomycin hydrochloride
lincture
linctus
lindane
Lindau's disease
Lindau-von Hippel disease
Lindholm operation
line, abdominal
line, absorption
line, alveolobasilar
line, alveolonasal
line, auriculobregmatic
line, base
line, basiobregmatic
line, Baudelocque's
line, biauricular
line, blue
line, canthomeatal
line, cement
line, cervical
line, costoarticular
line, costoclavicular
line of demarcation
line, Douglas'
line, epiphyseal
line of fibula, oblique
line of fixation
line, gingival
line, glabellomeatal
line, gum
line, iliopectineal
line of ilium,
  intermediate
line, incremental
line, incremental, of
  Retzius
line, incremental, of von
  Ebner
line, infraorbitomeatal
line, interauricular
line, intercondylar

line, interpupillary
line, intertrochanteric
line, intertuberal
line, lead
line, lip
line, mammillary
line of mandible, oblique
line, median
line, mentomeatal
line, milk
line, mucogingival
line, mylohyoid
line, nasobasilar
line, nuchal, superior
  and inferior
line, oblique, of fibula
line, oblique, of radius
line, parasternal
line, pectineal
line, popliteal, of tibia
line, resting
line, reversal
line, scapular
line, semilunar
line, Shenton's
line, sight
line, sternal
line, sternomastoid
line, supraorbital
line, temporal, of
  frontal bone
line, umbilicopubic
line, visual
lines, axillary
lines, Beau's
lines, cleavage
lines, gluteal
lines, Kerley's
lines of Owen
lines, supracondylar,
  medial and lateral
lines, Zöllner's
linea
linea alba
linea albicantes
linea aspera
linea costoarticularis
linea nigra

linea semilunaris
linea splendens
linea sternalis
linea striae atrophicae
linea terminalis
linea transversae ossis
  sacri
linear
linear accelerator
linear energy transfer
  (LET)
liner
liner, cavity
liner, soft
lingua
lingua frenata
lingua geographica
lingua nigra
lingua of mandible
lingua of sphenoid
lingua plicata
lingual
lingual frenum
lingual nerve
linguiform
lingula
lingula cerebelli
lingula of lung
lingulectomy
linguoclasia
linguoclination
linguodental
linguodistal
linguogingival
linguomesial
linguo-occlusal
linguopapillitis
linguopulpal
linguoversion
liniment
liniment, camphor
liniment, medicinal soft
  soap
linimentum
linitis
linitis plastica
linkage
linkage, sex

linseed
lint
lintin
Linton operation
Lioresal (baclofen)
liothyronine sodium
liotrix tablets
lip
lip, cleft
lip, double
lip, glenoid
lip, Hapsburg
lip reading
lip reading training
lip shave
lip, tympanic
lip, vestibule
lips, oral
lipacidemia
lipaciduria
liparocele
liparous
lipase
lipase, pancreatic
lipase, serum test
lipasuria
lipectomy
lipectomy, suction
lipedema
lipemia
lipemia, alimentary
lipemia retinalis
Lipex (natural lipotropic
  nutritional supplement)
lipid
lipid histiocytosis
lipid profile
lipide
lipidosis
lipiduria
lipin
Lipo-Nicin (nictonic acid
  supplement)
lipoarthritis
lipoatrophia
lipoatrophy
lipoblast
lipoblastoma

lipocardiac
lipocatabolic
lipocele
lipoceratous
lipocere
lipochondrodystrophy
lipochondroma
lipochrome
lipoclasis
lipoclastic
lipocyte
lipodieresis
lipodystrophy
lipodystrophy, insulin
lipodystrophy, intestinal
lipodystrophy,
  progressive
lipoferous
lipofibroma
lipofuscin
lipofuscinosis
lipogenesis
lipogenetic
lipogenic
lipogenous
lipogranuloma
lipogranulomatosis
lipoid
lipoidemia
lipoidosis
lipoidosis, arterial
lipoidosis, cerebroside
lipoiduria
lipolipoidosis
lipolysis
lipolytic
lipolytic digestion
lipolytic enzyme
lipoma
lipoma arborescens
lipoma, cystic
lipoma, diffuse
lipoma diffusum renis
lipoma durum
lipoma, hernial
lipoma, nasal
lipoma, osseous
lipoma telangiectodes

lipomatoid
lipomatous
lipomeningocele
lipomeria
lipometabolic
lipometabolism
lipomyoma
lipomyxoma
lipopectic
lipopenia
lipopenic
lipopeptid
lipopeptide
lipopexia
lipophage
lipophagia, granulomatous
lipophagic
lipophagy
lipophanerosis
lipophil
lipophilia
lipopolysaccharide
lipoprotein
lipoproteins
lipoproteins, high-
  density (HDL)
lipoproteins, low-density
  (LDL)
lipoproteins, very low
  density (VLDL)
liposarcoma
liposis
liposoluble
liposome
lipostomy
liposuction
lipothymia
lipotrophy
lipotropic
lipotropic factors
lipotropism
lipotropy
lipovaccine
lipoxeny
lipoxidase
lipoxygenase
Lippes Loop (intrauterine
  device)

lipping
lippitude
lipsis
lipsis animi
lipuria
Liquaemin (heparin
  sodium)
liquefacient
liquefaction
liquescent
liqueur
Liqui-Char (activated
  charcoal)
liquid air therapy
liquid crystals
liquid diet
liquid measure
Liquid Prep Syrup
  (prednisone)
Liquiprin
liquor
liquor amnii
liquor folliculi
liquor sanguinis
liquor solutions
Lisfranc operation
Lisfranc's ligament
lisping
lissencephalous
lissotrichy
Lister, Baron Joseph
listeriosis
listerosis
lisuride
liter (L)
lithagogue
Lithane (lithium
  carbonate)
lithecbole
lithectasy
lithectomy
lithemia
lithiasis
lithiasis biliaris
lithiasis nephritica
lithiasis renalis
lithic acid
lithicosis

lithium (Li)
lithium carbonate
lithium carbonate syrup
lithium level test
Lithobid (lithium
  carbonate)
lithocenosis
lithoclast
lithoclasty
lithoclysmia
lithocystotomy
lithodialysis
lithogenesis
lithokelyphopedion
lithokelyphos
litholabe
litholapaxy
litholapaxy, bladder
lithology
lithometer
lithometra
lithomyl
lithonephritis
lithonephrotomy
lithontriptic
lithopedion
lithophone
lithoscope
Lithostat
  (acetohydroxamic acid)
lithotome
lithotomy
lithotomy position
lithotony
lithotresis
lithotripsy
lithotripsy, bladder
lithotriptic
lithotriptor
lithotriptoscopy
lithotrite
lithotrity
lithous
lithoxiduria
lithuresis
lithureteria
lithuria

litmus
litmus paper
litter
Little's disease
Littlewood operation
Littre's glands
littritis
Litzmann's obliquity
livedo
livedo reticularis
liver
liver, abscess of
liver, acute yellow
  atrophy of
liver, biliary cirrhotic
liver biopsy
liver, cirrhosis of
liver, cysts of
liver failure
liver, fatty
liver flap
liver, floating
liver fluke, human
liver, foamy
liver, hobnail
liver, kidney, and spleen
  (LK&S)
liver lactic
  dehydrogenase (LLDH)
liver, lardaceous
liver, nutmeg
liver spots
liver, wandering
liver, waxy
livid
lividity
living will
livor
livor mortis
lixiviation
Lloyd-Davies operation
Lo/Ovral (norgestrel and
  ethinyl estradiol)
Lo/Ovral-28 (norgestrel
  and ethinyl estradiol)
Loa loa
loading test

loaiasis
lobar
lobar pneumonia
lobe
lobe, anterior, of
  hypophysis
lobe, azygos
lobe, caudate, of liver
lobe, central
lobe, flocculonodular
lobe, frontal
lobe, insular
lobe, limbic
lobe, occipital
lobe of ear
lobe of mamma
lobe of parotid,
  accessory
lobe, olfactory
lobe, parietal
lobe, posterior, of
  hypophysis
lobe, prefrontal
lobe, pyramidal, of
  thyroid
lobe, quadrate, of liver
lobe, Riedel's
lobe, spigelian
lobe, temporal
lobes, hepatic
lobes, lateral, of
  prostate
lobes, lateral, of
  thyroid gland
lobes, of cerebrum
lobes, of lungs
lobes, of pancreas
lobes, of prostate
lobes, orbital
lobectomy
lobelia
lobeline
lobi
lobitis
Lobo's disease
Loboa loboi
lobotomy
Lobstein's disease

lobular
lobulate
lobulated
lobule
lobule, paracentral
lobuli
lobulus
lobus
local
localization
localization, placenta
localized
localizer
locator
lochia
lochia alba
lochia cruenta
lochia purulenta
lochia rubra
lochia serosa
lochial
lochiocolpos
lochiometra
lochiometritis
lochiorrhagia
lochiorrhea
lochioschesis
lochometritis
Locke's solution
Locke-Ringer's solution
locked-in syndrome
lockjaw
Lockwood's ligament
loco
Locoid (hydrocortisone
  butyrate)
locomotion
locomotor
locomotor ataxia
locomotorium
locular
loculated
loculi
loculus
locum tenens
locus
locus ceruleus
locus niger

locus of control
Loeffler's bacillus
Loestrin (norethindrone
  acetate and ethinyl
  estradiol)
Lofenalac (low
  phenylalanine food)
Löffler's endocarditis
logadectomy
logaditis
logagnosia
logagraphia
logamnesia
logaphasia
logasthenia
logoklony
logokophosis
logomania
logoneurosis
logopathia
logopedia
logoplegia
logorrhea
logospasm
loiasis
loin
lolism
Lombard test
Lomotil (diphenoxylate
  HCl with atropine
  sulfate)
lomustine
Lonalac powder (low
  sodium, high protein
  beverage mix)
loneliness
long arm splint
  application
Long, Crawford Williamson
long GI tube introduction
long leg cast application
long leg cast brace
  application
long leg splint
  application
long-acting thyroid
  stimulation (LATS)

longevity
longing
longissimus
longitudinal
Longmire operation
longsightedness
long-term care (LTC)
longus
Loniten (minoxidil)
loop
loop ileal stoma
loopogram
looposcopy (ileal
  conduit)
loose body removal
loosening of associations
lophotrichea
lophotrichous
Lopid (gemfibrozil)
Lopressor (metoprolol
  tartrate)
Lopressor HCT (metoprolol
  tartrate and
  hydrochlorothiazide)
Loprox (ciclopirox
  olamine)
Lopurin (allopurinol)
Lorcet (propoxyphene HCl
  and acetaminophen)
Lorcet-HD (hydrocodone
  bitartrate and
  acetaminophen)
Lord operation
lordoma
lordoscoliosis
lordosis
Lorelco (probucol)
Lortab (hydrocodone
  bitartrate and
  acetaminophen)
loss of motion (LOM)
lotio
lotio alba
lotion
Lotrimin (clotrimazole)

Lotrisone (clotrimazole and betamethasone dipropionate)
Lotusate (talbutal)
loudness
loudness balance test
Louis-Bar syndrome
loupe
louse
louse, body
louse, crab
louse, head
lousiness
lovastatin
love
Loven's reflex
low-density lipoprotein (LDL)
Lowe's syndrome
lower GI endoscopy
lower GI series
lower motor neuron lesion
Lowila Cake (soap-free skin cleanser)
Lowman balance board
low-protein diet
low-salt diet
lox
loxapine succinate
loxarthron
loxia
Loxitane (loxapine succinate)
Loxitane C (loxapine HCl)
Loxosceles
loxoscelism
loxotic
loxotomy
lozenge
Lozol (indapamide)
lubb-dupp
Lubraseptic Jelly (for urethral instillation)
lubricant
lubricating enema
Lubrin Vaginal Lubricating Inserts

Lucas and Murray operation
Lucas-Championnière's disease
lucid
lucidity
luciferase
luciferin
lucifugal
lucipetal
lucotherapy
Ludiomil (maprotiline HCl)
Ludwig's angina
Luer-Lok syringe
lues
luetic
Lufyllin (dyphylline)
Lufyllin-GG (dyphylline and guaifenesin)
Lugol's solution
lumbago
lumbar
lumbar analgesia
lumbar discography
lumbar epidural injection
lumbar hernia repair
lumbar laminectomy
lumbar nerves
lumbar plexus
lumbar puncture
lumbar reflex
lumbar region
lumbar shunt
lumbar spinal puncture
lumbar spine
lumbar subarachnoid shunt
lumbar sympathectomy
lumbar vertebrae
lumbarization
lumboabdominal
lumbocolostomy
lumbocolotomy
lumbodynia
lumboiliac
lumboinguinal
lumbosacral
lumbosacral manipulation

lumbosacral myelography
lumbosacral plexus
lumbosacral spine
lumbrical
lumbrical bar
lumbricalis
lumbricide
lumbricoid
lumbricosis
Lumbricus
lumbus
lumen
luminal
luminescence
luminiferous
luminophore
luminous
lumirhodopsin
lumpectomy
lunacy
lunar
lunate
lunate arthroplasty
lunate dislocation
lunatic
lunatomalacia
lung
lung abscess
lung cancer
lung collapse
lung fluke
lung maturity profile
lung surfactant
lung transplantation
lungs
lungmotor
lungworm
lunula
lupiform
lupoid
lupous
Lupron (leuprolide
  acetate)
lupus
lupus erythematosus (LE)
lupus erythematosus,
  discoid (DLE)

lupus erythematosus,
  systemic
lupus pernio
lupus test (LE PREP)
lupus vulgaris
Luride (sodium fluoride)
Lust's reflex
lusus naturae
luteal
luteal hormone
lutein
lutein cells
luteinic
luteinization
luteinizing hormone (LH)
luteinizing hormone-
  releasing factor (LHRF)
Lutembacher's syndrome
luteohormone
luteolysin
luteoma
luteotropic hormone (LTH)
luteotropin
lutetium (Lu)
luteum, corpus
lutin
Lutz-Splendore-Almeida
  disease
lux
luxation
luxus
Luy's body
lyase
lycanthropy
lycopene
lycopenemia
lycoperdonosis
lycopodium
lycorexia
lye
lying-in
Lyme arthritis
Lyme disease (LD)
lymph
lymph node
lymph nodule
lymph sinus
lymphadenectasis

lymphadenectomy
lymphadenia
lymphadenia ossea
lymphadenitis
lymphadenocele
lymphadenogram
lymphadenography
lymphadenoid
lymphadenoptathy
lymphadenoptathy,
  dermatopathic
lymphadenosis benigna
  cutis
lymphadenotomy
lymphadenovarix
lymphagioendothelioma
lymphagogue
lymphangial
lymphangiectasis
lymphangiectomy
lymphangiitis
lymphangiofibroma
lymphangiogram
lymphangiography
lymphangiology
lymphangioma
lymphangioma, cavernous
lymphangioma, cystic
lymphangiophlebitis
lymphangioplasty
lymphangiorrhaphy
lymphangiosarcoma
lymphangiotomy
lymphangitis
lymphatic
lymphatic blockade
lymphatic capillary
lymphatic system
lymphatic vessels
lymphaticostomy
lymphatism
lymphatology
lymphatolysis
lymphatolytic
lymphedema
lymphemia
lymphendothelioma
lymphenteritis

lymphization
lymphnoditis
lymphoblast
lymphoblastic
lymphoblastoma
lymphoblastomatosis
lymphoblastosis
lymphocele
lymphocyte
lymphocyte, B.
lymphocyte culture
lymphocyte, T.
lymphocytes B-cell
  evaluation
lymphocytes test
lymphocythemia
lymphocytoblast
lymphocytoma
lymphocytopenia
lymphocytopoiesis
lymphocytosis
lymphocytosis-promoting
  factor (LPF)
lymphocytotoxin
lymphoduct
lymphoepithelioma
lymphogenesis
lymphogenous
lymphoglandula
lymphogonia
lymphogram
lymphogranuloma inguinale
lymphogranuloma skin test
lymphogranuloma venereum
  (LGV)
lymphogranulomatosis
lymphography
lymphoid
lymphoid interstitial
  pneumonitis (LIP)
lymphoidectomy
lymphoidocyte
lymphokine-activated
  killer (LAK)
lymphokine-activated
  killer (LAK) cells 1,2
lymphokines
lymphokinesis

lymphology
lymphoma
lymphoma, African
lymphoma, Burkitt's
lymphoma, clasmocytic
lymphoma, giant
  follicular
lymphoma granulomatous
lymphoma, lymphoblastic
lymphoma, lymphocytic
lymphoma, malignant,
  poorly differentiated
  diffuse lymphocytic
lymphoma, malignant,
  mixed cell
lymphoma, malignant,
  undifferentiated
lymphoma, malignant,
  well-differentiated
  diffuse lymphocytic
lymphomatoid
lymphomatosis
lymphomatous
lymphomyxoma
lymphonodus
lymphopathia venereum
lymphopathy
lymphopenia
lymphoplasty
lymphopoiesis
lymphopoietic
lymphoproliferative
lymphoprotease
lymphorecticular
  disorders
lymphoreticular
lymphoreticular system
lymphoreticulosis,
  benign, of inoculation
lymphorrhagia
lymphorrhea
lymphorrhoid
lymphosarcoma
lymphosarcomatosis
lymphostasis
lymphotaxis
lymphotome
lymphotomy

lymphotoxin
lymphotrophy
lymphuria
lynestrenol
lyochrome
lyoenzyme
lyogel
Lyon hypothesis
lyophil
lyophile
lyophilic
lyophilization
lyophobe
lyophobic
lyosorption
lyotrope
lyotropic
lypressin
lyra
lysate
lyse
lysemia
lysergic acid
  diethylamide (LSD)
lysimeter
lysin
lysine
lysinogen
lysis
lysocephalin
Lysodren (mitotane)
lysogen
lysogenesis
lysogenic
lysogeny
lysolecithin
lysomes
lysosomal storage disease
lysosome
lysozyme
lyssa
Lyssavirus
lyssoid
lyssophobia
lyterian
lytic
lyze

M

M.V.I. Pediatric (multi-
vitamin infusion)
M.V.I.-12 (multivitamin
infusion)
M.V.M. (multi-
vitamin/mineral
formula)
M-M-R (measles, mumps and
rubella virus vaccine)
M-R-Vax II (measles and
rubella virus vaccine)
mace
macerate
maceration
Mache unit (Mu)
machine
Machover test
macies
macrencephalia
macrencephaly
macroamylase
macroamylasemia
macrobiosis
macrobiota
macroblepharia
macrobrachia
macrocardius
macrocephalia
macrocephalic
macrocephalous
macrocephaly
macrocheilia
macrocheiria
macrochemistry
macrocnemia
macrocolon
macroconidium
macrocornea
macrocyst
macrocyte
macrocythemia
macrocytosis

macrodactylia
Macrodantin
(nitrofurantoin
macrocrystals)
Macrodex (plasma volume
expander)
macrodontia
macroesthesia
macrofauna
macroflora
macrogamete
macrogametocyte
macrogenitosomia praecox
macrogingivae
macroglia
macroglobulin
macroglobulin
immunodiffusion
macroglobulinemia
macroglossia
macrognathia
macrography
macrogyria
macrolabia
macroleukoblast
macrolymphocyte
macromania
macromastia
macromelia
macromelus
macromere
macromethod
macromolecule
macromonocyte
macromyeloblast
macronormoblast
macronucleus
macronychia
macropathology
macrophage
macrophage activating
factor
macrophage migration
inhibiting factor
macrophagocyte
macrophagus
macrophallus
macrophthalmia

macroplasia
macropodia
macropolycyte
macropromyelocyte
macroprosopia
macropsia
macrorhinia
macroscelia
macroscopic
macroscopy
macrosigmoid
macrosis
macrosmatic
macrosomatia
macrosomia
macrospore
macrostereognosis
macrostomia
macrostructure
macrotia
macrotome
macrotooth
macula
macula albidae
macula atrophicae
macula caeruleae
macula, cerebral
macula corneae
macula cribrosa
macula densa
macula flava laryngis
macula folliculi
macula germinativa
macula gonorrhoeica
macula lutea retinae
macula sacculi
macula utriculi
maculae acusticae
macular
maculate
maculated
maculation
macule
maculocerebral
maculopapular
maculopathy
mad
madarosis

madder
Madelung's deformity
Madelung's disease
madescent
madidans
Madlener operation
Madura foot
maduromycosis
mafenide acetate
Mag-Ox 400 (magnesium
    oxide)
magaldrate
Magan (magnesium
    salicylate)
magenblase syndrome
Magendie's foramen
magenstrasse
magenta
maggot
magic thinking
magistery
magistral
magma
magnesia
magnesia and alumina
magnesium (Mg)
magnesium carbonate
magnesium chloride
magnesium citrate
magnesium gluconate
magnesium hydroxide
magnesium oxide
magnesium salicylate
magnesium stearate
magnesium sulfate
magnesium trisilicate
magnet
magnet, horseshoe
magnetic
magnetic field
magnetic lines of force
magnetic resonance
    imaging (MRI)
magnetism
magnetoelectricity
magnetometer
magneton
magnetotherapy

magnetropism
magnification
magnification airway
  study
magnum
Magnuson operation
Magsal (magnesium
  salicylate and
  phenytoloxamine
  citrate)
Mahaim fibers
maim
main en griffe
mainstreaming
maintainer
Majocchi's disease
Majocchi's granuloma
major histocompatibility
  gene complex (MHC)
mal de Cayenne
mal de mer
mal perforant
mal perforant palatin
mala
malabsorption
malabsorption panel
malabsorption syndrome
malacia
malacoma
malacoplakia
malacoplakia vesicae
malacosarcosis
malacosis
malacosteon
malacotic
malacotomy
malactic
maladay
maladie de Roger
maladjusted
malaise
malalignment
malar
malar area
malar bone
malaria
malaria, cephalgic
malaria, cerebral

malaria, estivoautumnal
malaria, falciparum
malaria, latent
malaria, quartan
malaria, quotidian
malaria, tertian
malaria, vivax
malariacidal
malarial
malariology
malariotherapy
malarious
Malassezia
malassimilation
malate
malate dehydrogenase
malathion
malaxate
malaxation
maldigestion
male
male genital system
male infertility profile
malemission
maleruption
malformation
malfunction
malic
malic acid
malice
malign
malignancy
malignant
malinger
malingerer
malinterdigitation
malleable
malleation
malleoincudal
malleolar
malleolus
malleolus fracture
malleostapediopexy
malleotomy
mallet
mallet finger
mallet toe
malleus

Mallophaga
Mallory-Weiss syndrome
malnutrition
malocclusion
malonylurea
malpighian capsule
malpighian corpuscle
malpighian layer
malpighian pyramid
malposition
malpractice
malrotation
Malström's vacuum
    extraction
malt
malt extract
malt sugar
Malta fever
maltase
maltose
maltosuria
Maltsupex (malt soup
    extract)
malturned
malum
malum articulorum senilis
malum coxae senilis
malum perforans pedis
malum venereum
malunion
mamanpian
mamelon
mamma
mammal
mammalgia
mammaplasty
mammary
mammary angiography
mammary ductogram
mammary glands
mammary lymph node biopsy
mammectomy
mammilla
mammillary
mammillated
mammillation
mammilliform
mammilliplasty

mammillitis
mammitis
mammogen
mammogram
mammography
mammoplasty
mammoplasty, augmentation
mammoplasty, reduction
mammose
mammotomy
mammotrophic
mammotropin
man
Manchester operation
manchette
manchineel
mancinism
Mandelamine (methenamine
    mandelate)
mandelic acid
mandible
mandibula
mandibular
mandibulectomy
mandibulopharyngeal
Mandol (cefamandole
    nafate)
mandrel
mandril
mandrin
maneuver, Crede's
maneuver, Heimlich
maneuver, Leopold's
maneuver, Mauriceau-
    Smellie-Veit
maneuver, Müller's
maneuver, Munro Kerr
maneuver, Pinard's
maneuver, Prague
maneuver, Scanzoni
maneuver, Valsalva's
manganese (Mn)
manganese poisoning
Mangatrace (manganese
    chloride)
mange
mania
mania, puerperal

mania, religious
mania, transitory
mania, unproductive
maniac
maniacal
manic
manic-depressive
  psychosis
manifest
manifest hyperopia (Hm)
manifest squint
manifestation
manikin
maniphalanx
manipulation
manipulative surgery
manna
mannans
mannerism
mannitol
Mannkopf's sign
mannose
mannoside
mannosidosis
manometer
manometric studies
manometry
Mansonella
Mansonella ozzardi
mansonelliasis
Mansonia
Mantadil Cream
mantle
Mantoux reaction
manual
manual arts therapy
manual muscle test
manubrium
manudynamometer
manus
Maolate (chlorphenesin
  carbamate)
Maox
map, genetic
map, linkage
maple bark disease
maple syrup urine disease
mapping

marantic
marantology
marasmic
marasmoid
marasmus
Marax (ephedrine sulfate,
  theophylline,
  hydroxyzine HCl)
marble bones
Marblen (calcium and
  magnesium carbonates)
Marburg virus disease
marc
Marcaine (bupivacaine HCl
  and epinephrine)
Marcaine Spinal
  (bupivacaine HCl in
  dextrose injection)
Marchiafava-Micheli
  syndrome
marcid
Marckwald operation
Marcus Gunn pupil
Marezine (cyclizine HCl)
Marfan's syndrome
margarine
margin
marginal
margination
marginoplasty
margo
margo acutus
margo obtusus
Marie's ataxia
Marie's disease
Marie's sign
marihuana
marijuana
Marinol (dronabinol)
mark
mark, birth
mark, port-wine
mark, strawberry
marker
Marlyn Formula 50 (amino
  acids and B_6)
Marplan (isocarboxazid)
marrow

marrow aspiration
marrow, gelatinous
marrow, red
marrow, spinal
marrow transplantation
marrow, yellow
marsh fever
marsh gas
Marsh's test
Marshall-Marchetti
operation
Marshall-Marchetti-Krantz
procedure
marsupialization
marsupium
maschaladenitis
maschaliatry
maschaloncus
masculation
masculine
masculinization
masculinovoblastoma
maser
mask, BLB
mask, death
mask, ecchymotic
mask, Hutchinson's
mask, luetic
mask, Parkinson's
mask of pregnancy
masked
masochism
masochism, sexual
masochist
mass
mass number
mass psychogenic illness
massa
massage
massage, auditory
massage, cardiac
massage, electrovibratory
massage, general
massage, introductory
massage, local
massage, physical therapy
massage, tremolo
massage, vapor

massage, vibratory
Masse (breast cream)
Massengill Douches
masseter
masseter muscle reduction
masseur
masseuse
massive collapse of the
lung
massotherapy
mast cells
mastadenitis
mastadenoma
mastalgia
mastatrophia
mastatrophy
mastauxe
mastectomy
master (M)
Master two-step test
Masters' stress test
masthelcosis
mastic
mastication
masticatory
Mastigophora
mastigote
mastitis
mastitis, cystic
mastitis, interstitial
mastitis, parenchymatous
mastitis, puerperal
mastitis, stagnation
masto-occipital
mastocarcinoma
mastochondroma
mastocyte
mastocytoma
mastocytosis
mastodynia
mastography
mastoid
mastoid antrum
mastoid cells
mastoid fistula
mastoid obliteration
mastoid polytomography

mastoid portion of
    temporal bone
mastoid process
mastoidal
mastoidalgia
mastoidectomy
mastoideocentesis
mastoiditis
mastoiditis, Bezold's
mastoiditis externa
mastoiditis, sclerosing
mastoidotomy
mastoidotympanectomy
mastology
mastomenia
mastoncus
mastoparietal
mastopathy
mastopexy
mastoplasia
mastoplasty
mastoptosis
mastorrhagia
mastorrhaphy
mastoscirrhus
mastosquamous
mastostomy
mastotomy
masturbate
masturbation
Matas operation
match
match poisoning
matching
mate
mater
mater, dura
mater, pia
materia alba
materia medica
material
Materna (prenatal vitamin
    and mineral tablets)
maternal
maternal deprivation
    syndrome
maternity

maternity care and
    delivery
mating
matrilineal
matrix
matrixitis
matter, gray
matter, white
Matulane (procarbazine
    HCl)
maturate
maturation
mature
maturity
matutinal
matzoon
Maurer's dots
Maxepa (omega-3
    polyunsaturates)
Maxiflor (diflorasone
    diacetate)
maxilla
maxillary
maxillary artery
maxillary sinus
maxillectomy
maxillitis
maxillodental
maxillofacial
maxillofacial CAT
maxillofacial fixation
maxillomandibular
maxillopalatine
maxillotomy
maxima
maximal
maximal breathing
    capacity (MBC)
maximal inspiratory
    pressure (MIP)
maximal voluntary
    ventilation (MVV)
maximum
maximum allowable
    concentration (MAC)
maximum permissible dose
    (MPD)

Maxovite (pre-menstrual
syndrome-multi-
vitamin/mineral)
May-Vita Elixir (vitamins
and minerals)
Mayo operation
Mayo-Robson's point
Mazanor (mazindol)
maze
Mazet operation
mazopexy
mazoplasia
McArdle's disease
McBride operation
McBurney operation
McBurney's incision
McBurney's point
McBurney's sign
McCall operation
McCannel suture
McCarthy's reflex
McCauley operation
McCormac's reflex
McDonald operation
McIndoe operation
McKeever operation
McMurray's sign
McReynolds operation
MCT Oil (medium chain
triglycerides oil)
McVay operation
MDR (fitness tabs)
meal
mean
mean corpuscular
hemoglobin (MCH)
mean corpuscular
hemoglobin (MCH) test
mean corpuscular
hemoglobin
concentration (MCHC)
mean corpuscular volume
(MCV)
measles
measles and mumps virus
vaccine
measles and rubella
immunization

measles and rubella virus
vaccine
measles, black
measles, German
measles, hemorrhagic
measles, mumps and
rubella virus
immunization (MMR)
measles, mumps, and
rubella virus vaccine
measles virus vaccine,
live
measly
measure
meat
meat fibers, feces
meatal
meatometer
meatoplasty
meatorrhaphy
meatoscope
meatoscopy
meatotome
meatotomy
meatus
meatus acusticus externus
meatus acusticus internus
meatus, external auditory
meatus, inferior
meatus, internal auditory
meatus, middle
meatus nasi communis
meatus nasi inferior
meatus nasi medius
meatus nasi superior
meatus nasopharyngeus
meatus, superior
meatus urinarius
Mebaral (mephobarbital)
mebendazole
mebutamate
mecamylamine
hydrochloride
mechanical rectifier
mechanics
mechanism
mechanism, countercurrent
mechanism, defense

mechanism, Duncan's
mechanocyte
mechanoreceptor
mechanotherapy
mechlorethamine
mecism
Meckel, Johann Friedrich
Meckel's cartilage
Meckel's diverticulum
Meckel's ganglion
Meckel's space
meckelectomy
Meclan (meclocycline
  sulfosalicylate)
meclizine hydrochloride
meclocycline
  sulfosalicylate
Meclomen (meclofenamate
  sodium)
meconium
meconium ileus
mecystasis
media
mediad
medial
medialis
median
median line
median nerve
median plane
mediastinal
mediastinectomy
mediastinitis
mediastinography
mediastinopericarditis
mediastinoscopy
mediastinotomy
mediastinum
mediate
mediation
mediator
Mediatric (steroids,
  nutritional supplement,
  antidepressant)
medic
Medic Alert
medicable
Medicaid

medical
medical assistant (MA)
medical audit
medical corpsman
medical examiner (ME)
medical history
medical informatics
medical intensive care
  unit (MICU)
medical jurisprudence
medical preparations
medical record
medical record, problem-
  oriented (POMR)
medical records
  department (MRD)
medical records librarian
Medical Subject Headings
  (MESH)
medicament
medicamentosus
Medicare
medicate
medication
medication route
medicinal
medicinal enema
medicine (M)
medicine, aerospace
medicine, clinical
medicine, community
medicine, dental
medicine, disaster
medicine, emergency
medicine, environmental
medicine, family
medicine, folk
medicine, forensic
medicine, group
medicine, industrial
medicine, internal
medicine, legal
medicine man
medicine, nuclear
medicine, occupational
medicine, patent
medicine, physical
medicine, preclinical

medicine, preventive
medicine, proprietary
medicine, psychosomatic
medicine, socialized
medicine, sports
medicine, tropical
medicine, veterinary
medicinerea
medicochirurgical
medicolegal
medicomechanical
Medicone (rectal
  ointment)
Medicone (rectal
  suppositories)
Medicone Derma (ointment)
Medicone Derma-HC
  (ointment)
Medicone Dressing (cream)
Mediconet (medicated
  rectal wipes)
medicopsychology
medicopter
medicornu
Medigesic Plus
  (butalbital,
  acetaminophen, and
  caffeine)
Medihaler Ergotamine
  (ergotamine tartrate)
Medihaler-ISO
  (isoproterenol sulfate)
Medina worm
mediocarpal
mediocarpal joint
mediolateral
mediopontine
mediotarsal
Medipren (ibuprofen)
medisect
Mediterranean anemia
Mediterranean fever,
  familial
medium
medium, clearing
medium, contrast
medium, culture
medium, defined

medium, nutrient
medium, radiopaque
medium, refracting
medium, separating
medium-chain
  triglycerides
medius
MEDLARS
MEDLINE
medrogestone
Medrol
  (methylprednisolone)
medroxyprogesterone
  acetate
medrysone
medtotomy
medulla
medulla, adrenal
medulla nephrica
medulla oblongata
medulla of hair
medulla of kidneys
medulla of ovary
medulla ossium
medulla spinalis
medullary
medullary canal
medullary tractotomy
medullated
medullated nerve fiber
medullation
medullectomy
medullitis
medullization
medulloadrenal
medulloarthritis
medulloblast
medulloblastoma
medulloepithelioma
Mees lines
mefenamic acid
Mefoxin (cefoxitin
  sodium)
mega electron volt (MeV)
Mega-B (vitamin B
  complex)
megabladder
megabucks

megacardia
Megace (megestrol acetate)
megacephalic
megacolon
megacurie (Mc)
megadontia
Megadose (multiple mega-vitamin formula with minerals)
megadyne
megaesophagus
megahertz (MHz)
megakaryoblast
megakaryocyte
megakaryocytosis
megalencephaly
megalgia
megaloblast
megaloblastic anemia
megalocardia
megalocephalic
megalocephaly
megalocheiria
megalocornea
megalocystis
megalocyte
megalodactylous
megalodontia
megaloesophagus
megalogastria
megaloglossia
megalographia
megalohepatia
megalokaryocyte
megalomania
megalomelia
megalonychosis
megalopenis
megalophthalmus
megalopodia
megalopsia
megaloscope
megalosplenia
megalospore
megalosyndactyly
megaloureter

Megamor (acetaminophen and hydrocodone bitartrate)
megaprosopous
megarectum
megaseme
megavitamin
megavolt
megavoltage
megestrol acetate
meglumine
meglumine antimonate
megohm
megophthalmos
megrim
meibomian cyst
meibomian gland
meibomitis
meiogenic
meiosis
Meissner's corpuscles
Meissner's plexus
melagra
melalgia
melancholia
melancholia, affective
melancholia agitata
melancholia, involutional
melancholia, panphobic
melancholia, sexual
melancholia, simplex
melancholia stuporosa
melancholia, suicidal
melanedema
melanemia
melanephidrosis
Melanex (hydroquinone)
melanidrosis
melaniferous
melanin
melanism
melanoameloblastoma
melanoblast
melanoblastoma
melanocarcinoma
melanocyte-release-inhibiting factor (MIF)

melanocyte-releasing
　factor (MRF)
melanocyte-stimulating
　hormone (MSH)
melanocytoma
melanoderm
melanoderma
melanodermatitis
melanoepithelioma
melanogen
melanogenesis
melanoglossia
melanoid
melanoleukoderma
melanoma
melanomatosis
melanonychia
melanopathy
melanophage
melanophore
melanoplakia
melanorrhagia
melanorrhea
melanosarcoma
melanoscirrhus
melanosis
melanosis lenticularis
melanosome
melanotic
melanotrichia linguae
melanotroph
melanuria
melasma
melasma gravidarum
melatonin
melena
melena neonatorum
melenic
Melfiat IOS
　(phendimetrazine
　tartrate)
melicera
meliceris
melioidosis
melissophobia
melitagra
melitemia
melitensis

melitis
melitoptyalism
melituria
Mellaril (thioridazine
　HCl)
Mellaril-S (thioridazine
　HCl)
mellitum
melomelus
meloncus
melonoplasty
meloplasty
meloplasty, facial
melorheostosis
melosalgia
meloschisis
melotia
melphalan
melting point
member
membrane, alveodental
membrane,
　alveolocapillary
membrane, arachnoid
membrane, atlanto-
　occipital
membrane, basement
membrane, basilar
membrane, Bowman's
membrane, Bruch's
membrane, buccopharyngeal
membrane, cell
membrane, choroid
membrane, costocoracoid
membrane, cricothyroid
membrane, croupous
membrane, decidual
membrane, Descemet's
membrane, diphtheritic
membrane, drum
membrane, egg
membrane, elastic
membrane, enamel
membrane, fenestrated
membrane, fetal
membrane, fibrous
membrane, glassy
membrane, glial cell

membrane, Henle's elastic
membrane, homogeneous
membrane, Huxley's
membrane, hyaline
membrane, hyaloid
membrane, hyoglossal
membrane, interosseous
membrane, Krause's
membrane, laryngeal
  mucous
membrane, limiting,
  external
membrane, lingual mucous
membrane, masticatory
  mucous
membrane, medullary
membrane, mucous
membrane, nasal mucous
membrane, Nasmyth's
membrane, nictitating
membrane, nuclear
membrane, obturator
membrane, olfactory
membrane, oral
membrane, oronasal
membrane, otolithic
membrane, palatal mucous
membrane, peridental
membrane, periodontal
membrane, permeable
membrane, pharyngeal
membrane, pharyngeal
  mucous
membrane, placental
membrane, plasma
membrane potential
membrane, pseudoserous
membrane, pupillary
membrane, pyogenic
membrane, quadrangular
membrane, Reissner's
membrane, Ruysch's
membrane, Scarpa's
membrane, schneiderian
membrane, Schwann's
membrane, selectively
  permeable
membrane, semipermeable

membrane, serous
membrane, Shrapnell's
membrane, submucous
membrane, synovial
membrane, tectorial
membrane, thyrohyoid
membrane, tympanic
membrane, unit
membrane, vestibular
  mucous
membrane, virginal
membrane, vitelline
membrane, vitreous
membrane, yolk
membranectomy
membranella
membraniform
membranocartilaginous
membranoid
membranous
membrum muliebre
memory
memory, anterograde
memory, long-term
memory, retrograde
menacme
menadiol sodium
  diphosphate
menadione
menadione sodium
  bisulfite
menarche
Mendel's laws
Mendel's reflex
mendelevium (Md)
mendelism
Ménétrier's disease
menhidrosis
menidrosis
Ménière's disease
menigotyphoid
meningeal
meningeocortical
meningeorrhaphy
meninges
meningioma
meningiomatosis
meningism

meningismus
meningitic
meningitis
meningitis, acute
meningitis, acute aseptic
meningitis, basilar
meningitis, cerebral
meningitis, cerebrospinal
meningitis, listeria
meningitis, pneumococcal
meningitis, serosa
  circumscripta
meningitis, serous
meningitis, spinal
meningitis, sterile
meningitis, traumatic
meningitis, tuberculous
meningitophobia
meningo-osteophlebitis
meningoarteritis
meningocele
meningococcal
meningococcal
  polysaccharide vaccine
  group A
meningococcal
  polysaccharide vaccine
  group C
meningococcemia
meningococci
meningococcidal
meningococcus
meningocortical
meningocyte
meningoencephalitis
meningoencephalopathy
meningoencephalomyelitis
meningoencephalocele
meningomalacia
meningomyelitis
meningomyelocele
meningomyeloradiculitis
meningopathy
meningoradicular
meningoradiculitis
meningorrhachidian
meningorrhagia
meningorrhea

meningosis
meningovascular
meninguria
meninx
meniscectomy
menisci
meniscitis
meniscocyte
meniscocytosis
meniscorrhesis
meniscus
menometrorrhagia
Menomune-A/C/Y/W-135
  (meningococcal
  polysaccharide vaccine)
menopause
menopause, artificial
menopause, male
menopause, premature
menopause, surgical
menophania
menoplania
menorrhagia
menorrhea
menostasis
menostaxis
menotropins
menoxenia
Menrium 10-4
  (chlordiazepoxide and
  esterified estrogen)
Menrium 5-2
  (chlordiazepoxide and
  esterified estrogen)
Menrium 5-4
  (chlordiazepoxide and
  esterified estrogen)
menses
menstrual
menstrual cycle
menstrual epilepsy
menstrual extraction
menstrual regulation
menstruant
menstruate
menstruation
menstruation, anovulatory
menstruation, retrograde

menstruation, suppressed
menstruation, vicarious
menstruous
menstruum
mensual
mensuration
mentagrophyton
mental
mental age (MA)
mental deficiency
mental disorder
mental fog
mental health
mental hygiene
mental illness
Mental Measurements
  Yearbook
mental nerve destruction
mental retardation (MR)
mental status
mental status exam
mentality
mentation
Mentha
Mentha piperita
Mentha pulegium
Mentha viridis
menthol
menton
mentoplasty
mentulagra
mentulate
mentulomania
mentum
meocoxalgia
mepacrine hydrochloride
mepazine
mepenzolate bromide
Mepergan (meperidine HCl
  and promethazine HCl)
meperidine hydrochloride
mephenesin
mephentermine sulfate
mephenytoin
mephitic
mephobarbital
Mephyton (phytonadione
  [vitamin K_1])

mepivacaine hydrochloride
meprednisone
meprobamate
Meprospan (meprobamate)
meprylcaine hydrochloride
meralgia
meralgia paresthetica
merbromin
mercaptan
mercaptomerin sodium
  injection
mercaptopurine
Mercier's bar
mercurial
mercurial diuretics
mercurial palsy
mercurial rash
mercurialism
mercurialized
mercuric
mercuric chloride
mercuric chloride
  poisoning
mercuric oxide, yellow
Mercurochrome (merbromin)
mercurous
mercurous chloride
mercurous chloride
  poisoning
mercury (Hg)
mercury ammoniated
mercury bichloride
mercury chloride
mercury poisoning
mercy
meridian
merinthophobia
merispore
meristic
meroacrania
meroblastic
merocele
merocrine
merodiastolic
meroergasia
merogenesis

merogony
meromelia
meromicrosomia
meromyosin
meronecrosis
meropia
merorrhachischisis
merosmia
merosystolic
merotomy
merozoite
merozygote
Merrskey hemagglutination
  inhibition
Merthiolate (thimerosal)
Meruvax (rubella virus
  vaccine, live)
mesad
mesal
mesangium
Mesantoin (mephenytoin)
mesaortitis
mesaraic
mesareic
mesarteritis
mesaticephalic
mesatipellic
mesatipelvic
mescaline
mescalism
mesectoderm
mesencephalic tractotomy
mesencephalitis
mesencephalon
mesencephalotomy
mesenchyme
mesenchymoma
mesenterectomy
mesenteric
mesenteric artery
mesenteriolum
mesenteriopexy
mesenteriorrhaphy
mesenteriplication
mesenteritis
mesenterium
mesentery
mesiad

mesial
mesial drift
mesiobuccal
mesiobucco-occlusal
mesiobuccopulpal
mesiocervical
mesioclusion
mesiodens
mesiodistal
mesiogingival
mesiolabial
mesiolinguo-occlusal
mesiolinguopulpal
mesion
mesiopulpal
mesioversion
mesiris
mesmeric
mesmerism
meso-ontomorph
mesoappendicitis
mesoappendix
mesoarium
mesoblast
mesobronchitis
mesocardia
mesocardium
mesocarpal
mesocecum
mesocephalic
mesocephalon
mesocolic
mesocolon
mesocolopexy
mesocoloplication
mesocord
mesocuneiform
mesoderm
mesoderm, axial
mesoderm, extraembryonic
mesoderm, intermediate
mesoderm, lateral
mesoderm, paraxial
mesoderm, somatic
mesoderm, splanchnic
mesodiastolic
mesodont
mesoduodenum

mesoepididymis
mesogastric
mesogastrium
mesoglia
mesogluteal
mesogluteus
mesognathion
mesognathous
mesohyloma
mesoileum
mesojejunum
mesolymphocyte
mesomere
mesometritis
mesometrium
mesomorph
meson
mesonasal
mesonephric
mesonephric duct
mesonephric tubules
mesonephroma
mesonephros
mesoneuritis
mesopexy
mesophilic
mesophlebitis
mesophragma
mesophryon
mesopic
mesopneumon
mesoporphyrin
mesoprosopic
mesopulmonum
mesorchium
mesorectum
mesoridazine besylate
mesoropter
mesorrhachischisis
mesorrhaphy
mesorrhine
mesosalpinx
mesoseme
mesosigmoid
mesosigmoiditis
mesosigmoidopexy
mesoskelic
mesosome

mesosternum
mesosystolic
mesotarsal
mesotendineum
mesotendon
mesothelial
mesothelioma
mesothelium
mesothenar
mesothorium
mesotron
mesouranic
mesovarium
Mestinon (pyridostigmine
  bromide)
mestranol
meta-analysis
metabiosis
metabolic
metabolic balance
metabolic body size
metabolic equivalent
  (MET)
metabolic failure
metabolic gradient
metabolic panel
metabolic rate (MR)
metabolimeter
metabolism
metabolite
metabolize
metacarpal
metacarpectomy
metacarpophalangeal
metacarpophalangeal joint
  (MPJ)
metacarpus
metacentric
metacercaria
metachromasia
metachromatic
metachromatic
  leukodystrophy
metachromatism
metachromophil
metachrosis
metacone

metaconid
metaconule
metacyesis
metagenesis
metagglutinin
Metagonimus
Metagonimus yokogawai
Metahydrin
  (trichlormethiazide)
metaicteric
metainfective
metakinesis
metal fume fever
metalbumin
metallesthesia
metallic
metallic tinkling
metalloenzyme
metalloid
metallophilia
metallophobia
metalloporphyrin
metalloprotein
metalloscopy
metallotherapy
metallurgy
metamer
metamere
metameric
metamerism
metamorphopsia
metamorphosis
Metamucil (psyllium
  hydrophilic mucilloid)
metamyelocyte
Metandren
  (methyltestosterone)
metanephrine
metanephrogenic
metanephros
metaneutrophil
metaphase
metaphrenia
metaphysis
metaphysitis
metaplasia
metaplasm
metaplastic

metapneumonic
metapophysis
Metaprel (metaproterenol
  sulfate)
metaprotein
metaproterenol sulfate
metapsychology
metaraminol bitartrate
metarubricyte
metastable
metastasis
metastasize
metastatic
metasternum
metatarsal
metatarsalgia
metatarsectomy
metatarsophalangeal
metatarsophalangeal joint
metatarsus
metatarsus primus varus
metatarsus varus
Metatensin
  (trichlormethiazide and
  reserpine)
metathalamus
metathesis
metatrophia
metatrophic
metatypical
metaxalone
Metchnikoff's theory
metencephalon
meteorism
meteoropathy
meteorotropic
meteorotropism
meter (m)
meter-kilogram-second
  (MKS)
metergasis
metestrus
methacholine bronchial
  challenge test
methacholine chloride
methacycline
  hydrochloride
methadone hydrochloride

Methalgen (external
  analgesic cream)
methallenestril
methamphetamine
  hydrochloride
methandriol
methandrostenolone
methane (CH_4)
methanol
methantheline bromide
methapyrilene fumarate
methaqualone
  hydrochloride
metharbital
methazolamide
methdilazine
methemalbumin
methemoglobin
methemoglobin reductase
methemoglobinemia
methemoglobinuria
methenamine
methenamine mandelate
Methergine
  (methylergonovine
  maleate)
methicillin sodium
methimazole
methiodal sodium
methionine
methisazone
methixene hydrochloride
methocarbamol
methodology
methohexital sodium
methomania
methotrexate
methotrexate sodium
methotrimeprazine
methoxamine hydrochloride
methoxsalen
methoxyflurane
methoxyphenamine
  hydrochloride
methscopolamine bromide
methsuximide
methyclothiazide
methy alcohol poisoning

methylate
methylation
methylatropine nitrate
methylbenzethonium
  chloride
methylcellulose
methyldopa
methyldopa hydrochloride
methyldopa-
  hydrochlorothiazide
methylene
methylene blue
methylenophil
methylergonovine maleate
methylmalonic acidemia
methylparaben
methylphenidate
  hydrochloride
methylprednisolone
methylrosaniline chloride
methyltestosterone
methylthiouracil
methyltransferase
methyprylon
methysergide maleate
Metimyd (prednisolone
  acetate and
  sulfacetamide sodium)
metmyoglobin
metocurine iodide
metonymy
metopagus
metopic
metopion
Metopirone (metyrapone)
metopism
metopodynia
metoprolol tartrate
metoxenous
metoxeny
metralgia
metratome
metratomy
metratonia
metratrophia
metrectasia
metrectopia
metreurynter

metreurysis
metria
metriocephalic
metritis
metrizamide
metrocarcinoma
metrocele
metrocolpocele
metrocystosis
Metrodin (urofollitropin)
metrodynia
metromalacia
metromalacosis
metronidazole
metronome
metronoscope
metroparalysis
metropathia hemorrhagica
metropathic
metropathy
metroperitoneal
metroperitonitis
metrophlebitis
metroplasty
metroptosis
metrorrhagia
metrorrhea
metrorrhexis
metrosalpingitis
metrosalpingography
metrostaxis
metrostenosis
metrotherapy
metrotome
metrotomy
metrourethrotome
Metubine Iodide
   (metocurine iodide)
metyrapone
metyrapone test
Mevacor (lovastatin)
Mexate (methotrexate
   sodium)
Mexate-AQ (methotrexate
   sodium)
Mexitil (mexiletine HCl)
Meynert's commissure
Meynet's nodosities

Mezlin (mezlocillin
   sodium)
miasm
miasma
miasmatic
mica
mication
micella
miconazole nitrate
micra
micracusia
micrencephalon
micrencephalous
micrencephaly
MICRhoGAM (Rho(D) immune
   globulin [human])
Micro-Guard
   (antimicrobial skin
   cream)
Micro-K Extencaps
   (potassium chloride)
Micro-K 10 Extencaps
   (potassium chloride)
microabscess
microaerophilic
microanalysis
microanatomy
microaneurysm
microangiitis
microangiopathy
microbalance
microbe
microbial
microbic
microbicidal
microbicide
microbiology
microbiophobia
microbiota
microbiotic
microbism
microblast
microblepharism
microblephary
microbodies
microbrachia
microbrachius
microcalorie

microcardia
microcaulia
microcentrum
microcephalia
microcephalic
microcephalous
microcephalus
microcephaly
microcheilia
microcheiria
microchemistry
microchiria
microcinematography
microcirculation
Micrococcaceae
Micrococcus
Micrococcus albus
Micrococcus melitensis
microcolon
microcoria
microcornea
microcoulomb
microcrystalline
microcurie
microcurie-hour
microcyst
microcytase
microcyte
microcythemia
microcytic anemia
microcytosis
microdactylia
microdactylia repair
microdetermination
microdissection
microdissection, nervous
   system
microdont
microdontia
microdontism
microdose
microdosimetry
microelectrophoresis
microembolus
microencephaly
microenvironment
microerythrocyte
microfarad

microfauna
microfibril
microfibrillar collagen
   hemostat
microfiche
microfilament
microfilaremia
microfilaria
microfilm
microflora
microgamete
microgametocyte
microgamy
microgastria
microgenia
microgenitalism
microglia
microgliacyte
microglioma
microglobulin, beta-2
microglossia
micrognathia
micrognathism
microgonioscope
microgram (mcg)
micrograph
micrography
microgyria
microgyrus
microhematocrit
microhepatia
microhm
microincineration
microinjection
microinvasion
microleakage
microlens
microlentia
microlesion
microleukoblast
microliter
microlith
microlithiasis
micromanipulator
micromastia
micromazia
micromelia
micromelus

micromere
micrometer (μm)
micromethod
micrometry
micromicrogram (μμg)
micromicron (μμ, μμm)
micromillimeter (μmm)
micromole
micromolecular
Micromonospora
micromyces
micromyelia
micromyeloblast
micromyelolymphocyte
micron (μ, μm)
Micronase (glyburide)
microne
microneedle
micronize
micronodular
micronucleus
micronutrient
micronychia
microorganism
microparasite
micropathology
micropenis
microphage
microphagocyte
microphagus
microphakia
microphallus
microphobia
microphone
microphonia
microphonoscope
microphotograph
microphthalmia
microphthalmus
microphysics
microphyte
micropia
micropipette
microplasia
microplethysmography
micropodia
micropolariscope
microprobe

microprojection
microprosopia
micropsia
micropuncture
micropus
micropyle
microradiography
microrefractometer
microrespirometer
microrhinia
microscelous
microscope
microscope, binocular
microscope, compound
microscope, dark-field
microscope, electron
microscope, light
microscope, operating
microscope, phase
microscope, polarization
microscope, scanning
   electron (SEM)
microscope, simple
microscope, slit-lamp
microscope, stereoscopic
microscope, ultraviolet
microscope, x-ray
microscopic
microscopical
microscopy
microsecond
microseme
microsmatic
microsomal antibody
   (thyroid; RIA)
microsomal antibody test
microsome
microsomia
microspectrophotometry
microspectroscope
microspheres
microspherocyte
microspherocytosis
microsphygmia
microsplanchnic
microsplenia
microsporid
Microsporon

microsporosis
Microsporum
Microsporum audouini
Microsporum canis
microstomia
microstrabismus
microsurgery
microsyringe
microthelia
microtia
microtome
microtomy
microtonometer
microtrauma
microtropia
microtubule
microtus
microvascular
microvascular anastomosis
microvilli
microvolt
microwave
microwave, physical
  therapy
microxycyte
microxyphil
microzoon
micrurgy
miction
micturate
micturition
micturition syncope
Midamor (amiloride HCl)
midarm muscle
  circumference (MAMC)
midazolam hydrochloride
midbody
midbrain
midcarpal
middle lobe syndrome
midface hypoplasia
midge
midget
midgut
midgut volvulus reduction
midline
midoccipital
Midol 200 (ibuprofen)

Midol PMS
midpain
midplane
midriff
Midrin
midsagittal plane
midsection
midsternum
midstream specimen
midtarsal
midtarsal amputation
midtarsal arthrodesis
midtarsal osteotomy
midwife
midwifery
migraine
Migralam (isometheptene
  mucate, caffeine,
  acetaminophen)
migration
migration inhibitory
  factor test (MIF)
migratory
Mikulicz resection
Mikulicz's drain
Mikulicz's mask
Mikulicz's pad
Mikulicz's syndrome
mildew
milia
miliaria
miliary
miliary fever
miliary tubercles
miliary tuberculosis
milieu
milieu therapy
military antishock
  trousers (MAST)
milium
milk
milk, acidophilus
milk, casein
milk fever
milk leg
milk, ropy
milk teeth
milk tumor

milk, uviol
milk, witch's
milk-alkali syndrome
milker's nodules
milking
Milkman's syndrome
Miller procedure
Miller-Abbott tube
Miller-Abbott tube
  introduction
milliammeter
milliampere (ma)
milliampere minute
milliampere-seconds
millibar
millicoulomb
millicurie (mc)
milligram (mg)
millilambert
milliliter (ml)
millimicrocurie
millimicrogram
millimole (mM)
Millin-Read suspension
milling-in
millinormal
million electron volts
  (Mev)
milliosmole
millipede
millisecond
millivolt
Milontin (phensuximide)
milphae
milphosis
Milroy's disease
Miltown (meprobamate)
Milwaukee brace
mimesis
mimetic
mimic
mimmation
mimosis
Minamata disease
mind
mineral
mineral acid
mineral compounds

mineral oil
mineral spring
mineral water
mineralization
mineralocorticoid
Minerva cast
Mini-Gamulin Rh (Rho(D)
  immune globulin,
  [human])
minification
minim (m̞)
minimal
minimal air
minimal brain damage
  (MBD)
minimal brain dysfunction
  (MBD)
minimal cerebral
  dysfunction
minimal change disease
minimal dose
minimum
minimum daily
  requirements (MDR)
minimum lethal dose
minimum reacting dose
  (MRD)
Minin light
Minipress (prazosin HCl)
Minizide (prazosin HCl
  and polythiazide)
Minocin (minocycline HCl)
minocycline hydrochloride
Minot-Murphy diet
minoxidil
Mintezol (thiabendazole)
minute volume
miocardia
miodidymus
miolecithal
mionectic
mioplasmia
miopragia
miopus
miosis
miotic
miracidium
miracle, medical

mire
mirror
miryachit
misanthropia
miscarriage
misce (M)
misce bene (mb)
miscegenation
miscible
misocainia
misogamy
misogynist
misogyny
misologia
misoneism
misopedia
Mission Prenatal
  (vitamins-iron-calcium-
  folic acid)
mister
mistura
Mitchell procedure
Mitchell's disease
mite
mite, follicle
mite, itch
mite, mange
mite, red
mitella
Mithracin (plicamycin)
mithramycin
mithridatism
miticide
mitigated
mitis
mitochondria
mitogen
mitogen culture
mitogenesis
mitoma
mitome
mitomycin
mitoplasm
mitosis
mitosome
mitotane
mitotic
mitral commissurotomy

mitral disease
mitral murmur
mitral orifice
mitral regurgitation
mitral stenosis
mitral valve
mitral valve prolapse
mitralization
Mitrolan (calcium
  polycarbophil)
mittelschmerz
Mittendorf's dot
mix
mixed
mixoscopia
Mixtard (U-100 isophane
  purified pork insulin)
mixture
mnemasthenia
mnemic
mnemonics
Moban (molindone HCl)
Mobigesic (analgesic
  tablet)
mobile
mobile arm support
mobile intensive care
  unit (MICU)
mobile spasm
mobility
mobility training
mobilization
mobilize
Mobisyl (analgesic creme)
Möbius' disease
modal
modality
Modane (phenolphthalein)
Modane Plus
  (phenolphthalein and
  docusate sodium)
Modane Soft (docusate
  sodium)
Modane Versabran
  (psyllium and bran)
mode
model
modeling

modem
moderated
Moderil (rescinnamine)
Modicon 21 (combination oral contraceptive)
Modicon 28 (combination oral contraceptive)
modification
modiolus
modulation
modulus
Moduretic (amiloride HCl hydrochlorothiazide)
modus
modus operandi
mogilalia
mogiphonia
Mohrenheim's space
Mohs technique
Mohs' chemosurgery technique
moiety
moist
Moisturel (skin lubricant-moisturizer)
mol (m)
molal
molality
molar
molar solution
molariform
molarity
mold
molding
mole (m)
mole, blood
mole, Breus
mole, carneous
mole, false
mole, fleshy
mole, hydatid
mole, pigmented
mole, stone
mole, true
mole, vascular
mole, vesicular
molecular
molecular biology

molecular disease
molecular layer
molecular lesion
molecular weight (mol. wt.)
molecular weight assay
molecule
molimen
Moll's glands
mollities
mollities ossium
mollusc
Mollusca
molluscous
molluscum
molluscum contagiosum
molluscum fibrosum
mollusk
molt
molybdenum (Mo)
momentum
monad
monamide
monamine
monarthric
monarthritis
monarticular
monaster
monathetosis
monatomic
monaural
monaxonic
Mondonesi's reflex
Mondor's disease
monecious
monesthetic
monestrous
mongolian spots
mongolism
mongoloid
monilethrix
Monilia
monilial
moniliasis
moniliform
moniliid
moniliosis
Monistat (miconazole)

**Monistat 3 Vaginal
   Suppositories**
   (miconazole nitrate)
Monistat 7 Vaginal Cream
   (miconazole nitrate)
**Monistat 7 Vaginal
   Suppositories**
   (miconazole nitrate)
Monistat Dual Pak
   (miconzole nitrate)
Monistat-Derm (miconzole
   nitrate)
monitor
monitor, blood pressure
monitor, cardiac
monitor, fetal
monitor, Holter
monitor, personal
   radiation
monitor, temperature
monitoring test
Mono spot test
Mono-Vacc Test (O.T.)
   (old tuberculin)
monoacidic
monoamide
monoamine
monoamine oxidase
   inhibitors (MAO)
monoanesthesia
monobacillary
monobacterial
monobasic
monobenzone
monoblast
monoblastoma
monoblepsia
monobrachius
monobromated
monocalcic
monocardian
monocelled
monocephalus
monochord
monochorea
monochorionic
monochromasy
monochromatic

monochromatism
monochromatophil
monochromator
Monocid (cefonicid
   sodium)
Monoclate (factor VIII:C)
monoclinic
monoclonal
monoclonal antibodies
monococcus
monocontaminated
monocrotic
monocular
monoculus
monocyclic
monocyte
monocytic
monocytosis
monodactylism
monodal
monodermoma
monodiplopia
monodromia
monoecious
monogamy
monogenesis
monogerminal
monogony
monograph
monohydrated
monohydric
monoideaism
monoideism
monoinfection
monoiodotyrosine
monolayer
monolocular
monomania
monomaniac
monomastigote
monomelic
monomer
monomeric
monometallic
monomicrobic
monomolecular
monomorphic
monomyoplegia

monomyositis
mononeural
mononeuritis
mononeuropathy
mononoea
mononuclear
mononuclear phagocyte
  system (MPS)
mononucleosis
mononucleosis, infectious
mononucleotide
monoparesis
monoparesthesia
monopathy
monophagia
monophasia
monophobia
monophthalmus
monophyletic
monophyletism
monophyodont
monoplasmatic
monoplast
monoplegia
monopodia
monopolar
monops
monopsychosis
monopus
monorchia
monorchid
monorchidism
monorchism
monorhinic
monosaccharide
monosodium glutamate
  (MSG)
monosome
monosomy
monospasm
monospermy
monostotic
monostratal
monosubstituted
monosymptomatic
monosynaptic
monoterminal
monothermia

monotocous
Monotricha
monotrichous
monovalent
monoxenous
monoxide
monozygotic
monozygotic twins
Monro's foramen
Monro's sulcus
mons
mons pubis
mons veneris
monster
monstriparity
monstrosity
Monteggia's fracture
Montgomery straps
Montgomery's glands
monticulus
monticulus cerebelli
mood
mood disorders
moon face
Moore's lightning streaks
Moraxella
morbid
morbidity
morbidity rate
morbific
morbilli
morbilliform
morbillous
morbus
morbus caeruleus
morbus miseriae
morcellation
morcellement
mordant
mores
Morgagni
Morgagni's caruncle
Morgagni's cataract
Morgagni's hydatid
Morgagni's hyperostosis
Morgagni's ventricle
morgagnian
morgagnian cyst

morgue
moria
moribund
morioplasty
morning (a.m., AM)
morning care
morning sickness
morning stiffness
Moro reflex
moron
morphea
morpheme
morphia
morphine poisoning
morphine sulfate (MS)
morphinism
morphinomania
morphiomania
morphogenesis
morphogenetic
morphogenetic processes
morphogenetic substance
morphography
morphology
morphometric analysis
morphometry
morphon
morphosis
morpio
morpion
Morquio's syndrome
morrhuate sodium
  injection
mors
mors putativa
mors subita
morsal
morsulus
mortal
mortality
mortar
mortician
mortification
mortinatality
mortise joint
Morton's disease
Morton's foot syndrome
Morton's neuralgia

Morton's neuroma
Morton's syndrome
mortuary
morula
morulation
moruloid
Morvan's disease
mosaic
mosaic bone
mosaicism
mosquito
mosquito forceps
mosquitocide
moss
moss, sphagnum
mossy cell
mossy fibers
mother
mother cell
mother cyst
mother liquor
mother's mark
motile
motility
motion
motion, active
motion, passive
motion sickness
motivation
motive
motofacient
motoneuron
motor
motor aphasia
motor area
motor endplate
motor fibers
motor nerve
motor neuroma
motor neuron
motor neuron disease
  (MND)
motor points
motor sense
motor speech area
motor unit
motorial
motoricity

motorium
motorius
motorpathy
Motrin (ibuprofen)
mottled enamel
mottling
moulage
mounding
mount
mount, x-ray
mountain fever
mountain sickness,
  chronic
mountant
mounting
mourning
mouse
mouse, joint
mouse unit
mouth (os)
mouth, biopsy
mouth, floor
mouth, trench
mouthrinse
mouthstick
mouthwash
movement
movement, active
movement, ameboid
movement, angular
movement, associated
movement, autonomic
movement, bodily
movement, brownian
movement, ciliary
movement, circus
movement, disorders of
movement, gliding
movement, hinge
movement, jaw
movement, masticatory
movement, molecular
movement of restitution
movement, orthodontic
movement, passive
movement, peristaltic
movement, respiratory
movement, rotational

movement, segmenting
movement, tipping
movement, vermicular
movement, vibratile
movements, fetal
movements, pendular
movements, saccadic
moxa
moxalactam disodium
moxibustion
MS Contin (morphine
  sulfate)
MSIR (morphine sulfate)
MSTA (mumps skin test
  antigen)
Mubamycin (mitomycin)
mucedin
muciferous
muciform
mucigen
mucigenous
mucilage
mucilaginous
mucilago
mucilloid
mucilloid, psyllium
  hydrophilic
mucin
mucinase
mucinemia
mucinogen
mucinoid
mucinolytic
mucinuria
muciparous
mucocele
mucocolpos
mucocutaneous
mucocutaneous lymph node
  syndrome
mucodermal
mucoenteritis
mucofistula, creation
mucoglobulin
mucoid
mucomembranous
Mucomyst (acetylcysteine)
mucoperiosteum

mucopolysacchariduria
mucopolysaccharidase
mucopolysaccharide
mucopolysaccharidosis
  (MPS)
mucopolysaccharide, acid
mucoprotein
mucoprotein, Tamm-
  Horsfall
mucopurulent
mucopus
Mucor
mucoriferous
mucorin
mucormycosis
mucorrhea
mucosa
mucosa, alveolar
mucosa, lingual
mucosa, masticatory
mucosa, nasal
mucosa, oral
mucosal
mucosanguineous
mucosectomy, rectal
mucosedative
mucoserous
mucosin
mucositis
mucosocutaneous
mucostatic
mucous
mucous colitis
mucous membrane
mucous polypus
mucoviscidosis
mucro
mucus
Mudrane
Mudrane GG Elixir
Mudrane GG Tablets
Mudrane GG-2 Tablets
Mudrane-2 Tablets
mulatto
muliebria
muliebrity
mull
Müller, Heinrich

Müller, Johannes P.
Müller's ducts
Müller's fibers
Müller's muscle
Müller's ring
Müller's trigone
Müller's tubercle
Müllerian duct cyst
multangular
multangular bone, greater
multangular bone, lesser
multiarticular
multicapsular
multicellular
Multiceps
multicuspid
multicuspidate
multifactorial
multifamilial
multifid
multifocal
multiform
multiglandular
multigravida
multi-infection
multilobular
multilocular
multimammae
multinodal
multinodular
multinuclear
multinucleate
multipara
multiparity
multiparous
multipartial
multiphasic screening
multiple
multiple drug resistance
multiple endocrine
  neoplasia (MEN)
multiple endocrine
  neoplasia syndrome type
  I (MEN-I)
multiple gated
  acquisition (MUGA)
multiple myeloma
multiple personality

multiple sclerosis (MS)
multiple systems organ
  failure (MSOF)
multiplexor
multipolar
multirooted
multisynaptic
multiterminal
Multitest CMI (skin test
  antigens for cellular
  hypersensitivity)
Multitrace (trace element
  mixture)
Multitrace Pediatric
  (trace element mixture)
multivalent
Mulvidren-F Softab
  (fluoride with
  multivitamins)
Mumford operation
mummification
mumps
mumps immunization
mumps skin test antigen
mumps virus vaccine live
mumps virus vaccine live
  attenuated
Mumpsvax (mumps virus
  vaccine)
Münchhausen syndrome
mural
muramidase
Murchison-Pel-Ebstein
  fever
murdering while asleep
muriate
muriatic acid
Murine
murine
Murine Ear Drops
**Murine Ear Wax Removal
  System**
Murine Plus
murmur
murmur, aneurysmal
murmur, aortic
  obstructive

murmur, aortic
  regurgitant
murmur, apex
murmur, arterial
murmur, Austin flint
murmur, bronchial
murmur, cardiac
murmur, cardiopulmonary
murmur, continuous
murmur, crescendo
murmur, Cruveilhier-
  Baumgarten
murmur, diastolic
murmur, Duroziez'
murmur, ejection
murmur, endocardial
murmur, exocardial
murmur, Flint's
murmur, friction
murmur, functional
murmur, Gibson
murmur, Graham Steell's
murmur, heart
murmur, hemic
murmur, machinery
murmur, mitral
murmur, musical
murmur, organic
murmur, pansystolic
murmur, pericardial
murmur, physiologic
murmur, prediastolic
murmur, pulmonary
murmur, regurgitant
murmur, seagull
murmur, Still's
murmur, systolic
murmur, to-and-fro
murmur, tricuspid
murmur, vascular
murmur, vesicular
Murphy's button
Murphy's sign
Mus
Mus musculus
Musca
Musca domestica
muscae volitantes

muscarine
muscegenetic
muscicide
muscle
muscle, abductor digiti
 minimi manus
muscle, abductor digiti
 minimi pedis
muscle, abductor hallucis
muscle, abductor pollicis
 brevis
muscle, abductor pollicis
 longus
muscle, adductor brevis
muscle, adductor hallucis
muscle, adductor longus
muscle, adductor magnus
muscle, adductor pollicis
muscle, anconeus
muscle, antagonistic
muscle, antitragicus
muscle, appendicular
muscle, arrectores
 pilorum
muscle, articularis genus
muscle, aryepiglotticus
muscle, arytenoideus
muscle, auricularis
 anterior
muscle, auricularis
 posterior
muscle, auricularis
 superior
muscle, axial
muscle, biceps brachii
muscle, biceps femoris
muscle, biopsy
muscle, bipennate
muscle, brachialis
muscle, brachioradialis
muscle, buccinator
muscle, bulbospongiosus
muscle, ciliaris
muscle, coccygeus
muscle compartment
 syndrome
muscle, constrictor
 pharyngis inferior

muscle, constrictor
 pharyngis medius
muscle, constrictor
 pharyngis superior
muscle, coracobrachialis
muscle, corrugator cutis
 ani
muscle, corrugator
 supercilii
muscle cramps
muscle, cremaster
muscle, cricoarytenoideus
 lateralis
muscle, cricoarytenoideus
 posterior
muscle, cricothyroideus
muscle, deltoideus
muscle, debridement
muscle, depressor anguli
 oris
muscle, depressor labii
 inferioris
muscle, depressor septi
 nasi
muscle, depressor
 urethrae
muscle, diaphragma
muscle, digastricus
muscle, dilatator naris
 anterior
muscle, dilatator naris
 posterior
muscle, extensor carpi
 radialis brevis
muscle, extensor carpi
 radialis longus
muscle, extensor carpi
 ulnaris
muscle, extensor digiti
 minimi
muscle, extensor
 digitorum brevis
muscle, extensor
 digitorum communis
muscle, extensor
 digitorum longus
muscle, extensor hallucis
 longus

muscle, extensor indicis
  proprius
muscle, extensor pollicis
  brevis
muscle, extensor pollicis
  longus
muscle, extrinsic
muscle, fixation
muscle, flexor carpi
  radialis
muscle, flexor carpi
  ulnaris
muscle, flexor digiti
  quinti brevis manus
muscle, flexor digiti
  quinti brevis pedis
muscle, flexor digitorum
  brevis
muscle, flexor digitorum
  longus
muscle, flexor digitorum
  profundus
muscle, flexor digitorum
  superficialis
muscle, flexor hallucis
  brevis
muscle, flexor hallucis
  longus
muscle, flexor pollicis
  brevis
muscle, flexor pollicis
  longus
muscle, fusiform
muscle, gastrocnemius
muscle, gemellus inferior
muscle, gemellus superior
muscle, genioglossus
muscle, geniohyoideus
muscle, glossopalatinus
muscle, gluteus maximus
muscle, gluteus medius
muscle, gluteus minimus
muscle, gracilis
muscle, helicis major and
  minor
muscle, hyoglossus
muscle, iliacus

muscle, iliocostalis
  cervicis
muscle, iliocostalis
  lumborum
muscle, iliocostalis
  thoracis
muscle, infraspinatus
muscle, intercostalis
  externus
muscle, intercostalis
  internus
muscle, interossei
  dorsales manus
muscle, interossei
  dorsales pedis
muscle, interossei
  plantares
muscle, interossei
  volares
muscle, interspinales
muscle,
  intertransversarii
muscle, intrinsic
muscle, involuntary
muscle, ischiocavernosus
muscle, latissimus dorsi
muscle, levator anguli
  oris
muscle, levator ani
muscle, levator labii
  superioris
muscle, levator labii
  superioris alaeque nasi
muscle, levator palpebrae
  superioris
muscle, levator scapulae
muscle, levator veli
  palatini
muscle, levatores
  costarum
muscle, linguae
muscle, longissimus
  capitis
muscle, longissimus
  cervicis
muscle, longissimus
  thoracis
muscle, longus capitis

muscle, longus colli
muscle, lumbricales manus
muscle, lumbricales
   plantar
muscle, masseter
muscle, mentalis
muscle, multifidus
muscle, multipennate
muscle, mylohyoideus
muscle, nasalis
muscle, nonstriated
muscle, obliquus
   auriculae
muscle, obliquus capitis
   superior
muscle, obliquus externus
   abdominis
muscle, obliquus inferior
   oculi
muscle, obliquus internus
   abdominis
muscle, obliquus superior
   oculi
muscle, obturatorius
   internus
muscle, occipitofrontalis
muscle, omohyoideus
muscle, opponens digiti
   quinti
muscle, oppenens pollicis
muscle, orbicularis oculi
muscle, orbicularis oris
muscle, palmaris brevis
muscle, palmaris longus
muscle panel
muscle, papillary
muscle, pectineus
muscle, pectoralis major
muscle, pectoralis minor
muscle, peroneus brevis
muscle, peroneus longus
muscle, peroneus tertius
muscle, pharyngopalatinus
muscle, piriformis
muscle, plantaris
muscle, platysma
muscle, popliteus
muscle, postaxial

muscle, preaxial
muscle, procerus
muscle, pronator
   quadratus
muscle, pronator teres
muscle, psoas major
muscle, psoas minor
muscle, pterygoideus
   lateralis
muscle, pterygoideus
   medialis
muscle, pyramidalis
muscle, quadratus femoris
muscle, quadratus
   lumborum
muscle, quadratus plantae
muscle, quadriceps
   femoris
muscle, rectus abdominis
muscle, rectus capitis
   anterior
muscle, rectus capitis
   lateralis
muscle, rectus capitis
   posterior major
muscle, rectus capitis
   posterior minor
muscle, rectus externus
   or lateralis
muscle, rectus femoris
muscle, rectus inferior
muscle, rectus internus
   or medialis
muscle, rectus superior
muscle, rhomboideus major
muscle, risorius
muscle, rotatores
muscle, sacrospinalis
muscle,
   salpingopharyngeus
muscle, sartorius
muscle, scalenus anterior
muscle, scalenus medius
muscle, scalenus
   posterior
muscle, semimembranosus
muscle, semispinalis
   capitis

muscle, semispinalis
cervicis
muscle, semispinalis
thoracis
muscle, semitendinosus
muscle, serratus anterior
muscle, serratus
posterior inferior
muscle, serratus
posterior superior
muscle, skeletal
muscle, soleus
muscle, smooth
muscle, somatic
muscle soreness
muscle, sphincter
muscle, sphincter ani
externus
muscle, sphincter ani
internus
muscle, sphincter
urethrae membranaceae
muscle, sphincter of
urinary bladder
muscle, sphincter vesicae
muscle, spinalis capitis
muscle, spinalis cervicis
muscle, spinalis thoracis
muscle, splenius capitis
muscle, splenius cervicis
muscle, stapedius
muscle,
sternocleidomastoideus
muscle, sternohyoideus
muscle, sternothyroideus
muscle, striated
muscle, styloglossus
muscle, stylohyoideus
muscle, stylopharyngeus
muscle, subclavius
muscle, subcostales
muscle, subscapularis
muscle, supinator
muscle, supraspinatus
muscle, suspensorius
duodeni
muscle, temporalis

muscle, tensor fasciae
latae
muscle, tensor tympani
muscle, tensor veli
palatini
muscle, teres major
muscle, teres minor
muscle, testing
muscle, thyroarytenoideus
muscle, thyroepiglotticus
muscle, thyrohyoideus
muscle, tibialis anterior
muscle, tibialis
posterior
muscle, tragicus
muscle, transversus
abdominis
muscle, transversus
auriculae
muscle, transversus
perinei profundus
muscle, transversus
perinei superficialis
muscle, transversus
thoracis
muscle, trapezius
muscle, triceps brachii
muscle, unipennate
muscle, unstriated
muscle, uvulae
muscle, vastus
intermedius
muscle, vastus lateralis
muscle, vastus medialis
muscle, voluntary
muscle, zygomaticus major
muscle, zygomaticus minor
muscles, antigravity
muscles, extraocular eye
muscles, mastication
muscles, mimetic
muscles, synergistic
muscles electromyography
muscular
muscular dystrophy
muscularis
muscularis mucosae
muscularity

musculature
musculin
musculoaponeurotic
musculocutaneous
musculofascial
musculomembranous
musculophrenic
musculoplasty
musculoskeletal (MS)
musculotendinous
musculotendinous cuff
  repair
musculotropic
musculus
mushbite
mushroom
mushroom and toadstool
  poisoning
music therapy
musicogenic
musicogenic epilepsy
musicomania
musicotherapy
musk
mussel
mussel poisoning
Musset's sign
mussitation
mustard
mustard, nitrogen
mustard repair
Mustargen
  (mechlorethamine HCl)
mutacism
mutagen
mutagenesis
mutagenicity
mutant
mutase
mutation
mute
mute, deaf
mutiallelic
mutilate
mutilation
mutism
mutualism
mutualist

myalgia
Myambutol (ethambutol
  HCl)
myasis
myasthenia
myasthenia,
  angiosclerotic
myasthenia cordis
myasthenia gastrica
myasthenia gravis
myasthenic
myatonia
myatrophy
Mycelex (clotrimazole)
Mycelex G (clotrimazole)
mycelioid
mycelium
mycetes
mycethemia
mycetism
mycetismus
mycetogenetic
mycetoma
Myciguent (antibiotic
  ointment)
Mycitracin (triple
  antibiotic ointment)
mycobacteria culture
mycobacteriosis
Mycobacterium
Mycobacterium, atypical
Mycobacterium balnei
Mycobacterium bovis
Mycobacterium kansasii
Mycobacterium leprae
Mycobacterium marinum
*Mycobacterium
  tuberculosis*
mycocidin
mycoderma
mycodermatitis
mycodermomycosis
mycohemia
mycoid
Mycolog-II (nystatin and
  triamcinolone
  acetonide)
mycology

mycomyringitis
mycophthalmia
mycoplasma culture
mycoplasmas
mycoprecipitin
mycosis
mycosis fungoides
mycostasis
mycostat
Mycostatin Ointment
(nystatin)
Mycostatin Pastilles
(nystatin)
Mycostatin Vaginal
Tablets (nystatin)
mycotic
mycotoxicosis
mycotoxin
mycotoxinization
mycotoxins
mycterophonia
mydaleine
mydriasis
mydriatic
myectomy
myectopia
myelalgia
myelanalosis
myelapoplexy
myelasthenia
myelatelia
myelatrophy
myelauxe
myelemia
myelencephalon
myelic
myelin
myelin basic protein,
CSF, RIA
myelination
myelinic
myelinization
myelinoclasis
myelinogenesis
myelinogenetic
myelinolysis
myelinosis
myelitic

myelitis
myelitis, acute
myelitis, ascending,
acute
myelitis, bulbar
myelitis, central
myelitis, compression
myelitis, descending
myelitis, disseminated
myelitis, focal
myelitis, hemorrhagic
myelitis, sclerosing
myelitis, transverse
myelitis, traumatic
myelobastemia
myeloblast
myeloblastoma
myeloblastosis
myelocele
myelocyst
myelocystocele
myelocystomeningocele
myelocyte
myelocythemia
myelocytic
myelocytosis
myelodiastasis
myelodysplasia
myeloencephalic
myeloencephalitis
myelofibrosis
myelogenesis
myelogenic
myelogenous
myelogeny
myelogram
myelography
myeloid
myeloidosis
myelolymphangioma
myelolymphocyte
myelolysis
myeloma
myelomalacia
myelomatosis
myelomenia
myelomeningitis
myelomeningocele

myelomere
myelomyces
myeloneuritis
myelopathy
myelopetal
myelophage
myelophthisis
myeloplast
myeloplax
myeloplaxoma
myeloplegia
myelopoiesis
myelopoiesis, ectopic
myelopoiesis,
  extramedullary
myelopore
myeloproliferative
myeloradiculitis
myeloradiculodysplasia
myeloradiculopathy
myelorrhagia
myelorrhaphy
myelosarcomatosis
myeloschisis
myelosclerosis
myelosis
myelospongium
myelosuppressive
myelosyphilis
myelosyringosis
myelotome
myelotomy
myelotoxic
myelotoxin
myenteric
myenteric reflex
myenteron
Myerson's sign
myesthesia
myiasis
myiocephalon
myiodesopsia
myiosis
myitis
Mylanta (antacid/anti-
  gas)
Mylanta-II (antacid/anti-
  gas)

Myleran (busulfan)
Mylicon (simethicone)
mylodus
mylohyoid
myoalbumin
myoalbumose
myoarchitectonic
myoatrophy
myoblast
myoblastoma
myocardial
myocardial infarction
  (MI)
myocardial insufficiency
myocardial perfusion
myocardial repair of
  septal defect
myocardial resection
myocardial scan
myocardial
  scintiphotography
myocardiectomy
myocardiograph
myocardiopathy
myocardiosis
myocardiotomy
myocarditis
myocarditis, acute
  primary
myocarditis, acute
  secondary
myocarditis, acute septic
myocarditis, chronic
myocarditis,
  fragmentation
myocarditis, indurative
myocardium
myocardosis
myocele
myocelialgia
myocelitis
myocellulitis
myoceptor
myocerosis
myochorditis
myochrome
myochronoscope

Myochrysine (gold sodium
  thiomalate)
myocinesimeter
myoclasis
myoclonia
myoclonus multiplex
myoclonus, palatal
myocoele
myocolpitis
myocomma
myocrismus
myocutaneous flap
myocyte
myocytoma
myodemia
myodesopsia
myodiastasis
myodiopter
myodynamia
myodynamometer
myodynia
myodystonia
myodystrophy
myoedema
myoelastic
myoelectric
myoelectric prosthesis
myoendocarditis
myoepithelial
myoepithelioma
myofasciitis
myofibril
myofibrilla
myofibroma
myofibrosis
myofibrositis
myofilament
myofunctional
myogelosis
myogen
myogenesis
myogenetic
myogenic
myoglia
myoglobin
myoglobinuria
myoglobulin
myognathus

myogram
myograph
myographic
myography
myohematin
myohemoglobin (MHb)
myohysterectomy
myoid
myoidema
myoischemia
myokerosis
myokinase
myokinesimeter
myokinesis
myokymia
myolemma
myolipoma
myology
myolysis
myoma
myoma, nonstriated
myoma striocellulare
myoma telangiectodes
myoma uteri
myomalacia
myomalacia cordis
myomatosis
myomatous
myomectomy
myomectomy, anorectal
myomectomy, uterine
myomelanosis
myomere
myometer
myometritis
myometrium
myomohysterectomy
myomotomy
myonecrosis
myonephropexy
myoneural
myoneuralgia
myoneurasthenia
myoneuroma
myonosus
myonymy
myopachynsis
myoparalysis

myoparesis
myopathic
myopathic facies
myopathy
myopathy, centronuclear
myopathy, cortisone
myopathy, distal
myopathy, facial
myopathy, metabolic
myopathy, myotubular
myopathy, nemaline
myopathy, ocular
myopathy, thyrotoxic
myope
myopericarditis
myophage
myophone
myopia (MY)
myopia, axial
myopia, chronic
myopia, curvature
myopia, index
myopia, malignant
myopia, pernicious
myopia, prodromal
myopia, progressive
myopia, stationary
myopia, transient
myopic
myopic crescent
myoplamus
myoplasm
myoplastic
myoplasty
myopolar
myoporthosis
myoprotein
myopsis
myopsychopathy
myorrhaphy
myorrhexis
myosalgia
myosalpingitis
myosarcoma
myosclerosis
myoseism
myosin
myosinase

myosinogen
myosinose
myosinuria
myositis, epidemic
myositis, fibrosa
myositis, interstitial
myositis, multiple
myositis ossificans
myositis, parenchymatous
myositis purulenta
myositis, traumatic
myositis, trichinosa
myospasm
myosteoma
myosthenometer
myostroma
myosuria
myosuture
myosynizesis
myotactic
myotasis
myotatic
myotatic reflex
myotenontoplasty
myotenoplasty
myotenositis
myotenotomy
myothermic
myotic
myotility
myotome
myotomy
myotomy, cricopharyngeal
Myotonachol (bethanechol chloride)
myotonia
myotonia atrophica
myotonia congenita
myotonia dystrophica
myotonic
myotonoid
myotonometer
myotonus
myotony
myotrophy
myotropic
myotube
myovascular

myriachit
Myriapoda
myriapodiasis
myricin
myringa
myringectomy
myringitis bullosa
myringodectomy
myringomycosis
myringoplasty
myringoscope
myringotome
myringotomy
myrmecia
myrrh
Mysoline (primidone)
mysophilia
mysophobia
Mysteclin-F (tetracycline
  and amphotericin B)
mytacism
mythomania
mythophobia
mytilotoxin
Mytrex (nystatin-
  triamcinolone
  acetonide)
myxadenitis
myxadenitis labialis
myxadenoma
myxangitis
myxasthenia
myxedema
myxedematoid
myxedematous
myxemia
myxiosis
myxoadenoma
Myxobacterales
myxochondrofibrosarcoma
myxochondroma
myxocystoma
myxocyte
myxoedema
myxoenchondroma
myxofibroma
myxofibrosarcoma
myxoglioma

myxoid
myxoinoma
myxolipoma
myxoma
myxoma, cartilaginous
myxoma, cystic
myxoma, enchondromatous
myxoma, erectile
myxoma, fibrous
myxoma, intracanalicular,
  of mamma
myxoma, odontogenic
myxoma, telangiectatic,
  vascular
Myxomycetes
myxomyoma
myxoneuroma
myxopapilloma
myxopoiesis
myxorrhea
myxosarcoma
myxosarcomatous
myxospore
Myxosporidia
myxoviruses
myzesis
Myzomyia
Myzorhynchus

N

nabothian cysts
nacreous
NADH-diaphorase
Naegele's obliquity
Naegele's pelvis
Naegele's rule
nafcillin sodium
nail
nail bed
nail biting
nail debridement
nail, eggshell
nail fold
nail groove

nail, hang
nail, ingrown
nail, intermedullary
nail matrix
nail plate
nail, reedy
nail removal
nail root
nail, Smith-Petersen
nail, spoon
nail wall
nail-patella syndrome
nailbed
Naja-naja
naked
Nalfon (fenoprofen calcium)
nalidixic acid
nalorphine hydrochloride
nandrolone decanoate
nandrolone phenpropionate
nanism
nanocephalism
nanocephalous
nanocormia
nanocurie (nc)
nanogram
nanoid
nanomelus
nanometer
nanophthalmos
nanosecond
nanosoma
nanosomia
nanosomus
nanous
nanukayami
nanus
nap
napalm
napalm burn
nape
napex
naphazoline hydrochloride
Naphcon-A (naphazoline HCl and pheniramine maleate)
naphtha

naphthalene
naphthol
napiform
naprapathy
Naprosyn (naproxen)
Naqua (trichlormethiazide)
Naquival (trichlormethiazide, reserpine)
Narcan (naloxone HCl)
narcissism
narcissistic
narcissistic object choice
narcoanalysis
narcoanesthesia
narcohypnia
narcohypnosis
narcolepsy
narcoleptic
narcomatous
narcosis
narcosynthesis
narcotic
narcotic addict
narcotic poisoning
narcotism
narcotize
Nardil (phenelzine sulfate)
naris, anterior
naris, posterior
narrowing
nasal abscess
nasal bleeding
nasal bones
nasal cavity
nasal concha
nasal douche
nasal endoscopy
nasal feeding
nasal fossa
nasal fracture
nasal function studies
nasal gavage
nasal graft
nasal height

nasal hematoma
nasal hemorrhage
nasal index
nasal line
nasal meatus
nasal mucous membrane
 test
nasal obstruction
nasal polyp, excision
nasal reflex
nasal septal perforations
 repair
nasal septum
nasal sinuses, accessory
nasal smear for
 eosinophils
nasal tip, rhinoplasty
nasal turbinate
nasal width
Nasalide (flunisolide)
nascent
nasioiniac
nasion
nasitis
Nasmyth's membrane
nasoantral
nasoantritis
nasociliary
nasoethmoid fracture
nasofrontal
nasogastric tube
nasolabial
nasolabial fistula repair
nasolacrimal
nasolacrimal duct
nasology
nasomaxillary fracture
nasomental
nasomental reflex
naso-oral
nasopalatine
nasopharyngeal
nasopharyngeal hemorrhage
 control
nasopharyngeal lesion
 excision
nasopharyngitis
nasopharyngography

nasopharyngoscope
nasopharynx
nasorostral
nasoscope
nasoseptitis
nasosinusitis
nasospinale
nasotracheobronchial
 aspiration
nasus
Natabec Kapseals (vitamin
 and mineral formula)
Natabec Rx Kapseals
 (vitamin and mineral
 formula with folic
 acid)
Natafort Filmseal
 (vitamin and mineral
 formula)
natal
Natalins (multivitamin
 and multimineral
 supplement)
Natalins RX
 (multivitamin,
 multimineral, folic
 acid and iron)
natality
natamycin
natant
nates
natimortality
National Cancer Institute
 (NCI)
National Dental
 Association (NDA)
National Formulary (NF)
National Institute of
 Arthritis and Metabolic
 Diseases (NIAMD)
National Institute of
 General Medical
 Sciences (NIGMS)
National Institutes of
 Health (NIH)
National Institute of
 Allergy and Infectious
 Diseases (NIAID)

National Institute of
Child Health and Human
Development (NICHHD)
National Institute of
Dental Research (NIDR)
National Institute of
Mental Health (NIMH)
National Institute of
Neurological Diseases
and Blindness (NINDB)
National League for
Nursing (NLN)
National Multiple
Sclerosis Society
(NMSS)
National Organization for
Rare Diseases (NORD)
National Organization for
Rare Disorders (NORD)
native
Native American
natremia
natrium
natriuresis
natriuretic
natron
natural
natural chilbirth
natural killer cells (NK
cells)
natural selection
nature and nurture
Nature's Remedy
(laxative)
Naturetin-5
(bendroflumethiazide)
Naturetin-10
(bendroflumethiazide)
naturopath
naturopathy
nausea
nausea and vomiting (N&V)
nausea gravidarum
nausea navalis
nausea, vomiting, and
diarrhea (NVD)
nauseant
nauseate

nauseous
Naval Medical Research
Institute (NMRI)
Navane Capsules
(thiothixene)
Navane Concentrate
(thiothixene HCl)
navel
navicula
navicular
navicular fossa
navicular-cuneiform
arthrodesis
near point (np)
near visual acuity (NVA)
near-death experience
nearsight
nearsighted
nearsightedness
nearthrosis
Nebcin (tobramycin
sulfate)
nebula
nebulization
nebulizer
Necator
Necator americanus
necatoriasis
neck
neck, anatomical, of
humerus
neck conformer
neck, Madelung's
neck of femur
neck of mandible
neck of tooth
neck of uterus
neck, surgical, of
humerus
neck vein distension
(NVD)
neck, wry
neck-righting reflex
necklace, Casal's
necrectomy
necrobiosis
necrobiosis lipoidica
diabeticorum

necrobiotic
necrocytosis
necrocytotoxin
necrogenic
necrogenous
necrologist
necrology
necrolysis
necromania
necrometer
necromimesis
necronectomy
necroparasite
necrophagous
necrophile
necrophilia
necrophilic
necrophilism
necrophilous
necrophobia
necropneumonia
necropsy
necrosadism
necroscopy
necrose
necrosin
necrosis
necrosis, anemic
necrosis, aseptic
necrosis, Balser's fatty
necrosis, caseous
necrosis, central
necrosis, cheesy
necrosis, coagulation
necrosis, colliquative
necrosis, dry
necrosis, embolic
necrosis, fat
necrosis, fibrinous
necrosis, focal
necrosis, gummatous
necrosis, ischemic
necrosis, liquefactive
necrosis, medial
necrosis, moist
necrosis, postpartum
  pituitary
necrosis, putrefactive

necrosis, subcutaneous
  fat, of newborn
necrosis, superficial
necrosis, thrombotic
necrosis, total
necrosis, ustilaginea
necrosis, Zenker's
necrospermia
necrotic
necrotizing
necrotomy
necrotoxin
need
needle
needle, aneurysm
needle, aspirating
needle, atraumatic
needle, cataract
needle, discission
needle, Hagedorn
needle, hypodermic
needle, knife
needle, ligature
needle, obturator
needle, Reverdin's
needle, stop
Neer arthroplasty
negation
negative (NEG)
negative culture
negative electrode
negative glow
negative sign
negativism
negatron
NegGram (nalidixic acid)
Negri bodies
Neisseria
Neisseria catarrhalis
Neisseria gonorrhoeae
Neisseria meningitidis
Neisseria sicca
Neisseriaceae
Nélaton's line
nemathelminth
Nemathelminthes
nematocide
nematocyst

Nematoda
nematode
nematodiasis
nematoid
nematology
nematospermia
Nembutal (pentobarbital
sodium)
Neo-Synalar (neomycin
sulfate, fluocinolone
acetonide)
Neo-Synephrine
(phenylephrine HCl)
Neo-Synephrine 12 Hour
(oxymetazoline HCl)
neoantigen
neoarthrosis
neobiogenesis
neoblastic
neocerebellum
neocinetic
neocortex
Neodecadron (neomycin,
sulfate-dexamethasone
sodium phosphate)
neodymium (Nd)
neofetus
neoformation
neogala
neogenesis
neogenetic
neohymen
neolalism
neologism
Neoloid (emulsified
castor oil)
neomembrane
neomorph
neomycin sulfate
neon (Ne)
neonatal
neonatal diaphragmatic
hernia
neonatal gastrostomy
neonate
neonatologist
neopallium
neopathy

neophobia
neophrenia
neoplasia
neoplasm
neoplasm, benign
neoplasm, histoid
neoplasm, malignant
neoplasm, mixed
neoplasm, multicentric
neoplasm, organoid
neoplasm, unicentric
neoplastic
neoplastic disease
neoplasty
Neosar (cyclophosphamide)
Neosporin
Neosporin G.U. Irrigant
(neomycin sulfate-
polymyxin B sulfate)
Neosporin Ointment
(polymyxin B-
bacitracin-neomycin)
**Neosporin Ophthalmic
Ointment**
**Neosporin Ophthalmic
Solution**
Neosporin Cream
(polymyxin B-neomycin)
neostigmine
neostigmine bromide
neostigmine methylsulfate
neostomy
neostriatum
neoteny
neothalamus
nephelometer
nephelometry
nephelopia
nephradenoma
nephralgia
nephralgic
nephrapostasis
nephratony
nephrauxe
nephrectasis
nephrectasy
nephrectomize
nephrectomy

nephrectomy, abdominal
nephrectomy,
  paraperitoneal
nephrelcosis
nephrelcus
nephremia
nephremphraxis
nephric
nephridium
nephritic
nephritis
nephritis, acute
nephritis, chronic
nephritis, glomerular
nephritis, interstitial
nephritis, salt-losing
nephritis, scarlatinal
nephritis, suppurative
nephritis, transfusion
nephritogenic
nephroabdominal
nephroblastoma
nephrocalcinosis
Nephrocaps (dialysis
  vitamin supplement)
nephrocapsectomy
nephrocardiac
nephrocele
nephrocolic
nephrocolopexy
nephrocoloptosis
nephrocutaneous fistula
  closure
nephrocystanastomosis
nephrocystitis
nephrocystosis
nephroerysipelas
nephrogenetic
nephrogenic
nephrogenous
nephrogram
nephrography
nephrohydrosis
nephrohypertrophy
nephrolith
nephrolithiasis
nephrolithotomy
nephrologist

nephrology
nephrolysine
nephrolysis
nephroma
nephromalacia
nephromegaly
nephromere
nephron
nephroncus
nephroparalysis
nephropathy
nephropathy, analgesic
nephropathy,
  hypercalcemic
nephropathy, hypokalemic
nephropathy, membranous
nephropexy
nephrophthisis
nephroptosis
nephropyelitis
nephropyelography
nephropyeloplasty
nephropyosis
nephrorrhagia
nephrorrhaphy
nephrosclerosis
nephrosis, lipoid
nephrospasis
nephrostogram
nephrostoma
nephrostomy
nephrotic
nephrotic syndrome (NS)
nephrotome
nephrotomogram
nephrotomography
nephrotomy
nephrotoxin
nephrotresis
nephrotropic
nephrotuberculosis
nephrotyphoid
nephroureterectomy
nephrourography
nephrovisceral fistula
Nephrox Suspension
  (aluminun hydroxide)
Neptazane (methazolamide)

neptunium (Np)
nerve
nerve, abducent (6th cranial)
nerve, accessory (11th cranial)
nerve, acoustic
nerve, adrenergic
nerve, anterior, crural
nerve, auditory (8th cranial)
nerve, auricular, great
nerve, auricular, posterior
nerve, auriculotemporal
nerve, autonomic
nerve block
nerve, buccal
nerve cell
nerve, cerebrospinal
nerve, cervical, superficial
nerve, cholinergic
nerve, chorda tympani
nerve, ciliary, long
nerve, ciliary, short
nerve, circumflex (axillary)
nerve, coccygeal
nerve, cochlear (vestibulocochlear)
nerve conduction studies
nerve conduction velocity (NCV)
nerve, cranial
nerve, cutaneous, cervical
nerve, cutaneous, medial
nerve, cutaneous, lesser medial
nerve, dental, inferior
nerve, dental, superior
nerve, depresssor
nerve, digastric
nerve, efferent
nerve ending
nerve entrapment syndrome
nerve, excitatory

nerve, excitoreflex
nerve, external respiratory of Bell
nerve, facial (7th cranial)
nerve, femoral
nerve fiber
nerve fiber, adrenergic
nerve fiber, arcuate
nerve fiber, association
nerve fiber, cholinergic
nerve fiber, collateral
nerve fiber, commissural
nerve fiber, myelinated
nerve fiber, nonmedullated
nerve fiber, postganglionic
nerve fiber, preganglionic
nerve fiber, projection
nerve fiber's, climbing, of cerebellum
nerve fibril
nerve, frontal
nerve, gangliated
nerve, genitocrural
nerve, genitofemoral
nerve, glossopharyngeal (9th cranial)
nerve, gluteal, inferior
nerve, gluteal, superior
nerve, great sciatic
nerve growth factor (NGF)
nerve, hypogastric
nerve, hypoglossal (12th cranial)
nerve, iliohypogastric
nerve, ilioinguinal
nerve impulse
nerve, infraorbital
nerve, infratrochlear
nerve, inhibitory
nerve, intercostal
nerve, intercostobrachial
nerve, interosseous, anterior

nerve, interosseous,
    posterior
nerve, Jacobson's
nerve, lacrimal
nerve, laryngeal,
    inferior
nerve, laryngeal
    recurrent
nerve, laryngeal,
    superior
nerve, lingual
nerve, lumbar
nerve, mandibular
nerve, masseteric
nerve, maxillary
nerve, median
nerve, mental
nerve, mixed
nerve, motor
nerve, musculocutaneous
nerve, mylohyoid
nerve, nasal
    (nasociliary)
nerve, nasopalatine
nerve, obturator
nerve, occipital, greater
nerve, occipital, lesser
nerve, occipital, third
nerve, oculomotor (3rd
    cranial)
nerve, olfactory (1st
    cranial)
nerve, ophthalmic
nerve, optic (2nd
    cranial)
nerve, palatine,
    anterior, middle, and
    posterior
nerve, parasympathetic
nerve, perineal
nerve, peroneal, common
nerve, peripheral
nerve, phrenic
nerve, pilomotor
nerve plexus
nerve, pneumogastric
nerve, popliteal, lateral
nerve, pressor

nerve, pterygoid
nerve, pterygoid canal
nerve, pudendal
nerve, radial
nerve, sacral
nerve, saphenous,
    external or short
nerve, saphenous,
    internal or long
nerve, sciatic
nerve, secretory
nerve, sensory
nerve, somatic
nerve, sphenopalatine
nerve, spinal
nerve, spinal accessory
    (11th cranial)
nerve, splanchnic
nerve, stapedial
nerve, stylohyoid
nerve, suboccipital
nerve, subscapular
nerve, sudomotor
nerve, supra-acromial
nerve, supraclavicular,
    anterior
nerve, supraclavicular,
    intermediate
nerve, supraclavicular,
    lateral
nerve, supraclavicular,
    medial (middle)
nerve, supraclavicular,
    posterior
nerve, supraorbital
nerve, suprascapular
nerve, suprasternal
nerve, supratrochlear
nerve, sural
nerve, sympathetic
nerve, temporal, deep
nerve, thoracic
nerve, thoracic, anterior
nerve, thoracic, long
nerve, tibial
nerve, transverse of neck
nerve, trigeminal (5th
    cranial)

nerve, trochlear (4th
  cranial)
nerve, trophic
nerve trunk
nerve, tympanic
nerve, ulnar
nerve, vagus (10th
  cranial)
nerve, vasoconstrictor
nerve, vasodilator
nerve, vasomotor
nerve, vasosensory
nerve, vestibulocochlear
  (8th cranial)
nerve, vidian
nerve, volar interosseous
nerve, zygomatic
nerves, accelerator
nerves, olfactory
nervi
nervi terminales
nervimotility
nervimotor
nervous
nervous breakdown
nervous debility
nervous impulse
nervous prostration
nervousness
nervus
nervus erigens
nervus intermedius
nervus nervorum
nervus vasorum
Nesacaine (chloroprocaine
  HCl)
nesidiectomy
nesidioblastoma
Nessler's reagent
nesslerize
nest, cancer
nest, cell
Nestabs FA
nesteostomy
nestiatria
net reproductive rate
  (NRR)

Netromycin (netilmicin
  sulfate)
nettle rash
network
Neumann's disease
neurad
neuragmia
neural
neural crest
neural fold
neural plate
neural tube defects (NTD)
neuralgia
neuralgia, cardiac
neuralgia, degenerative
neuralgia, facial
neuralgia, facialis vera
neuralgia, Fothergill's
neuralgia, geniculate
neuralgia,
  glossopharyngeal
neuralgia, hallucinatory
neuralgia, Hunt's
neuralgia, idiopathic
neuralgia, intercostal
neuralgia, mammary
neuralgia, Morton's
neuralgia, nasociliary
neuralgia, occipital
neuralgia, otic
neuralgia, reminiscent
neuralgia, sphenopalatine
neuralgia, stump
neuralgia, symptomatic
neuralgia, trifacial
neuralgic
neuralgiform
neuramebimeter
neuraminidase
neuranagenesis
neurapophysis
neurapraxia
neurarchy
neurarthropathy
neurasthenia
neurasthenic
neuratrophia

neuratrophy
neuraxis
neuraxitis
neuraxon
neuraxone
neurectasis
neurectasy
neurectomy
neurectopia
neurectopy
neurenteric
neurenteric canal
neurepithelium
neurergic
neurexeresis
neuriatry
neurilemmitis
neurilemmoma
neurilemoma
neurimotility
neurimotor
neurinoma
neurinomatosis
neurite
neuritis
neuritis, adventitial
neuritis, ascending
neuritis, axial
neuritis, degenerative
neuritis, descending
neuritis, dietetic
neuritis, diphtheritic
neuritis, disseminated
neuritis, endemic
neuritis, interstitial
neuritis, intraocular
neuritis, migrans
neuritis, multiple
neuritis, nodosa
neuritis, optic
neuritis, parenchymatous
neuritis, peripheral
neuritis, retrobulbar
neuritis, rheumatic
neuritis, sciatic
neuritis, segmental
neuritis, senile
neuritis, sympathetic

neuritis, tabetic
neuritis, toxic
neuro-ophthalmology
neuro-optic
neuroallergy
neuroanastomosis
neuroanatomy
neuroarthritism
neuroarthropathy
neuroastrocytoma
neurobiology
neurobiotaxis
neuroblast
neuroblastoma
neurocanal
neurocardiac
neurocele
neurocentral
neuroceotrum
neurochorioretinitis
neurochoroiditis
neurocirculatory asthenia
neurocladism
neuroclonic
neurocoele
neurocranium
neurocrine
neurocutaneous
neurocyte
neurocytolysis
neurocytoma
neurodealgia
neurodegenerative
neurodendrite
neurodendron
neurodermatitis
neurodermatosis
neurodermatrophia
neurodiagnosis
neurodynamic
neurodynia
neuroectoderm
neuroencephalomyelopathy
neuroendocrine
neuroendocrinology
neuroenteric
neuroepidermal
neuroepithelioma

neuroepithelium
neurofibril
neurofibrilla
neurofibroma
neurofibromatosis
neurofibrosarcoma
neurofibrositis
neurogangliitis
neuroganglion
neurogastric
neurogenesis
neurogenetic
neurogenic
neurogenous
neuroglia
neurogliacyte
neuroglial
neuroglioma
neuroglioma, ganglionare
neurogliomatosis
neurogliosis
neurogram
neurography
neurohematology
neurohistology
neurohormone
neurohumor
neurohypophysis
neuroid
neuroinduction
neurokeratin
neurokyme
neurolemma
neurolemmitis
neurolemmoma
neurolemmoma excision
neuroleptanesthesia
neuroleptic
neuroleptic anesthesia
neuroleptic drugs
neuroleptic malignant
  syndrome (NMS)
neuro-linguistic
  programming (NLP)
neurologic
neurological
neurologist
neurology

neurolymphomatosis
neurolysin
neurolysis
neurolytic
neurolytic destruction
neuroma
neuroma, acoustic
neuroma, amputation
neuroma, amyelinic
neuroma, appendiceal
neuroma, cutis
neuroma, cystic
neuroma, false
neuroma, ganglionated
neuroma, multiple
neuroma, myelinic
neuroma, plexiform
neuroma, telangiectodes
neuroma, traumatic
neuromalacia
neuromatosis
neuromatous
neuromechanism
neuromere
neuromimesis
neuromuscular
neuromyasthenia
neuromyelitis
neuromyopathic
neuromyositis
neuron, afferent
neuron, associative
neuron, bipolar
neuron, central
neuron, commissural
neuron, efferent
neuron, motor
neuron, multipolar
neuron, peripheral
neuron, preganglionic
neuron, sensory
neuron, unipolar
neuronal
neurone
neuronephric
neuronevus
neuronitis
neuronophage

neuronophagia
neuronophagy
neurons
neuropacemaker
neuropapillitis
neuroparalysis
neuropathic
neuropathogenesis
neuropathogenicity
neuropathology
neuropathy
neuropharmacology
neurophilic
neurophonia
neurophthalmology
neuro-ophthalmology
neurophthisis
neurophysiological
  treatment approach
neurophysiology
neuropil
neuroplasm
neuroplasty
neuropodia
neuropore
neuropotential
neuropraxia
neuropsychiatrist
neuropsychiatry
neuropsychopathy
neuropsychopharmacology
neuro-optic
neuroradiography
neuroradiology
neurorelapse
neuroretinitis
neuroretinopathy
neuroroentgenography
neurorrhaphy
neurosarcokleisis
neurosarcoma
neuroscience
neurosclerosis
neurosecretion
neurosensory
neurosis
neurosis, accident
neurosis, anxiety

neurosis, association
neurosis, cardiac
neurosis, compensation
neurosis, compulsion
neurosis, craft
neurosis, expectation
neurosis, fatigue
neurosis, obsessional
neurosis, occupational
neurosis, pension
neurosis, sexual
neurosis, traumatic
neurosis, war
neuroskeletal
neuroskeleton
neurosome
neurospasm
neurosplanchnic
neurospongioma
Neurospora
neurostimulator
neurosurgeon
neurosurgery
neurosuture
neurosyphilis
neurosyphilis,
  asymptomatic
neurosyphilis,
  meningovascular
neurosyphilis, paretic
neurosyphilis, tabetic
neurotendinous
neurotension
neurothecitis
neurothele
neurotherapeutics
neurotherapy
neurotic
neurotic disorder
neuroticism
neurotization
neurotmesis
neurotome
neurotomy
neurotonic
neurotoxicity
neurotoxin
neurotransmitter

neurotrauma
neurotripsy
neurotrophasthenia
neurotrophy
neurotropism
neurotropy
neurotrosis
neurotubule
neurovaccine
neurovaricosis
neurovascular
neurovascular dissection
neurovegetative
neurovescular pedicle
  flap graft
neurovirus
neurovisceral
neurtology
Neurtra-Phos (phosphorus
  dietary supplement)
neurula
neurulation
neutophilic
neutral
neutral fat
neutral point
neutralization
neutralize
neutrino
neutroclusion
neutrocyte
neutrocytopenia
neutrocytosis
neutron
neutron capture analysis
neutropenia
neutrophil
neutrophilia
neutrophilous
neutrophils test
neutrotaxis
nevocarcinoma
nevoid
nevolipoma
nevose
nevoxanthoendothelioma
nevus angiectodes
nevus angiomatodes

nevus araneus
nevus, blue
nevus, blue rubber bleb
nevus, capillary
nevus comedonicus
nevus, connective tissue
nevus, cutaneous
nevus, epidermal
nevus flammeus
nevus, hairy
nevus, halo
nevus, intradermal
nevus, Ito's
nevus, juction
nevus lipomatodes
nevus maternus
nevus, melanocytic
nevus, nevocytic
nevus, Ota's
nevus pigmentosus
nevus pilosus
nevus, sebaceous
nevus, spider
nevus spilus
nevus spongiosus albus
  mucosae
nevus, strawberry
nevus, telangiectatic
nevus unius lateris
nevus vascularis
nevus venosus
nevus verrucosus
nevus, white sponge
newborn
Newcastle disease
newton (N)
newton meter (Nm)
nexus
niacin
niacinamide
Niaplus (niacin)
nib
niche
nickel (Ni)
nickel carbonyl
nicking
Niclocide (niclosamide)
niclosamide

Nico-400 (nicotinic acid)
Nicolar (niacin)
Nicolas-Favre disease
Nicorette (nicotine
  polacrilex)
nicotinamide
nicotinamide adenine
  dinucleotide-diaphorase
  (NADH-diaphorase)
nicotinamide adenine
  dinucleotide (NAD+)
nicotinamide adenine
  dinucleotide phosphate
  (NADP)
nicotinamide adenine
  diphosphate
nicotine
Nicotinex (nicotinic
  acid)
nicotinic acid (NA)
nicotinism
nictation
nictitate
nictitating
nictitation
nidal
nidation
nidus
nidus avis cerebelli
nidus hirundinis
Niemann-Pick disease
Niferex
night blindness
Night Cast (sulfur,
  salicylic acid, and
  alcohol)
**Night Cast Special
  Formula** (sulfur,
  resorcinol, and
  alcohol)
night sweat
night terrors
night vision
Nightingale, Florence
Nightingale Pledge
nightmare
nightshade
nightwalking

nigra
nigricans
nigrities
nigrities linguae
nigrosin
nigrostriatal
nihilism
nikethamide
Nikolsky's sign
Nilstat (nystatin)
ninth cranial nerve
niobium (NB)
niphablepsia
niphotyphlosis
nipple
nipple, crater
nipple, retracted
nipple shield
Nipride (sodium
  nitroprusside)
Nissen esophagogastric
  fundoplasty
Nissl bodies
nisus
nit
niter
niton
nitrate
nitrated
nitration
nitre
nitremia
nitric acid
nitridation
nitride
nitrification
nitrifying
nitrifying bacteria
nitrile
nitritoid
nitrituria
Nitro-Bid (nitroglycerin)
Nitro-Dur II
  (nitroglycerin)
nitrobenzene
nitroblue tetrazolium dye
  test (NTD)
nitrocellulose

Nitrocine Timecaps
(nitroglycerin)
Nitrocine Transdermal
System (nitroglycerin)
Nitrodisc (nitroglycerin
transdermal system)
nitrofurantoin
nitrofurazone
Nitrogard (transmucosal
controlled release
nitroglycerin)
nitrogen (N)
nitrogen balance
nitrogen cycle
nitrogen equilibrium
nitrogen fixation
nitrogen lag
nitrogen monoxide
nitrogen mustards
nitrogen narcosis
nitrogenase
nitrogenous
Nitroglyn (nitroglycerin)
Nitrol IV (nitroglycerin)
Nitrolingual Spray
(nitroglycerin lingual
aerosol)
nitromersol
nitrometer
nitromuriatic acid
Nitron EMS (electrical
muscle stimulator)
Nitron TENS
(transcutaneous
electrical nerve
stimulator)
Nitrong (nitroglycerin)
Nitropress (sodium
nitroprusside)
Nitrosomonas
Nitrospan (nitroglycerin)
Nitrostat (nitroglycerin)
nitrous
nitrous acid
nitrous oxide
Nix (permethrin)
Nizoral (ketoconazole)
NMR spectroscopy

no acute disease (NAD)
no appreciable disease
(NAD)
no complaints (N/C)
no diagnosis
No Doz
Nobel prize
nobelium
Nocardia
Nocardia asteroides
Nocardia brasiliensis
nocardial
nocardiosis
nociassociation
nociceptive
nociceptive impulses
nociceptive reflex
nociceptor
noci-influence
nociperception
"no code" orders
noctalbuminuria
noctambulation
noctambulism
noctiphobia
nocturia
nocturnal
nocturnal emission
nocturnal enuresis
nocturnal penile
tumescence (NPT)
nocuous
nodal
nodal points
nodal rhythm
nodding
nodding spasm
node
node, A-V
node, Aschoff's
node, atrioventricular
node, Bouchard's
node, Flack's
node, hemal
node, Hensen's
node, lymph
node, piedric
node, Schmorl's

node, sentinel
node, signal
node, singer's
node, sinoatrial
node, sinoauricular
node, sinus
node, syphilitic
node, teacher's
node, Troisier's
node, Virchow
nodes, Haygarth's
nodes, Heberden's
nodes, Meynet's
nodes of Ranvier
nodes, Osler's
nodes, Parrot's
nodi
nodose
nodosity
nodular
nodulation
nodule
nodule, apple jelly
nodule, Aschoff's
nodule, lymph
nodule, milker's
nodule of semilunar valve
nodule, rheumatic
nodule, Schmorl's
nodule, Sister Mary
  Joseph
nodule, solitary
nodules, aggregate
nodules, Albini's
nodules, Arantius
nodules, cortical
nodules, Gamna
nodules, Morgagni
nodules, siderotic
nodules, subcutaneous
nodules, surfer's
nodules, typhoid
nodules, typhus
nodulus
nodus
noematachograph
noematachometer
noematic

noesis
Noguchia
noise
Nolahist (phenindamine
  tartrate)
Nolamine
noli me tangere
Noludar (methyprylon)
Nolvadex (tamoxifen
  citrate)
noma
nomadism
nomenclature
Nomina Anatomica (NA)
nomogram
nomography
nomotopic
non compos mentis
non repetat
non-invasive vascular
  diagnostic studies
non-nucleated
nonan
noncompliance
nonconductor
nondisjunction
nonelectrolyte
nonesterified fatty acids
  (NEFA)
nonigravida
noninvasive neoplasm
nonipara
nonlaxative diet
nonmedullated
nonmyelinated
nonocclusion
nonopaque
nonose
nonoxynol
nonparous
nonpolar
nonpolar compound
nonproprietary name
nonprotein
nonprotein nitrogen (NPN)
nonrestraint
nonrotation
nonsecretor

nonseptate
nonsexual
nonspecific
nonspecific urethritis
nonsteroidal anti-
   inflammatory drugs
   (NSAIDs)
nonstress test
nontoxic
nonunion
nonus
nonvalent
nonviable
nonyl
nookleptia
Noonan's syndrome
noopsyche
Nor-QD (norethindrone)
noradrenalin
noradrenalin bitartrate
Norcuron (vecuronium
   bromide)
Nordette-21
   (levonorgestrel and
   ethinyl estradiol)
norepinephrine
norethandrolone
norethindrone
norethynodrel
Norflex (orphenadrine
   citrate)
norflurane
Norgesic (aspirin,
   caffeine)
Norgesic Forte (aspirin,
   caffeine)
norgestrel
Norinyl 1 + 35
   (norethindrone and
   ethinyl estradiol)
Norinyl 2 mg
   (norethindrone and
   ethinyl estradiol)
Norisodrine Aerotrol
   (isoproterenol HCl)
Norlestrin (norethindorne
   acetate and ethinyl
   estradiol)

Norlutate (norethindrone
   acetate)
Norlutin (norethindrone)
norm
norma
norma, anterior
norma basilaris
norma facialis
norma frontalis
norma, inferior
norma lateralis
norma occipitalis
norma sagittalis
norma, superior
norma ventralis
norma verticalis
normal
normal intraocular
   tension (TN)
normal saline solution
   (NSS)
normal salt solution
   (NSS)
normal sinus rhythm (NSR)
normal solution
normalization
normergic
normetanephrine
normoblast
normoblastoma
normocapnia
normocapnic
normocholesterolemia
normochromasia
normochromia
normocyte
normocytosis
Normodyne (labetalol HCl)
normoerythrocyte
normoglycemia
normokalemia
normo-orthocytosis
normoskeocytosis
normospermic
normosthenuria
normotensive
normothermia
normotonic

normotopia
normovolemia
Normozide (labetalol HCl
  and
  hydrochlorothiazide)
Noroxin (norfloxacin)
Norpace (disopyramide
  phosphate)
Norpramin (desipramine
  HCl)
Norrie's disease
nortriptyline
  hydrochloride
Norwalk agent
Norwegian itch
NoSalt
noscapine
nose
nose, hammer
nose, saddle
nosebleed
Nosema
nosepiece
nosetiology
nosh
nosochthonography
nosocomial
nosocomial infection
nosogenesis
nosogeny
nosogeography
nosography
nosohemia
nosology
nosomania
nosomycosis
nosonomy
nosophilia
nosophobia
nosopoietic
Nosopsyllus
Nosopsyllus fasciatus
nosotaxy
nosotherapy
nosotoxic
nosotoxicosis
nosotrophy
nosotropic

nostalgia
nostomania
nostril
nostril reflex
nostrils
nostrum
not applicable (NA)
not sufficient (NS)
notal
notalgia
notancephalia
notanencephalia
notch
notch, acetabular
notch, aortic
notch, cardiac
notch, cerebellar
notch, clavicular
notch, costal
notch, cotyloid
notch, ethmoidal
notch, frontal
notch, interclavicular
notch, jugular
notch, labial
notch, mandibular
notch, manubrial
notch, nasal
notch of Rivinus
notch, pancreatic
notch, parotid
notch, radial
notch, scapular
notch, sciatic
notch, semilunar
notch, sphenopalatine
notch, tentorial
notch, thyroid
notch, tympanic
notch, ulnar
notch, umbilical
notch, vertebral
note
note blindness
notencephalocele
notencephalus
nothing by mouth (NPO)
notifiable diseases

notochord
notogenesis
notomelus
noumenal
noumenon
nourishment
Novafed (pseudoephedrine
HCl)
Novahistine DH
(antitussive-
decongestant-
antihistamine)
Novahistine DMX
(antitussive-
decongestant-
expectorant)
Novahistine Elixir
(decongestant-
antihistaminic)
Novahistine Expectorant
(antitussive-
decongestant-
expectorant)
novobiocin sodium
Novocain (procaine HCl)
noxious
NPH Iletin I (isophane
insulin suspension)
NPH Insulin (isophane
insulin suspension)
Nu-Iron (polysaccharide-
iron complex)
Nubain (nalbuphine HCl)
nubecula
nubile
nubility
nubleotidase
nucha
nuchal
Nuck's canal
nuclear
nuclear antigen
nuclear arc
nuclear envelope
nuclear family
nuclear magnetic
resonance (NMR)

nuclear magnetic
resonance imaging
(NMRI)
nuclear medicine
nuclear winter
nuclear-bone scans
nuclear-brain scans
nuclear-heart scans
nuclear-kidney scans
nuclear-liver scans
nuclear-lung scans
nuclear-thyroid scans
nuclease
nucleate
nucleic acid
nucleic acid probe
nucleiform
nuclein
nucleinase
nucleocapsid
nucleochylema
nucleochyme
nucleofugal
nucleohistone
nucleoid
nucleolar
nucleoli
nucleoliform
nucleoloid
nucleolonema
nucleolus
nucleomicrosome
nucleons
nucleopetal
nucleophilic
nucleoplasm
nucleoplasmic
nucleoplasmic index
nucleoprotein
nucleosidase
nucleoside
nucleospindle
nucleotidase
5-nucleotidase
nucleotide
nucleotidyl
nucleotidyltransferase

nucleotoxin
nucleus, abducens
nucleus, ambiguous
nucleus, amygdaloid
nucleus, angular
nucleus, anterior
nucleus, arcuate
nucleus, atomic
nucleus, auditory
nucleus, Bechterew's
nucleus, Bekhterev's
nucleus, caudate
nucleus, centromedian
nucleus, cerebellar
nucleus, cochlear
nucleus, cornucommissural
nucleus, cuneate
nucleus, Deiters'
nucleus, dentate
nucleus, diploid
nucleus, dorsal
nucleus, ectoblastic
nucleus, Edinger-Westphal
nucleus, emboliform
nucleus, facial motor
nucleus, fastigial
nucleus, fertilization
nucleus, free
nucleus funiculi gracilis
nucleus, germinal
nucleus, globose
nucleus, gonad
nucleus gracilis
nucleus, habenular
nucleus, haploid
nucleus, hypoglossal
nucleus, hypothalamic
nucleus, interpeduncular
nucleus, interstitial, of
  Cajal
nucleus, intraventricular
nucleus, lenticular
nucleus lentis
nucleus, masticatory
nucleus, mesencephalic
  tract
nucleus, mother
nucleus, motor

nucleus, oculomotor
nucleus of Burdach
nucleus of origin
nucleus of termination
nucleus, olivary
nucleus, paraventricular
nucleus, pontine
nucleus, principal
  trigeminal sensory
nucleus, pulposus
nucleus, pyramidal
nucleus, red
nucleus, reproductive
nucleus, reticular
nucleus ruber
nucleus, salivatory
nucleus, segmentation
nucleus, sensory
nucleus, sperm
nucleus, subthalamic
nucleus, supraoptic
nucleus, thalamic
nucleus, thoracic
nucleus, trigeminal
  spinal
nucleus, vesicular
nucleus, vestibular
nucleus, vitelline
nucleus, white
nucleus, yolk
nuclide
Nucofed (codeine
  phosphate and
  pseudoephedrine HCl)
nude
nude mice
nudism
nudomania
nudophobia
Nuel's space
Nuhn's glands
null hypothesis
nulla per os (NPO)
nulligravida
nullipara
nulliparity
nulliparous
nullisomatic

numb
number (No)
number, atomic
number, Avogadro's
number, hardness
number, mass
numbness
numeral
numerical aperture (NA)
nummiform
nummular
nummulation
Numorphan (oxymorphone HCl)
nunnation
Nupercainal (hemorrhoidal and anesthetic cream)
Nupercainal (hemorrhoidal and anesthetic ointment)
Nupercainal Suppositories
Nuprin (ibuprofen)
nurse, charge
nurse, clinical specialist
nurse clinician
nurse, community health
nurse, dental
nurse, epidemiologist
nurse, flight
nurse, general duty
nurse, graduate
nurse, head
nurse, health
nurse, infection control
nurse, licensed practical
nurse, practical
nurse practitioner
nurse, prescribing
nurse, private duty
nurse, public health
nurse, registered
nurse, school
nurse, scrub
nurse, special
nurse, specialist
nurse, student
nurse, trained

nurse, visiting
nurse, wet
nurse's aide (NA)
nurses, probationer
nursemaid elbow
nurse-midwife
nursery
Nurses' Educational Funds (NEF)
nursing
nursing assessment
nursing assistant (NA)
nursing audit
nursing diagnosis
nursing histories
nursing intervention
nursing process
Nursoy (soy protein formula)
nutation
nutgall
Nutracort (hydrocortisone)
Nutraderm (skin-lubricant-moisturizer)
Nutramigen (iron fortified protein hydrolysate formula)
nutrient
nutrilite
nutriment
nutrition
nutritional
nutritional adequacy
nutritional anemia
nutritious
nutritive
nutritive enema
nutriture
Nutrox (antioxidant formulation)
nux vomica
nuyclein bases
nyctalbuminuria
nyctalgia
nyctalopia
nyctamblyopia
nyctaphonia

nycterine
nycthemerus
nyctohemeral
nyctophilia
nyctophobia
nyctotyphlosis
nycturia
nylidrin hydrochloride
nymph
nympha
nymphectomy
nymphitis
nymphocaruncular sulcus
nymphohymenal sulcus
nympholepsy
nymphomaniac
nymphoncus
nymphotomy
nystagmic
nystagmiform
nystagmograph
nystagmoid
nystagmus
nystagmus, aural
nystagmus, Cheyne's
nystagmus, convergence
nystagmus, dissociated
nystagmus, end-position
nystagmus, fixation
nystagmus, jerk
nystagmus, labyrinthine
nystagmus, latent
nystagmus, lateral
nystagmus, miner's
nystagmus, opticokinetic
nystagmus, pendular
nystagmus, retraction
nystagmus, rhythmic
nystagmus, rotatory
nystagmus, vertical
nystagmus, vestibular
nystagmus, voluntary
nystatin
nystaxis
Nysten's law
Nystex (nystatin)
nysthymia
nyxis
NZB mouse

O

oakum
oarialgia
oasis
oasthouse urine disease
oat
oath
oatmeal
obcecation
obdormition
obduction
obelion
Ober fasciotomy
Ober-Yount fasciotomy
obese
obesity
obesity, endogenous
obesity, exogenous
obesity, hypethalamic
obesity, morbid
obex
obfuscation
object
object blindness
object film distance
    (OFD)
object relations
objective, achromatic
objective, apochromatic
objective, immersion
objective sign
objective symptoms
obligate
oblique
oblique computerized
    tomography
oblique muscles
obliquity
obliquity, Litzmann's
obliquity, Naegele's
obliquity, Roederer's
obliquity of pelvis

obliquus
obliquus reflex
obliteration
obliterative sinusotomy
Oblomov syndrome
oblongata
obmutescence
obscure
observerscope
obsession, impulsive
obsession, inhibitory
obsessional neurosis
obsessive-compulsive
obsessive-compulsive
  disorder (OCD)
obsolescence
obstetric profile
obstetrician
obstetrics (OB)
obstetrics and gynecology
  (OB-GYN)
obstipation
obstruction, aortic
obstruction, intestinal
obstruent
obtund
obtundent
obturation
obturator
obturator foramen
obturator membrane
obturator muscles
obturator nerve
obturator nodes
obturator sign
obtuse
obtusion
Occam's razor
occipital bone
occipital lobe
occipital nerve
occipitalis
occipitalization
occipito laevo anterior
  (OLA)
occipitoatloid
occipitoaxoid
occipitobregmatic

occipitocervical
occipitofacial
occipitofrontal
occipitolaevas posterior
  (OLP)
occipitomastoid
occipitomental
occipitoparietal
occipitotemporal
occipitothalamic
occiput
occiput position (OP)
occlude
occlusal
Occlusal (salicylic acid)
occlusal plane
occlusal surface
occlusal wear
Occlusal-HP (salicylic
  acid [high potency])
occlusion
occlusion, abnormal
occlusion, adjusted
occlusion, balanced
occlusion, centric
occlusion, coronary
occlusion, eccentric
occlusion, habitual
occlusion, traumatic
occlusion, working
occlusive
occlusive dressing
occlusometer
occult
occult blood
occult blood test
occupational neurosis
occupational safety and
  health administration
  (OSHA)
occupational therapist
  (OT)
occupational therapist
  assistant (OTA)
occupational therapy (OT)
occupational therapy aide
  (OTA)

Ocean Mist (buffered isotonic saline)
Ocean-A/S (nasal spray)
ochlesis
ochlophobia
ochrometer
ochronosis
octahedron
octamethyl pyrophosphoramide
Octamide (metoclopramide HCl)
octan
octane
octapeptide
octaploid
octaploidy
octarius (O)
octavalent
octigravida
octipara
octogenarian
Ocuclear
ocular
ocular cavity
ocular evisceration
ocular foreign body removal
ocular photography
ocular plethysmography
oculi
oculi unitas (OU)
oculinium
oculist
oculocardiac reflex
oculocephalogyric reflex
oculocerebrorenal syndrome
oculocutaneous
oculofacial
oculogyration
oculogyria
oculogyric
oculogyric crisis
oculomotor nerve (III)
oculomotorius
oculomycosis
oculonasal

oculoplethysmography (OPG)
oculopupillary
oculoreaction
oculozygomatic
oculozygomatic line
oculus
oculus dexter (OD)
oculus laevus (OL)
oculus sinister (OS)
oculus sinistern (OS)
oculus uterque
odaxesmus
odaxetic
Oddi sphincterotomy
Oddi's sphincter
odditis
odogenesis
odonpic
odontagra
odontatrophy
odontectomy
odonterism
odontia
odontitis
odontoblast
odontoblastoma
odontobothrion
odontobothritis
odontocele
odontochirurgical
odontoclasis
odontoclast
odontodynia
odontogenesis
odontogeny
odontograph
odontography
odontoid
odontoid process
odontolith
odontologist
odontology
odontolysis
odontoma
odontoma, ameloblastic
odontoma, composite
odontoma, coronary

odontoma, follicular
odontoma, radicular
odontonecrosis
odontonomy
odontopathy
odontophobia
odontoprisis
odontorrhagia
odontoschism
odontoscopy
odontosis
odontotherapy
odontotripsis
odor
odorant
odoriferous
odorimetry
odoriphore
odorography
odorous
odynacusis
odynometer
odynophagia
odynophobia
Oedipus complex
oenology
oersted
oervomuscular
oesophagostomiasis
Oesophagostomum
Oesophagostomum
  apiostomum
oestrus
Oestrus ovis
office call (OC)
official
officinal
Ogen (estropipiate)
Ogilvie's syndrome
Oguchi's disease
ohm
Ohm's law
ohmammeter
ohmmeter
oikofugic
oikomania
oikophobia
oil

oil immersion field (OIF)
ointment
olea
oleaginous
oleander
oleate
oleatum
olecranal
olecranarthritis
olecranarthrocace
olecranarthropathy
olecranoid
olecranon
olecranon bursa
oleic
oleic acid
olein
oleo
oleoarthrosis
oleogranuloma
oleoinfusion
oleoma
oleomargarine
oleometer
oleoresin
oleosaccharum
oleostearate
oleotherapy
oleothorax
oleovitamin
oleum (ol)
oleum morrhuae
oleum olivea
oleum percomorphum
oleum ricini
olfactie
olfaction
olfactive
olfactology
olfactory
olfactory area
olfactory bulb
olfactory cortex
olfactory esthesioneuroma
olfactory lobe
olfactory membrane
olfactory nerve (I)
olfactory nerves

olfactory organ
olfactory striae
olfactory tract
olfactory trigone
olfactory tubercle
oligemia
oligergasia
oligoamnios
oligocholia
oligochromemia
oligochylia
oligochymia
oligoclonal immune
  globulin (Ig)
oligocystic
oligodactylia
oligodendroblast
oligodendroblastoma
oligodendroglia
oligodendroglioma
oligodipsia
oligodontia
oligodynamic
oligogalactia
oligohemia
oligohydramnios
oligolecithal
oligoleukocythemia
oligomastigate
oligomenorrhea
oligomorphic
oligonucleotide
oligophosphaturia
oligophrenia
oligoplastic
oligopnea
oligoposy
oligoptyalism
oligoria
oligosaccharide
oligosialia
oligospermia
oligosynaptic
oligotrichia
oligotrophy
oligozoospermatism
oligozoospermia
oliguresis

oliguria
oliva
olivary
olivary body
olive
olive oil
olivifugal
olivipetal
olivopontocerebellar
Ollier layer
Ollier, Léopold L.X.E.
Ollier's disease
Ollier-Thiersch graft
olophonia
Olshausen suspension
omagra
omalgia
omasitis
omasum
ombrophobia
omega-3 fatty acids
omenta
omental
omental bursa
omentectomy
omentitis
omentofixation
omentopexy
omentoplasty
omentorrhaphy
omentosplenopexy
omentum, gastrocolic
omentum, gastrohepatic
omentum, greater
omentum, lesser
omentumectomy
omitis
Ommaya reservoir
Omnipen (ampicillin)
omnipotence of thought
omnivorous
omoclavicular
omodynia
omohyoid
omophagia
omphalectomy
omphalelcosis
omphalic

omphalitis
omphaloangiopagus
omphalocele
omphalochorion
omphalomesenteric
omphalomesenteric duct
  excision
omphaloncus
omphalopagus
omphalophlebitis
omphalorrhagia
omphalorrhea
omphalorrhexis
omphalos
omphalosite
omphalospinous
omphalotomy
omphalotripsy
omphalus
onanism
onanist
Onanoff's reflex
Onchocerca
Onchocerca volvulus
onchocerciasis
Oncocerca
oncocercosis
oncocyte
oncocytoma
oncofetal
oncogene
oncogenesis
oncogenic
oncogenic virus
oncograph
oncoides
oncologist
oncology
oncolysis
oncolytic
oncometer
oncometric
oncometry
oncosis
oncosphere
oncotherapy
oncothlipsis
oncotic

oncotic pressure,
  colloidal
oncotomy
oncotropic
Oncovin (vincristine
  sulfate)
oncovirus
Ondine's curse
One-A-Day Stressgard
oneiric
oneirism
oneirodynia
oneirology
oneiroscopy
oniomania
onion
onkinocele
onlay
onomatology
onomatomania
onomatophobia
onomatopoiesis
ontogenesis
ontogenetic
ontogeny
onychalgia
onychatrophia
onychauxis
onychectomy
onychia
onychia craquele
onychia lateralis
onychia maligna
onychia parasitica
onychia, piannic
onychia punctata
onychitis
onychocryptosis
onychodystrophy
onychogenic
onychograph
onychogryposis
onychoheterotopia
onychoid
onycholysis
onychoma
onychomadesis
onychomalacia

onychomycosis
onycho-osteodysplasia
onychopathology
onychopathy
onychophagia
onychophosis
onychophyma
onychoptosis
onychorrhexis
onychoschizia
onychosis
onychotillomania
onychotomy
onychotrophy
onyx
onyxis
onyxitis
ooblast
oocyesis
oocyst
oocytase
oocyte
oocytin
oogenesis
oogenetic
oogonium
ookinesis
ookinete
oolemma
oophagy
oophoralgia
oophorauxe
oophorectomy
oophoritis
oophorocystectomy
oophorocytosis
oophorohysterectomy
oophoroma
oophoron
oophoropathy
oophoropeliopexy
oophoropexy
oophoroplasty
oophorosalpingectomy
oophorosalpingitis
oophorostomy
oophorotomy
oophorrhagia

oophorrhaphy
ooplasm
oosperm
oosporangium
oospore
ootheca
oothecohysterectomy
ootid
opacification
opacity
opalescent
opaque
open heart surgery
open reduction
opening
opening, aortic
opening, cardiac
opening, pyloric
operable
operant conditioning
operate
operating room (OR)
operation
operation, ablative
operation, cosmetic
operation, exploratory
operation, flap
operation, major
operation, minor
operation, plastic
operation, radical
operation, reconstructive
operation, subtotal
operative
operative dentistry
operative procedure (OP)
operator
opercular
operculectomy
operculitis
operculum
operculum, dental
operculum, trophoblastic
operon
ophiasis
ophidiasis
ophidiophobia
ophidism

ophiotoxemia
ophritis
ophryitis
ophryon
ophryosis
ophthalmagra
ophthalmalgia
ophthalmatrophy
ophthalmectomy
ophthalmencephalon
ophthalmia
ophthalmia, catarrhal
ophthalmia, Egyptian
ophthalmia, electric
ophthalmia, gonorrheal
ophthalmia, granular
ophthalmia, metastatic
ophthalmia neonatorum
ophthalmia,
    neuroparalytic
ophthalmia, phlyctenular
ophthalmia, purulent
ophthalmia, scrofulous
ophthalmia, spring
ophthalmia, sympathetic
ophthalmia, varicose
ophthalmiatrics
ophthalmic
ophthalmic biometry
ophthalmic echography
ophthalmic mucous
    membrane test
ophthalmic nerve
ophthalmic reaction
ophthalmic ultrasonic
    foreign body
    localization
ophthalmitis
ophthalmoblennorrhea
ophthalmocele
ophthalmocopia
ophthalmodesmitis
ophthalmodiagnosis
ophthalmodiaphanoscope
ophthalmodonesis
ophthalmodynamometer
ophthalmodynamometry
ophthalmodynia

ophthalmoeikonometer
ophthalmofundoscope
ophthalmography
ophthalmogyric
ophthalmolith
ophthalmological
    examination
ophthalmologist
ophthalmology
ophthalmomalacia
ophthalmometer
ophthalmomycosis
ophthalmomyiasis
ophthalmomyitis
ophthalmomyositis
ophthalmomyotomy
ophthalmoneuritis
ophthalmopathy
ophthalmophlebotomy
ophthalmophthisis
ophthalmoplasty
ophthalmoplegia
ophthalmoplegia externa
ophthalmoplegia interna
ophthalmoplegia, nuclear
ophthalmoplegia,
    Parinaud's
ophthalmoplegia partialis
ophthalmoplegia
    progessiva
ophthalmoplegia totalis
ophthalmoptosis
ophthalmoreaction
ophthalmorrhagia
ophthalmorrhea
ophthalmorrhexis
ophthalmoscope
ophthalmoscopy
ophthalmostasis
ophthalmostat
ophthalmostatometer
ophthalmosynchysis
ophthalmothermometer
ophthalmotomy
ophthalmotonometer
ophthalmotoxin
ophthalmotrope
ophthalmotropometer

ophthalmovascular
ophthalmoxerosis
ophthalmoxyster
ophthalometry
Ophthochlor
  (chloramphenicol
  ophthalmic solution)
Ophthocort
  (chloramphenicol,
  polymyxin B sulfate,
  hydrocortisone)
opiate
opiate abstinence
  syndrome
opiate poisoning
opiate receptor
opididymus
opioid
opioid peptides,
  endogenous
opiomania
opiophagism
opisthenar
opisthiobasial
opisthion
opisthionasial
opisthognathism
opisthoporeia
opisthorchiasis
Opisthorchis
Opisthorchis felineus
Opisthorchis sinensis
opisthotic
opisthotonoid
opisthotonos
opium
opium poisoning
opiumism
opocephalus
Oppenheim's gait
oppilation
opponens
opponens plasty
opponens splint
opportunistic infections
opposition
opsialgia
opsin

opsinogen
opsinogenous
opsiometer
opsiuria
opsoclonus
opsogen
opsomania
opsonic
opsonification
opsonin
opsonin, immune
opsonization
opsonize
opsonocytophagic
opsonometry
opsonophilia
opsonophilic
opsonotherapy
optesthesia
opthalmospasm
optic
optic chiasm
optic disk
optic foramen
optic foramina
optic nerve (II)
optic neuropathy
optic papilla
optic tract
optical
optical activity
optician
opticianry
opticist
opticociliary
opticokinetic
opticonasion
opticopupillary
Opticrom (cromolyn
  sodium)
Optilets-500 (high
  potency multivitamin)
optimal immunomodulating
  dose (OID)
Optimine (azatadine
  maleate)
optimum
optimum temperature

optogram
optokinetic
optokinetic nystagmus
  test
optomeninx
optometer
optometrist
optometry
optomyometer
optophone
optostriate
optotype
ora
ora serrata retinae
Orabase HCA (topical
  dental paste)
orad
oral cholecystogram (OC)
oral contraceptive (OC)
oral diagnosis
oral glucose tolerance
  test
oral polio vaccine (OPV)
oral rehydration
  solutions (ORS)
oral rehydration therapy
  (ORT)
orale
orality
oralogy
orange juice (OJ)
orange, methyl
Orap (pimozide)
orb
orbicular
orbicular bone
orbicular muscle
orbicular process
orbiculare
orbicularis oculi reflex
orbiculus
orbiculus ciliaris
orbiculus oculi
orbiculus oris
orbit
orbita
orbital

orbital advancement,
  skull
orbital floor fracture
orbital hypertelorism
  correction
orbital implant
orbital repositioning
orbital venography
orbitale
orbitocraniofacial
  reconstruction
orbitomeatal line (OML)
orbitonasal
orbitonometer
orbitonometry
orbitopagus
orbitotomy
orcein
orchectomy
orcheoplasty
orchialgia
orchichorea
orchidalgia
orchidectomy
orchidic
orchiditis
orchidoncus
orchidopexy
orchidoplasty
orchidoptosis
orchidorrhaphy
orchidotomy
orchiectomy
orchiepididymitis
orchilytic
orchiocele
orchiodynia
orchioncus
orchioneuralgia
orchiopathy
orchiopexy
orchioplasty
orchiorrhaphy
orchioscheocele
orchioscirrhus
orchiotomy
orchis
orchitic

orchitis
orchitis, gonorrheal
orchitis, metastatic
orchitis, syphilitic
orchitis, tuberculous
orchotomy
orcin
orcinol
ordinate
ordure
Oretic
  (hydrochlorothiazide)
Oreticyl
  (hydrochlorothiazide
  and deserpidine)
Oreton Methyl
  (methyltestosterone)
orexia
orexigenic
oreximania
Orexin Softab
  (therapeutic vitamin
  supplement)
orf
organ
organ panels
organ perfusion system
organ transplantation
  tissue typing
organ-specific
organelle
organic
organic acid
organic brain syndrome
organic chemistry
organic disease
organic dust toxic
  syndrome (ODTS)
organic psychoses
organicism
organicist
Organidin (iodinated
  glycerol)
organism
organization
organization center
organize
organoferric

organogel
organogenesis
organogeny
organography
organoid
organoleptic
organology
organoma
organomegaly
organomercurial
organometallic
organon
organonomy
organopathy
organopexy
organophilic
organoscopy
organotherapy
organotrope
organotrophic
organotropic
organotropism
organum
organum auditus
organum gustus
organum olfactus
organum spirale
organum
  vestibulocochleare
organum visus
organum vomeronasale
orgasm
Oriental score
orientation
orifice, anal
orifice, atrioventricular
orifice, cardiac
orifice, mitral
orifice, oral
orifice, pyloric
orifice, ureteric
orifice, urethral
orificial
orificium
origin
Orimune (poliovirus
  vaccine)
Orinase (tolbutamide)

Ormond's disease
Ornade Spansule
ornithine
ornithine carbamyl
  transferase (OCT)
Ornithodoros
ornithosis
orodiagnosis
orofacial
orofaciodigital syndrome
orolingual
oromaxillary fistula
  repair
oromeningitis
oronasal
oronasal fistula repair
oropharynx
orosomucoid
orotherapy
orotic acid
orotic aciduria
Oroya fever
orphan drugs
orphenadrine citrate
orrhology
orrhomeningitis
orrhoreaction
orrhorrhea
orrhotherapy
orris root
orthergasia
orthesis
orthetics
orthetist
Ortho Diaphragm Kits
Ortho Dienes
Ortho Disposable
  Applicator
Ortho Personal Lubricant
Ortho-Creme
  (contraceptive cream)
Ortho-Gynol
  (contraceptive jelly)
Ortho-Novum
  (norethindrone/
  mestranol)

Ortho-Novum 1/35
  (combination oral
  contraceptive)
Ortho-Novum 1/50
  (combination oral
  contraceptive)
Ortho-Novum 1/80
  (combination oral
  contraceptive)
Ortho-Novum 10/11
  (combination oral
  contraceptive)
Ortho-Novum 7/7/7
  (combination oral
  contraceptive)
orthoacid
orthobiosis
orthocephalic
orthochorea
orthochromatic
orthochromophil
Orthoclone OKT
  (muromonab-CD3)
orthocytosis
orthodentin
orthodiagraph
orthodigita
orthodontic cephalogram
orthodontics
orthodontist
orthodromic
orthogenesis
orthogenic
orthogenics
orthograde
orthokinetic cuff
orthokinetics
orthomelic
orthometer
orthomolecular
orthomolecular psychiatry
orthomyxoviruses
orthopantogram
orthopedia
orthopedic
orthopedic surgery

orthopedics
orthopedist
orthopercussion
orthophoria
orthophrenia
orthopnea
orthopneic position
Orthopoxvirus
orthopraxis
orthopsia
orthopsychiatry
orthoptic
orthoptic training
orthoptics
orthoroentgenography
orthoroentgenogram
orthoscopic
orthoscopy
orthosis
orthostatic
orthostatic hypotension
orthostatism
orthotast
orthotic
orthotic "check-out"
orthotics
orthotics training
orthotist
orthotonos
orthotonus
orthotopic
orthovoltage
orthuria
Orudis (ketoprofen)
os
os calcis
os coxae
os hamatum
os hyoideum
os ilii
os innominatum
os magnum
os orbiculare
os peroneum
os planum
os pubis
os scaphoideum
os temporale

os trigonum
os unguis
os uteri
os uteri externum
os uteri internum
os ventriculi
os vesalianum
Os-Cal 500 (calcium
  supplement)
osazone
oscedo
oscheal
oscheitis
oschelephantiasis
oscheocele
oscheohydrocele
oscheolith
oscheoma
oscheoncus
oscheoplasty
oschitis
oscillating tracking test
oscillation
oscillator
oscillogram
oscillograph
oscillometer
oscillometry
oscillopsia
oscilloscope
Oscinidae
oscitation
osculation
osculum
Osgood-Schlatter disease
Osler, Sir William
Osler's disease
Osler's maneuver
Osler's nodes
Osler-Vaquez disease
Osler-Weber-Rendu disease
osmate
osmatic
osmesis
osmesthesia
osmic acid
osmicate
osmics

osmidrosis
osmiophilic
osmiophobic
osmium (Os)
osmodysphoria
osmolagnia
osmolality, blood
osmolality test
osmolality, urine
osmolar
osmolarity
Osmolite HN (high
  nitrogen isotonic
  liquid nutrition)
osmology
osmometer
osmonosology
osmophilic
osmophore
osmoreceptor
osmoregulation
osmose
osmosis
osmotherapy
osmotic
osmotic fragility, RBC
osmotic pressure
osphresiolagnia
osphresiology
osphresiometer
osphresis
osphretic
osphus
osphyalgia
osphyitis
osphyomyelitis
ossa
ossein
osseocartilaginous
osseofibrous
osseointegration
osseomucin
osseous
osseous survey,
  radiological
osseous tissue
osseous tuberosities
  excision

ossicle
ossicula
ossicular chain
  reconstruction
ossiculectomy
ossiculotomy
ossiculum
ossiferous
ossific
ossification
ossification,
  endochondral
ossification,
  intramembranous
ossification, pathologic
ossification, periosteal
ossifluence
ossiform
ossify
ostalgia
osteal
ostealgia
osteanagenesis
ostearthrotomy
ostectomy
osteectomy
osteectopia
osteitis
osteitis, condensing
osteitis deformans
osteitis fibrosa cystica
  generalistata
osteitis fragilitans
osteitis, gummatous
osteitis, rarefying
osteitis, sclerosing
ostembryon
ostemia
ostempyesis
osteoanagenesis
osteoanesthesia
osteoaneurysm
osteoarthritis
osteoarthropathy
osteoarthropathy,
  hypertrophic pulmonary
osteoarthrosis
osteoarthrotomy

osteoblast
osteoblastoma
osteocampsia
osteocarcinoma
osteocartilaginous
osteocele
osteocephaloma
osteochondral
osteochondritis
osteochondritis deformans
  juvenilis
osteochondritis dissecans
osteochondrodystrophy
osteochondrolysis
osteochondroma
osteochondromatosis
osteochondrosarcoma
osteochondrosis
osteochondrosis deformans
  tibiae
osteochondrous
osteoclasia
osteoclast
osteoclast activating
  factor (OAF)
osteoclastic
osteoclastoma
osteoclasty
osteocope
osteocopic
osteocranium
osteocyte
osteocytoma
osteodensitometer
osteodentin
osteodermia
osteodesmosis
osteodiastasis
osteodynia
osteodystrophia
osteodystrophy
osteoectomy
osteoepiphysis
osteofibroma
osteogen
osteogenesis
osteogenic
osteogenic sarcoma

osteogeny
osteography
osteohalisteresis
osteoid
osteolipochondroma
osteologist
osteology
osteolysis
osteolytic
osteoma
osteoma, cancellous
osteoma, cavalryman's
osteoma cutis
osteoma, dental
osteoma durum, eburneum
osteoma medullare
osteoma, osteoid
osteoma spongiosum
osteomalacia
osteomalacic
osteomatoid
osteomatosis
osteomere
osteometry
osteomyelitis
osteomyelodysplasia
osteon
osteoncus
osteonecrosis
osteonectin
osteoneuralgia
osteopath
osteopathic
osteopathology
osteopathy
osteopecilia
osteopedion
osteopenia
osteoperiosteal
osteoperiostitis
osteopetrosis
osteophage
osteophagia
osteophlebitis
osteophone
osteophony
osteophore
osteophyma

osteophyte
osteophytectomy (spine)
osteoplaque
osteoplast
osteoplastic
osteoplastic flap
osteoplasty
osteopoikilosis
osteoporosis
osteoporosis
  circumscripta cranii
osteoporosis of disuse
osteoporosis,
  posttraumatic
osteoporotic
osteoradionecrosis
osteorrhagia
osteorrhaphy
osteosarcoma
osteosarcomatous
osteosclerosis
osteoscope
osteoseptum
osteosis
osteosis cutis
osteospongioma
osteosteatoma
osteostixis
osteosuture
osteosynovitis
osteotabes
osteotelangiectasia
osteothrombosis
osteotome
osteotomies
osteotomoclasis
osteotomy
osteotomy, cuneiform
osteotomy, linear
osteotomy, Macewen's
osteotomy,
  subtrochanteric
osteotomy,
  transtrochanteric
osteotribe
osteotrophy
osteotylus
osteotympanic

Osti-Derm Lotion
ostial
ostitis
ostium
ostium abdominale tubae
  uterinae
ostium arteriosum
ostium internum
ostium pharyngeum
ostium primum
ostium primum defect
ostium secundum
ostium secundum defect
ostium tympanicum
ostium urethrae externum
ostium uteri
ostium uterinum tubae
ostium vaginae
ostomate
ostomy
ostosis
ostraceous
ostreotoxismus
otacoustic
otalgia
otantritis
otectomy
othelcosis
othematoma
othemorrhea
othygroma
otic
Otic-H.C. (ear drops)
oticodinia
otitic
otitis, aero-
otitis, aviation
otitis externa
otitis, furuncular
otitis interna,
  labyrinthica
otitis labyrinthica
otitis mastoides
otitis media (OM)
otitis media with
  effusion
otitis mycotica
otitis parasitica

otitis sclerotica
otoantritis
Otobiotic (polymixin B
  sulfate and
  hydrocortisone)
otoblennorrhea
otocatarrh
otocephalus
otocephaly
otocleisis
otoconium
otocyst
otodynia
otoganglion
otogenic
otogenous
otography
otolaryngologist
otolaryngology
otolith
otological
otologist
otology
otomassage
otomucormycosis
otomyasthenia
otomyces
otomycosis
otoncus
otonecrectomy
otonecronectomy
otoneuralgia
otoneurasthenia
otoneurology
otopathy
otopharyngeal
otopharyngeal tube
otoplasty
otopolypus
otopyorrhea
otopyosis
otorhinolaryngology
otorhinolaryngologist
otorhinology
otorrhagia
otorrhea
otosalpinx
otoscleronectomy

otosclerosis
otoscope
otoscopy
otosis
otosteal
ototomy
ototoxic
Otrivin (xylometazoline
  HCl)
Otto pelvis
ouabain
oulitis
oulorrhagia
outflow, craniosacral
outflow, thoracolumbar
outflow tract
  augmentation
outpatient (OP)
outpatient clinic (OPC)
outpatient department
  (OPD)
outpocketing
output, cardiac
output, energy
output, stroke
output, urinary
outrigger
ova
ova and parasites (O&V)
oval
oval window
oval window fistula
  repair
ovalbumin
ovalocyte
ovalocytosis
ovaralgia
ovarialgia
ovarian
ovarian abscess drainage
ovarian cyst
ovarian cyst drainage
ovarian cystectomy
ovarian lesions
ovarian medulla
ovarian pregnancy
ovarian vein syndrome
ovariectomy

ovaries
ovariocele
ovariocentesis
ovariocyesis
ovariodysneuria
ovariogenic
ovariohysterectomy
ovariolysis
ovariopathy
ovariopexy
ovariorrhexis
ovariosalpingectomy
ovariosteresis
ovariostomy
ovariotexy
ovariotomy
ovariotubal
ovaritis
ovarium
Ovcon 50 (nerethindrone and ethinyl estradiol)
overbite
overclosure
overcompensation
overcorrection
overdenture
overdetermination
overeruption
overexertion
overextension
overflow
overgrowth
overhang
overhydration
overjet
overlap
overlay
overproduction
overresponse
overriding
overtoe
overtone
overvalued idea
overventilation
ovi albumin
ovicide
oviduct
oviferous

oviform
ovigenesis
ovigerm
ovination
ovine
ovinia
oviparity
oviparous
oviposition
ovipositor
ovisac
ovocenter
ovocyte
ovoflavin
ovogenesis
ovoglobulin
ovogonium
ovoid
ovomucin
ovomucoid
ovoplasm
ovotestis
ovovitellin
ovoviviparous
Ovral (norgestrel and ethinyl estradiol)
Ovrette (norgestrel)
ovula
ovular
ovulation
ovulatory
ovule
Ovulen-21 (ethynodiol diacetate with mestranol)
Ovulen-28 (ethynodiol diacetate with mestranol)
ovulogenous
ovulum
ovum
ovum, alecithal
ovum, centrolecithal
ovum, holoblastic
ovum, human
ovum, isolecithal
ovum, meroblastic
ovum, permanent

ovum, primordial
ovum, telolecithal
ovum transfer
Owren prothrombin-
  proconvertin (P&P)
Owren's disease
ox-19 agglutinins
oxa
oxalacetic acid
oxalate
oxalate, potassium
oxalemia
oxalic acid
oxalic acid poisoning
oxalism
oxalosis
oxaluria
oxalylurea
oxandrolone
oxazepam
oxidant
oxidase
oxidase, copper
  (ceruloplasmin)
oxidase, cytochrome
oxidation
oxidation-reduction
  reaction
oxide
oxidize
oxidoreductase
oxim
oxime
oximeter
oximetry, blood gases
oxonemia
oxophenarsine
  hydrochloride
Oxsoralen (methoxsalen)
Oxsoralen-Ultra
  (methoxsalen)
oxtriphylline
Oxy Clean
oxyacoia
oxyacusis
oxybenzene
oxybenzone
oxyblepsia

oxybutyria
oxybutyric acid, beta
oxycalcium
oxycephalous
oxychloride
oxychromatic
oxychromatin
oxycinesia
oxyecoia
oxyesthesia
oxygen (O_2)
oxygen capacity
oxygen debt
oxygen dissociation cure
oxygen radicals
oxygen saturation
oxygen tent
oxygen therapy
oxygen toxicity
oxygen uptake, expired
  gas analysis
oxygen-hemoglobin
  affinity
oxygenase
oxygenate
oxygenation, hyperbaric
oxygenator
oxygenator, bubble
oxygenator, rotating disk
oxygenator, screen
oxygenic
oxygenize
oxygeusia
oxyhematin
oxyhematoporphyrin
oxyhemoglobin
oxyhemoglobinometer
oxyhydrocephalus
oxyiodide
oxylalia
oxymetazoline
  hydrochloride
oxymetholone
oxymorphone hydrochloride
oxymyoglobin
oxyntic
oxyopia
oxyopter

oxyosmia
oxyosphresia
oxypathia
oxypathy
oxyperitoneum
oxyphenbutazone
oxyphil
oxyphile
oxyphilous
oxyphonia
oxypurine
oxyrhine
oxytalan
oxytetracycline
oxytocia
oxytocic
oxytocic principle
oxytocin
oxytocin challenge test
   (OCT)
oxytocinase
oxyuriasis
oxyuricide
oxyurid
Oxyuris
Oxyuris vermicularis
Oxyuroidea
oyster
ozena
ozochrotia
ozonator
ozone
ozonization
ozonize
ozonometer
ozonoscope

P

P-V-Tussin
PA catheter
Pabalate
Pabalate-SF
pabular
pabulum

pacchionian bodies
pacchionian depressions
pacemaker
pacemaker, cardiac,
   artificial
pacemaker, demand
pacemaker, dual-chamber
   analysis
pacemaker, ectopic
pacemaker, electronic
   analysis
pacemaker, external
pacemaker, fixed rate
pacemaker, insertion
pacemaker, mediastinal
pacemaker, permanent
pacemaker, programmable
pacemaker, removal
pacemaker, repair
pacemaker, single chamber
   analysis
pacemaker, temporary
pacemaker, transthoracic
pacemaker, transvenous
pacemaker wandering
pacer
pachismus
pachyacria
pachyakria
pachyblepharon
pachyblepharosis
pachycephalic
pachycephalous
pachycephaly
pachycheilia
pachycholia
pachychromatic
pachycolpismus
pachydactylia
pachydactyly
pachyderma
pachyderma circumscripta
pachyderma laryngis
pachyderma
   lymphangiectatica
pachyderma, occipital
pachyderma vesicae
pachydermatocele

pachydermatosis
pachydermatous
pachyemia
pachyglossia
pachygnathous
pachygyria
pachyhematous
pachyleptomeningitis
pachylosis
pachymenia
pachymeningitis
pachymeningitis, external
pachymeningitis,
  hemorrhagic
pachymeningitis, internal
pachymeningitis, spinal
pachymeningopathy
pachymeninx
pachynema
pachynsis
pachyonychia
pachyonychia congenita
pachyostosis
pachyotia
pachypelviperitonitis
pachyperiostitis
pachyperitonitis
pachypleuritis
pachypodous
pachyrhinic
pachysalpingitis
pachysalpingoovaritis
pachysomia
pachytene
pachytrichous
pachyvaginalitis
pachyvaginitis
pacifier
pacing
pacing code
pacing wire
pacinian corpuscles
pack
pack, cold
pack, dry
pack, full
pack, half
pack, hot

pack, ice
pack, one-sheet
pack, partial
pack, periodontal
pack, three-quarter
pack, umbrella
pack, wet-dry
pack, wet-sheet
package insert
packed cell volume (PCV)
packed cells
packed red cells (PRC)
packer
packing
pad
pad, abdominal
pad, dinner
pad, fat
pad, kidney
pad, Malgaigne's
pad, Mikulicz's
pad, perineal
pad, sucking
pad, surgical
pads, knuckle
page turner
Paget's disease
pagetoid
Pagitane Hydrochloride
  (cycrimine HCl)
pagophagia
pain
pain, abdominal
pain, aching
pain, acute
pain, agonizing
pain, angina pectoris
pain, appendicitis
pain, boring
pain, Brodie's
pain, burning
pain, cardiac
pain, causalgic
pain, central
pain, cephalgic
pain, chest
pain, chronic
pain, chronic intractable

pain, cramplike
pain, dental
pain, dull
pain, ear
pain, eccentric
pain epigastric
pain, false
pain, fulgurant
pain, gallbladder
pain, gas
pain, gastralgic
pain, girdle
pain, head
pain, heterotopic
pain, homotopic
pain, hunger
pain, hypogastric
pain, imperative
pain, inflammatory
pain, intermenstrual
pain, intractable
pain, lancinating
pain, lightning
pain, lingual
pain, lung
pain, menstrual
pain, mental
pain, middle
pain, migraine
pain, mind
pain, mobile
pain, movement
pain, neuralgic
pain, night
pain, noise
pain, objective
pain, organic
pain, osteocopic
pain, paresthesic
pain, phantom limb
pain, postprandial
pain, precordial
pain, premonitory
pain, pseudomyelic
pain, psychic
pain, psychogenic
pain, psychosomatic
pain, pulmonary

pain, rectal, constant
pain, referred
pain, remittent
pain, rest
pain, root
pain, shifting
pain, subdiaphragmatic
pain, subjective
pain, sympathetic
pain, tenesmic
pain, terebrant
pain, thermalgesic
pain, thoracic
pain, throbbing
pain, tongue
pain tracheal
pain wandering
pains, bearing-down
pains, dilating
pains, expulsive
pains, growing
pains, labor
pains, spot
pains, starting
paint
paint, Castellani's
painters' colic
pair
pair, base
palatable
palatal
palatal reflex
palate
palate, artificial
palate bones
palate, bony
palate, cleft
palate, falling
palate, gothic
palate, hard
palate, pendulous
palate, primary
palate, secondary
palate, soft
palatiform
palatine
palatine arches
palatine artery, greater

palatine bone
palatine tonsils
palatitis
palatoglossal
palatoglossus
palatognathous
palatograph
palatography
palatomaxillary
palatomyograph
palatonasal
palatopharyngeal
palatopharyngeus
palatopharyngoplasty
palatoplasty
palatoplasty for cleft
  palate
palatoplegia
palatorrhaphy
palatosalpingeus
palatoschisis
palatum
palebral cartilages
paleencephalon
paleocerebellum
paleoencephalon
paleogenesis
paleogenetic
paleokinetic
paleontology
paleopathology
paleostriatal
paleostriatum
paleothalamus
palikinesia
palilalia
palinal
palindromia
palindromic
palindromic rheumatism
palinesthesia
palingenesis
palingraphia
palinopsia
paliphrasia
palladium
pallanesthesia
pallescence

pallesthesia
palliate
palliative
pallid
pallidal
pallidectomy
pallidoansotomy
pallidotomy
pallidum
pallidus, globus
  stereotactic lesion
pallium
pallor
palm
palm-chin reflex
palm tendon excision
palm tendon sheath
  drainage
palm tendon sheath
  synovectomy
palm tenolysis, flexor
palm tenotomy, flexor
palma
palmar
palmar bursa drainage
palmar cuff
palmar fasciectomy
palmar fasciotomy
palmar grasp reflex
palmar reflex
palmar tendon transfer
palmaris
palmaris tendon graft
palmature
palmic
palmitic acid
palmitin
palmomental reflex
palmoplantar
palmus
palpable
palpate
palpation
palpation, light-touch
palpatopercussion
palpebra
palpebra inferior
palpebra superior

palpebrae
palpebral
palpebral commissure
palpebral fissure
palpebral ligament
palpebral muscles
palpebral wound closure
palpebrate
palpebritis
palpitant
palpitate
palpitation
palpitation, arterial
palsy
palsy, Bell's
palsy, birth
palsy, bulbar
palsy, cerebral
palsy, crutch
palsy, diver's
palsy, Erb's
palsy, facial
palsy, lead
palsy, night
palsy, progressive
   supranuclear
palsy, Saturday night
palsy, scrivener's
palsy, shaking
palsy, wasting
paludal
paludism
palynology
Pamelor (nortriptyline
   HCl)
Pamine (methscopolamine
   bromide)
pampiniform
pampiniform plexus
pampinocele
panacea
Panadol
Panafil
panagglutinable
panagglutinin
**Panalgesic Liniment and
   Cream**
panangiitis

panaris
panarteritis
panarthritis
Panas operation
panasthenia
panatrophy
panblastic
pancarditis
panchreston
panchromia
Pancoast syndrome
pancolectomy
pancreas
pancreas, accessory
pancreas, annular
pancreas biopsy
pancreas cyst
   marsupialization
pancreas divisum
pancreas, dorsal
pancreas, lesser
pancreas pseudocyst
   drainage
pancreas transplant
pancreas, transplantation
   of
pancreas, ventral
pancreas, Willis'
Pancrease (pancrelipase)
pancreatalgia
pancreatectomy
pancreatemphraxis
pancreathelcosis
pancreatic
pancreatic cyst
   anastomosis
pancreatic duct
pancreatic juice
pancreatic juice
   collection
pancreatic panel
pancreaticicalculus
   removal
pancreaticochole-
   cystostomy
pancreaticocysto-
   enterotomy

pancreaticocysto-
gastrostomy
pancreaticocysto-
duodenostomy
pancreaticocysto-
jejunostomy
pancreaticoduodenal
pancreaticoduodenectomy
pancreaticoduodenostomy
pancreaticoenterostomy
pancreaticogastrostomy
pancreaticoileostomy
pancreaticojejunostomy
pancreatin
pancreatitis
pancreatitis, acute
pancreatitis, acute
  hemorrhagic
pancreatitis, calcareous
pancreatitis, centrilobar
pancreatitis, chronic
pancreatitis,
  interstitial
pancreatitis, perilobar
pancreatitis, purulent
pancreatitis, suppurative
pancreatoduodenectomy
pancreatoduodenostomy
pancreatogenic
pancreatogenous
pancreatogram
pancreatography
pancreatolith
pancreatolithectomy
pancreatolithiasis
pancreatolithotomy
pancreatolysis
pancreatolytic
pancreatomy
pancreatoncus
pancreatopathy
pancreatotomy
pancreatotropic
pancreectomy
pancreolithotomy
pancreolysis
pancreolytic
pancreopathy

pancreoprivic
pancreozymin-
  cholecystokinin
pancreozymin-secretin
  test
pancuronium bromide
pancytopenia
pandemia
pandemic
pandiculation
Pándy (spinal fluid
  protein)
panel
panel agglutinins
panel antibody
  identification
panencephalitis
panendoscope
panendoscopy
panesthesia
Paneth, cells of
pang
pangamic acid
pangenesis
panglossia
Panhematin (hemin, I.V.)
panhidrosis
panhyperemia
panhypopituitarism
panhysterectomy
panhysterocolpectomy
panhystero-oophorectomy
panhysterosalpingectomy
panhysterosalpingo-
  oophorectomy
panic
panic attack
panic disorder
panic, homosexual
panimmunity
panis
panmyeloid
panmyelophthisis
panmyelosis
panneuritis
panneuritis epidemica
panniculectomy

panniculitis
panniculitis, nodular
  nonsuppurative
panniculitis, relapsing
  febrile nodular
  nonsuppurative
panniculus
panniculus adiposus
panniculus carnosus
pannus
pannus carateus
pannus carnosus
pannus crassus
pannus degenerativus
pannus, phlyctenular
pannus siccus
pannus tenuis
panodic
panography
panophobia
panophthalmia
panophthalmitis
panoptic
panoptic stain
panoptosis
pan-oral radiography
panosteitis
panotitis
Panoxyl 5 (benzoyl
  peroxide)
panphobia
panplegia
pansclerosis
pansinusitis
pansphygmograph
Panstrongylus
Panstrongylus megistus
pansystolic
pant
pantabasic
pantachromatic
pantalar arthrodesis
pantalgia
pantaloon operation
pantamorphia
pantanencephaly
pantankyloblepharon
pantatrophia

pantatrophy
pantetheine
panthodic
panting
pantograph
pantomography
pantomorphia
pantophobia
Pantopon (hydrochlorides
  of opium alkaloids)
pantoscopic
pantoscopic glasses
pantothenate
pantothenic acid
pantothermia
pantropic
panturbinate
Panwarfin (warfarin
  sodium)
panzootic
pap
Pap smear
Pap test
papain
Papanicolaou test (Pap
  smear)
papaverine hydrochloride
papaya
paper
paper, articulating
paper, bibulous
paper, blistering
paper chromatography
paper, filter
paper, indicator
paper, litmus
paper, occluding
paper, test
papilla
papilla, acoustic
papilla, Bergmeister's
papilla, circumvallate
papilla, clavate
papilla, conical
papilla, dental
papilla, dermal
papilla, douodenal
papilla, filiform

papilla, foliate
papilla, fungiform
papilla, gingival
papilla, gustatory
papilla, incisive
papilla, interdental
papilla, interproximal
papilla, lacrimal
papilla, lenticular
papilla, lingual
papilla, mammae
papilla of corium
papilla of hair
papilla of Vater
papilla, optic
papilla, palatine
papilla, parotid
papilla pili
papilla, renal
papilla, tactile
papilla, taste
papilla, urethral
papilla, vallate
papillae
papillary
papillary ducts of
  Bellini
papillary layer
papillary muscles
papillary tumor
papillate
papillectomy
papillectomy, anal
papilledema
papilliform
papillitis
papilloadenocystoma
papillocarcinoma
papilloma
papilloma durum
papilloma,
  fibroepithelial
papilloma, hard
papilloma, Hopmann's
papilloma, intracystic
papilloma molle
papilloma, soft
papilloma, villous

papillomatosis
papillomaviruses
papilloretinitis
papovaviruses
pappataci fever
pappose
pappus
paprika
papula
papular
papular fever
papulation
papule
papule, dry
papule, moist
papule, mucous
papules, split
papuliferous
papuloerythematous
papulopustular
papulosis
papulosquamous
papulovesicular
papyraceous
Paquin operation
par
para
para-actinomycosis
para-aminobenzoic acid
  (PABA)
para aminohippurate (PAH)
para-aminosalicylic acid
  (PAS)
para-anesthesia
para-aortic bodies
para-appendicitis
para-aortic
  lymphadenectomy
parabionts
parabiosis
parabiotic
parablepsia
parablepsis
parabulia
paracanthoma
paracasein
Paracelsus
paracenesthesia

paracentesis
paracentesis capitis
paracentesis cordis
paracentesis pericardii
paracentesis pulmonis
paracentesis thoracis
paracentesis tunicae
　vaginalis
paracentesis tympani
paracentesis vesicae
paracentetic
paracentral
paracentral lobule
paracephalus
paracervical (uterine)
　nerve injection
parachlorophenol
parachlorophenol,
　camphorated
paracholera
paracholia
parachordal
parachordal cartilage
parachromatism
parachromatopsia
parachute reflex
　(reaction)
paracinesia
paracinesis
paracme
paracoagulation,
　protamine (PPP)
Paracoccidioides
Paracoccidioides
　brasiliensis
paracoccidioidomycosis
paracolitis
paracolostomy hernia
paracolpitis
paracolpium
paracone
paraconid
paracousis
paracrine control
paracrisis
paracusia
paracusia acris
paracusia duplicata

paracusia loci
paracusia willisiana
paracusis
paracystic
paracystitis
paracystium
paracytic
paradenitis
paradental
paradentium
paradidymal
paradidymis
Paradione
　(paramethadione)
paradipsia
paradox, Weber's
paradoxic
paradoxical
paradoxical respiration
paraequilibrium
paraffin
paraffin bath
paraffin, hard
paraffin, liquid
paraffin, soft
paraffin, white soft
paraffin, yellow soft
paraffinoma
paraffinum
Paraflex (chlorzoxazone)
Parafon Forte DSC
　(chlorzoxazone)
paraformaldehyde
paragammacism
paraganglia
paraganglioma
paraganglion
parageusia
parageusis
paraglossa
paraglossia
paragnathus
paragonimiasis
Paragonimus
Paragonimus westermani
paragrammatism
paragranuloma
paragraphia

parahemophilia
parahepatic
parahepatitis
parahormone
parahypnosis
parahypophysis
parainfection
parainfluenza viruses
parakeratosis
parakeratosis ostracea
parakeratosis
  psoriasiformis
parakinesia
paralalia
paralalia literalis
paralambdacism
paralbumin
paraldehyde
paraldehyde poisoning
paraldehydism
paralepsy
paralexia
paralgesia
paralgia
parallactic
parallagma
parallax
parallax, binocular
parallax, heteronymous
parallax, homonymous
parallelism
parallelometer
parallergic
parallergy
paralogia
paralogy
paralysis
paralysis, acoustic
paralysis, acute
  ascending spinal
paralysis, acute atrophic
paralysis, acute
  infectious
paralysis agitans
paralysis, alcoholic
paralysis, anesthesia
paralysis, anterior
  spinal

paralysis, arsenical
paralysis, ascending
paralysis, association
paralysis, asthenic
  bulbar
paralysis, atrophic
  spinal
paralysis, Bell's
paralysis, birth
paralysis, brachial
paralysis, brachiofacial
paralysis, bulbar
paralysis, central
paralysis, cerebral
  spastic, infantile
paralysis, complete
paralysis, compression
paralysis, conjugate
paralysis, crossed
paralysis, crutch
paralysis, decubitus
paralysis, diphtheritic
paralysis, diver's
paralysis, Duchenne-Erb
paralysis, Duchenne's
paralysis, exhaustion
paralysis, facial
paralysis, familial
  periodic
paralysis, flaccid
paralysis, general
paralysis, ginger
paralysis, glossolabial
paralysis, Gubler's
paralysis, histrionic
paralysis, hyperkalemic
  periodic
paralysis, hypokalemic
  periodic
paralysis, hysteric
paralysis, immunological
paralysis, incomplete
paralysis, infantile
paralysis, infantile
  cerebral ataxic
paralysis, infantile
  spinal

paralysis, infectious
  bulbar
paralysis, ischemic
paralysis, jake
paralysis, Jamaica ginger
paralysis, Klumpke's
paralysis, Kussmaul's
paralysis, labial
paralysis, Landry's
paralysis, lead
paralysis, local
paralysis, mimetic
paralysis, mixed
paralysis, muscular
paralysis, musculospiral
paralysis, normokalemic
  periodic
paralysis, nuclear
paralysis, obstetrical
paralysis, ocular
paralysis of
  accommodation
paralysis periodica
  paramyotonia
paralysis, phonetic
paralysis,
  postdiphtheritic
paralysis, posticus
paralysis, Pott's
paralysis, primary
  periodic
paralysis, progressive
  bulbar
paralysis, pseudobulbar
paralysis,
  pseudohypertropic
  muscular
paralysis, radial
paralysis, Saturday night
paralysis, sensory
paralysis, sleep
paralysis, spastic
paralysis, spinal
paralysis, supranuclear
paralysis, tick-bite
paralysis, Todd's
paralysis, tourniquet
paralysis vasomotor

paralysis Volkmann's
paralysis, wasting
paralytic
paralytic dementia
paralytic ileus
paralyzant
paralyze
paralyzer
paramagnetic
paramania
paramastigote
paramastitis
paramastoid
paramedian
paramedian incision
paramedic
paramedical
paramedical personnel
paramenia
paramesial
parameter
paramethadione
paramethasone acetate
parametric
parametritic
parametritis
parametrium
paramimia
paramnesia
paramolar
paramorphia
paramucin
paramusia
paramyloidosis
paramyoclonus multiplex
paramyosinogen
paramyotonia
paramyotonia ataxia
paramyotonia congenita
paramyotonia, symptomatic
paramyotonus
paramyxoviruses
paranalgesia
paranasal
paranasal sinuses
paraneoplastic syndromes
paranephric
paranephritis

paranephros
paranesthesia
paraneural
paranoia
paranoiac
paranoid
paranoid ideation
paranoid reaction type
paranomia
paranormal
paranuclear
paranucleate
paranucleolus
paranucleus
paraomphalic
paraoperative
paraosteoarthropathy
parapancreatic
paraparesis
parapedesis
parapeptone
paraperitoneal
parapestis
parapharyngeal abscess
paraphasia
paraphemia
paraphia
paraphilia
paraphimosis
paraphimosis oculi
paraphobia
paraphonia
paraphonia puberum
paraphora
paraphrasia
paraphrenitis
paraphronia
paraphyseal
paraphysis
paraplasm
paraplastic
paraplectic
paraplegia
paraplegia, alcoholic
paraplegia, ataxic
paraplegia, cerebral
paraplegia, congenital
  spastic

paraplegia dolorosa
paraplegia, infantile
  spastic
paraplegia, peripheral
paraplegia, Pott's
paraplegia, senile
paraplegia, spastic
paraplegia, spastic,
  primary
paraplegia, superior
paraplegia, tetanoid
paraplegic
paraplegiform
parapleuritis
parapoplexy
parapraxia
paraproctitis
paraproctium
paraprostatitis
paraprotein
paraproteinemia
parapsia
parapsis
parapsoriasis
parapsoriasis en plaque
parapsoriasis lichenoides
  chronica
parapsychology
paraquat
pararectal
parareflexia
pararenal
pararrhythmia
pararthria
parasacral
parasalpingitis
parasecretion
parasexuality
parasigmatism
parasinoidal
parasite
parasite, accidental
parasite, external
parasite, facultative
parasite, incidental
parasite, intermittent
parasite, internal
parasite, malarial

parasite, obligate
parasite, occasional
parasite, periodic
parasite, permanent
parasite, specific
parasite, temporary
parasitemia
parasites
parasitic
parasitic disease drug
  service
parasiticide
parasitism
parasitize
parasitogenic
parasitologist
parasitology
parasitophobia
parasitosis
parasitotropic
parasitotropism
parasitotropy
parasomnias
paraspadia
paraspasm
paraspinal
  electromyography
paraspinal muscle
  transfer
parasteatosis
parasternal
parasternal line
parasternal region
parasthenia
parastruma
parasympathetic
parasympathetic nervous
  system
parasympathicotonia
parasympatholytic
parasympathomimetic
parasynapsis
parasynovitis
parasystole
paratarsium
paratenon
paratenon tissue grafts
paratereseomania

parathion
parathion poisoning
parathormone (PTH)
parathymia
parathyroid
parathyroid extract (PTE)
parathyroid glands
parathyroid injection
parathyroid panel
parathyroidectomy
parathyroprivia
parathyroprivic
parathyrotropic
paratonsillar
paratope
paratrichosis
paratripsis
paratrophic
paratrophy
paratyphlitis
paratyphoid
paratyphoid fever
paratypic
paraumbilical
paraurethral
parauterine
paravaccinia
paravaginal
paravaginitis
paravenous
paravertebral
paravertebral anesthesia
paravertebral facet joint
  nerve destruction
paravertebral nerve
  injection
paravertebral sympathetic
  injection
paravesical
paravitaminosis
paraxial
paraxon
parazoon
parched
Paré, Ambroise
parectasia
parectasis
parectropia

Paredrine 1%
  (hydroxyamphetamine
  hydrobromide)
paregoric
paregoric poisoning
parelectronomic
parencephalia
parencephalocele
parencephalous
parenchyma
parenchyma testis
parenchymatitis
parenchymatous
parent
parenteral
parenteral digestion
parenteral nutrition
parenterally
parenting
parenting, surrogate
Parepectolin
parepididymus
parepithymia
paresis
paresis, juvenile
paresthesia
paresthesia, Berger's
pargyline hydrochloride
pari passu
paridrosis
paries
parietal
parietal bone
parietal cells
parietal lobe
parietes
parietography
parieto-occipital
parietosplanchnic
parietosquamosal
parietotemporal
parietovisceral
Parinaud, Henri
Parinaud's oculoglandular
  syndrome
Parinaud's
  ophthalmoplegia
parity

"Parking"
park and repair
Parkinson, James
Parkinson's disease
Parkinson's facies
Parkinson's mask
parkinsonism
Parlodel (bromocriptine
  mesylate)
Parnate (tranylcypromine
  sulfate)
paroccipital
parodontitis
parodontium
parodynia
parodynia perversa
parolivary
parolivary bodies
paromomycin sulfate
paromphalocele
paroniria
paroniria ambulans
paroniria salax
paronychia
paronychia tendinosa
paronychomycosis
paronychosis
paroophoritis
paroophoron
parophthalmia
parophthalmoncus
parorchidium
parorchis
parorexia
parosmia
parosphresia
parosphresis
parosteal
parosteosis
parostetis
parostitis
parostosis
parotic
parotid
parotid abscess drainage
parotid duct
parotid duct diversion
parotid gland

parotid sialolithotomy
parotid tumor excision
parotidectomy
parotiditis
parotidoscirrhus
parotitis
parous
parovarian
parovariotomy
parovaritis
parovarium
paroxysm
paroxysmal
paroxysmal atrial
  tachycardia (PAT)
paroxysmal cold
  hemoglobinuria
paroxysmal tachycardia
  (PT)
paroxysmal ventricular
  tachycardia (PVT)
parrot fever
Parrot, Jules Marie
Parrot's disease
Parrot's nodes
Parrot's sign
Parrott's pseudoparalysis
Parrott's ulcer
Parry's disease
pars
pars basilaris ossis
  occipitalis
pars buccalis hypophyseos
pars caeca oculi
pars caeca retinae
pars cephalica et
  cervicalis systematis
  autonomici
pars ciliaris retinae
pars distalis
  adenohypophyseos
pars flaccida membranae
  tympani
pars intermedia
  adenohypophyseos
pars iridica retinae
pars mastoidea ossis
  temporalis

pars membranacea urethrae
  masculinae
pars nervosa hypophyseos
pars optica hypothalami
pars optica retinae
pars petrosa ossis
  temporalis
pars plana corporis
  ciliaris
pars planitis
pars radiata lobuli
  corticalis renis
pars spongiosa urethrae
  masculinae
pars squamosa ossis
  temporalis
pars tensa membranae
  tympani
pars tuberalis
  adenohypophyseos
pars tympanica ossis
  temporalis
Parsidol (ethopropazine
  HCl)
partes
parthenogenesis
parthenophobia
partial thromboplastin
  time (PTT, APTT)
partial weight-bearing
  (PWB)
particle
particle agglutination
  rapid test
particle, alpha
particle, beta
particle, Dane
particle, elementary
particle, elementary of
  the mitochondria
particulate
parts per million (PPM)
Partsch operation
parturient
parturifacient
parturiometer
parturiphobia
parturition

parulis
parumbilical
paruria
parvicellular
parvoline
parvovirus
parvule
pascal
Paschen bodies
passage
passion
passional
passive
passive congestion
passive exercise
passive hyperemia
passive motion
passive movement
passive smoking
passivism
passivity
past history (PH)
past menstrual period
   (PMP)
past-pointing
paste
Pasteur, Louis
Pasteur effect
Pasteur treatment
Pasteurella
Pasteurella multocida
pasteurellosis
pasteurization
pastille
patagia
patagium
patch
patch closure atrial
   septal defect
patch closure endocardial
   cushion defect
patch closure sinus
   venosus
patch closure ventricular
   septal defect
patch, cotton wool
patch esophagogastric
   fundoplasty

patch graft repair of
   aneurysm
patch graft
   thromboendarterectomy
patch, herald
patch, Hutchinson's
patch, mucous
patch, opaline
patch, Peyer's
patch photo tests
patch, salmon
patch skin test
patch, smoker's
patch, soldier's
patch test
patch tympanic membrane
patchydermoperiostosis
patefaction
patella
patella, bipartite
patella, floating
patella, fracture of
patella, rider's painful
patella, slipping
patellapexy
patellar
patellar ligament
patellar reflex
patellar tendon bearing
   (PTB)
patellectomy
patelliform
patellofemoral
patellometer
patency
patent
patent ductus arteriosus
patent medicine
paternal
paternity test
path, condyle
path, incisor
path of closure
pathema
pathergasia
pathergia
pathergy
pathetic

pathetism
pathfinder
Pathilon (tridihexethyl
  chloride)
pathoamine
pathoanatomy
pathobiology
Pathocil (dicloxacillin
  sodium monohydrate)
pathoclisis
pathocrine
pathodixia
pathodontia
pathoformic
pathogen
pathogenesis
pathogenetic
pathogenic
pathogenicity
pathogeny
pathognomonic
pathognomy
pathognostic
pathography
pathologic
pathological
pathological reaction to
  alcohol
pathologist
pathology (path)
pathology, anatomic
pathology, cellular
pathology, chemical
pathology, clinical
pathology, comparative
pathology, dental
pathology, experimental
pathology, functional
pathology, geographical
pathology, humoral
pathology, medical
pathology, molecular
pathology, oral
pathology, surgical
pathomimesis
pathomimicry
pathomorphism
pathonomia

pathophilia
pathophobia
pathophoric
pathophysiology
pathopoiesis
pathopsychology
pathotropism
pathway
pathway, afferent
pathway, biosynthetic
pathway, central
pathway, conduction
pathway, efferent
pathway, Embden-Myerhof
pathway of incidence
pathway, metabolic
pathway, motor
pathway, pentose
  phosphate
pathway, sensory
patient (pt)
patient advocate
patient-controlled
  analgesia (PCA)
patient day
patient delay
patient dumping
patient mix
patricide
Patrick's test
patrilineal
Pattee operation
patten
pattern
pattern, occlusal
pattern, wear
patterning
patulous
paucisynapic
Paul-Bunnell test
pause
pause, compensatory
Pavabid (papaverine HCl)
pavementing
Pavlik harness
Pavlov, Ivan Patrovich
pavor
pavor diurnus

pavor nocturnus
Pavulon (pancuronium bromide)
Paxipam (halazepam)
PBZ-SR (tripelennamine HCl)
PCE (erythromycin)
peak expiratory flow rate (PEF)
peak inspiratory flow (PIF)
peanut oil
pearl
pearl, epithelial
pearl, gouty
pearl, Laënnec's
pearl's enamel
peau d'orange
peccant
peccatiphobia
pecten
pectenosis
pectenotomy
pectic acid
pectin
pectinase
pectinate
pectineal
pectineal line
pectineus
pectiniform
pectization
pectora
pectoral
pectoral mastectomy
pectoralgia
pectoralis
pectoralis major
pectoralis minor
pectoriloquy
pectoriloquy, aphonic
pectoriloquy, whispering
pectorophony
pectose
pectunculus
pectus
pectus carinatum
pectus excavatum

pectus recurvatum
pedal
Pedameth (racemethionine)
pedarthrocace
pedatrophia
pedatrophy
pederast
pederasty
pedes
pedesis
Pedi-Bath Salts
Pedi-Boro Soak Paks
Pedi-Cort V Creme
Pedi-Dri Foot Powder
Pedi-Pro Foot Powder
Pedi-Vit A Creme
PediaCare (cold formula)
Pediaflor Drops (sodium fluoride oral solution)
pedialgia
Pedialyte (oral electrolyte maintenance solution)
Pediamycin (erythromycin ethylsuccinate)
Pediapred (prednisolone sodium phosphate)
pediatric
Pediatric Nurse Practitioner (PNP)
pediatric pneumogram
pediatrician
pediatrics (peds)
pediatrist
pediatry
Pediazole (erythromycin ethylsuccinate and sulfisoxazole acetyl)
pedicel
pedicellation
pedicle
pedicle flap
pedicle flap attachment
pedicle flap cross lip
pedicle flap delay
pedicle flap eyelid repair
pedicle flap transfer

pedicle graft island
pedicle graft
  neurovascular flap
pedicle nerve
pedicle tube formation
pedicterus
pedicular
pediculate
pediculation
pediculicide
Pediculidae
pediculophobia
pediculosis
pediculosis capitis
pediculosis corporis
pediculosis palpebrarum
pediculosis pubis
pediculosis vestimenti
pediculous
pediculus
Pediculus
Pediculus humanus capitis
Pediculus humanus
  corporis
pedicure
pediform
pedigree
pediluvium
pedionalgia
pediophobia
pediphalanx
pedobaromacrometer
pedodontia
pedodontics
pedodontist
pedodynamometer
pedograph
pedologist
pedology
pedometer
pedomorphism
pedophilia
peduncle
peduncle, cerebellar,
  inferior
peduncle, cerebellar,
  middle

peduncle, cerebellar,
  superior
peduncle, cerebral
peduncle, mamillary
peduncle of flocculus
peduncle of superior
  olive
peduncle, olfactory
peduncle, pineal
peduncle, thalamic
peduncular
pedunculate
pedunculated
pedunculotomy
pedunculus
peel acid, of skin
peeling
peenash
peer
peer review (PR)
Peet operation
Peganone (ethotoin)
pejorative
pelade
pelage
Pel-Ebstein fever
Pelger-Huët anomaly
pelioma
peliosis
pellagra
pellagra sine pellagra
pellagrazein
pellagrin
pellagroid
pellagrous
pellant
Pellegrini-Stieda disease
Pellegrini's disease
pellet
pellet, cotton
pellet, foil
pellicle
pellicle, salivary
pellotine
pellucid
pellucid zone
pelotherapy

pelvectomy
pelvic
pelvic abscess drainage
pelvic anastomosis
  colectomy
pelvic angiography
pelvic bone
pelvic colpotomy
pelvic diameter
pelvic echography
pelvic examination
pelvic exenteration
pelvic floor repair
pelvic girdle
pelvic inflammatory
  disease (PID)
pelvic inlet
pelvic laparoscopy
pelvic lymphangiography
pelvic outlet
pelvic relaxation
pelvicephalography
pelvicephalometry
pelvifixation
pelvilithotomy
pelvimeter
pelvimetry
pelviolithotomy
pelvioplasty
pelvioscopy
pelviostomy
pelviotomy
pelviperitonitis
pelvirectal
pelvirectal abscess
  drainage
pelvis
pelvis aequabiliter justo
  major
pelvis aequabiliter justo
  minor
pelvis, android
pelvis, anthropoid
pelvis, assimilation
pelvis, beaked
pelvis bone imaging
pelvis, brachypellic
pelvis, brim of

pelvis computer
  tomography
pelvis, contracted
pelvis, cordate
pelvis, coxalgic
pelvis cyst
pelvis, dolichopellic
pelvis, dwarf
pelvis, elastic
pelvis excision, tumor,
  soft tissue
pelvis, extrarenal
pelvis, false
pelvis fissa
pelvis, fissured
pelvis, flat
pelvis, frozen
pelvis, funnel-shaped
pelvis, giant
pelvis, gynecoid
pelvis, halisteretic
pelvis, infantile
pelvis, justo major
pelvis, justo minor
pelvis, juvenile
pelvis, Kilian's
pelvis, kyphoscoliotic
pelvis, kyphotic
pelvis, large
pelvis, lordotic
pelvis major
pelvis, malacosteon
pelvis, masculine
pelvis, mesatipellic
pelvis, minor
pelvis, Naegele's
pelvis nana
pelvis obtecta
pelvis, osteomalacic
pelvis, Otto
pelvis plana
pelvis, platypellic
pelvis, Prague
pelvis,
  pseudo-osteomalacic
pelvis, rachitic
pelvis, reduced
pelvis, renal

pelvis, reniform
pelvis resection, tumor,
  soft tissue
pelvis, Robert's
pelvis Rokitansky
pelvis, rostrate
pelvis rotunda
pelvis, round
pelvis, rubber
pelvis, scoliotic
pelvis, simple flat
pelvis, small
pelvis spinosa
pelvis, split
pelvis, spondylolisthetic
pelvis spuria
pelvis, triangular
pelvis, true
pelvitherm
pelvi-ureteroplasty
pelvoscopy
pelvospondylitis
pelvospondylitis
  ossificans
Pemberton osteotomy,
  iliac or acetabular
pemoline
pemphigoid
pemphigoid, benign
  musocal
pemphigold, bullous
pemphigold, cicatricial
pemphigus
pemphigus acutus
pemphigus, benign
  familial
pemphigus circinatus
pemphigus, erythematous
pemphigus foliaceus
pemphigus neonatorum
pemphigus, ocular
pemphigus vegetans,
  Hallopeau type
pemphigus vegetans,
  Neumann type
pemphigus vulgaris
pendular
pendulous

Penecort (hydrocortisone)
penetrance
penetrate
penetrating
penetrating power
penetrating wound
penetration
penetrometer
penicillamine
penicillic acid
penicillin
penicillin,
  beta-lactamase
  resistant
penicillin G benzathine
penicillin V potassium
Penicillin VK
penicillinase
penicillinase-producing
  Neisseria gonococcus
  (PPNG)
penicilliosis
penicilloyl-polylysine
Penicillium
penicillus
penile
penile foreign body
  removal
penile plaque excision
penile prosthesis
penile prosthesis
  insertion
penile reflex
penile ring
penile specimen
penile tumescence test
penile urethroplasty
penile urethrorrhaphy
penis
penis amputation
penis biopsy
penis captivus
penis, clubbed
penis destruction of
  lesion
penis, double
penis incision and
  drainage

penis lunatus
penis palmatus
penis plethysmography
penis priapism operation
penis prosthesis
  operation
penis repair
penis surgery
penis, webbed
penischisis
penitis
pennate
penniform
pennyroyal
pennyweight
penoscrotal
penoscrotal urethroplasty
pension neurosis
pentachlorophenol
pentad
pentadactyl
pentaerythritol
  tetranitrate
pentagastrin
pentagastrin, gastric
  stimulation
pentalogy
Pentam 300 (pentamidine
  isethionate)
pentamethylenediamine
pentamidine
pentane
pentapeptide
pentaploid
pentastomiasis
pentatomic
pentavalent
pentazocine
Penthrane
  (methoxyflurane)
Pentids (pencillin G
  potassium)
Pentids for Syrup
  (penicillin G
  potassium)
pentobarbital
pentobarbital sodium
pentosazon

pentose
pentosemia
pentoside
pentostam
pentosuria
Pentothal (thiopental
  sodium)
pentoxide
Pentrax (tar shampoo with
  Fractar)
peonin
peotillomania
peotomy
Pepcid (famotidine)
pepo
pepper
peppermint spirit
pepsic
pepsin
pepsinogen
pepsinuria
peptic
peptic ulcer (PU)
peptidase
peptidase, cystine amino
peptide
peptidoglycan
peptidolytic
peptinotoxin
peptization
Pepto-Bismol
Peptococcus
peptogenic
peptogenous
peptoid
peptolysis
peptolytic
peptone
peptonemia
peptonization
peptonize
peptonolysis
peptonuria
Peptostreptococcus
peptotoxin
per anum
per contiguum
per continuum

per diem cost
per os (PO)
per primam intentionem
per rectum
per secundarm intentionem
per tertiam intentionem
per tubam
per vaginam
per vias naturales
peracephalus
peracid
peracidity
peracute
perarticulation
peratodynia
percent
percentile
percept
perception
perception, extrasensory
  (ESP)
perception, stereognostic
perceptivity
Percocet (oxycodone HCl
  and acetaminophen)
Percodan (oxycodone HCl,
  oxycodone terephthalate
  and aspirin)
Percogesic (acetaminophen
  and phenyltoloxamine
  citrate)
percolate
percolation
percolator
Percorten acetate
  (desoxycorticosterone
  acetate)
Percorten pivalate
  (desoxycorticosterone
  pivalate)
percuss
percussible
percussion
percussion and
  auscultation (P&A)
percussion, auscultatory
percussion, bimanual
percussion, deep

percussion, direct
percussion, finger
percussion, immediate
percussion, indirect
percussion, mediate
percussion of chest wall
percussion, palpation
percussion, threshold
percussor
percutaneous
percutaneous
  cholecystostomy
percutaneous endoscopic
  gastrotomy (PEG)
percutaneous
  nephrocystolithotomy
percutaneous nephrostomy
  tract
percutaneous tests
percutaneous transhepatic
  cholangiography (PTHC)
percutaneous transluminal
  angioplasty (PTA)
percutaneous transluminal
  coronary angioplasty
  (PTCA)
percutaneous ultrasonic
  lithotripsy (PUL)
percutaneous ultrasonic
  lithotriptor
perencephaly
Pereyra hysterectomy
Pereyra urethropexy
Pereyra vesical neck
  suspension
perfectionism
perflation
perforans
perforate
perforation
perforation, Bezold's
perforation of stomach or
  intestine
perforation, tooth
perforator
perforator, tympanum
perforatorium
perforators, ligation

performance
perfrication
perfrigeration
perfusate
perfusion
perfusion myocardium
  imaging
perfusion pulmonary
  imaging
perfusion test, acid
perfusionist
Pergonal (menotropins)
  perhydrocyclo-
  pentanophenanthrene
Peri-Colace (casanthranol
  and docusate sodium)
periacinal
periacinous
Periactin (cyproheptadine
  HCl)
periadenitis
periadenitis mucosa
  necrotica recurrens
perialienitis
periamygdalitis
perianal
perianal abscess
periangiitis
periangiocholitis
periaortic
periaortitis
periapex
periapical
periappendicitis
periappendicitis
  decidualis
periappendicular
periarterial
periarteritis
periarteritis gummosa
periarteritis nodosa
periarthric
periarthritis
periarticular
periatrial
periauricular
periaxial
periaxillary

periaxonal
periblast
peribronchial
peribronchiolar
peribronchiolitis
peribronchitis
peribulbar
peribursal
pericanalicular
pericardiac
pericardial
pericardial cyst or
  tumor excision
pericardial effusion
pericardial fluid
  analysis
pericardial partial
  resection
pericardial rub
pericardial window for
  drainage
pericardicentesis
pericardiectomy
pericardiocentesis
pericardiolysis
pericardiomediastinitis
pericardiopexy
pericardiophrenic
pericardioplasty
pericardiopleural
pericardiorrhaphy
pericardiostomy
pericardiosymphysis
pericardiotomy
pericarditic
pericarditis
pericarditis, acute
  fibrinous
pericarditis, acute
  nonspecific
pericarditis, adhesive
pericarditis,
  constrictive
pericarditis, external
pericarditis, fibrinous
pericarditis, hemorrhagic
pericarditis, idiopathic
pericarditis, ischemic

pericarditis, neoplastic
pericarditis obliterans
pericarditis, serofibrinous
pericarditis, uremic
pericardium
pericardium, adherent
pericardium, bread-and-butter
pericardium externum
pericardium, fibrous
pericardium internum
pericardium, parietal
pericardium, serous
pericardium, shaggy
pericardium, visceral
pericardotomy
pericecal
pericecitis
pericellular
pericemental
pericementitis
pericementitis, apical
pericementoclasia
pericementum
pericentral
pericholangitis
pericholecystitis
perichondral
perichondrial
perichondritis
perichondrium
perichondroma
perichord
perichordal
perichorioidal
perichoroidal
pericolic
pericolitis
pericolonitis
pericolpitis
periconchal
pericorneal
pericoronal
pericoronal tissues excision
pericoronitis
pericranial

pericranitis
pericranium
pericranium internum
pericystic
pericystitis
pericystium
pericyte
pericytial
peridectomy
peridendritic
peridens
peridental
peridentitis
peridentium
periderm
peridesmitis
peridesmium
Peridex (chlorhexidine gluconate)
perididymis
perididymitis
peridiverticulitis
periductal
periduodenitis
peridural
periencephalitis
periencephalomenigitis
periendothelioma
perienteric
perienteritis
perienteron
periependymal
periesophagitis
perifistular
perifocal
perifollicular
perifolliculitis
perigangliitis
periganglionic
perigastric
perigastritis
perigemmal
periglandulitis
periglottic
Perihemin (hematinic capsules)
perihepatic
perihepatitis

perihernial
perijejunitis
perikaryon
perikeratic
perikymata
perilabyrinthitis
perilaryngeal
perilaryngitis
perilenticular
periligamentous
perilimbal section
perilimbal suction
perilymph
perilympha
perilymphangeal
perilymphangitis
perimastitis
perimeningitis
perimeter
perimetric
perimetritic
perimetritis
perimetrium
perimetry
perimyelis
perimyelitis
perimyelography
perimyoendocarditis
perimyositis
perimysia
perimysial
perimysiitis
perimysium
perinatal
perinatalogy
perineal
perineal abscess drainage
perineal body
perineal colostomy
perineal fascia
perineal hernia
perineal prostatectomy
perineal section
perineal transplant
perineal urethra
perineal urethroplasty
perineal urethrorrhaphy

perineal urinary
  extravasation
perineocele
perineocolpo-
  rectomyomectomy
perineogram
perineometer
perineoplasty
perineorrhaphy
perineorrhaphy, anterior
perineorrhaphy, colpo-
perineorrhaphy, posterior
perineoscrotal
perineotomy
perineovaginal
perinephrial
perinephric
perinephric cyst excision
perinephritis
perinephrium
perineum
perineum biopsy
perineum
  colpoperineorrhaphy
perineum perineoplasty
perineum, tears of the
perineural
perineurial
perineuritis
perineurium
perinuclear
periocular
period
period, absolute
  refractory
period, childbearing
period, critical
period, effective
  refractory
period, ejection
period, fertile
period, gestation
period, incubation
period, isoelectric
period, isometric
period, latency
period, latent
period, menstrual

period, missed
period, monthly
period, neonatal
period, patent
period, postsphygmic
period, presphygmic
period, puerperal
period, relative
  refractory
period, safe
period, silent
period, sphygmic
period, Wenckebach
periodic
periodic law
periodic table
periodicity
periodontal
periodontal abscess
periodontal disease
periodontal ligament
periodontal mucosal
  grafting
periodontal pocket
periodontia
periodontics
periodontitis
periodontium
periodontoclasia
periodontology
periodontosis
periodoscope
periomphalic
periontogenic
perionychia
perionychium
perionyx
perionyxis
perioophoritis
perioophorosalpingitis
perioothecitis
perioothecosalpingitis
perioperative
periophthalmic
perioptometry
perioral
periorbita
periorbital

periorbital hypertelorism
  correction
periorbital osteotomies
periorbital
  photoplethysmography
periorbititis
periorchitis
periorchitis,
  hemorrhagica
periosteal
periosteitis
periosteoedema
periosteoma
periosteomyelitis
periosteophyte
periosteorrhaphy
periosteosis
periosteotome
periosteotomy
periosteous
periosteum
periosteum, alveolar
periosteum externum
periosteum internum
periostitis
periostitis, albuminous
periostitis, alveolar
periostitis, dental
periostitis, diffuse
periostitis, hemorrhagic
periostoma
periostomedullitis
periostosis
periostosteitis
periostotome
periostotomy
periotic
periotic bone
periovaritis
periovular
peripachymeningitis
peripancreatitis
peripapillary
peripatetic
peripenial
periphacitis
periphakus
peripharyngeal

peripherad
peripheral
peripheral artery
  angioplasty
peripheral blood sex
  chromatin
  identification
peripheral blood smear
peripheral imaging
peripheral iridectomy
peripheral nerve
  neurofibroma
peripheral nervous system
  (PNS)
peripheral resistance
  (PR)
peripheral vascular
  arteriography
peripheral vascular
  disease (PVD)
peripheral vascular
  occlusive disease
  (PVOD)
peripheraphose
peripherocentral
peripherophose
periphery
periphlebitis
periphoria
periphrastic
periphrenitis
Periplaneta
Periplaneta americana
Periplaneta australasiae
periplasmic vesicles
periplast
peripleural
peripleuritis
peripolar
peripolesis
periporitis
periportal
periproctic
periproctitis
periprostatic
periprostatitis
peripylephlebitis
peripyloric

periradicular
perirectal
perirectitis
perirectofistulectomy
perirenal
perirhinal
perirhizoclasia
perisalpingitis
perisalpingoovaritis
perisalpinx
perisclerium
periscopic
perish
perisigmoiditis
perisinous
perisinusitis
perispermatitis
perispermatitis serosa
perisplanchnic
perisplanchnitis
perisplenic
perisplenitis
perisplenitis
  cartilaginea
perispondylic
perispondylitis
perissodactylous
peristalsis
peristalsis, mass
peristalsis, reverse
peristaltic
peristaphyline
peristasis
peristomatous
peristome
peristrumitis
peristrumous
perisynovial
perisystole
peritectomy
peritendineum
peritendinitis
peritendinitis calcarea
peritendinitis serosa
peritenon
peritenonitis
perithelioma
perithelium

perithelium, Elberth's
perithoracic
perithyroiditis
Peritinic (hematinic with
  vitamins and fecal
  softner)
peritomy
peritoneal
peritoneal cavity
peritoneal dialysis
peritoneal dialysis
  continuous ambulatory
peritoneal fluid
peritonealgia
peritonealize
peritoneocentesis
peritoneoclysis
peritoneopathy
peritoneopericardial
peritoneopexy
peritoneoplasty
peritoneoscope
peritoneoscopy
peritoneotomy
peritoneum
peritoneum, parietal
peritoneum, visceral
peritoneumectomy
peritonism
peritonitic
peritonitis
peritonitis, acute
  diffuse
peritonitis, adhesive
peritonitis, aseptic
peritonitis, benign
  paroxysmal
peritonitis, bile
peritonitis, chemical
peritonitis, chronic
peritonitis,
  circumscribed
peritonitis, deformans
peritonitis,
  diaphragmatic
peritonitis, diffuse
peritonitis, encapsulans
peritonitis, fibrocaseous

peritonitis, gas
peritonitis, generalized
peritonitis, localized
peritonitis meconium
peritonitis, pelvic
peritonitis, periodic
peritonitis, primary
peritonitis, puerperal
peritonitis, secondary
peritonitis, septic
peritonitis, serous
peritonitis, silent
peritonitis, talc
peritonitis, traumatic
peritonitis, tuberculous
peritonize
peritonsillar
peritonsillitis
peritracheal
Peritrate SA
  (pentaerythritol
  tetranitrate)
Peritricha
peritrichal
peritrichic
peritrichous
peritrochanteric
perityphlic
perityphlitis
periumbilical
periungual
periureteral
periureteritis
periurethral
periurethritis
periuterine
periuvular
perivaginal
perivaginitis
perivascular
perivasculitis
perivenous
perivertebral
perivesical
perivesiculitis
perivisceral
perivisceritis
perivitelline

perixenitis
perle
perlèche
perlingual
permanent
permanent and total
  disability (PTD)
permanent teeth
permanganate
permeability
permeability, capillary
permeable
permeation
permissible exposure
  limits
Permitil (fluphenazine
  HCl)
permutation
perniciosiform
pernicious
pernicious anemia
pernicious trend
pernio
perobrachius
perocephalus
perochirus
perocormus
perodactylia
perodactylus
peromelia
peromelus
perone
peroneal
peroneal artery bypass
  graft
peroneal sign
peroneotibial
peroneus
peronia
peropus
peroral
peroral biopsy of
  intestine
peroral biopsy of stomach
perosomus
perosplanchnia
perosseous
peroxidase

peroxidase stain
peroxide
peroxisome
perphenazine
perplication
Persa-Gel (benzoyl
  peroxide)
Persa-Gel W (benzoyl
  peroxide)
persalt
Persantine (dipyridamole)
perserveration
person
persona
personal
personality
personality, alternating
personality, antisocial
personality, borderline
personality, compulsive
personality, double
personality, dual
personality, extroverted
personality, histrionic
personality, inadequate
personality, introverted
personality, multiple
personality, neurotic
personality,
  obsessive-compulsive
personality, paranoid
personality,
  passive-aggressive
personality, psychopathic
personality, schizoid
persons in need of
  supervision (PINS)
perspiration
perspiration, insensible
perspiration, sensible
perspire
persuasion
persulfate
Perthes disease
Pertofrane (desipramine
  HCl)
pertrochanteric femoral
  fracture

perturbation
pertussis
pertussis immune globulin
pertussis vaccine
pertussoid
perversion
perversion, sexual
pervert
pervious
pes
pes abductus
pes adductus
pes anserinus
pes anserinus advancement
pes cavus
pes contortus
pes equinovalgus
pes equinovarus
pes equinus
pes gigas
pes hippocampi
pes infraorbital
pes planus
pes valgus
pes varus
pessary
pessary, cup
pessary, diaphragm
pessary, Gariel's
pessary, Hodge's
pessary, lever
pessary, Menge's
pessary, ring
pessary, stem
pessimism
pessimism, therapeutic
pest
pesticemia
pesticide
pesticide residue
pestiferous
pestilence
pestilential
pestis
pestis ambulans
pestis fulminans
pestis major
pestis minor

pestis siderans
pestis variolosa
pestle
petechiae
petechial
pethidine hydrochloride
petiole
petiolus
petiolus epiglottidis
Petit, François Pourfour
   du
Petit, Jean Louis
petit mal
Petit's canal
Petit's ligament
Petit's sinuses
Petit's triangle
Petri dish
petrifaction
petrified
petrify
pétrissage
petro occipital
petrolatoma
petrolatum
petrolatum, liquid
petrolatum, white
petroleum
petromastoid
petropharyngeus
petrosa
petrosal
petrosalpingostaphylinus
petrositis
petrosomastoid
petrosphenoid
petrosquamous
petrostaphylinus
petrous
petrous ganglion
Peutz-Jeghers syndrome
pexin
Peyer's patch
peyote
Peyronie's disease
Pfeiffer, Emil
Pfeiffer, Richard F.
Pfeiffer's bacillus

Pfeiffer's disease
Pfeiffer's phenomenon
Pfizerpen (penicillin G
  potassium)
Pfizerpen-AS (penicillin
  G procaine)
phacitis
phacoanaphylaxis
phacocele
phacocyst
phacocystectomy
phacocystitis
phacoemulsification
phacoerysis
phacofragmentation
phacoglaucoma
phacohymenitis
phacoid
phacoiditis
phacoidoscope
phacolysis
phacoma
phacomalacia
phacomatosis
phacometachoresis
phacometer
phacoplanesis
phacosclerosis
phacoscope
phacoscotasmus
phacotoxic
Phaedra complex
phage
phage typing
phagedena
phagedena, sloughing
phagedenic
phagocyte
phagocytic
phagocytic index
phagocytize
phagocytoblast
phagocytolysis
phagocytolytic
phagocytose
phagocytosis
phagocytosis, induced
phagocytosis, spontaneous

phagodynamometer
phagokaryosis
phagolysis
phagolysosome
phagomania
phagophobia
phagopyrism
phagosome
phagotherapy
phagotype
phakitis
phakolysis
phakoma
phalacrosis
phalacrotic
phalacrous
phalangeal
phalangeal cells, inner
phalangeal cells, outer
phalangeal condylectomy
phalangeal fracture
phalangeal shaft fracture
phalangectomies
phalangectomy
phalangectomy hammertoe
  operation
phalanges
phalangette
phalangette, drop
phalangitis
phalangization
phalanx
phalanx, distal
phalanx, metacarpal
phalanx, metatarsal
phalanx, middle
phalanx, proximal
phalanx, terminal
phalanx, ungual
phallalgia
phallectomy
phallic
phalliform
phallitis
phallocampsis
phallocrypsis
phallodynia
phalloid

phalloidin
phalloncus
phalloplasty
phallorrhagia
phallus
phanerogenic
phaneromania
phanerosis
phanic
phantasia
phantasm
phantasmology
phantasy
phantogeusia
phantom
phantom corpuscle
phantom limb
phantom tumor
phantom vision
phantosmia
pharmacal
pharmaceutical
pharmaceutical chemistry
pharmaceutics
pharmacist
pharmacochemistry
pharmacodiagnosis
pharmacodynamics
pharmacoendocrinology
pharmacognetics
pharmacognosy
pharmacography
pharmacokinetics
pharmacologist
pharmacology
pharmacomania
pharmacopedia
pharmacopeia
Pharmacopeia, United
   States (USP)
pharmacophilia
pharmacophobia
pharmacophore
pharmacopsychosis
pharmacotherapy
pharmacy
pharyngalgia
pharyngeal

pharyngeal bursa
pharyngeal flap operation
pharyngeal flap
   palatoplasty
pharyngeal hypophysis
pharyngeal reflex
pharyngeal tonsil
pharyngectomy
pharyngemphraxis
pharyngismus
pharyngitis
pharyngitis, acute
pharyngitis, atrophic
pharyngitis, chronic
pharyngitis, croupous
pharyngitis, diphtheritic
pharyngitis, follicular
pharyngitis, gangrenous
pharyngitis, granular
pharyngitis herpetica
pharyngitis, hypertrophic
pharyngitis, membranous
pharyngitis sicca
pharyngitis ulcerosa
pharyngo-oral
pharyngoamygdalitis
pharyngocele
pharyngoceratosis
pharyngoconjunctival
   fever, acute (APC)
pharyngodynia
pharyngoepiglottidean
pharyngoepiglottic
pharyngoesophageal repair
pharyngoespoghageal
pharyngoglossal
pharyngogram
pharyngography
pharyngokeratosis
pharyngolaryngeal
pharyngolaryngitis
pharyngolith
pharyngology
pharyngolysis
pharyngomaxillary
pharyngomycosis
pharyngonasal
pharyngopalatine

pharyngoparalysis
pharyngopathy
pharyngoperistole
pharyngoplasty
pharyngoplegia
pharyngorhinitis
pharyngorhinoscopy
pharyngorrhaphy
pharyngorrhea
pharyngoscleroma
pharyngoscope
pharyngoscopy
pharyngospasm
pharyngostenosis
pharyngotherapy
pharyngotome
pharyngotomy
pharyngotonsillitis
pharyngoxerosis
pharynx
phase
phase, continuous
phase, disperse
phasic
phatnorrhagia
Phazyme (simethicone)
Phazyme-PB (simethicone
  and phenobarbital)
phenacaine hydrochloride
phenacemide
phenacetin
phenakistoscope
phenanthrene
Phenaphen with Codeine
  (codeine phosphate and
  acetaminophen)
phenate
phenazopyridine
  hydrochloride
phencyclidine (PCP)
phencyclidine
  hydrochloride
phenelzine sulfate
Phenergan (promethazine
  HCl)
phenethicillin potassium
phenformin hydrochloride

phengophobia
phenic acid
phenindione
pheniramine maleate
phenmetrazine
  hydrochloride
phenobarbital
phenobarbital, sodium
phenocopy
phenol
phenolemia
phenology
phenolphthalein
phenolsulfonphthalein
  (PSP)
phenoluria
phenomenology
phenomenon
phenomenon, Bell's
phenopeel (skin)
phenothiazine
phenotype
phenoxybenzamine
  hydrochloride
phenozygous
phenprocoumon
phensuximide
phentermine
phentolamine
  hydrochloride
phentolamine injection
Phenurone (phenacemide)
phenyl
phenylalanine
phenylamine
phenylbutazone
phenylephrine
  hydrochloride
phenylethyl alcohol
phenylhydrazine
phenylhydrazine, Heinz
  bodies
phenylketones
phenylketonuria (PKU)
phenylmercuric acetate
phenylmercuric nitrate
phenylpropanolamine

phenylpropanolamine
  hydrochloride
phenylpyruvic acid
phenylpyruvic acid
  oligophrenia
phenylthiocarbamide (PTC)
phenylthiourea
phenytoin
phenytoin (Dilantin)
  toxicology test
pheochrome
pheochromoblast
pheochromoblastoma
pheochromocyte
pheochromocytoma
pheomelanins
pheromone
phial
Philadelphia chromosome
philiater
Phillips' Laxcaps
  (phenolphthalein and
  docusate sodium)
**Phillips' Milk of
  Magnesia** (magnesium
  hydroxide)
philoneism
philoprogenitive
philter
philtre
philtrum
phimosis
pHisoDerm
pHisoHex (hexachlorophene
  detergent cleanser)
phlebalgia
phlebangioma
phlebarteriectasia
phlebarteriodialysis
phlebectasia
phlebectasis
phlebectomy
phlebectopia
phlebemphraxis
phlebismus
phlebitis
phlebitis, adhesive
phlebitis, migrating

phlebitis nodularis
  necrotisans
phlebitis, obliterative
phlebitis, plastic
phlebitis, proliferative
phlebitis, puerperal
phlebitis, sclerosing
phlebitis, sinus
phlebitis, suppurative
phlebogoniostomy
phlebogram
phlebograph
phlebography
phleboid
phlebolite
phlebolith
phlebolithiasis
phlebology
phlebomanometer
phlebometritis
phlebomyomatosis
phlebopexy
phlebophlebostomy
phleboplasty
phleborrhagia
phleborrhaphy
phleborrhexis
phlebosclerosis
phlebostasia
phlebostasis
phlebostenosis
phlebothrombosis
phlebotome
phlebotomist
phlebotomize
Phlebotomus
Phlebotomus argentipes
Phlebotomus chinensis
Phlebotomus fever
Phlebotomus papatasil
Phlebotomus sergenti
Phlebotomus verrucarum
phlebotomy
phlegm
phlegmasia
phlegmasia alba dolens
phlegmasia, cellulitic
phlegmasia, malabarica

phlegmatic
phlegmon
phlegmonous
phlogistic
phlogogenic
phlogogenous
phlorhizin
phlyctena
phlyctenar
phlyctenoid
phlyctenosis
phlyctenula
phlyctenular
phlyctenule
phlyctenulosis
phobia
phobic
phobic desensitization
phobophobia
phocomelia
phocomelus
phonacoscope
phonacoscopy
phonal
phonasthenia
phonation
phonatory
phonautograph
phone
phoneme
phonendoscope
phonendoskiascope
phonetics
phoniatrics
phonic
phonism
phonocardiogram
phonocardiography
phonocardiography,
  carotid
phonocatheter
phonogram
phonograph
phonology
phonomania
phonomassage
phonometer
phonomyoclonus

phonomyogram
phonomyography
phonopathy
phonophobia
phonophotography
phonopsia
phonoreceptor
phonorenogram
phonoscope
phonoscopy
Phormia
phorotone
phorozoon
Phos-Flur (acidulated
  phosphate fluoride)
pHos-pHaid (urinary
  acidifier)
Phoschol
  (phosphatidylcholine)
phose
phosgene
phosphagen
phosphatase
phosphatase, acid
phosphatase, alkaline
phosphate
phosphate, acid
phosphate-bond energy
phosphate, calcium
phosphate, creatine
phosphate, normal
phosphatemia
phosphates, tubular
  reabsorption (TRP)
phosphatide
phosphatoptosis
phosphaturia
phosphene
phosphene, accommodation
phosphide
phosphite
phosphoamidase
phosphocreatine
phosphofructokinase
phosphoglucomutase
phosphogluconate
phosphokinase, creatine
  (CPK)

Phospholine Iodide
  (echothiophate iodide)
phospholipase
phospholipid
phospholipid test
phospholipids
phospholipin
phosphonerosis
phosphonuclease
phosphopenia
phosphoprotein
phosphor
phosphor, rare earth
phosphorated
phosphorescence
phosphorhidrosis
phosphoribosyltransferase
phosphoric acid
phosphoridrosis
phosphorism
phosphorolysis
phosphorous acid
phosphoruria
phosphorus (P)
phosphorus (P) test
phosphorus poisoning
phosphoryl
phosphorylase
phosphorylation
phosphuria
photalgia
photaugiaphobia
photechy
photegenic
photesthesis
photic
photic driving
photic epilepsy
photic sneezing
photism
photo-ophthalmia
photo patch test
photoactinic
photoallergic contact
  dermatitis
photoallergy
photobacterium
photobiology

photobiotic
photocatalysis
photoceptor
photochemistry
photochemotherapy (PUVA)
photochromic glass
photochromogen
photocoagulation
photodermatitis
photodynamic
photodynamic action
photodynia
photodysphoria
photoelectricity
photoelectron
photoerythema
photofluorography
photogastroscope
photogene
photogenic epilepsy
photogenous
photographic radiometer
photography
photohemotachometer
photokinetic
photokymograph
photolabile
photoluminescence
photolysis
photolyte
photolytic
photomania
photometer
photometry
photomicrograph
photomotor
photon
photonosus
photopathy
photoperceptive
photoperiod
photoperiodism
photophilic
photophobia
photophone
photophthalmia
photopia
photopic

photoplethysmography
photopsia
photopsin
photopsy
photoptarmosis
photoptometer
photoptometry
photoradiometer
photoreaction
photoreactivation
photoreception
photoreceptive
photoreceptor
photoretinitis
photoscan
photoscope
photoscopy
photosensitivity
photosensitization
photosensitizer
photostable
photosynthesis
phototaxis
phototherapy
photothermal
photothermal radiation
phototimer
phototonus
phototopia
phototoxic
phototoxis
phototrophic
phototropism
photuria
phren
phrenalgia
phrenectomy
phrenemphraxis
phrenetic
phrenic
phrenic avulsion
phrenic nerve
phrenicectomy
phreniclasia
phrenicoexeresis
phreniconeurectomy
phrenicotomy
phrenicotripsy

Phrenilin
Phrenilin with codeine
  No.3
phrenitis
phrenocolic
phrenocolopexy
phrenodynia
phrenogastric
phrenoglottic
phrenograph
phrenohepatic
phrenologist
phrenology
phrenopericarditis
phrenoplasty
phrenoplegia
phrenoptosis
phrenosin
phrenospasm
phrenosplenic
phrenotropic
phrictopathic
phronesis
phrynoderma
phthalylsulfathiazole
phthiriasis
phthiriophobia
Phthirus
Phthirus pubis
phthisic
phthisical
phthisis
phthisis, abdominal
phthisis, black
phthisis bulbi
phthisis, fibroid
phthisis, grinders'
phthisis, miner's
phthisis, pulmonary
phthisis, stonecutter's
phycobilin
phycochrome
phycocyanin
phycoerythrin
phycology
Phycomycetes
phycomycosis
phylactic

phylaxis
phyletic
phylloquinone
phylogenesis
phylogenetic
phylogeny
phylum
phyma
phymatoid
phymatorrhysin
phymatosis
physaliform
physaliphore
physaliphorous
physalis
physalliform
Physaloptera
physiatrics
physiatrist
physic
physical
physical activity and
    exercise
physical examination (PE)
physical fitness
physical medicine (PM)
physical medicine and
    rehabilitation (PMR)
physical sign
physical therapist
physical therapy (PT)
physician
physician accountability
physician, attending
physician, family
physician, primary care
physician, resident
physician shortage area
physician's assistant
    (PA)
Physicians' Desk
    Reference (PDR)
physicist
physicochemical
physics
physiochemical
physiocogenic
physiocopyrexia

physiognomy
physiognosis
physiological
physiological saline
    solution (PSS)
physiological salt
    solution (PSSA)
physiological tooth
    movement
physiologicoanatomical
physiologist
physiology
physiology, cell
physiology, comparative
physiology, general
physiology, pathologic
physiology, special
physiomedical
physiopathologic
physiotherapy
physique
physis
physocele
physocephaly
physohematometra
physohydrometra
physometra
physopyosalpinx
physostigmine salicylate
phytalbumose
phytase
phytin
phytoagglutinin
phytoalexins
phytobezoar
phytochemistry
phytocholesterol
phytogenesis
phytogenous
phytohemagglutinin (PHA)
phytohemoglutination
phytoid
phytomenadione
phytomitogen
phytonadione
phytoparasite
phytopathogenic
phytopathology

phytophagous
phytopharmacology
phytophotodermatitis
phytoplankton
phytoplasm
phytoprecipitin
phytosis
phytosterol
phytotoxic
phytotoxin
pia
pia-arachnitis
pia-arachnoid
pia mater
Piaget, Jean
pial
pian
pianists' cramp
piarachnitis
piarachnoid
pica
piceous
pick
Pick, Arnold
Pick, Friedel
Pick, Ludwig
Pick's cells
Pick's disease
pickling
pickwickian syndrome
picogram (pg)
picornaviruses
picrate
picric acid
picrocarmine
picroformal
picrotoxin
pictograph
piebald skin
piedra
piercing ear, external
  (pinna)
Pierre Robin syndrome
piesesthesia
piesimeter
piesometer
pieurodesis
piezochemistry

piezoelectricity
piezogenic pedal papules
piezometer
pigeon breast
pigeon-breeder's disease
pigeon-toed
pigment
pigment, blood
pigment, endogenous
pigment, exogenous
pigment, hematogenous
pigment, hepatogenous
pigment, respiratory
pigment, skin
pigment, urinary
pigment, uveal
pigments, bile
pigments, intradermal
  tattooing
pigmentary
pigmentation
pigmentation,
  hematogenous
pigmented
pigmenting, skin
pigmentolysin
pigmentophage
pigmentophore
pigmentum nigrum
piitis
Pik retrograde lavage
  colonoscopy
pila
pilar
pilary
pilaster
pile
pile, sentinel
pileous
piles
pileum
pileus
pili
pili annulata
pili incarnati
pili tactiles
pili torti
piliation

piliform
pilimiction
pill
pill, morning after
pillar
pillar cells
pillars, anterior, of
  fornix
pillars of Corti
pillars of diaphragm
pillars of fauces
pillet
pillion
pilobezoar
pilocarpine hydrochloride
pilocarpine nitrate
pilocystic
piloerection
pilojection
pilomatrixoma
pilomotor
pilomotor muscle
pilomotor nerve
pilomotor reflex
pilonidal
pilonidal cyst
pilonidal fistula
pilonidal sinus
pilose
pilosebaceous
pilosis
pilosity
pilous
Piltz's reflex
pilula
pilular
pilule
pilus
pilus cuniculatus
pilus incarnatus
pilus tortus
Pima Syrup (potassium
  iodide)
pimelitis
pimeloma
pimelopterygium
pimelorrhea
pimelorthopnea

pimelosis
pimeluria
pimple
pin
pin, endodontic
pin insertion
pin removal of implant
pin, self-threading
pin, Steinmann
Pinard maneuver
pincement
pinch
pinch graft, single or
  multiple
pinch meter
pindolol
pine tar
pineal
pineal body
pineal gland
pinealectomy
pinealism
pinealoblastoma
pinealocyte
pinealoma
pinealopathy
Pinel, Philippe
pineoblastoma
ping-ponging
pinguecula
pinhole
pinhole os
pinhole pupil
piniform
pink disease
pinkeye
pinna
pinna nasi
pinnal
pinocyte
pinocytosis
pinosome
Pins' sign
Pinsker operation
pint (pt)
pinta
pintid
pinus

pinworm
pioepithelium
pion therapy
pionemia
piorthopnea
Piper
piperacetazine
piperazine
piperoxan
pipet
pipette
pipobroman
Pipracil (piperacillin
  sodium)
piptonychia
piriform
Pirogoff's amputation
Pirquet's test
piscicide
pisiform
pit
pit, anal
pit, auditory
pit, costal
pit, gastric
pit, lens
pit, nasal
pit of stomach
pit, olfactory
pit, primitive
pitch
pitchblende
pith
pithecoid
pithiatic
pithiatism
pithiatric
pithiatry
pithing
pithode
Pitocin (oxytocin)
Pitres' sections
Pitressin (vasopressin)
Pitressin Tannate in Oil
  (vasopressin tannate)
pitting
pitting edema
pituicyte

pituita
pituitarism
pituitarium
pituitary
pituitary, anterior
pituitary gland
pituitary growth hormone
  (PGH)
pituitary, posterior
pituitary, whole
pituitous
pityriasis
pityriasis alba
pityriasis amiantacea
pityriasis capitis
pityriasis lichenoides,
  acute
pityriasis linguae
pityriasis nigra
pityriasis rosea
pityriasis rubra pilaris
pityriasis versicolor
pityroid
pivot
pix
placebo
placenta
placenta, abruption of
placenta, accessory
placenta accreta
placenta, adherent
placenta, annular
placenta, battledore
placenta, bidiscoidal
placenta, bilobate
placenta, bipartite
placenta, chorioallantoic
placenta, circinate
placenta, circumvallata
placenta, cirsoid
placenta, cordiform
placenta, deciduate
placenta, dimidiate
placenta, discoid
placenta, double
placenta, duplex
placenta,
  endotheliochorial

placenta,
  epitheliochorial
placenta fenestrata
placenta, fetal
placenta, fundal
placenta, hemochorial
placenta, hemoendothelial
placenta, horseshoe
placenta, incarcerated
placenta, increta
placenta, lateral
placenta, maternal
placenta, membranous
placenta, multilobate
placenta, nondeciduate
placenta percreta
placenta previa
placenta previa partialis
placenta reflexa
placenta, reniform
placenta, retained
placenta spuria
placenta, succenturiate
placenta, trilobate
placenta, tripartite
placenta, triple
placenta uterina
placenta, velamentous
placenta, villous
placenta, zonary
placental
placental estradiol
placental estriol
placental lactogen
placental pelvimetry
placental radiologic exam
placental souffle
placentation
placentitis
placentogram
placentography
placentography, indirect
placentoid
placentolysin
placentoma
placentotherapy
Placido's disk
Placidyl (ethchlorvynol)

placing reflex
placode
placode, auditory
placode, lens
placode, olfactory
placoid
pladaroma
pladarosis
plage, bite
plagiocephalic
plagiocephalism
plagiocephaly
plague
plague, ambulatory
plague, black
plague, bubonic
plague, glandular
plague, hemorrhagic
plague immunization
plague, larval
plague, murine
plague, pneumonic
plague, septicemic
plague, sylvatic
plague vaccine
plague, white
plan
plan, medical care
plan, nursing care
planaria
planchet
plane
plane, Aeby's
plane, alvecolocondylar
plane, axiolabiolingual
plane, axiomesiodistal
plane, Baer's
plane, bite
plane, coccygeal
plane, coronal
plane, datum
plane, Daubenton's
plane, Frankford
  horizontal
plane, frontal
plane, Hodge's
plane, horizontal
plane, Listing's

plane, Meckel's
plane, median
plane, midsagittal
plane, Morton's
plane, occlusal
plane of refraction
plane of regard
plane, sagittal
plane, subcostal
plane, transverse
plane, vertical
plane, visual
planes, Addison's
planes, focal
planes inclined, of
  pelvis
planes, intertubercular
planes of pelvis
planes parallel, of
  pelvis
planigram
planigraphy
planimeter
planing
planing, skin
plankton
planned parenthood
planning
planocellular
planoconcave
planoconvex
planography
planomania
Planorbis
planotopokinesia
plant
planta pedis
plantago seed
plantalgia
plantar
plantar arch
plantar digital nerve
  decompression
plantar fascia division
plantar fasciectomy
plantar fasciotomy
plantar flexion
plantar grasp reflex

plantar reflex
plantar wart
plantaris
plantation
plantation, tooth
plantigrade
planula
planum
planum, nuchal
planum, occipital
planum, orbital
planum, popliteal
planum, sternal
planum, temporal
planuria
plaque
plaque, atheromatous
plaque, bacterial
plaque, dental
plaque, Hollenhorst
plaque, mucous
plaque, penile, excision
plaque vaccine
Plaquenil Sulfate
  (hydroxychloroquine
  sulfate)
plasm
plasma
plasma, antihemophilic
  factor
plasma, blood
plasma exchange
plasma exchange therapy
plasma, fresh frozen
plasma, hyperimmune
plasma, lymph
plasma, normal human
plasma protein fraction
plasma renin activity
  (PRA)
plasma volume (PV)
plasma volume extender
Plasma-Plex (plasma
  protein fraction
  [human])
plasmablast
plasmacyte
plasmacytoma

plasmacytosis
plasmagel
plasmagene
plasmalemma
plasmapheresis
plasmasome
Plasmatein 5% (plasma
  protein fraction
  [human])
plasmatherapy
plasmatic
plasmatogamy
plasmatorrhexis
plasmic
plasmid
plasmin
plasminogen
plasminogen activator
  inhibitor number 1
  (PnAI-1)
plasmocyte
plasmocytoma
plasmodesma
plasmodesmata
plasmodial
plasmodicidal
Plasmodium
Plasmodium falciparum
Plasmodium malariae
Plasmodium ovale
Plasmodium vivax
plasmodium
plasmogamy
plasmogen
plasmology
plasmolysis
plasmolyzable
plasmolyze
plasmoma
plasmon
plasmoptysis
plasmorrhexis
plasmoschisis
plasmotomy
plasson
plastein
plaster
plaster, adhesive

plaster, blistering
plaster cast
plaster, mustard
plaster of paris
plaster, porous
plaster, resin
plaster, salicylic acid
plaster, warming
plastic
plastic bronchitis
plastic closure
plastic implant removal
  penis
plastic operation
plastic reconstruction
plastic repair
plastic revision hymen
plastic surgery
plasticity
plastid
plastogamy
plastron
plate
plate, approximation
plate, auditory
plate, axial
plate, blood
plate, bone
plate, cortical
plate, deck
plate, dental
plate, dorsal
plate, end
plate, epiphyseal
plate, equatorial
plate, floor
plate, foot
plate, medullary
plate, muscle
plate, nail avulsion
plate, neural
plate, polar
plate, removal of implant
plate, roof
plate, tarsal
plate, tarsal
  transposition
plate, tympanic

plate, ventral
plateau
plateau, ventricular
platelet
platelet concentrate
platelet count
plateletpheresis
plating
platinic
Platinol (cisplatin)
platinosis
platinous
platinum (Pt)
platybasia
platycelous
platycepalic
platycephalous
platycephaly
platycnemia
platycnemic
platycnemism
platycoria
platycoriasis
platycrania
platyglossal
platyhelminth
Platyhelminthes
platyhieric
platymeric
platymorphia
platyopia
platyopic
platypellic
platypelvic
platypnea
platypodia
platyrrhine
platysma myoides
platysmal reflex
platyspondylia
platyspondylisis
platystencephaly
play
play, psychotherapy
play, therapy
pleasure principle
pledget
plegaphonia

Plegine (phendimetrazine
  tartrate)
pleiotropia
pleiotropism
pleochroic
pleochroism
pleochromatic
pleocytosis
pleomastia
pleomazia
pleomorphic
pleomorphism
pleomorphous
pleonasm
pleonexia
pleonosteosis
pleonosteosis, Leri's
pleoptics
pleroceroid
plerosis
plesiomorphism
plesiomorphous
plesiopia
plessesthesia
plessimeter
plessor
plethora
plethoric
plethysmograph
plethysmographic
plethysmographic,
  arterial study
plethysmography
pleura
pleura cavity
pleura, costal
pleura, diaphragmatica
pleura, mediastinal
pleura, parietal
pleura, pericardiaca
pleura, phrenica
pleura pulmonalis
pleura, visceral
pleuracentesis
pleuracotomy
pleural
pleural cavity
pleural fibrosis

pleural scarification
pleural thoracentesis
pleuralgia
pleurapophysis
pleurectomy
pleurisy
pleurisy, acute
pleurisy, adhesive
pleurisy, diaphragmatic
pleurisy, dry
pleurisy, encysted
pleurisy, fibrinous
pleurisy, hemorrhagic
pleurisy, interlobar
pleurisy, plastic
pleurisy, pulmonary
pleurisy, purulent
pleurisy, sacculated
pleurisy, serofibrinous
pleurisy, serous
pleurisy, suppurative
pleurisy, tuberculous
pleurisy, typhoid
pleurisy, visceral
pleurisy, wet
pleurisy with effusion
pleuritic
pleuritis
pleuritogenous
pleurocele
pleurocentesis
pleurocetrum
pleurocholecystitis
pleuroclysis
pleurodesis
pleurodynia
pleurodynia, epidemic
pleurogenic
pleurogenous
pleurography
pleurohepatitis
pleurolith
pleurolysis
pleuromelus
pleuroparietopexy
pleuropericardial
pleuropericarditus
pleuroperitoneal

pleuroperitoneal cavity
pleuropexy
pleuropneumonia
pleuropneumonia-like
  organisms (PPLO)
pleuropneumonolysis
pleuropulmonary
pleurorrhea
pleuroscopy
pleurosoma
pleurothotonos
pleurotomy
pleurotyphoid
pleurovisceral
plexal
plexectomy
plexiform
pleximeter
plexitis
plexometer
plexor
plexus
plexus, autonomic
plexus, brachial
plexus, cavernous
plexus, celiac
plexus, cervical
plexus, choroid
plexus, enteric
plexus, lumbar
plexus, myenteric
plexus, nerve
plexus, pampiniform
plexus, prevertebral
plexus, sacral
pliability
plica
plica, circular
plica, epiglottic
plica, lacrimal
plica, palmate
plica polonica
plica, semilunar, of
  colon
plica, semilunar, of
  conjunctiva
plica, semilunar,
  synovial

plica, transverse, of
  rectum
plicamycin
plicate
plication
plicotomy
plicotomy, tympanum
plinth
ploidy
plombage
plombage, lung
plototoxin
plug
plug, Dittrich's
plug, epithelial
plug, mucous
plug, Traube's
plug, vaginal
plugger
plugger, automatic
plugger, back-action
plugger, foot
plumbic
plumbism
plumbum
Plummer-Vinson syndrome
plumose
plumper
pluriceptor
pluridyscrinia
pluriglandular
plurigravida
plurilocular
plurinuclear
pluripara
pluriparity
pluripotent
pluripotential
pluripotentiality
pluriresistant
plutomania
plutonium (Pu)
PMB 200 (Premarin and
  meprobamate)
pneocardiac reflex
pneodynamics
pneogram
pneograph

pneometer
pneopneic reflex
pneoscope
pneumarthrogram
pneumarthrography
pneumarthrosis
pneumascope
pneumatic
pneumatics
pneumatinuria
pneumatization
pneumatized
pneumatocardia
pneumatocele
pneumatocele,
  extracranial
pneumatocele,
  intracranial
pneumatodyspnea
pneumatogram
pneumatograph
pneumatology
pneumatometer
pneumatometry
pneumatorrhachis
pneumatoscope
pneumatosis
pneumatosis abdominis
pneumatosis cystoides
  intestinalis
pneumatotherapy
pneumatothorax
pneumaturia
pneumatype
pneumectomy
pneumoangiography
pneumoarthrography
pneumobulbar
pneumocardial
pneumocele
pneumocentesis
pneumocephalus
pneumocholecystitis
pneumocisternogram
pneumococcal
pneumococcal immunization
pneumococcal vacine,
  polyvalent

pneumococcemia
pneumococci
pneumococcidal
pneumococcolysis
pneumococcus
pneumocolon
pneumoconiosis
pneumocranium
Pneumocystis carinii
pneumocystis carinii
  pneumonia (PCP)
pneumocystis pneumonia
pneumocystography
pneumocystosis
pneumoderma
pneumodyamics
pneumoemphyema
pneumoencephalitis
pneumoencephalogram
pneumoencephalography
  (PEG)
pneumoenteritis
pneumofasciogram
pneumogalactocele
pneumogastric
pneumogastric nerve
pneumogastrography
pneumogram
pneumograph
pneumography
pneumography, pelvic
pneumogynecography
pneumohemia
pneumohemopericardium
pneumohemorrhagica
pneumohemothorax
pneumohydrometra
pneumohydropericardium
pneumohydrothorax
pneumohypoderma
pneumokidney
pneumolith
pneumolithiasis
pneumology
pneumolysin
pneumolysis
pneumomalacia
pneumomassage

pneumomediastinum
pneumomelanosis
pneumometer
pneumomycosis
pneumomyelography
pneumonectasia
pneumonectasis
pneumonectomy
pneumonia
pneumonia, abortive
pneumonia, acute lobar
pneumonia, alba
pneumonia, anthrax
pneumonia, apex, apical
pneumonia, aspiration
pneumonia, atypical
pneumonia, bronchial
pneumonia, caseous
pneumonia, catarrhal
pneumonia, central
pneumonia, congenital
  aspiration
pneumonia, contusion
pneumonia, croupous
pneumonia, deglutition
pneumonia, desquamative
  interstitial
pneumonia, double
pneumonia, Eaton agent
pneumonia, fibrinous
pneumonia, fibrous
pneumonia, Friedländer's
pneumonia, gangrenous
pneumonia, giant cell
pneumonia, hypostatic
pneumonia, influenza
pneumonia, interstitial
pneumonia, interstitial
  plasma cell
pneumonia, intrauterine
pneumonia, Legionella
pneumonia, lipid
pneumonia, lobar
pneumonia, migratory
pneumonia, pneumocystis
pneumonia, primary
  atypical
pneumonia, secondary

pneumonia, staphylococcal
pneumonia, streptococcal
pneumonia, terminal
pneumonia, traumatic
pneumonia, tuberculous
pneumonia, tularemic
pneumonia, typhoid
pneumonia, varicella
pneumonia, viral
pneumonia, woolsorter's
pneumonic
pneumonic, embolic
pneumonic, eosinophilic
pneumonitis
pneumonitis,
  hypersensitivity
pneumonocele
pneumonocentesis
pneumonoconiosis
pneumonograph
pneumonography
pneumonolysis
pneumonolysis,
  extrapleural
pneumonolysis,
  intrapleural
pneumonomelanosis
pneumonomycosis
pneumonopathy
pneumonoperitonitis
pneumonopexy
pneumonopleuritis
pneumonorrhaphy
pneumonosis
pneumonostomy
pneumonotherapy
pneumonotomy
pneumopathy
pneumopericardium
pneumoperitoneography
pneumoperitoneum
pneumoperitonitis
pneumopexy
pneumopleuritis
pneumopleuroparietopexy
pneumopyelography
pneumopyopericardium
pneumopyothorax

pneumoradiography
pneumoretroperitoneum
pneumorrhachis
pneumorrhagia
pneumoserothorax
pneumosilicosis
pneumotachograph
pneumotachometer
pneumotaxic
pneumotherapy
pneumothermomassage
pneumothorax
pneumothorax, artificial
pneumothorax,
  extrapleural
pneumothorax, open
pneumothorax, spontaneous
pneumothorax, tension
pneumothorax, therapeutic
pneumothorax, valvular
pneumotomy
pneumotyphus
pneumouria
Pneumovax 23
  (pneumococcal vaccine)
pneumoventricle
pneumoventriculogram
pneumoventriculography
pneusis
pneuumotoxin
pnigophobia
PNU-Imune 23
  (pneumococcal vaccine,
  polyvalent)
pock
pocket
pocket, gingival
pocket, pseudo-
pocketing
pockmarked
poculum diogenis
Pod-Ben-25 (C&M)
podagra
podalgia
podalic
podalic version
podarthritis
podedema

podencephalus
podiatrist
podiatry
podium
podobromidrosis
podocyte
pododynamometer
pododynia
podogram
podograph
podology
podophyllum
podophyllum resin
pogoniasis
pogonion
poikiloblast
poikilocyte
poikilocytosis
poikilodentosis
poikiloderma
poikiloderma atrophicans
  vasculare
poikiloderma of Civatte
poikilonymy
poikilotherm
poikilothermal
poikilothermic
poikilothermy
poikilothrombocyte
point
point, absorbent
point, auricular
point, Boas'
point, boiling
point, Broca's
point, cold rigor
point, contact
point, convergence
point, craniometric
point, critical, of gases
point, critical, of
  liquids
point, dew
point, Erb's
point, external orbital
point, far
point, fixation
point, flash

point, focal
point, freezing
point, fusion
point, Guéneau de Mussy's
point, gutta-percha
point, Halle's
point, hot
point, ice
point, isoelectric
point, isoionic
point, jugal
point, lacrimal
point, Lanz's
point, Lian's
point, malar
point, maximum occipital
point, McBurney's
point, median mandibular
point, melting
point, mental
point, metopic
point, motor
point, Munro's
point, nasal
point, near
point, occipital
point of maximal impulse
  (PMI)
point of regard
point, preauricular
point, spinal
point, subnasal
point, supra-auricular
point, supraorbital
point, thermal death
point, trigger
point, triple
point, vital
point, Voillemier's
points, Capuron's
points, cardinal
points, corresponding
points, deaf, of ear
points, disparate
points, hysterogenic
points, identical retinal
points, nodal
points, painful

points, pressure
points, principal
points, Trousseau's
  apophysiary
points, Valleix's
Point-Two (sodium
  fluoride)
pointillage
pointing
poise
Poiseuille's law
Poiseuille's space
poison
poison, cellular
poison control center
poison ivy
poison ivy dermatitis
poison oak
poison, pesticidal
poison sumac
poisoning
poisoning, arsenic
poisoning, blood
poisoning, convulsive
poisoning, corrosive
poisoning, fish
poisoning, food
poisoning, lead
poisoning, mushroom
poisoning, potato
poisoning, unknown
  substances
poisonous
poisonous plants
poker back
pokeroot
pokeroot poisoning
polar
Polaramine
  (dexchlorpheniramine
  maleate)
polarimeter
polarimetry
polariscope
polariscopy
polarity
polarization
polarizer

poldine methylsulfate
pole
pole, animal
pole, frontal
pole, occipital
pole, pelvic
pole, placental, of
  chorion
pole, temporal
pole, vegetal
poles of eye
poles of kidney
poles of testicle
policlinic
polio
polioclastic
polioencephalitis
polioencephalitis,
  anterior superior
polioencephalitis,
  hemorrhagica
polioencephalitis,
  posterior
polioencephalo-
  meningomyelitis
polioencephalomyelitis
polioencephalopathy
poliomyelencephalitis
poliomyelitis
poliomyelitis, abortive
poliomyelitis, acute
  anterior
poliomyelitis, anterior
poliomyelitis, bulbar
poliomyelitis,
  nonparalytic
poliomyelitis, paralytic
poliomyelopathy
polioplasm
poliosis
poliovirus
poliovirus vaccine,
  inactivated (IPV)
poliovirus vaccine
  inactivated (Salk type)
poliovirus vaccine, live
  oral (OPV)
polishing

Politano-Leadbetter
  operation
Politzer bag
politzerization
politzerization,
  eustachian tube
pollakiuria
pollen
pollenogenic
pollenosis
pollex
pollex extensus
pollex valgus
pollex varus
pollicization
pollinosis
pollodic
pollution
Polocaine (mepivacaine
  HCl)
polocyte
polonium (Po)
poloychondritis
poltophagy
polus
poly
Poly I:C
Poly-Histine DM Syrup
Poly-Vi-Flor
  (multivitamin and
  fluoride)
polyacid
polyadenitis
polyadenomatosis
polyadenopathy
polyadenous
polyalgesia
polyandry
polyangitis
polyarteritis (nodosa)
polyarthric
polyarthritis
polyarthritis, chronic
  villous
polyarthritis,
  rheumatica, acute
polyarticular
polyatomic

polyavitaminosis
polybasic
polyblast
polyblennia
polycarbophil
polycentric
polycheiria
polychemotherapy
polychlorinated biphenyls
  (PCBs)
polycholia
polychondritis, chronic
  atrophic relapsing
polychrest
polychromasia
polychromatic
polychromatocyte
polychromatophilia
polychromatophil(e)
polychromophilia
polychylia
Polycitra (tricitrate)
Polycitra-K (potassium
  citrate and citric
  acid)
polyclinic
polyclonal
polyclonia
polycoria
Polycose (glucose
  polymers)
polycrotic
polycrotism
polycyesis
polycystic
polycystic ovary syndrome
polycythemia
polycythemia,
  compensatory
polycythemia, myelopathic
polycythemia, primary
polycythemia, relative
polycythemia, rubra
polycythemia, rubra vera
polycythemia, secondary
polycythemia,
  splenomegalic
polycythemia vera (PV)

polycytotropic
polydactylism
polydactyly
polydentia
polydipsia
polydysplasia
polydystrophic
polydystrophy
polyemia
polyendocrine
polyendocrine deficiency
  syndromes
polyene
polyergic
polyesthesia
polyesthetic
polyestrous
polyethylene
polyethylene, glycol 400
polyethylene, glycol 4000
polygalactia
polygalacturonase
polygamy
polyganglionic
polygastria
polygen
polygenic
polyglandular
polyglycolic acid
polygnathus
polygram
polygraph
polygyny
polygyria
polyhedral
polyhemia
polyhidrosis
polyhistor
polyhybrid
polyhydramnios
polyhydric
polyhydruria
polyhypermenorrhea
polyhypomenorrhea
polyidrosis
polyinfection
polykaryocyte
polyleptic

polylysine
polymastia
polymastigote
polymath
polymazia
polymelia
polymelus
polymenia
polymenorrhea
polymer
polymer fume fever
polymerase
polymeria
polymeric
polymerid
polymerism
polymerization
polymerize
polymicrobial
polymicrobic infections
polymicrogyria
polymitus
polymorph
polymorphic
polymorphism
polymorphocellular
polymorphonuclear
polymorphonuclear
  "drumsticks" sex
  chromatin
polymorphonuclear
  leukocyte
polymorphous
polymyalgia arteritica
polymyalgia rheumatica
polymyoclonus
polymyopathy
polymyositis
polymyxin
polymyxin B
polymyxin B sulfate
polynesic
polyneural
polyneuralgia
polyneuritic
polyneuritis
polyneuritis, acute
  idiopathic

polyneuritis, Jamaica
  ginger
polyneuritis, metabolic
polyneuritis, toxic
polyneuromyositis
polyneuropathy
polyneuropathy, amyloid
polyneuropathy, buckthorn
polyneuropathy,
  erythredema
polyneuropathy, porphyric
polyneuropathy,
  progressive
  hypertrophic
polyneuroradiculitis
polynuclear
polynucleate
polynucleotidase
polynucleotide
polyodontia
polyomavirus
polyonychia
polyopia
polyopsia
polyorchidism
polyorchis
polyorchism
polyostotic
polyotia
polyovulatory
polyoxyl stearate
polyp
polyp, adenomatous
polyp, aural
polyp, bleeding
polyp, cardiac
polyp, cervical
polyp, choanal
polyp, colon
polyp, fibrinous
polyp, fleshy
polyp, gelatinous
polyp, Hopmann's
polyp, hydatid
polyp, juvenile
polyp, laryngeal
polyp, lymphoid
polyp, maxillary sinus

polyp, mucous
polyp, nasal
polyp, placental
polyp, removal
polyp, retention
polyp, sphenoid sinus
polyp, urethral
polyp, vascular
polypapilloma
polyparesis
polypathia
polypectomy
polypeptidase
polypeptide
polypeptidemia
polypeptidorrhachia
polyphagia
polyphalangism
polypharmacy
polyphenoloxidase
polyphobia
polyphrasia
polyphyletic
polyphyodont
polypiform
polyplastic
polyplegia
polyploid
polyploidy
polypnea
polypodia
polypoid
polyporous
polyposia
polyposis
polyposis, coli
polyposis, familial
polyposis, ventriculi
polypotome
polypotrite
polypsychotropia
polyptychial
polypus
polyradiculitis
polyradiculoneuropathy
polyradiculoneuritis
polyribosome
polyrrhea

polyrrhoea
polysaccharide
polysaccharides, immune
polysaccharose
polyscelia
polyscelus
polyserositis
polyserositis, familial
  paroxysmal
polysialia
polysinuitis
polysinusitis
polysomaty
polysome
polysomia
polysomnography
polysorbates
polyspermia
polyspermism
polyspermy
Polysporin Ointment
  (polymyxin B-
  bacitracin)
Polysporin Ophthalmic
  Ointment (polymyxin B-
  bacitracin)
Polysporin Powder
  (polymyxin B-
  bacitracin)
Polysporin Spray
  (polymyxin B-
  bacitracin)
polystichia
polystomatous
polystyrene
polysynaptic
polysyndactyly
polytendinitis
polytene
polyteny
polythelia
polythelism
polythiazide
polytocous
polytrichia
polytrichosis
polytrophia
polytrophy

polytropic
polyunguia
polyunsaturated
polyuria
polyvalent
polyvalent serum
polyvalent vaccine
polyvinyl alcohol
polyvinyl chloride (PVC)
polyvinylpyrrolidone
  (PVP)
pomade
pomatum
Pomeroy operation
Pompe's disease
pompholyx
pomphus
pomum
pomum, adami
Ponaris
Poncet operation
ponderal
ponderal index
Pondimin (fenfluramine
  HCl)
ponograph
ponophobia
pons
pons, cerebelli
pons hepatis
pons varolii
Ponstel (mefenamic acid)
pontic
ponticulus
pontile
pontile hemiplegia
pontile nuclei
pontine
pontobulbar
Pontocaine (tetracaine
  HCl)
Pontocaine Hydrochloride
  (tetracaine HCl)
pool
pool, abdominal
pool, gene
pool, metabolic
pool therapy

pool, vaginal
poples
popliteal
popliteal artery
popliteal arthrotomy
popliteal neurectomy
popliteal space
popliteal
  thromboendarterectomy
popliteal-tibial bypass
  graft
popliteal-tibio-peroneal
  embolectomy
popliteal-tibio-peroneal
  thrombectomy
popliteal venipuncture
popliteus
poppy
population dynamics
population of world
poradenitis
porcelain
porcelaneous
porcelanous
porcine
pore
pore, alveolar
pore, gustatory
pore, taste
porencephalia
porencephalitis
porencephalous
porencephaly
pori
poriomania
porion
pornography
porocele
porocephaliasis
porocephalosis
Porocephalus
porokeratosis
poroma
poroma, cerebral
poroma, eccrine
porosis
porosity
porotomy

porous
porphin
porphobilinogen
porphobilinogen, urinary
  test
porphyria
porphyria, acute
  intermittent
porphyria, congenital
  erythropoietic
porphyria, cutanea tarda
  hereditaria
porphyria,
  erythropoietica
porphyria, hepatica
porphyria, South African
  genetic
porphyria, variegate
porphyrin
porphyrin, urinary test
porphyrins
porphyrinuria
porphyrization
porphyruria
Porro operation
Porro's operation
port
port-wine mark, stain
porta
porta, hepatis
porta, lienis
porta, pulmonis
porta, renis
portacaval
portacaval anastomosis
portacaval shunt
Portagen (iron fortified
  powder with medium
  chain triglyceride)
portal
portal circulation
portal hypertension
portal, intestinal
portal of entry
portal system
portal vein
portio
portio dura

portio intermedia
portio vaginalis
portoenterostomy
portogram
portography
portography, portal
portography, splenic
portography, transhepatic
portosystemic
Portuguese man-of-war
porus
porus acusticus externus
porus acusticus internus
porus gustatorious
porus lactiferous
porus opticus
porus sudoriferus
position
position, anatomic
position Bonnet's
position, Bozeman's
position, Brickner
position, centric
position, decubitus
position, dorsal
position, dorsal elevated
position, dorsal
  recumbent
position, dorsosacral
position, Edebohls
position, Elliot's
position, English
position, Fowler's
position, genucubital
position, genupectoral
position, horizontal
position, horizontal
  abdominal
position, jacknife
position, knee-chest
position, knee-elbow
position, laterosemiprone
position, left lateral
  recumbent
position, lithotomy
position, Noble's
position, obstetrical
position, orthograde

position, orthopneic
position, PA
position, physiologic
  rest
position, prone
position, reclining
position, rest
position, Rose's
position, side, semiprone
position, Simon's
position, Sims'
position, Trendelenburg
position, unilateral
  recumbent
position, Walcher
positional change of
  finger
positioner
positive (pos)
positive end-expiratory
  pressure (PEEP)
positive pressure
  ventilation (PPV)
positrocephalogram
positron
positron-emission
  tomography (PET)
posological
posology
possessed
possession
possession, demoniacal
Possum (patient operated
  selector mechanism)
post mortem
post partum
postabortal
postacetabular
postadolescent
postanal
postanesthetic
postapoplectic
postauricular fistula
postauricular incision
postaxial
postbrachial
postcapillary
postcardial

postcardiotomy
postcaval
postcentral
postcibal
postclavicular
postclimacteric
postcoital
postconnubial
postconvulsive
postdiastolic
postdicrotic
postdicrotic wave
postdiphtheritic
postencephalitis
postepileptic
posterior
posterior capsular
  release
posterior central gyrus
posterior colporrhaphy
posterior compartment
  decompression leg
posterior drawer sign
posterior fossa
posterior nasal packs
posterior pituitary
  injection
posterior rhizotomy
posterior sclerotomy
posterior segment, eye
  foreign body removal
posterior synechiae
  incision
posterior talotibial
  capsulotomy
posterior tibial nerve
  decompression
posterior tibial tendon
  advancement
posterior urethra
  resection
posterior vesical neck
  wedge resection
posterior vestibuloplasty
posteroanterior (PA)
posteroexternal
posteroinferior
posterointernal

posterolateral
posteromedial
posteromedian
posteroparietal
posterosuperior
posterotemporal
postesophageal
postethmoid
postfebrile
postganglionic
postganglionic fiber
postganglionic neuron
posthemiplegic
posthemorrhagic
posthepatitic
posthetomy
posthioplasty
posthitis
posthumous
posthypnotic
posthypnotic suggestion
postictal
posticteric
postidenoidectomy
  nasopharyngeal-
  hemorrhage
postmalarial
postmature
postmaturity
postmediastinal
postmenopausal
postmortem (PM)
postmortem examination
postnasal
postnasal drip (PND)
postnatal
postnecrotic
postneuritic
postocular
postocular neuritis
postolivary
postoperative (PO)
postoperative care
postoperculum
postoral
postorbital
postpalatine
postpallium

postpaludal
postparalytic
postpartum (PP)
postpartum blues
postpartum depression
postpartum fallopian tube
  transection
postpartum hemorrhage
postpartum pituitary
  necrosis
postpartum psychosis
postpharyngeal
postpneumonic
postpoliomyelitis
  muscular atrophy (PPMA)
postprandial (PP)
postprandial blood sugar
  (PPBS)
postpubertal
postpuberty
postpubescent
postpyramidal
postpyramidal nucleus
postradiation
postsacral
postscapular
postscarlatinal
postsphygmic
postsplenic
poststenotic
postsynaptic
post-tarsal
post-term infant
post-tibial
post-tonsillectomy
  oropharyngeal
  hemorrhage
post-tranfusion syndrome
post-traumatic
post-traumatic stress
  syndrome
postulate
postural
postural drainage
postural hypotension
posture
Posture (calcium
  supplement)

posture, coiled
posture, dorsal rigid
posture, orthopnea
posture, orthotonos
posture, prone
posture, semireclining
Posture-D (calcium with
  vitamin D)
postuterine
postvaccinal
postviral fatigue
  syndrome
Potaba (aminobenzoate
  potassium)
potable
Potain's apparatus
Potain's sign
potamophobia
potash
potash, caustic
potash, sulfurated
potassemia
potassic
potassium (K)
potassium acetate
potassium alum
potassium aminosalicylate
potassium arsenite
  solution
potassium bicarbonate
potassium bitartrate
potassium bromide
potassium carbonate
potassium chlorate
potassium chloride
potassium chromate
potassium citrate
potassium cyanide
potassium gluconate
potassium
  guaiacolsulfonate
potassium hydroxide
potassium iodide
potassium nitrite
potassium permanganate
potassium phosphate,
  dibasic

potassium sodium,
  tartrate
potassium sulfate
potassium tartrate
potbelly
potency
potent
potentia coeundi
potential
potential action (AP)
potential demarcation
potential of hydrogen
  (ph)
potential resting
potentiate
potentiation
potentiometer
potion
Pott's disease
Pott's fracture
Potter-Bucky diaphragm
Potts bimalleolar ankle
  fracture
Potts-Smith shunt
pouch
pouch, abdominovesical
pouch, branchial
pouch, Broca's
pouch, Heidenhain
pouch, laryngeal
pouch of Douglas
pouch, Pavlov
pouch, pharyngeal
pouch, Prussak's
pouch, Rathke's
pouch, rectouterine
pouch, rectovesical
poudrage
poultice
pound (lb)
pound, avoirdupois
pound, troy
Poupart's ligament
poverty
poverty of thought
povidone
povidone-iodine
powder

power
pox
poxvirus
practical nurse (PN)
practice
practitioner
praecox
praevia
praevius
pragmatagnosia
pragmatamnesia
pragmatic
pragmatism
pragmatist
Prague maneuver
pralidoxime chloride
Pramegel (pramoxine HCl
  and menthol)
Pramilet FA (prenatal
  vitamin/mineral
  preparation)
Pramosone
pramoxine hydrochloride
prandial
Prantal (diphemanil
  methylsulfate)
praseodymium (Pr)
Prausnitz-Küstner
  reaction
praxinoscope
praxiology
praxis
Prayer of Maimonides
prazepam
praziquantel
prazosin hydrochloride
pre-excitation
pre-kallikrein-assay
pre-martial profile
Pre-Pen
  (benzylpenicilloyl
  polylysine)
preadmission
  certification
preagonal
prealbuminuric
preanal
preanesthesia

preanesthetic
preantiseptic
preaortic
preataxic
preauricular
preaxial
precancer
precancerous
precapillary
precava
precentral convolution
prechordal
precipitable
precipitant
precipitate
precipitation
precipitation test
precipitin
precipitin culture,
  typing
precipitin test
precipitinogen
precipitinoid
precipitophore
precipitum
preclinical
preclinical dental
  training
preclinical technique
preclival
precocious
precocity
precocity, sexual
precognition
precoital
precoma
preconscious
preconvulsive
precordia
precordial
precordialgia
precordium
precornu
precostal
precritical
precuneus
precursor
predentin

prediabetes
prediastole
prediastolic
predicrotic
prediction rules
predigestion
predisposing
predisposition
Prednicen-M (prednisone)
prednisolone
prednisone
predormition
preeclampsia
preeclamptic toxemia
  (PET)
preeruptive
preexisting condition
preferred provider
  organization (PPO)
Prefrin Liquifilm
  (phenylephrine HCl)
prefrontal
preganglionic
preganglionic fiber
preganglionic neuron
pregenital
Pregestimil (iron
  fortified protein
  hydrolysate)
pregnancy
pregnancy, abdominal
pregnancy, ampullar
pregnancy, bigeminal
pregnancy, cervical
pregnancy, cornual
pregnancy, ectopic
pregnancy, extrauterine
pregnancy, false
pregnancy, heterotopic
pregnancy, hydatid
pregnancy, interstitial
pregnancy,
  intraligamentary
pregnancy, intramural
pregnancy, mask of
pregnancy, membranous
pregnancy, mesenteric
pregnancy, molar

pregnancy, multiple
pregnancy, mural
pregnancy, ovarian
pregnancy, phantom
pregnancy, postdate
pregnancy test
pregnancy, tubal
pregnancy, tuboabdominal
pregnancy,
  tuboligamentary
pregnancy, tubo-ovarian
pregnancy, uteroabdominal
pregnane
pregnanediol
pregnanediol test
pregnanetriol
pregnant (pg)
pregnene
pregneninolone
pregnenolone
Pregnyl (chorionic
  gonadotropin)
pregravidic
prehallux
prehemiplegic
prehensile
prehension
prehormone
prehyoid
prehypophysis
preictal
preicteric
preimmunization
preinvasive
Preiser's disease
preleukemia
preload
Prelu-2 (phendimetrazine
  tartrate)
Preludin (phenmetrazine
  HCl)
premaniacal
Premarin (conjugated
  estrogens)
premature
premature arterial
  contractions (PAC)
premature beat

premature ejaculation
premature infant
premature labor
premature rupture of
  membranes (PROM)
premature ventricular
  contraction (PVC)
prematurity
premaxilla
premaxillary
premedication
premenarchal
premenstrual
premenstrual syndrome
  (PMS)
premenstrual tension
  syndrome
premenstruum
premolar
premonition
premonitory
premonocyte
premorbid
premunition
premyeloblast
premyelocyte
prenarcosis
prenares
prenatal
prenatal care
prenatal diagnosis
Prenate 90 (vitamin-
  mineral supplement)
preneoplastic
preoperative care
preoptic area
preoral
prep
prepalatal
preparalytic
preparation
Preparation H
  (hemorrhoidal ointment
  and suppositories)
prepare (prep)
prepatellar
prepatellar bursa
  excision

prepatellar bursitis
prepatent
prepatent period
preperception
preperitoneal
preplacental
prepotent
preprandial
prepuberal
prepubertal
prepubescent
prepuce
preputial
preputial adhesions lysis
preputial glands
preputiotomy
preputium
prepyloric
prerectal
prerenal
preretinal
presacral
presacral neurectomy
presacral sympathectomy
presacral tumor excision
presbyacousia
presbyacusia
presbyatrics
presbyatry
presbycardia
presbycusis
presbykousis
presbyope
presbyopia (Pr)
presbyopic
presbytiatrics
prescribing nurse
prescription (Rx)
presenile
presenium
presentation
presentation, breech
presentation, brow
presentation, cephalic
presentation, compound
presentation, face
presentation, footling
presentation, funic

presentation, funis
presentation, longitudinal
presentation, oblique
presentation, pelvic
presentation, placental
presentation, shoulder
presentation, transverse
presentation, vertex
preservative
presomite
presphenoid
presphygmic
prespinal
prespondylolisthesis
pressor
pressor base
pressor nerves
pressoreceptive
pressoreceptor
pressosensitive
pressure
pressure palsy
pressure paralysis
pressure points
pressure sore
pressure speech
pressure ulcer
pressure ventilation assist and management
pressurization
presternum
Presun 8, 15 (sunscreen)
presuppurative
presylvian fissure
presymptomatic
presynaptic
presystole
presystolic
pretarsal
preterm
pretibial
pretibial fever
pretympanic
preurethritis
prevalence
preventive
preventive dentistry

preventive medicine
preventive nursing
prevertebral
prevertebral ganglia
prevertiginous
prevesical
prevesical space abscess
  drainage
previable
Prevident (neutral sodium
  fluoride)
prevocational evaluation
prezonular
prezygotic
priapism
priapism corpora
  cavernosa
priapitis
priapus
Price-Jones red blood
  cell size
prickle cell
prickly heat
prilocaine hydrochloride
primal scene
primaquine phosphate
primary
primary bubo
primary care
primary cell
primary hemorrhage
primary lateral sclerosis
  (PLS)
primary lesion
primary nursing
primary physician
primary radiation
primary site
primary sore
primate
Primatene (theophylline
  anhydrous and ephedrine
  HCl)
Primatene Mist
  (epinephrine)
Primatene Mist Suspension
  (epinephrine
  bitartrate)

Primates
Primaxin (imipenem-
  cilastatin sodium)
prime
prime mover
Primer (Unna boot)
primidone
primigravida (grav I)
primipara
primiparity
primiparous
primitiae
primitive
primitive groove
primitive streak
primordial
primordium
primum non nocere
princeps
principal
principal fibers of the
  periodontal ligament
  (PDL)
**Principen '125' for Oral
  Suspension** (ampicillin)
Principen '250' Capsules
  (ampicillin)
Principen with Probenecid
  (ampicillin and
  probenecid)
principle
Printen and Mason
  operation
Prinzmetal's angina
prion
Priscoline HCl
  (tolazoline HCl)
prism (Pr)
prismatic
prismoid
prismoptometer
privacy
private (pv)
privileged communication
Privine (naphazoline HC)
pro re nata (prn)
proaccelerin

proaccelerin clotting
  factor V
proactinomycin
proactivator
proagglutinoid
proal
proamnion
proantithrombin
proatlas
probability
proband
probang
Pro-Banthine
  (propantheline bromide)
probationary
probationer
probe
Probec-T (vitamin B
  complex supplement)
probenecid
probing
probing lacrimal
  canaliculi
probing nasolacrimal duct
problem-oriented medical
  record (POMR)
problem-oriented record
  (POR)
procainamide
procainamide
  hydrochloride
procaine hydrochloride
Procan SR (procainamide
  HCl)
procarbazine
  hydrochloride
procarboxypeptidase
Procardia (nifedipine)
procaryote
procatarctic
procatarxis
procedure
procelous
procentriole
procephalic
Pro-Ception
procercoid
procerus muscle

process
processus
procheilon
prochlorperazine
prochondral
prochordal
procidentia
procollagen
proconvertin
proconvertin clotting
  factor VII
procreate
procreation
procreative
proctagra
proctalgia
proctatresia
proctectasia
proctectasis
proctectomy
proctenclisis
procteurynter
proctitis
proctocele
proctoclysis
Proctofoam-HC
  (hydrocortisone acetate
  and pramoxine HCl)
proctologist
proctology (proct)
proctopexy
proctoplasty
proctorrhaphy
proctoscope
proctoscopy
proctosigmoidopexy
proctosigmoidoscopy
proctostomy
proctotomy
products of conception
  (POC)
Proetz displacement
  therapy
Profasi (human chorionic
  gonadotropin)
Professional Standards
  Review Organization
  (PSRO)

Profilate Heat-Treated
  (antihemophilic
  [human], factor VIII)
Profilnine Heat-Treated
  (factor IX complex)
profundus tendon
  advancement
progeria
Progestasert
  (intrauterine
  progesterone
  contraceptive system)
progesterone
progesterone receptor
  assay
Proglycem (diazoxide)
prognathic recession
prognathism
prognosis (Px, prog)
progressive bulbar palsy
  (PBP)
progressive muscular
  atrophy (PMA)
progressive retinopathy
progressive systemic
  sclerosis (PSS)
proinsulin
prolactin hormone (PRL)
prolactin releasing-
  inhibiting factor (PIF)
prolactin RIA test
prolapse
proliferation
proliferous
prolific
Prolixin (fluphenazine
  HCl)
Prolixin Decanoate
  (fluphenazine
  decanoate)
Prolixin Enanthate
  (fluphenazine
  enanthate)
Proloid (thyroglobulin)
Proloprim (trimethoprim)
promethium (Pm)
promine
prominence

prominentia
Promod (protein
  supplement)
promonocyte
promontory
promoter
promyelocyte
pronaeus
pronate
pronation
pronator
pronator syndrome
pronaus
prone
Pronemia (hematinic
  capsules)
Pronestyl (procainamide
  HCl)
Pronestyl-SR
  (procainamide HCl)
prong
pronometer
pronucleus
pronunciation
propagation
propagative
Propagest
  (phenylpropanolamine
  HCl)
properitoneal fat
prophylactic
prophylaxis
Prophyllin
Proplex SX-T (factor IX
  complex)
Proplex T (factor IX
  complex)
propoxyphene
propoxyphene napsylate
proprapolol
proprietary
prosection
prosector
Prosobee (iron fortified
  soy protein formula)
prostaglandins (PG)
prostatalgia
prostate

prostate gland
prostate-specific antigen
  (PSA)
prostatectomy
prostatectomy perineal,
  radial
prostatectomy perineal,
  subtotal
prostatectomy retropubic,
  radial
prostatectomy retropubic,
  subtotal
prostatectomy suprapubic,
  subtotal
prostatic abscess
prostatic acid
  phosphatase (PAP)
prostatic calculus
prostatic fossa
  fulguration
prostatic fraction
prostatic panel
prostatic urethroplasty
prostatitis
prostatocystitis
prostatocystotomy
prostatolithotomy
prostatomembranous
  urethrorrhaphy
prostatotomy
prostatovesiculectomy
prosthesis
prosthetic
Prostigmin (neostigmine
  bromide)
Prostin VR Pediatric
  (alprostadil)
prostration
protactinium (Pa)
protamine
protamine paracoagulation
  product (PPP)
Protamine sulfate
**Protamine, Zinc & Iletin
  I** (protamine zinc
  insulin suspension)
protease inhibitor typing
  (PI)

protein
protein C
protein-calorie
  malnutrition
protein loss, GI
protein, quantitative
protein, total test
protein-bound iodine
  (PBI)
protein-bound thyroxine
  (PBT_4)
proteinemia
proteinuria
Protenate (plasma protein
  fraction [human])
proteolysin
proteolysis
proteolytic
proteometabolism
proteose
proteosuria
proteuria
proteus agglutinins
Proteus
Proteus mirabilis
Proteus morganii
Proteus vulgaris
prothrombin
prothrombin clotting
  factor II
prothrombin time (PT, Pro
  time)
prothrombin utilization
prothrombin-proconvertin
  (P&P)
prothrombinase
prothrombinemia
prothrombinogenic
prothrombinopenia
Protista
protobiology
protoblast
protoblastic
Proto-Chol (natural fish
  oils)
protocol
Protocort
  (hydrocortisone)

protodiastole
protoduodenum
protogaster
protoleukocyte
Protomastigida
proton
Protopam Chloride
  (pralidoxime chloride)
protoplasm
protoporphyria
protoporphyrin
Protostat (metronidazole)
prototype
Protozoa
protozoa
protozoal
protozoal disease
protozoan
protozoiasis
protozoology
protozoon
protozoophage
protraction
protractor
protriptyline
  hydrochloride
Protropin (somatrem for
  injection)
protrude
protrusion
protuberance
proud flesh
Proventil (albuterol
  sulfate)
Proventil Inhaler
  (albuterol)
Provera
  (medroxyprogesterone
  acetate)
provocative test
  (allergy)
provocative tests for
  glaucoma
Provocholine
  (methacholine chloride)
proximal
proximal gastric vagotomy

proximal interphalangeal
  (PIP)
proximate
proximoataxia
proximobuccal
proximolabial
proximolingual
prozone
Prulet (white
  phenolphthalein N.F.)
prune
prune-belly defect
pruriginous
prurigo
pruritus
Prussak's space
prussic acid
psalterium
psammoma
psammoma bodies
psammosarcoma
psammotherapy
psammous
pselaphesia
pselaphesis
psellism
psellismus
pseudarthrosis, tibia
  repair
pseudarthrosis, wrist
  arthroplasty
pseudocyesis
pseudocyst, pancreas
  external drainage
pseudoisochromatic plates
Pseudomonas
Pseudomonas aeruginosa
Pseudomonas mallei
Pseudomonas pseudomallei
pseudopod
pseudopodium
psilocin
psilocybin
psittacosis
psoas
psora
psoralen

Psorcon (diflorasone
diacetate)
psoriasis
psychedelic
psychiatric diagnostic
interview
psychiatric environmental
intervention
psychiatric preparation
of report
psychiatric procedure
narcosynthesis
psychiatrist
psychiatry (psy, psych)
psychoanalysis
psychodrama
psychological
psychology
psychometric tests
psychomotor
psychoneurosis
psychoneurotic
psychoparesis
psychopath
psychopathia
psychopathic
psychopathology
psychopathy
psychopharmacology
psychophysical
psychophysics
psychophysiologic
psychophysiology
psychosexual
psychosis
psychosomatic
psychotherapy
psychotic
psychotropic drugs
psyllium seed
pterygium
ptergoid
ptergoid process
ptergomaxillary fossa
surgery
ptilosis
ptomaine
ptosis correction

ptyalin
ptyalogogue
ptyalography
ptyalolith
ptyalolithiasis
ptyalolithotomy
puberty
pubes
pubescence
pubescent
pubetrotomy
pubic
pubic bone
pubic fracture
pubic hair
pubiotomy
public health (PH)
public relations (PR)
pubococcygeoplasty
pudenda
pudendal
pudendal nerve
pudendum
puerpera
puerperal
puerperal eclampsia
puerperalism
puerperal period
puerperal sepsis
Puestow operation
Puestow
pancreaticojejunostomy
pulley, tendon
reconstruction
Pulmocare (specialized
nutrition for pulmonary
patients)
pulmometer
pulmometry
pulmonary
pulmonary alveolar
proteinosis
pulmonary angiography
pulmonary artery
pulmonary artery
diastolic pressure
(PADP)

pulmonary artery systolic pressure (PASP)
pulmonary artery wedge pressure
pulmonary circulation
pulmonary compliance study
pulmonary decortication
pulmonary disease
pulmonary edema
pulmonary embolism
pulmonary emphysema
pulmonary function tests
pulmonary insufficiency
pulmonary intensive care unit (PICU)
pulmonary mucociliary clearance
pulmonary panel
pulmonary perfusion imaging
pulmonary peripheral vascular (PV)
pulmonary shunt
pulmonary stenosis
pulmonary stress testing
pulmonary surfactant
pulmonary valve
pulmonary valvotomy
pulmonary vein
pulmonary ventilation imaging
pulmonectomy
pulmonic
pulmonitis
pulmotor
pulp
pulpa
pulpal
pulpalgia
pulp amputation
pulp capping
pulpectomy
pulpotomy
pulsate
pulsatile
pulsation
pulse (P)

pulse, abdominal
pulse, accelerated
pulse, alternating
pulse, anacrotic
pulse, apical
pulse, asymmetrical radial
pulse, bigeminal
pulse, bounding
pulse, brachial
pulse, capillary
pulse, carotid
pulse, catadicrotic
pulse, central
pulse, collapsing
pulse, Corrigan's
pulse, coupled
pulse, deficit
pulse, dicrotic
pulse, dorsalis pedis
pulse, entoptic
pulse, febrile
pulse, femoral
pulse, filiform
pulse, formicant
pulse, full
pulse, hard
pulse, hepatic
pulse, high-tension
pulse, incident
pulse, intermediate
pulse, intermittent
pulse, irregular
pulse, jerky
pulse, jugular
pulse, Kussmaul's
pulse, long
pulse, low-tension
pulse, monocrotic
pulse, nail
pulse, paradoxical
pulse, peripheral
pulse, pistol-shot
pulse, plateau
pulse, popliteal
pulse, Quincke's
pulse, radial
pulse, rapid

pulse, regular
pulse, respiratory
pulse, Riegel's
pulse, running
pulse, senile
pulse, short
pulse, slow
pulse, soft
pulse, tense
pulse, thready
pulse, tremulous
pulse, tricrotic
pulse, trigeminal
pulse, triphammer
pulse, undulating
pulse, unequal
pulse, vagus
pulse, venous
pulse, vermicular
pulse, waterhammer
pulse, wiry
pulse generator insertion
pulse generator
  replacement
pulse pressure (PP)
pulse rate (PR)
pulse wave
pulsimeter
pulsing electromagnetic
  field (PEMF)
pulsion
pulsus
pulsus, alternans
pulsus, bigeminus
pulsus celer
pulsus differens
pulsus paradoxus
pulsus parvus et tardus
pulsus tardus
pulverulent
pulvinar
pulvinate
pulvis
pumice
pump
pump-oxygenator, for
  extracorporeal
  circulation

punch biopsy
punchdrunk
punch graft for hair
  transplant
punch operation
punch sclerectomy
punctum
punctum caecum
punctum lacrimale
punctum nasale inferius
punctum proximum (PP)
punctum remotum (PR)
puncture
puncture, cisternal
puncture, diabetic
puncture, exploratory
puncture, lumbar
puncture, Quincke's
puncture, spinal
puncture, sternal
puncture, ventricular
puncture wound
pungency
pungent
pupil
pupil, Adie's
pupil, Argyll Robertson
pupil, artificial
pupil, bounding
pupil, Bumke's
pupil, cat's-eye
pupil, cornpicker's
pupil, fixed
pupil, Hutchinson's
pupil, keyhole
pupil, Marcus Gunn
pupil, occlusion of
pupil, pinhole
pupil, stiff
pupil, tonic
pupilla
pupillary
pupillary reflex
pupillometer
pupillomotor reflex
pupilloplegia
pupilloscopy
pupillostatometer

pupillotomy
pupils equal, react to
 light and accommodation
 (PERLA)
pure
pure line
purgation
purgative
purgative, cholagogue
purgative, drastic
purgative, saline
purgative enema
purge
Purge (flavored castor
 oil)
Puri-Clens (wound
 deodorizer and
 cleanser)
purified protein
 derivative (PPD)
purine
purine-free diet
purine-low diet
purinemia
Purinethol
 (mercaptopurine)
Purkinje, Johannes E. von
Purkinje cells
Purkinje fibers
Purkinje figures
Purkinje network
Purkinje phenomenon
Purkinje-Sanson images
Purkinje vesicle
purposeful movement
purpura
purpura, allergic
purpura, anaphylactoid
purpura annularis
 telangiectodes
purpura, fibrinolytic
purpura fulminans
purpura, hemorrhagic
purpura, Henoch
purpura, idiopathic
 thrombocytopenic (ITP)
purpura nervosa

purpura,
 nonthrombocytopenic
purpura rheumatica
purpura, Schönlein-Henoch
purpura, senile
purpura simplex
purpura, thrombocytopenic
purpura, thrombotic
 thrombocytopenic
purpureaglycosides A and
 B
purse string conjunctival
 flap
purpuru
purring thrill
purulence
purulency
purulent
puruloid
pus
pus cells
push transfusion, blood
push-back operation
pustula
pustulant
pustular
pustulation
pustule
Putti-Platt
 capsulorrhaphy
putrefaction
putrefactive
putrefy
putrescence
putrescine
putrid
PUVA therapy
pyarthrosis
pycnemia
pyecchysis
pyelectasia
pyelectasis
pyelitic
pyelitis
pyelocaliectasis
pyelocutaneous fistula
pyelocutaneous fistula
 closure

pyelocystitis
pyelocystostomosis
pyelogram
pyelography
pyelolithotomy
pyelonephritis
pyelonephrosis
pyelopathy
pyeloplasty
pyeloplication
pyeloscopy
pyelostomy
pyelotomy
pyeloureterogram
pyeloureteroplasty
pyemesis
pyemia
pyemic
Pyemotes
Pyemotes ventricosus
pyencephalus
pyesis
pygal
pygalgia
pygmy
pygodidymus
pygomelus
pyknic
pyknodysostosis
pyknometer
pyknomorphous
pyknophrasia
pyknosis
pylephlebectasia
pylephlebectasis
pylephlebitis
pylethrombophlebitis
pylethrombosis
pylon
pyloralgia
pylorectomy
pyloric
pyloric antrum
pyloric canal
pyloric cap
pyloric gland
pyloric obstruction and
  dilatation

pyloric orifice
pyloric stenosis
pyloristenosis
pyloritis
pylorodiosis
pyloroduodenitis
pylorogastrectomy
pyloromyotomy
pyloroplasty
pyloroplasty and vagotomy
  (P&V)
pyloroscopy
pylorospasm
pylorostenosis
pylorostomy
pylorotomy
pylorus
pyocele
pyocelia
pyocephalus
pyochezia
Pyocidin-Otic (polymyxin
  B-hydrocortisone)
pyococcus
pyocolpocele
pyocolpos
pyoculture
pyocyanic
pyocyst
pyoderma
pyodermatitis
pyodermatosis
pyodermia
pyofecia
pyogenesis
pyogenic
pyogenic microorganisms
pyohemia
pyohemothorax
pyoid
pyolabyrinthitis
pyometra
pyometritis
pyonephritis
pyonephrolithiasis
pyonephrosis
pyoovarium

Pyopen
  (carbenicillin
  disodium)
pyopneumothorax
pyopoiesis
pyorrhagia
pyorrhea
pyosalpingitis
pyosalpingo-oophoritis
pyosalpinx
pyothorax
pyramid
pyramidal
pyramidal cell
pyramidal tract
pyrantel pamoate
pyretic
pyretic therapy
Pyridium (phenazopyridine
  HCl)
pyridoxine (vitamin B_6)
pyrogenic
pyrogens, endotoxin,
  bacterial
pyromania
pyrophosphate crystals
pyrosis
Pyrroxate
pyruvate
pyruvic acid
pyruvic transaminase,
  glutamic (SGPT)
pyuria

Q

Q angle
Q disk
Q fever
Q law
Q wave
Q-T segment
QRS complex
QRST complex
Quaalude (methaqualone

HCl)
quack
quadrangular
quadrangular lobe
quadrangular membrane
quadrant
quadrant resection of
  breast
quadrantanopia
quadrantanopsia
quadrate
quadrate lobe
quadrate lobule
quadribasic
quadriceps
quadriceps femoris
quadriceps reflex
quadricepsplasty
quadricuspid
quadridigitate
quadrigemina
quadrigeminal
quadrigeminum
quadrigeminus
quadrilateral
quadrilocular
Quadrinal (ephedrine HCl
  and phenobarbital)
quadripara
quadripartite
quadriplegia
quadripolar
quadrisect
quadrisection
quadritubercular
quadrivalent
quadruped
quadrupedal reflex
quadruplet
quale
qualimeter
qualitative
qualitative analysis
quality
quality assurance
quality of life
quanta
quanti-Pirquet

quantitative
quantitative analysis
quantity
quantity not sufficient
  (QNS)
quantivalence
quantum
quantum libet (ql)
quantum sufficit (qs)
quantum theory
quarantine
quart (qt)
quartan
quartile
quartipara
quartisect
quartz
quartz applicator
quartz glass
Quarzan (clidinium
  bromide)
quassation
quassia
Quatelet index
quater in die (q.i.d.)
quaternary
Queckenstedt's sign
quenching
quenching, fluorescence
querulent
Quervain's disease
Questran (cholestyramine
  resin)
Quibron (theophylline-
  guaifenesin)
Quibron-T (theophylline,
  anhydrous)
quick
Quick's test
quickening
quicklime
quicksilver
quiet (qt)
quinacrine hydrochloride
Quinaglute (quinidine
  gluconate)

Quinalan (quinidine
  gluconate)
Quinamm (quinine sulfate)
Quinchke's puncture
Quincke's disease
Quincke's pulse
Quine (quinine sulfate)
quinestrol
quinethazone
quingestanol acetate
quinic acid
Quinidex Extentabs
  (quinidine sulfate)
quinidine gluconate
quinidine sulfate
quinine
quinine and urea
  hydrochloride
quinine bisulfate
quinine dihydrochloride
quinine hydrochloride
quinine sulfate
quinine tannate
quininism
quinoline
quinone
Quinora (quinidine
  sulfate)
Quinquaud's disease
quinquetubercular
quinquevalent
quinquina
quinsy
quintan
quintipara
quintuplet
quotidian
quotidian fever
quotient
quotient, achievement
quotient, intelligence
quotient, respiratory

R

R&C Spray (lice control
  insecticide)
rabbetting
rabbit fever
rabbitpox
rabiate
rabic
rabicidal
rabid
rabies
rabies immune globulin
  (RIG)
rabies immunization
rabies virus group
rabiform
racemase
racemate
racemic
racemization
racemose
rachial
rachialbuminimeter
rachialgia
rachianalgesia
rachianesthesia
rachicele
rachicentesis
rachidial
rachidian
rachigraph
rachilysis
rachiocampsis
rachiocentesis
rachiodynia
rachiometer
rachiomyelitis
rachiopagus
rachiopathy
rachioplegia
rachioscoliosis
rachiotome
rachiotomy
rachis

rachischisis
rachitic
rachitis
rachitism
rachitogenic
rachitome
rachitomy
raclage
rad
radectomy
radiability
radiad
radial
radial artery
radial artery surgery
radial head arthroplasty
radial head dislocation
radial head excision
radial head fracture
radial head implant
  removal
radial head partial
  excision
radial head resection
radial head
  sequestrectomy
radial head subluxation
radial nerve
radial reflex
radial styloid tendon
  sheath incision
radial styloidectomy
radialis
radian
radiant
radiate
radiatio
radiation
radiation absorbed dose
  (RAD; rad)
radiation, acoustic
radiation, auditory
radiation, corpuscular
radiation, destruction of
  eye lesion
radiation,
  electromagnetic
radiation, heterogeneous

radiation, homogeneous
radiation, infrared
radiation, interstitial
radiation, ionizing
radiation, irritative
radiation, occipitothalamic
radiation of corpus callosum
radiation, optic
radiation, photochemical
radiation physics
radiation, pyramidal
radiation, striatomesencephalic
radiation, striatosubthalamic
radiation, striatothalamic
radiation, thalamic
radiation therapy (RT)
radiation, ultraviolet
radiation, visible
radiations, solar
radiator
radical
radical neck dissection (RND)
radices
radiciform
radicle
radicotomy
radicula
radiculalgia
radicular
radiculectomy
radiculitis
radiculoganglionitis
radiculomedullary
radiculomeningomyelitis
radiculomyelopathy
radiculoneuritis
radiculoneuropathy
radiculopathy
radiectomy
radiferous
radii

radio-cobalt B_{12} Schilling
radioactinium
radioactive
radioactive carbon (C_{14})
radioactive decay
radioactive fibrinogen
radioactive interstitial colloid therapy
radioactive intracavitary colloid therapy
radioactive iodine (RAI)
radioactive iodine uptake test (RAI)
radioactive serum iron
radioactive substance
radioactive tracer
radioactivity
radioallergosorbent test (RAST)
radioanaphylaxis
radioautogram
radioautography
radiobicipital
radiobiology
radiocalcium
radiocarbon
radiocardiogram
radiocardiography
radiocarpal
radiocarpal joint arthrotomy
radiocarpal joint dislocation
radiochemistry
radiochroism
radiochrometer
radiochromium
radiocinematograph
radiocurable
radiocystitis
radiode
radiodense
radiodermatitis
radiodiagnosis
radiodigital
radiodontia
radioecology

radioelectrocardiogram
radioelement
radioencephalogram
radioencephalography
radioepidermitis
radioepitheliitis
radiofrequency
radiofrequency
  electrophrenic
  respiration
radiofrequency neurolysis
radiogenesis
radiogenic
radiogold
radiogram
radiograph
radiographer
radiography
radiohumeral
radioimmunity
radioimmunoassay (RIA)
radioimmunodiffusion
radioimmuno-
  electrophoresis
radioiodinated GI fat
  absorption study
radioiodinated liver
  function test
radioiodinated placenta
  localization
radioiodine
radioiron
radioisotope
radiolead
radiolesion
radioligand
radiologic examination
radiologic monitoring
radiologist
radiology
radiolucency
radiolucent
radiolunar
radiolus
radiometer
radiomicrometer
radiomimetic
radiomuscular

radiomutation
radion
radionecrosis
radioneuritis
radionitrogen
radionuclide
radionuclide volume-
  dilution
radiopacity
radiopaque
radioparency
radioparent
radiopelvimetry
radiopharmaceuticals
radiophobia
radiophosphorus
radiopotassium
radiopotentiation
radiopraxis
radiopulmonography
radioreaction
radioreceptor
radioresistant
radioresponsive
radioscopy
radiosensibility
radiosensitive
radiosensitivity
radiosodium
radiostrontium
radiosulfur
radiosurgery
radiotelemetry
radiotherapeutics
radiotherapist
radiotherapy
radiothermy
radiothorium
radiotoxemia
radiotransparent
radiotropic
radioulnar arthrotomy
radioulnar joint, distal
  repair
radium (Ra)
radius
radix
radon (Rn)

raffinose
rage
ragsorters' disease
ragweed (RW)
Raillietina
*Raillietina
  demerariensis*
railway sickness
Raimiste's phenomenon
raised
raising, pedicle graft
rale
Ramadier operation
ramal
rami
rami, ventral
ramicotomy
ramification
ramify
ramisection
ramisectomy
ramitis
ramollissement
ramose
Ramstedt operation
ramulus
ramus
rancid
rancidify
randomization
range
range of motion (ROM)
ranine
Rankin operation
ranula
ranula excision
ranula marsupialization
Ranvier's nodes
rape
rape, date
rape, marital
rape, prison
rape, statutory
rapeseed
raphania
raphe
rapid eye movement (REM)
raptus

rarefaction
rarefy
rarefying osteitis
rash
rash, butterfly
rash, cable
rash, diaper
rash, ecchymotic
rash, gum
rash, heat
rash, hemorrhagic
rash, macular
rash, maculopapular
rash, mulberry
rash, nettle
rash, red
rash, rose
rash, serum
rash, sunburnlike
rash, tooth
rash, wandering
Rashkind operation
rasion
raspatory
Rastafarian cult
Rastelli repair
rasura
rat
rat-bite fever
rate
Rathke's pouch
ratio albumin/globulin
ratio galvanic/tetanus
ratio ketogenic steroids
ratio ketosteroids
ratio lecithin-
  sphingomyelin (L/S)
ration
rational
rationale
rationalization
rattle, death
raucous
Raudixin (rauwolfia
  serpentina)
Rauscher leukemia virus
Rauwiloid (alseroxylon)
rauwolfia serpentina

Rauzide (rauwolfia
  serpentina and
  bendroflumethiazide)
rave
raving
ray, alpha
Ray amputation metacarpal
ray, beta
ray, gamma
Raynaud's disease
rayon, purified
re-education
re-entry
re-exploration
reabsorb
reabsorption, tubular,
  phosphates (TRP)
reacher
react
reactant
reaction
reaction intracutaneous
  tests
reaction of degeneration
  (DR)
reaction of degeneration
  muscle
reactivate
reactivation
reactive depression
reactivity
read-only memory (ROM)
reading, lip
reagent
reagin
reaginic
realignment extensor
reality principle
reality testing
reality therapy
real-time scan
reamer
reamputation
reanastomosis
reanastomosis, surgical
reanimate
reapers' keratitis
rearrangement

reasonable charge
reattachment
rebase
rebound
recalcification
recalcification time
recanalization
recapitulation theory
receiver
receptaculum
receptaculum, chyli
receptor
receptosome
recess
recession
recessive
recessive gene
recessus
recidivation
recidivism
recidivist
recidivity
recipe
recipient
recipiomotor
reciprocal
reciprocal inhibition
reciprocation
reciprocity
Recklinghausen, Friedrich
  D. von
Recklinghausen's canals
Recklinghausen's disease
reclination
recline
Reclus' disease
recombinant DNA
recombinant TPA
recombination
Recombivax HB (hepatitis
  B vaccine
  [recombinant])
recommended daily
  allowance (RDA)
recomposition
recompression
recon
reconstruction

recontour, gingiva
record
recover
recovery
recovery room (RR)
recreational therapy (RT)
recrement
recrudescence
recrudescent
recruitment
rectal (R)
rectal alimentation
rectal anesthesia
rectal crisis
rectal feeding
rectal incontinence
rectal prolapse
rectal reflex
rectalgia
rectectomy
rectification
rectified
rectifier
rectoabdominal
rectocele
rectocele repair
rectoclysis
rectococcygeal
rectococcypexia
rectocolitis
rectocystotomy
rectolabial
rectoperineorrhaphy
rectopexy
rectophobia
rectoplasty
rectorectostomy
rectorrhaphy
rectoscope
rectoscopy
rectosigmoid
rectosigmoidectomy
rectostenosis
rectostomy
rectotomy
rectourethral
rectourethral fistula

rectourethral fistula
  closure
rectovaginal
rectovaginal fistula
rectovesical
rectovesical fistula
rectovesical fistula
  closure
rectovestibular
rectovulvar
rectum (R)
rectus
rectus muscle
recumbency
recumbent
recuperation
recurrence
recurrent dislocation
  capsulorrhaphy
recurrent femoral hernia
  repair
recurrent ganglion
  excision
recurrent ventral hernia
  repair
recurvation
recurve
red blindness
red blood cell volume
  (RBCV)
red blood cells (RBCs)
  test
red blood count (RBC)
red cell exchange
red cell sequestration
red cell survival studies
red cell survival study
red cell utilization,
  radioiron
red, Congo
red, cresol
red cross
red lead
red, methyl
red, neutral
red nucleus
red, phenol
red precipitate

red, scarlet
red, vital
redia
redifferentiation
redintegration
redirection muscle
Redisol (cyanocobalamine
  [vitamin B$_{12}$])
red-out
redox
redressement
reduce
reducible
reducing agent
reducing substances
reductant
reductase
reductase, glutathione
reduction
reduction division
reduction of fractures,
  closed
reduction of fractures,
  open
redundant
reduplicated
reduplication
Reduviidae
Reduvius
Reduvius personatus
Reed-Sternberg cells
reef
Rees-Ecker platelet count
Referon-A (interferon
  alpha-2a, recombinate)
referred pain
refine
reflection
reflector
reflex
reflex, Achilles
reflex acoustic, testing
reflex arc
reflex, Babinski's
reflex, Bainbridge
reflex, Brain's
reflex, Chaddock's
reflex, conditioned

reflex, cough
reflex, gag
reflex, Grünfelder's
reflex, Hering-Breuer
reflex, Hoffmann's
reflex, inborn
reflex, knee-jerk
reflex, Magnus-de Kleijn
reflex, Mayer's
reflex, Mendel-Bekhterev
reflex, Moro
reflex orbicularis oculi,
  testing
reflex, rooting
reflex, Rossolimo's
reflex, startle
reflex, sucking
reflex, swallowing
reflex, unconditioned
reflexogenic
reflexogenous
reflexograph
reflexology
reflexometer
reflexophil
reflexotherapy
reflux
reflux, hepatojugular
reflux, vesicoureteral
reformation, chamber of
  eye
refract
refracta dosi
refraction
refractionist
refractive
refractive power
refractivity
refractometry
refractory
refracture
refresh
refrigerant
refrigeration
refringent
Refsum's disease
refusion
refusion, spine

regainer
regel
regel kleine
regeneration
regimen
region
regional
regional blood blow study
register
registered care
  technologist (RCT)
registrant
registrar
registration
registry
Regitine (phentolamine
  mesylate)
Reglan (metoclopramide
  HCl)
Regonol (pyridostigmine
  bromide)
regression
regressive
regressive resistive
  exercise (RRE)
Regroton (chlorthalidone
  and reserpine)
Regular (Concentrated)
  Iletin II, U-500
  (insulin, purified
  pork)
Regular Iletin I (beef-
  pork insulin)
regular insulin (pork 100
  units/ml)
regular sinus rhythm
  (RSR)
regulation
regulation, menstrual
regulative
regulator
regurgitant
regurgitant index
regurgitation
rehabilitation (rehab)
rehabilitee
rehalation

Rehydralyte (oral
  electrolyte rehydration
  solution)
rehydration
Reichert's cartilage
Reid's base line
Reil's island
reimplantation
reimplantation, kidney
reimplantation, ureter(s)
  into bladder
reinfection
reinforcement
reinforcement, ocular
  implant
reinforcement, sclera
reinforcer
reinfusion
reinnervation
reinoculation
Reinsch heavy metal
  screen
reinsertion
reinsertion, ocular
  implant
reinsertion, ruptured
  biceps tendon
reinsertion, spinal
  device
reintegration
reinversion
Reissner's membrane
Reiter's syndrome
rejection
rejuvenation
rejuvenescence
relapse
relapsing fever
related living donor
  (RLD)
relative value schedule
  (RVS)
relax
relaxant
relaxation
relaxin
release
release of clubfoot

release-inhibiting
   hormone (RIH)
releasing hormone
relief
relieve
reline
Remak's axis cylinder
Remak's band
Remak's fibers
Remak's ganglion
Remak's sign
remedial
remedy
remineralization
remission
remittance
remittent
remittent fever
remobilization
remodeling
removal
ren
ren amyloidens
ren mobilis
ren unguliformis
Renacidin
renal
renal abscess
renal angiography
renal artery
renal autotransplantation
renal biopsy
renal calyx
renal clearance test
renal colic
renal corpuscle
renal cyst
renal echography
renal endoscopy
renal exploration
renal failure
renal function study
   (RFS)
renal hemodialysis
renal insufficiency
renal lymphadenectomy
renal panel
renal papillary necrosis

renal pelvis
renal pelvis aspiration
renal pelvis brush biopsy
renal pelvis catheter
   introduction
renal pelvis drainage
renal pelvis
   nephrolithotomy
renal pelvis
   ureteropyelostomy
renal scanning
renal transplant
renal transplantation
renal tubule
renal vein bypass graft
renal vessels, aberrant
   transection
renal vessels,
   repositioning
Rendu-Osler-Weber disease
Renese (polythiazide)
Renese-R (polythiazide
   and reserpine)
reniculus
renifleur
reniform
renin
renin furosemide test
renin test
renipelvic
reniportal
reniportal anastomosis
renipuncture
rennet
rennin
renninogen
renocutaneous
renogastric
renogram
renogram kidney imaging
renography
renointestinal
renopathy
renoprival
renotrophic
renotropic
Renshaw cells

Reocyl (sodium
   thiosalicylate)
reoperation strabismus
reovirus
repair
repair of peroneal tendon
repellent
repercolation
repercussion
repercussive
replacement
replacement, aortic valve
replacement, enterostomy
   tube
replacement, hearing
   device
replacement, total hip
replant, pulmonary artery
replantation
replantation, arm
replantation, digit
replantation, foot
replantation, forearm
replantation, hand
replantation, leg
replantation, thumb
repletion
replication
replicon
repolarization
reportable diseases
reposition
repositioning, aberrant
   renal vessels
repositioning, cardiac
   catheters
repositioning, orbit
repositioning,
   transvenous electrodes
repositioning, tricuspid
   valve
repositioning, ureter
repositioning, uveal
   tissue
repositor
repression
repressor
reproductive

reptilase test
repullulation
repulsion
res ipsa loquitur
rescinnamine
resect
resectable
resection
resection, annular
   ligament, elbow
resection, aortic
   subvalvular tissue
resection, bladder neck
resection, bladder tumor
resection, bowel
resection, bunion
resection, cervical rib
resection, elbow
resection, femoral head
resection, gastric
resection, head of
   phalanx, toe
resection, humeral head
resection, infundibulum
resection, intestine
   (Mikulicz)
resection, kidney
resection, lip
resection, liver
resection, long tendon of
   biceps
resection, lung
resection, myocardium
resection, nasal septum,
   submucous
resection, omentum
resection, ovary
resection, palate
resection, pelvic
   exenteration
resection, pericardium,
   partial
resection, pharyngeal
   wall
resection, radical, for
   malignant tumor, organ,
   or structure
resection, rectum, partial

resection, rib
resection, right
  ventricular
resection, scrotum
resection, small
  intestine
resection,
  sternocleidomastoid
  muscle
resection, temporal bone
resection, tongue
resection, transurethral
resection, tumor
resection, turbinate,
  submucous
resection, ulna
resection, uvea
resection, ventricular
  aneurysm
resection, vertebral body
resection, vertebral
  component, partial
resection, wedge
resection, window
resection, wrist capsule
resectoscope
resectoscopy
reserpine
reserve
reservoir
residency
resident
residual
residual functional
  capacity
residual lung capacity
  (RLC)
residual urine
residue
residuum
resilience
resilient
resin
resinoid
resinous
resistance
resolution
resolve

resolvent
resonance
resonant
resonating
resonator
resorb
resorcin
resorcinol
resorcinolphthalein
resorption
Respaire-SR
  (pseudoephedrine HCl
  and guaifenesin)
Respbid (theophylline)
respiration (R)
respiration, abdominal
respiration, accelerated
respiration, aerobic
respiration, amphoric
respiration, anaerobic
respiration, apneustic
respiration, artificial
respiration, Biot's
respiration, Cheyne-
  Stokes
respiration, cogwheel
respiration, costal
respiration, decreased
respiration,
  diaphragmatic
respiration,
  electrophrenic
respiration, external
respiration, fetal
respiration, forced
respiration, internal
respiration, interrupted
respiration, intrauterine
respiration, Kussmaul's
respiration, labored
respiration, paradoxical
respiration, periodic
respiration, placental
respiration, stertorous
respiration, stridulous
respiration, thoracic
respirator
respiratory

respiratory anemometer
respiratory arrest
respiratory distress
  syndrome (RDS)
respiratory failure
respiratory flow volume
  loop
respiratory insufficiency
respiratory myoclonus
respiratory quotient (RQ)
respiratory rate (RR)
respiratory syncytial
  virus
respiratory therapist
  (RT)
respirometer
response, anamnestic
response, conditioned
response, galvanic skin
response, immune
response, inflammatory
response, reticulocyte
response, triple
response, unconditioned
rest
restenosis
restiform
restiform body
resting pan splint
resting potential
restitutio ad integrum
restitution
restless legs
restoration
restorative
Restoril (temazepam)
restraint
restriction-fragment-
  length polymorphism
  (RFLP)
resuscitation
resuscitation, cardiac
resuscitation,
  cardiopulmonary (CPR)
resuscitator
ret
retainer
retardate

retardation
retarded (rtd)
retch
retching
rete
retention
retia
retial
reticula
reticular
reticular activating
  system (RAS)
reticular formation
reticular layer
reticulate
reticulated
reticulation
reticulin
reticulocyte
reticulocyte count
reticulocytopenia
reticulocytosis
reticuloendothelial
reticuloendothelioma
reticuloendotheliosis
reticuloendothelium
reticulohistiocytoma
reticulohistiocytosis
reticuloid
reticuloma
reticulopenia
reticulosarcoma
reticulosis
reticulum
retiform
Retin-A (tretinoin)
retina
retinaculum
retinaculum,
  transposition
retinal
retinal detachment
retine
retinene
retinitis
retinoblastoma
retinochoriditis
retinochoroid

retinocystoma
retinodialysis
retinoid
retinol
retinopapillitis
retinopathy
retinoschisis
retinoscope
retinosis
retisolution
retispersion
retoperithelium
retort
retothelium
retract
retractile
retraction
retractor
retrad
retreat
retrenchment
retrieval
retroaction
retroauricular
retrobucall
retrobulbar
retrobulbar injection
retrocaval ureterolysis
retrocecal
retrocedent
retrocervical
retroclusion
retrocolic
retrocollic
retrocollis
retrocursive
retrodeviation
retrodisplacement
retroesophageal
retrofilling
retroflexed
retroflexion
retrogasserian
retrognathia
retrognathism
retrograde pyelogram
  (RPG)
retrograde pyelography

retrography
retrogression
retroinfection
retroinsular
retroiridian
retrojection
retrolabyrinthine
retrolental fibroplasia
  (RLF)
retrolenticular
retrolingual
retromammary
retromandibular
retromastoid
retronasal
retroocular
retroparotid
retroperitoneal
retroperitoneal abscess
  drainage
retroperitoneal
  echography
retroperitoneal
  exploration
retroperitoneal
  lymphadenectomy
retroperitoneal mass
  biopsy
retroperitoneal tumor
  destruction
retroperitoneal tumor
  excision
retroperitoneal
  ureterolysis
retroperitoneum
retropharyngeal
retropharyngeal abscess
  drainage
retropharyngitis
retropharynx
retroplacental
retroplasia
retroposed
retroposition
retropubic prostatectomy
retropulsion
retrorectal abscess
  drainage

retrospective
retrospondylolisthesis
retrosternal
retrotarsal
retrouterine
retroversioflexion
retroversion
Retrovir (zidovudine)
retroviruses
retrude
retrusion
Retzius, lines of
Retzius, space of
Retzius, veins of
reunient
Reuss, August R. von
revaccination
revascularization
revellent
reverberation
Reverdin's needle
reversal
reverse transcriptase
  (RT)
reversible
reversion
revertant
review of systems (ROS)
revision, cleft palate
revision, colostomy
revision, enterostomy
  tube
revision, fenestration
revision, frenum
  (frenoplasty)
revision, gastroduodenal
  anastomosis
revision, gastrojejunal
  anastomosis
revision, hymen
revision, ileostomy
revision, mastoidectomy
revision, neurostimulator
  electrodes
revision, orbital implant
revision,
  orbitocraniofacial
  reconstruction

revision, rhinoplasty
revision, shunt
revision, tympanoplasty
revivescence
revivification
revolutions per minute
  (rpm)
revulsant
revulsion
revulsive
Reye's syndrome
Rh antibody titer
Rhabditis
rhabdoid
rhabdomyoblastoma
rhabdomyolysis
rhabdomyoma
rhabdomyosarcoma
rhabdophobia
rhabdosarcoma
rhabdovirus
rhachiocampsis
rhachioplegia
rhachioscoliosis
rhachitis
rhacoma
rhagades
rhagadiform
rhaphania
rhegma
rhegmatogenous
rhenium
rheobase
rheobasic
rheology
rheometer
rheostat
rheostosis
rheotachygraphy
rheotaxis
rheotropism
Rhesus factor (Rh)
Rhesus factor negative
  (Rh neg)
Rhesus factor positive
  (Rh pos)
rheum
rheuma

rheumatic
rheumatic fever (RF)
rheumatic heart disease
  (RHD)
rheumatid
rheumatism
rheumatismal
rheumatoid
rheumatoid arthritis
rheumatoid arthritis
  factor (RAF)
rheumatoid factor (RF)
rheumatoid factor (RF,RA)
  test
rheumatologist
rheumatology
rhexis
rhigosis
rhinal
rhinalgia
rhinectomy
rhinedema
rhinencephalon
rhinencephalus
rhinesthesia
rhineurynter
rhinion
rhinism
rhinitis, acute
rhinitis, allergic
rhinitis, atrophic
rhinitis, caseosa
rhinitis, chronic
  hyperplastic
rhinitis, chronic
  hypertrophic
rhinitis, fibrinous
rhinitis, hypertrophic
rhinitis, membranous
rhinitis, perennial
rhinitis, periodic
rhinitis,
  pseudomembranous
rhinitis, purulent
rhinitis, vasomotor
rhinoanemometer
rhinoantritis
rhinobyon

rhinocanthectomy
rhinocele
rhinocephalus
rhinocephaly
rhinocheiloplasty
rhinocleisis
rhinodacryolith
rhinodynia
Rhinoestrus
Rhinoestrus purpureus
rhinogenous
rhinokyphosis
rhinolalia
rhinolalia aperta
rhinolalia clausa
rhinolaryngitis
rhinolith
rhinolithiasis
rhinologist
rhinology
rhinomanometer
rhinomanometry
rhinometer
rhinomiosis
rhinommectomy
rhinomycosis
rhinonecrosis
rhinopathy
rhinopharyngeal
rhinopharyngitis
rhinopharyngocele
rhinopharyngolith
rhinopharynx
rhinophonia
rhinophycomycosis
rhinophyma
rhinoplasty
rhinopneumonitis
rhinopolypus
rhinorrhagia
rhinorrhaphy
rhinorrhea
rhinorrhea, cerebrospinal
rhinorrhea, gustatory
rhinosalpingitis
rhinoscleroma
rhinoscope
rhinoscopic

rhinoscopy
rhinoseptoplasty
rhinosporidiosis
Rhinosporidium
Rhinosporidium seeberi
rhinostenosis
rhinotomy
rhinotracheitis
rhinovaccination
rhinovirus
Rhipicephalus
Rhipicephalus sanguineus
rhitidectomy
rhitidosis
rhizodontropy
rhizodontrypy
rhizoid
rhizome
rhizomelic
rhizomeningomyelitis
Rhizopoda
rhizotomy
rhizotomy, anterior
rhizotomy, posterior
rhodium (Rh)
rhodogenesis
rhodophane
rhodophylaxis
rhodopsin
RhoGAM (Rh$_o$(D) immune globulin [human])
rhombencephalon
rhombocele
rhomboid
rhomboid fossa
rhomboideus
rhombomere
rhoncal
rhonchi
rhonchus
rhoncial
rhopheocytosis
rhotacism
rhubarb
Rhus Tox Antigen (poison ivy extract)
rhypophobia

rhythmic
rhythmicity
rhytid dermabrasion
rhytidectomy
rhytidoplasty
rhytidosis
rib
ribbon
riboflavin (vitamin B$_2$)
ribonuclease (RNase)
ribonucleic acid (RNA)
ribonucleoprotein
ribonucleotide
ribose
ribosome
ribosyl
rice, polished
Richardson operation
Richardson urethral meatoplasty
ricin
ricinine
ricinoleic acid
rickettsia
Rickettsia
rickettsialpox
rickettsicidal
rickettsiosis
rickettsiostatic
Rid (lice control spray)
Ridaura (auranofin)
riders' bone
ridge
ridgel
Riedel's lobe
Rifadin (rifampin)
Rifamate (rifampin and isoniazid)
rifampin
rifamycin
Riga-Fede's disease
Riggs' disease
right (rt)
right arm (RA)
right bundle branch block (RBBB)
right ear, AD (auris dextra)

right eye, OD (oculus dexter)
right lateral (rt lat)
right leg (RL)
right lower lobe (RLL)
right lower quadrant (RLQ)
right occiputs posterior (ROP)
right occiputs transverse (ROT)
right posterior oblique (RPO)
right to know law
right upper lobe (RUL)
right upper quadrant (RUQ)
right-handedness
rigid
rigidity
rigor
rigor mortis
rim
rima
Rimactane (rifampin)
rimose
Rimso-50 (dimethyl sulfoxide)
rimula
rind
Ringer, Sydney
ringworm
Rinkel test
Rinne test
Riolan's arch
Riolan's bouquet
Riolan's muscle
Riopan (magaldrate)
Riopan Plus (magaldrate and simethicone)
ripa
ripening
Ripstein operation
risk factors
risk-benefit analysis
risorius
ristocetin
risus

Ritalin (methylphenidate HCl)
Ritgen maneuver
Ritter's disease
ritual
ritualistic surgery
rivalry
Rivinus' canals
Rivinus' gland
Rivinus' incisure
Rivinus' ligament
rivus lacrimalis
riziform
RMS Suppositories (rectal morphine sulfate)
Robaxin (methocarbamol)
Robaxisal (methocarbamol and aspirin)
Robert's pelvis
Robertson's pupil
Robitussin
Robitussin-CF
Robitussin-DAC
Robitussin-DM
Robitussin-PED
Rocaltrol (calcitriol)
Rocephin (ceftriaxone sodium)
Rochelle salt
rocker knife
Rocky Mountain Spotted Fever (RMSF)
rodent
rodent ulcer
rodenticide
Rodney Smith operation
rodonalgia
rods and cones
roentgen (per) hour (at one) meter (rhm)
roentgen (R)
roentgen unit (RU)
roentgenography
Roentgen, Wilhelm Konrad
roentgenkymogram
roentgenkymograph
roentgenkymography
roentgenocinematography

roentgenogram
roentgenography
roentgenologist
roentgenology
roentgenometer
roentgenoscope
roentgenoscopy
roentgenotherapy
roeteln
roetheln
Roger's disease
Rokitansky's disease
rol Cream
Rolando's area
Rolando's fissure
role
role model
role playing
rolfing
rolitetracycline
roll
roll over protection
  structures (ROPS)
roller
rolling of conjunctiva
Roma-nol (iodine
  solution)
roman numerals
romanopexy
romanoscope
Romberg's sign
rombergism
Rondec Oral Drops
Rondec Syrup
Rondec Tablet
Rondec-DM Oral Drops
Rondec-DM Syrup
Rondec-TR Tablet
Rondomycin (methacycline
  HCl)
rongeur
ronula fistulization
roof nucleus
rooming-in
root
root angiography,
  coronary
root, aortography

root, apicoectomy
root, arteries
root, canal
root, irrigation
root, nerve,
  decompression
root, resection (tooth)
root, residual or
  retained
root resorption of teeth
root sheath
root zone
rooting reflex
Rorschach test
rosa
rosacea
rosaniline
rosary
rose bengal sodium I
  131
rose bengal test
rose fever
Rose, Frank A.
rose water
Rose's position
Rosenbach, Ottomar
Rosenmüller, Johann
  Christian
roseola
roseolous
rosette
rosin
Ross SLD (surgical liquid
  diet)
Ross' bodies
Rossolimo's reflex
rostellum
rostral
rostrate
rostriform
rostrum
rot, jungle
rotameter
rotate
rotating tourniquet
rotation
rotation, adjacent tissue
rotation of fetal head

rotational correction
  osteotomy
rotator
rotaviruses
röteln
rotenone
Roth's spots
rötheln
rotoextractor removal of
  vitreous
rotoxamine tartrate
Rouget's cells
rough
roughage
rouleau
round ligament
round window
roundworm
Roux-en-Y
Roux-en-Y anastomosis
Roux-en-Y operation
Roux-Goldthwait operation
Roux-Herzen-Judine
  operation
Roven's IMDC
Roxanol (morphine
  sulfate)
Roxicet (oxycodone and
  acetaminophen)
Roxicodon (oxycodone HCl)
Royal Free disease
rub
rub, pericardial
rub, pleural friction
rubber dam
rubefacient
rubella
rubella test
rubella titer
rubella virus vaccine,
  live
rubeola
rubeosis iridis
ruber
rubescent
rubidium (Rb)
rubigo
Rubin's test

Rubner's test
rubor
rubriblast
rubric
rubricyte
rubrospinal
rubrothalamic
rubrum
rubrum scarlatinum
ructus
rudiment
rudimentary
rudimentum
Rufen (ibuprofen)
Ruffini's corpuscles
rufous
ruga
rugae of vagina
Ruggeri's reflex
rugine
rugose
rugosity
rugous
Ruiz-Mora hammertoe
  operation
rule of nines
rum fits
Rum-K (potassium
  chloride)
ruminant
rumination
rump
Rumpf's symptom
run
runaround
runners' high
runround
rupia
rupioid
rupophobia
rupture
rupture of membranes
  (ROM)
rush
Russell bodies
Russell's viper venom
Russian bath
Rust's disease

rusts
rusty
rut
rut-formation
ruthenium (Ru)
rutherford
rutidosis
rutilism
rutin
rye
Rynatuss (antitussive
  /antihistamine
    /decongestant
    /bronchodilator)
rytidosis

S

SAAVE (nutritional
  supplement)
saber shin
Sabin vaccine
sabulous
saburra
sac
sac, air
sac, allantoic
sac, alveolar
sac, amniotic
sac, chorionic
sac, conjunctival
sac, dental
sac, endolymphatic
sac, heart
sac, hernial
sac, lacrimal
sac, lesser peritoneal
sac, vitelline
sac, yolk
saccades
saccadic
saccate
saccharase
saccharated
saccharic acid

saccharide
sacchariferous
saccharification
saccharin
saccharine
saccharogalactorrhea
saccharolytic
Saccharomyces
saccharomycosis
saccharorrhea
saccharose
saccharosuria
saccharum
sacciform
Saccomanno technique
saccular
sacculated
sacculation
saccule
sacculocochlear
sacculotomy
sacculus
saccus
saccus endolymphaticus
saccus lacrimalis
sacrad
sacral
sacral bone
sacral canal
sacral flexure
sacral index
sacral nerve
sacral nerves
sacral pressure ulcer
sacral spine
sacral vertebra
sacralgia
sacralization
sacrectomy
sacroadenoma
sacroanterior
sacrococcygeal
sacrococcygeal tumor
sacrococcygeus
sacrocoxalgia
sacrocoxitis
sacrodynia
sacroiliac

sacroiliac joint
sacroilitis
sacrolisthesis
sacrolumbar
sacroposterior
sacrosciatic
sacrospinal
sacrospinalis
sacrospinous ligament
　fixation
sacrotomy
sacrouterine
sacrovertebral
sacrum
sactosalpinx
saddle
saddle back
saddle block anesthesia
saddle joint
saddle nose
sadism
sadist
sadness
sadomasochism
sadomasochist
Saemisch corneal section
Saemisch's ulcer
safe sex
Safe Suds (hypo-
　allergenic detergent)
safelight
sagittal
sagittal plane
sagittal sinus
sagittal sulcus
sagittal suture
sagittalis
sago
Saint Vitus' dance
sal
sal ammoniac
sal soda
salaam convulsion
salabrasion
Salac (salicylic acid in
　a surfactant blend)
salacious
Salactic

Salflex (salsalate)
salicylamide
salicylanilide
salicylate
salicylate, methyl
salicylate, sodium
salicylate poisoning
salicylate toxicology
　test
salicylated
salicylazosulfapyridine
salicylic acid (SA)
salicylism
salicylsulfonic acid test
salicyluric acid
salifiable
salify
salimeter
saline
saline cathartic
saline enema
saline, hypertonic
saline, hypotonic
saline infusion test
saline load test, gastric
saline solution
Salinex (isotonic sodium
　chloride solution)
salinometer
saliva
saliva, artificial
salivant
salivary
salivary corpuscles
salivary cyst
salivary digestion
salivary fistula
salivary glands
salivation
salivatory
salivolithiasis
Salk vaccine
sallow
salmin
salmine
salmon patch
Salmonella
Salmonella choleraesuis

Salmonella enteritidis
Salmonella paratyphi
Salmonella schottmülleri
Salmonella typhi
Salmonella typhimurium
salmonellosis
salpingectomy
salpingemphraxis
salpingian
salpingion
salpingitis
salpingitis, eustachian
salpingitis, gonococcal
salpingocatheterism
salpingocele
salpingocyesis
salpingography
salpingolithiasis
salpingolysis
salpingoneostomy
salpingo-oophorectomy
  (SO)
salpingo-oophoritis
salpingo-oophorocele
salpingo-oophorostomy
salpingo-oophoroplasty
salpingo-oophororrhaphy
salpingo-oophorotomy
salpingo-oothecitis
salpingo-oothecocele
salpingo-ovariectomy
salpingoperitonitis
salpingopexy
salpingopharyngeal
salpingopharyngeus
salpingoplasty
salpingorrhaphy
salpingosalpingostomy
salpingoscope
salpingostenochoria
salpingostomatomy
salpingostomy
salpingotomy
salpingo-ureterostomy
salpingo-uterostomy
salpingysterocyesis
salt
salt, acid

salt, basic
salt, bile
salt, buffer
salt, double
salt, epsom
salt, Glauber's
salt, haloid
salt, iodized
salt, neutral
salt, Rochelle
salt, rock
salt, smelling
saltation
saltatory
saltatory conduction
saltatory spasm
Salter osteotomy
salt-free diet
salt glow
salting out
salt-losing syndrome
saltpeter
saltpetre
salt-poor diet
salt solution, normal
salt solution,
  physiological
salubrious
saluresis
saluretic
Saluron
  (hydroflumethiazide)
salutary
Salutensin
  (hydroflumethiazide and
  reserpine)
Salvarsan
salve
Samaritans
samarium (Sm)
sample
sample, biased
sampling
sampling, random
sanative
sanatorium
sanatory
sand

sand, auditory
sand, brain
sandflies
sandfly fever
Sandhoff's disease
Sandimmune (cyclosporine)
sandpapering (skin)
Sandril (reserpine)
Sandsert (methysergide maleate)
Sandwith's bald tongue
sane
Sanfilippo's disease
Sang-Park septostomy
sanguicolous
sanguifacient
sanguiferous
sanguification
sanguimotor
sanguimotory
sanguine
sanguineous
sanguinolent
sanguinopoietic
sanguinopurulent
sanguinous
sanguirenal
sanguis
sanguisuga
sanguivorous
sanies
saniopurulent
sanioserous
sanitarian
sanitarium
sanitary
sanitary napkin
sanitation
sanitization
sanitize
sanitizer
sanity
San Joaquin valley fever
SA node
Sanorex (mazindol)
Sansert (methysergide maleate)
santonin

Santyl (collagenase)
sap
sap, cell
sap, nuclear
saphena
saphenectomy
saphenous
saphenous nerve
saphenous opening
saphenous veins
sapid
sapo
saponaceous
saponatus
saponification
saponification number
saponify
saponin
sapophore
saporific
sapphism
saprobes
saprogen
saprogenic
saprophilous
saprophyte
saprophytic
saprozoic
Sarapin (*Sarracenia purpurea*, pitcher plant)
sarapus
Sarcina
sarcina
sarcitis
sarcoadenoma
sarcobiont
sarcoblast
sarcocarcinoma
sarcocele
sarcocyst
Sarcocystis
Sarcocystis lindemanni
Sarcodina
sarcogenic
sarcoid
sarcoid, Boeck's
sarcoidosis

sarcolemma
sarcology
sarcolysis
sarcolytic
sarcoma
sarcoma, alveolar soft part
sarcoma, botryoid
sarcoma, chondro-
sarcoma, endometrial
sarcoma, Ewing's
sarcoma, fibro-
sarcoma, giant cell
sarcoma, Kaposi's
sarcoma, lipo-
sarcoma, lymphangio-
sarcoma, myeloid
sarcoma, myxo-
sarcoma, osteogenic
sarcoma, reticulum cell
sarcoma, rhabdomyo-
sarcoma, spindle cell
sarcomatoid
sarcomatosis
sarcomatous
sarcomere
sarcomphalocele
sarcomyces
Sarcophagidae
sarcophagy
sarcoplasm
sarcoplasmic
sarcopoietic
Sarcoptes
Sarcoptidae
sarcosis
sarcosome
Sarcosporidia
sarcosporidiosis
sarcostosis
sarcostyle
sarcotic
sarcotubules
sarcous
sardonic laugh
sarin (GB)
sartorius
SAS-500 (sulfasalazine)

satellite
satellite, bacterial
satellite cells
satellitosis
satiety
saturated
saturated compound
saturated hydrocarbon
saturated solution
saturation
saturation index
saturation, oxygen
saturation time
Saturday night paralysis
saturnine
saturnine breath
saturnine gout
saturnism
satyriasis
satyromania
saucerization
Sauer-Bacon operation
sauna
savory
saw
saxifragant
saxitoxin
Sayre's jacket
scab
Scabene Lotion (lindane)
Scabene Shampoo (lindane)
scabicide
scabies
scabies, Norwegian
scabietic
scabieticide
scabiphobia
scabrities
scabrities, unguium
scala
scala, media
scala, tympani
scala, vestibuli
scald
scalded skin syndrome
scale
scale, absolute
scale, Baumé

scale, Celsius
scale, centigrade
scale, Fahrenheit
scale, French
scale, Kelvin
scale of contrast
scalene
scalene fat pad
scalene tubercle
scalenectomy
scaleniotomy
scalenotomy
scalenus
scalenus anticus repair
scalenus syndrome
scaler
scaling
scaling and polishing,
  dental
scall
scalp
scalpel
scalpriform
scalprum
scalp tourniquet
scalp vein
scaly
scan
scan, abdomen
scan, adrenal
scan, amniotic fluid
scan, bone
scan, bone marrow
scan, bowel
scan, brain
scan, cardiac output
scan, cardiovascular
scan, CAT (computerized
  axial tomography)
scan, cerebral
scan, circulation time
scan, CT (computerized
  tomography)
scan, eye
scan, gallium
scan, gastrointestinal
scan, head
scan, hematopoietic

scan, intestine
scan, iodine-131
scan, kidney
scan, liver
scan, lung
scan, lymphatic system
scan, myocardial
  infarction
scan, pancreatic
scan, parathyroid
scan, pituitary
scan, placenta
scan, protein-bound
  iodine
scan, radio-iodine uptake
scan, radioisotope
scan, renal
scan, skeletal
scan, spleen
scan, thermal
scan, thorax
scan, thyroid
scan, total body
scan, uterus
scandium (Sc)
scanning
scanning electron
  microscope (SEM)
scanning, radioisotope
scanning speech
scanogram
scanty
Scanzoni maneuver
scapha
scaphocephalic
scaphocephalism
scaphocephalous
scaphocephaly
scaphohydrocephaly
scaphoid
scaphoid bone
scaphoid fossa
scaphoiditis
scapula
scapula, winged
scapulalgia
scapular
scapular reflex

scapulary
scapulectomy
scapuloclavicular
scapulodynia
scapulohumeral
scapulohumeral reflex
scapulopexy
scapulothoracic
scapus
scapus penis
scapus pili
scar
scar, cicatricial
scar, keloid
scar, painful
scarabiasis
scarification
scarification,
   conjunctiva
scarification, nasal
   veins
scarification, pleura
scarification,
   pericardium
scarificator
scarifier
scarlatina
scarlatina anginosa
scarlatina hemorrhagica
scarlatina maligna
scarlatinal
scarlatinella
scarlatiniform
scarlatinoid
scarlet fever (SF)
scarlet rash
scarlet red
Scarpa's fascia
Scarpa's fluid
Scarpa's foramina
Scarpa's ganglion
Scarpa's membrane
Scarpa's triangle
scatemia
scatologic
scatology
scatoma
scatophagy

scatoscopy
scatter
scatter, back-
scattered radiation
scattergram
scavenger cell
scent
Schafer's method of
   artificial respiration
Schäffer's reflex
Schanz operation
Schatzki ring
Schauta hysterectomy
Schede thoracoplasty
Scheie's syndrome
schema
schematic
scheroma
Schick test
Schick test control
Schilder's disease
Schiller's test
Schilling's
   classification
Schilling test
schindylesis
Schirmer's test
schistocelia
schistocephalus
schistocormia
schistocystis
schistocyte
schistocytosis
schistoglossia
schistomelus
schistoprosopia
schistorachis
Schistosoma
Schistosoma haematobium
Schistosoma japonicum
Schistosoma mansoni
schistosome dermatitis
schistosomia
schistosomiasis
schistosomicide
schistosternia
schistothorax
schistotrachelus

schizamnion
schizaxon
schizencephaly
schizoblepharia
schizocyte
schizocytosis
schizogenesis
schizogony
schizogyria
schizoid
schizoid personality
  disorder
schizomycete
Schizomycetes
schizont
schizonticide
schizonychia
schizophasia
schizophrenia (schiz)
schizophrenia, catatonic
schizophrenia,
  disorganized
schizophrenia, paranoid
schizophrenia,
  undifferentiated
schizophrenic
schizoprosopia
schizotonia
schizotrichia
schizozoite
Schlatter operation
Schlatter-Osgood disease
Schlemm, canal of
Schmorl's disease
Schmorl's nodules
schneiderian membrane
Schönlein's disease
Schönlein-Henoch purpura
school phobia
Schroeder operation
Schuchardt operation
Schüffner's dots
Schüller's disease
Schultz reaction
Schultze's bundle
Schultze's cells
Schultze's granule masses
Schwabach test

Schwalbe's ring
Schwann's cells
Schwann's sheath
Schwann's white substance
schwannoma
schwannosis
sciage
sciatic
sciatica
sciatic nerve
science
science's, life
scieropia
scintigram
scintigraphy
scintillascope
scintillation
scintiphotography
scintiscan
scintiscanner
scirrhoid
scirrhoma
scirrhosarca
scirrhous
scirrhus
scission
scissor gait
scissor leg
scissors
scissura
sclera
sclera, blue
sclera reinforcement
scleradenitis
scleral
scleral buckling
scleral laceration
scleral shell
scleral trephination with
  iridectomy
scleratogenous
sclerectasia
sclerectoiridectomy
sclerectoiridodialysis
sclerectomy
sclerectomy, for retinal
  reattachment
sclerectomy, Holth's

sclerectomy, trephine
sclerectomy, with implant
scleredema
scleredema adultorum
scleredema, Buschke's
scleredema neonatorum
sclerema
sclerema adiposum
sclerema adultorum
sclerema neonatorum
sclerencephalia
scleriasis
scleriritomy
scleritis
scleritis, annular
scleritis, anterior
scleritis, posterior
scleroblastema
scleroblastemic
sclerocataracta
sclerochoroiditis
sclerochoroiditis,
  posterior
scleroconjunctival
sclerocornea
sclerodactylia
scleroderma
scleroderma,
  circumscribed
scleroderma neonatorum
sclerodermatitis
sclerodermatous
sclerogenic
sclerogenous
scleroid
scleroiritis
sclerokeratitis
sclerokeratoiritis
sclerokeratosis
scleroma
scleromalacia
scleromalacia perforans
Scleromate (morrhuate
  sodium)
scleromere
scleromyxedema
scleronychia
scleronyxis

sclero-oophoritis
sclerophthalmia
scleroplasty
scleroprotein
sclerosal
sclerosant
sclerose
sclerosed
sclerosing
sclerosis
sclerosis, Alzheimer's
sclerosis, amyotrophic
  lateral
sclerosis, annular
sclerosis, arterial
sclerosis, arteriolar
sclerosis, diffuse
sclerosis, disseminated
sclerosis, hyperplastic
sclerosis, insular
sclerosis, intimal
sclerosis, lateral
sclerosis, lobar
sclerosis, medial
sclerosis, multiple
sclerosis, neural
sclerosis, renal
sclerosis, tuberous
sclerosis, vascular
sclerosis, venous
scleroskeleton
sclerostenosis
sclerostenosis cutanea
sclerostomy
sclerotherapy
sclerotherapy,
  hemorrhoids
sclerothrix
sclerotic
sclerotica
sclerotic acid
sclerotic dentin
sclerotic teeth
scleroticectomy
scleroticochoroiditis
scleroticonyxis
scleroticopuncture
scleroticotomy

sclerotitis
sclerotium
sclerotome
sclerotomy
sclerotomy, anterior
sclerotomy, posterior
sclerotrichia
sclerous
scobinate
scoleciasis
scoleciform
scolecoid
scolecology
scolex
scoliokyphosis
scoliometer
scoliorachitic
scoliosiometry
scoliosis
scoliosis, cicatricial
scoliosis, congenital
scoliosis, coxitic
scoliosis, empyematic
scoliosis, habit
scoliosis, inflammatory
scoliosis, ischiatic
scoliosis, myopathic
scoliosis, ocular
scoliosis, osteopathic
scoliosis, paralytic
scoliosis, rachitic
scoliosis, rheumatic
scoliosis, sciatic
scoliosis, static
scoliosometry
scoliotic
scoliotone
scombrine
scombroid
scombroid poisoning
scoop
scoop, bone
scoop, bullet
scoop, cataract
scoop, ear
scoop, lithotomy
scoop, mastoid
scoop, renal

scoparius
scopolamine hydrobromide
scopometer
scopophilia
scopophobia
scopophobiac
scoracratia
scorbutic
scorbutigenic
scorbutus
scordinema
score
score, Apgar
scoretemia
scorpion
scorpion sting
scotochromogen
scotodinia
scotogram
scotograph
scotoma
scotoma, absolute
scotoma, annular
scotoma, arcuate
scotoma, central
scotoma, centrocecal
scotoma, color
scotoma, eclipse
scotoma, flittering
scotoma, negative
scotoma, peripheral
scotoma, physiological
scotoma, positive
scotoma, relative
scotoma, ring
scotoma, scintillating
scotomagraph
scotomata
scotomatous
scotometer
scotometry
scotomization
scotophilia
scotophobia
scotopia
scotopic
scotopic vision
scotopsin

scotoscopy
Scott operation
Scott-Tussin Cough & Cold Medicine
scout film
scraping
scratch
scratch percutaneous tests
scratch test
screatus
screen
screen, Bjerrum
screen, fluorescent
screen, intensifying
screen, tangent
screening
screening, multiphasic
Scribner shunt
scrobiculate
scrobiculus
scrofula
scrofulid
scrofulide
scrofuloderma
scrofulosis
scrofulous
scrotal
scrotal reflex
scrotectomy
scrotitis
scrotocele
scrotoplasty
scrotorrhaphy
scrotum
scrubbing
scrub nurse
scrub, posterior nasal
scrub typhus
scruple (scr)
sculpturing, heart valve
Scultetus bandage
Scultetus position
scum
scurf
scurvy
scurvy, infantile
scute

scutiform
scutular
scutulum
scutum
scybalous
scybalum
scyphoid
seabather's eruption
seal
seal, border
seal finger
seal, posterior palatal
seal, velopharyngeal
sealant
sealant, dental
sealant, pit and fissure
searcher
seasickness
seasonal affective disorder (SAD)
seat
seat, basal
seat, rest
Seattle foot
seatworm
sebaceous
sebaceous cyst
sebaceous gland
sebastomania
sebiferous
sebiparous
sebolite
sebolith
seborrhagia
seborrhea
seborrhea capiti
seborrhea congestiva
seborrhea corporis
seborrhea faciei
seborrhea furfuracea
seborrhea nigricans
seborrhea oleosa
seborrhea sicca
seborrheic
seborrheid
seborrhoic
Sebulex (antiseborrheic treatment shampoo)

sebum
sebum, palpebrale
Sebutone (antiseborrheic
  tar shampoo)
secernent
seclusion of pupil
seclusion pupillae
  siderosis bulbi
secobarbital
secobarbital sodium
secodont
Seconal (secobarbital)
Seconal Sodium
  (secobarbital sodium)
second (sec)
second cranial nerve
second intention
second look laparotomy
second opinion
  consultation
second sight
second stage of labor
second wind
secondary
secondary areola
secondary care
secondary gain
secondary hemorrhage
secondary nursing care
secondary radiation
secreta
secretagogue
secrete
secretin
secretinase
secretion
secretion, apocrine
secretion, external
secretion, holocrine
secretion, internal
secretion, merocrine
secretion, paralytic
secretogogue
secretoinhibitory
secretomotor
secretor
secretory
secretory capillaries

secretory fibers
sectarian
sectile
section
section, abdominal
section, cesarean
section, cesarean,
  postmortem
section, coronal
section, frontal
section, frozen
section, midsagittal
section, paraffin
section, perineal
section, Pitres'
section, sagittal
section, serial
section, vaginal
sectioning
sectioning, ultrathin
sector
sectorial
Sectral (acebutolol HCl)
secundigravida
secundina
secundines
secundipara
secundiparity
secundum artem
Sedapap #3
  (acetaminophen,
  butalbital and codeine
  phosphate)
Sedapap-10 (acetaminophen
  and butalbital)
sedation
sedative
sedative, cardiac
sedative, nervous
Seddon-Brooks tenoplasty
sedentary
sedentary living
sediment
sediment, urinary
sedimentation
sedimentation rate (sed
  rate)
sedimentator

seed
Seessel's pouch
Seffin (cephalothin
  sodium)
segment
segment, bronchopulmonary
segment, hepatic
segment, interannular
segment, mesodermal
segment, uterine
segmental
segmental reflex
segmental static
  reactions
segmentation
segmentation, rhythmic
segmented neutrophils
  (segs)
segmenter
segmentum
segregation
segregator
Segstaken-Blakemore tube
Séguin's signal symptom
SeHCAT (selenium-75
  artificial bile salt)
Seidlitz powder
  (effervescent
  cathartic)
seisesthesia
seismesthesia
seizure
seizure, absence
seizure, convulsive
seizure focus, cerebral
seizure, grand mal
seizure, jacksonian
seizure, petit mal
Seldane (terfenadine)
Seldinger technique
selection
selection, artificial
selection, natural
selection, sexual
selenium (Se)
selenoid cells
selenomethionine Se 75
  injection

selenomethionine tumor
  localization
self
self-acceptance
self-administered
  medication program
  (SAM)
self-conscious
self-contained underwater
  breathing apparatus
  (SCUBA)
self-defeating
  personality disorder
self-differentiation
self-digestion
self-hypnosis
self-infection
self-limited disease
self-tolerance
sellar
sella turcica
Selsun (selenium sulfide)
Selsun Blue (selenium
  sulfide lotion, 1%)
seltzer water
Selverstone clamp
semantics
Semb operation
semeiography
semeiology
semeiotics
semelincident
semen
semen test
semenarche
semenuria
semicanal
semicanalis
semicanalis musculi
  tensoris tympani
semicanalis tubae
  auditivae
semicartilaginous
Semicid (vaginal
  contraceptive inserts)
semicircular
semicircular canals
semicircular ducts

semicoma
semicomatose
semicrista
semicrista incisiva
semidecussation
semierection
semiflexion
semi-Fowler's position
Semilente Iletin I
  (prompt insulin zinc
  suspension)
Semilente Insulin (prompt
  insulin zinc
  suspension)
semilunar
semilunar bone
semilunar cartilages
semilunar cusps
semilunar ganglion
semilunar line
semilunar lobe
semilunar notch
semilunar valves
semilunare
semiluxation
semimembranosus
semimembranous
seminal
seminal duct
seminal emission
seminal fluid
seminal vesicle
semination
semination, artificial
seminiferous
seminiferous tubules
seminoma
seminormal
seminormal solution
seminose
seminuria
semiology
semiorbicular
semiotic
semiotics
semipenniform
semipermeable
semipronation

semiprone
semirecumbent
semis (half; ss)
semisideratio
semisideration
semisopor
semispinalis
semisulcus
semisupination
semisupine
semisynthetic
semitendinosus
semitendinous
senescence
Sengstaken tamponade
Sengstaken-Blakemore tube
senile
senilism
senility
senility, premature
senility, psychosis of
senium
senna
Senning operation
Senning repair
sennosides
Senokot (senna
  concentrate)
Senokot-S (senna
  concentrate and
  docusate sodium)
senopia
sensation
sensation, cincture
sensation, cutaneous
sensation, delayed
sensation, epigastric
sensation, external
sensation, girdle
sensation, gnostic
sensation, internal
sensation, palmesthetic
sensation, primary
sensation, proprioceptive
sensation, referred
sensation, reflex
sensation, somesthetic
sensation, subjective

sensation, tactile
sense
sense, color
sense, kinesthetic
sense, light
sense, muscular
sense, posture
sense, pressure
sense, proprioception
sense, sixth
sense, space
sense, special
sense, static
sense, stereognostic
sense, temperature
sense, time
sense, tone
sense, visceral
sensibility
sensibility, deep
sensibility, mesoblastic
sensibility, palmesthetic
sensibilization
sensible
sensiferous
sensigenous
sensimeter
sensing type pacemaker
sensitinogen
sensitive
sensitivity
sensitivity tests,
  antimicrobial
sensitivity studies
sensitivity training
sensitization
sensitization, active
sensitization,
  autoerythrocyte
sensitization, passive
sensitization, protein
sensitized
sensitized vaccine
sensitizer
sensitometer
sensomobile
Sensorcaine (bupivacaine
  HCl)

sensorial
sensoriglandular
sensorimetabolism
sensorimotor
sensorimotor exam
sensorimuscular
sensorineural
sensorineural acuity
  level test
sensorium
sensorivasomotor
sensory
sensory amusia
sensory aphasia
sensory area
sensory area, somesthetic
sensory deprivation
sensory ending
sensory epilepsy
sensory integration
sensory nerve
sensory unit
sensual
sensualism
sensuous
sentient
sentiment
sentinel gland
sentinel node
separation
separation, Siamese twins
separator
separatorium
sepsis
sepsis, puerperal
septa
septal
septal defect (SD)
septal defect repair
septan
septate
septectomy
septectomy, atrial
septemia
septic
septic fever
septic shock
septic sore throat

septicemia
septicemia,
  bronchopulmonary
septicemia, cryptogenic
septicemia, fungal
septicemia, puerperal
septicemic
septicophlebitis
septicopyemia
septigravida
septimetritis
septipara
septivalent
septomarginal
septometer
septonasal
septoplasty
septorhinoplasty
septostomy
septostomy, atrial
septotome
septotomy
septotomy, nasal
Septra (trimethoprim and
  sulfamethoxazole)
septula
septula testis
septulum
septum
septum, atrial
septum, atriorum cordis
septum, atrioventricular
septum, crural
septum, femoral
septum, interatrial
septum, interdental
septum, intermuscular
septum, interradicular
septum, interventricular
septum, lingual
septum lucidum
septum, mediastinal
septum, nasal
septum, orbital
septum pectiniforme
septum pellucidum
septum primum
septum, rectovaginal

septum, rectovesical
septum scroti
septum, ventricular
septuplet
sequel
sequela (seq)
sequence
sequester
sequestra
sequestral
sequestration
sequestration, pulmonary
sequestrectomy
sequestrotomy
sequestrum (seq)
Sequin's signal symptom
Ser-Ap-Es (reserpine,
  hydralazine HCl,
  hydrochlorothiazide)
sera
seralbumin
Serax (oxazepam)
serendipity
Serentil (mesoridazine
  besylate)
serial
serial sevens test
serialography
sericeps
series
series, aliphatic
series, aromatic
series, erythrocytic
series, fatty
series, granulocytic
series, homologous
series, leukocytic
series, monocytic
series, thrombocytic
serine
seriscission
seroalbuminuria
serocolitis
seroconversion
seroculture
serocystic
serodermatosis
serodiagnosis

seroenteritis
seroepidemiology
serofast
serofibrinous
seroflocculation
serohepatitis
seroimmunity
serolipase
serologic
serologic test for
  syphilis (STS)
serological
serologist
serology
serolysin
seroma
seromembranous
seromucous
seromuscular
Seromycin (cycloserine)
seronegative
seroperitoneum
Serophene (clomiphene
  citrate)
seropositive
seroprevention
seroprognosis
seroprophylaxis
seropurulent
seropus
seroreaction
seroresistance
seroresistant
serosa
serosamucin
serosanguineous
seroserous
serositis
serosity
serosynovial
serosynovitis
serotherapy
serotonin
serotype
serous
serous cavity
serous cell

serous effusion
serous exudate
serous glands
serous inflammation
serous membrane
serous otitis media (SOM)
serovaccination
serovar
serozymogenic
Serpasil (reserpine)
Serpasil-Apresoline
  (reserpine and
  hydralazine HCl)
Serpasil-Esidrix
  (reserpine and
  hydrochlorothiazide)
serpiginous
serrate
Serratia
Serratia marcescens
serration
serratus muscle
serrefine
serrenoeud
serrulate
Sertoli's cells
serum
serum albumin
serum, anticrotalus
serum, antidiphtheritic
serum, antilymphocytic
  (ALS)
serum, antimeningococcal
serum antimicrobial level
serum, antipneumococcal
serum, antitetanic
serum, antitoxic
serum, antityphoid
serum, bactericidal
serum bactericidal titer
serum, bacteriolytic
serum, blood
serum, convalescent
serum creatine
  phosphokinase (SCPK)
serum, foreign
serum globulin (SG)

serum glutamic
  oxaloacetic
  transaminase (SGOT)
serum glutamic pyruvic
  transaminase (SGPT)
serum hepatitis (SH)
serum, immune
serum
  immunoelectrophoresis
serum, polyvalent
serum, pooled
serum, pregnancy
serum, pregnant mare's
serum protein
serum protein
  electrophoresis (SPE)
serum protein-bound
  iodine (SPBI)
serum radioimmunoassay
serum sickness
servomechanism
sesame oil
sesamoid
sesamoid bone
sesamoid cartilage
sesamoidectomy
sesamoiditis
sesquihora
sesquioxide
sessile
set
seta
setaceous
Setchenov's inhibitory
  centers
setiferous
setigerous
seton
setose
set point weight
setup
seventh cranial nerve
seven-year itch
sever (sev)
Sever operation
severe combined immune
  deficiency (SCID)
severed (sev)

severing of
  blepharorrhaphy
sevum
Sewell operation
sewer gas
sex
sex, chromosomal
sex, morphological
sex, nuclear
sex, psychological
sex chromatin
sex chromosomes
sex clinic
sex determination
sex hormone (SH)
sexdigital
sexduction
sexism
sexivalent
sex-limited
sex-linked
sexology
sex ratio
sex surrogate
sextan
sextigravida
sextipara
sextuplet
sexual
sexual dysfunction
sexual health
sexual intercourse
sexuality
sexual reassignment
sexual reflex
sexually transmitted
  diseases (STDs)
Sézary cells
Sézary syndrome
shadow
shadow-casting
shadowgram
shadowgraph
shaft
shaft, hair
shake (agit)
shakes
shaking

shaking palsy
shaman
shamanism
shank
shape
sharkskin
Sharpey's intercrossing
  fibers
Sharpey's perforating
  fibers
shaving, bone
shaving, cornea
shaving, for smear or
  culture
shaving, patella
shear
sheath
sheath, arachnoid
sheath, axon
sheath, carotid
sheath, crural
sheath, dentinal
sheath, dural
sheath, femoral
sheath of Henle
sheath of Key and
  Retzius, connective
  tissue
sheath, lamellar
sheath, medullary
sheath, myelin
sheath, nerve
sheath of Neumann
sheath, pial
sheath, root
sheath of Schwann
sheath of Schweigger-
  Seidel
sheath, synovial
sheath, tendon
shedding
Sheehan's syndrome
sheep cell agglutination
  test (SCAT)
sheet
sheet, draw
sheet, lift
shelf

shelf, dental
Shelf operation
shelf-life
shell
shell shock
shellac
Shenton's line
shield
shield, embryonic
shield, gonadal
shield, nipple
shield, phallic
shift
shift, chloride
shift to the left
shift to the right
Shiga's bacillus
Shigella
Shigella boydii
Shigella dysenteriae
Shigella flexneri
Shigella sonnei
shigellosis
shin
shin, saber
shin spots
shingles
shinsplints
Shirodkar tracheloplasty
shiver
shock
shock, anaphylactic
shock, anesthesia
shock, cardiogenic
shock, deferred
shock, electric
shock, endotoxin
shock, epigastric
shock, hemorrhagic
shock, hypovolemic
shock, insulin
shock, mental
shock, peptone
shock, psychic
shock, secondary
shock, septic
shock, serum
shock, spinal

shock, surgical
shock, syndrome
shock therapy
shock, traumatic
shoemakers' cramp
Shohl's solution
short bowel syndrome
short increment
  sensitivity index
  (SISI)
shortening, bone
shortening, endopelvic
  fascia
shortening, extraocular
  muscle
shortening, eye muscle
shortening, eyelid margin
shortening, femur
shortening, finger
shortening, hand
shortening, heel cord
shortening, levator
  palpebrae muscle
shortening, ligament
shortening, sclera
shortening, tendon
shortening, tibia
shortening, ulna
shortening, ureter
shortness of breath (SOB)
shortsightedness
shot
shotgun prescription
shoulder (sh)
shoulder, dislocation of
shoulder blade
shoulder girdle
shoulder joint
show
Shrapnell's membrane
shreds
shrink
shudder
shunt
shunt, abdominovenous
shunt, aorta-coronary
  sinus
shunt, aorta-pulmonary

shunt, aortocarotid
shunt, aortoceliac
shunt, aortofemoral
shunt, aortoiliofemoral
shunt, aortomesenteric
shunt, aorto-myocardial
shunt, aortorenal
shunt, aortosubclavian
shunt, apicoaortic
shunt, arteriovenous
shunt, ascending aorta to
  pulmonary artery
shunt, axillary-femoral
shunt, cardiovascular
shunt, carotid-carotid
shunt, carotid-subclavin
shunt, caval-mesentéric
shunt, corpora cavernosa
  corpus spongiosum
shunt, descending aorta
  to pulmonary artery
shunt, dialysis
shunt, endolymph-
  perilymph
shunt, endolymphatic
shunt, femoroperoneal
shunt, femoropopliteal
shunt, iliofemoral
shunt, ilioiliac
shunt, intestinal, large-
  to-large
shunt, intestinal, small-
  to-large
shunt, intestinal, small-
  to-small
shunt, left subclavian to
  descending aorta
shunt, left-to-right
shunt, left ventricle and
  aorta
shunt, LeVeen
shunt, lienorenal
shunt, lumbar-
  subarachnoid
shunt, mesocaval
shunt, peritoneal-jugular
shunt, peritoneo-vascular
shunt, peritoneovenous

shunt, pleurothecal
shunt, portacaval
shunt, portal-systemic
shunt, postcaval
shunt, pulmonary vein to
atrium
shunt, renoportal
shunt, reversed
shunt, right atrium and
pulmonary artery
shunt, right-to-left
shunt, right ventricle
and pulmonary artery
shunt, salpingothecal
shunt, semicircular
subarachnoid
shunt, spinal
shunt, splenorenal
shunt, subarachnoid-
peritoneal
shunt, subarachnoid-
ureteral
shunt, tetralogy of
Fallot
shunt, vena cava to
pulmonary shunt, left-
to-right (systemic-
pulmonary artery)
shunt, ventriculoatrial
shunt, ventriculocaval
shunt,
ventriculocisternal
shunt, ventriculolumbar
shunt, ventriculomastoid
shunt, ventriculonaso-
pharyngeal
shunt, ventriculopleural
Shy-Drager syndrome
SI units (Système
International)
siagonantritis
sialaden
sialadenitis
sialadenoncus
sialagogue
sialaporia
sialectasia
sialectasis

sialemesis
sialic
sialic acid, blood
sialine
sialism
sialismus
sialitis
sialoadenectomy
sialoadenitis
sialoadenolithotomy
sialoadenotomy
sialoaerophagy
sialoangiectasis
sialoangiography
sialoangiitis
sialoangitis
sialocele
sialodochitis
sialodochitis fibrinosa
sialodochoplasty
sialoductitis
sialogenous
sialogogic
sialogogue
sialogram
sialography
sialolith
sialolithiasis
sialolithotomy
sialoncus
sialoporia
sialorrhea
sialoschesis
sialosemeiology
sialosis
sialostenosis
sialotic
Siamese twins
sib
sibilant
sibilation
sibilismus
sibilismus aurium
sibilus
sibling
sibling, half
sibship
siccant

siccative
sicchasia
siccolabile
siccostabile
siccus
sick
sick sinus syndrome (SSS)
sickle cell
sickle cell anemia
sickle cell crisis
sickle cell test
sickle hemoglobin
sicklemia
sickling
sickness
sickness, balloon
sickness, bleeding
sickness, car
sickness, falling
sickness, green
sickness, morning
sickness, motion
sickness, mountain
sickness, sea
sickness, serum
sickness, sleeping
side
side effect
side position
sideration
siderism
siderismus
sideroblast
siderocyte
sideroderma
siderodromophobia
siderofibrosis
siderogenous
sideropenia
sideropenic
siderophil
siderophilin
siderophilous
siderophone
siderophore
sideroscope
siderosis
siderosis, hepatic

siderosis, urinary
siderosome
siderotic
siemens
Siemens' syndrome
sieve
sieve, molecular
Sigault's operation
sigh
sight
sight, blind
sight, day
sight, far
sight, near
sight, night
sight, old
sight, second
sigma
sigmatism
sigmoid
sigmoidectomy
sigmoid flexure
sigmoiditis
sigmoidomyotomy
sigmoidopexy
sigmoidoproctostomy
sigmoidorectostomy
sigmoidorrhaphy
sigmoidoscope
sigmoidoscope, flexible
sigmoidoscopy
sigmoidosigmoidostomy
sigmoidostomy
sigmoidotomy
sigmoidovesical
sign
sign language
sign, objective
sign, physical
sign's, vital
signs and symptoms (SS)
signa (S or sig)
signal
signature
significance, statistical
significant
significant others
signing

Sigtab
Silain (simethicone)
Silastic (silicone
   material)
silent
silent disease
silent period
silica
silicate
siliceous
silicious
silicoanthracosis
silicofluoride
silicon (Si)
silicone
silicone, injectable
silicosiderosis
silicosis
silicotic
silicotuberculosis
siliqua olivae
siliquose
siliquose cataract
siliquose desquamation
silo-filler's disease
Silvadene (1% silver
   sulfadiazine)
silver (Ag)
silver amalgam
silver chloride (Ag Cl)
silver, colloidal
silver halide
silver nitrate (Ag NO$_3$)
silver nitrate, toughened
Silver operation
silver picrate
silver protein
silver sulfadiazine
silver fork deformity
silver nitrate poisoning
Silvester's method
Simeco (aluminum
   hydroxide gel,
   magnesium hydroxide,
   simethicone)
simesthesia
simethicone
simian crease

Similac
Similac PM 60/40
Similac with Iron
similia similibus
   curantur
similimum
Simmond's disease
Simon's position
simple
simple fracture
simple inflammation
simple mastectomy (SM)
simple reflex
Simplotan (tinedezole)
Simpson's forceps
Simpson's syndrome
Sims' position
simul
simulate
simulation
simulator
Simulium
Simulium damnosum
Simulium venustum
Sinapis
sinapism
Sinarest
sincipital
sinciput
Sine-Aid (sinus headache
   tablets)
Sinemet (carbidopa-
   levodopa)
Sinequan (doxepin HCl)
sinew
sinew, weeping
sing
singer's node
single-chamber pacemaker
   analysis
single photon
   absorptiometry
single proton emission
   computed tomography
   (SPECT)
Singlet (decongestant-
   antihistamine-
   analgesic)

singleton
singultation
singultus
sinister
sinistrad
sinistral
sinistraural
sinistrocardia
sinistrocerebral
sinistrocular
sinistrocularity
sinistrogyration
sinistromanual
sinistropedal
sinistrotorsion
sinistrous
sinoatrial (SA)
sinoatrial node (SA node)
sinoauricular
sinobronchitis
sinogram
sinter
Sinubid
Sinufed Timecelles
  (pseudoephedrine HCl
  and guaifenesin)
Sinulin
sinuitis
sinuotomy
sinuous
sinus
sinus, accessory nasal
sinus, anal
sinus, aortic
sinus, basilar
sinus, carotid
sinus, cavernosus
sinus, cerebral
sinus, circular
sinus, coccygeal
sinus, coronary, of heart
sinus, cranial
sinus, dermal
sinus, draining
sinus, ethmoidal
sinus, frontal
sinus, genitourinary

sinus, hair
sinus, inferior
  longitudinal
sinus, inferior petrosal
sinus, inferior sagittal
sinus, intercavernous
sinus, lateral
sinus, lymph
sinus, marginal
sinus, maxillary
sinus, occipital
sinus of the pulmonary
  trunk
sinus, paranasal
sinus, pilonidal
sinus, pleural
sinus, pocularis
sinus, rectus
sinus, renal
sinus, rhomboid
sinus rhythm
sinus, sigmoid
sinus, sphenoidal
sinus, sphenoparietal
sinus of spleen
sinus, straight
sinus, superior
  longitudinal
sinus, superior petrosal
sinus, superior sagittal
sinus, tarsal
sinus, tentorial
sinus, terminal
sinus, thyroglossal
sinus, transverse
sinus, transverse, of the
  dura mater
sinus, transverse, of the
  pericardium
sinus, tympanic
sinus, urachal
sinus, urogenital
sinus, uterine
sinus, uteroplacental
sinus of Valsalva
sinus of venal canal
sinus of venarum cavarum

sinus, venous
sinus, venous, of the
  dura mater
sinus, venous, of sclera
sinus, venography
sinus venosus
sinusitis
sinusitis, acute
  catarrhal
sinusitis, acute
  suppurative
sinusitis, chronic
  hyperplastic
sinusitis, chronic
  hypertrophic
sinusoid
sinusoidal
sinusoidal current
sinusoidalization
sinusotomy
Sioux alarm
siphon
siphonage
Siphonaptera
siphonoma
Sipple syndrome
Sippy diet
sirenomelia
siriasis
sister
Sister Mary Joseph nodule
site
site, active
site, binding
site, receptor
sitieirgia
sitology
sitomania
sitophobia
sitosterols
sitotaxis
sitotherapy
sitotoxin
sitotoxism
sitotropism
situation
situs
situs inversus viscerum

situs perversus
sitz bath
sixth cranial nerve
size reduction, abdominal
  wall
size reduction, arms
size reduction, breasts
size reduction, buttocks
size reduction, skin
size reduction,
  subcutaneous tissue
size reduction, thighs
Sjögren's syndrome (SS)
SK-65 (propoxyphene HCl)
SK-Apap (acetaminophen
  with codeine)
skateboard
skatol
skatole
skatoxyl
SK-Bamate (meprobamate)
SK-Chlorothiazide
  (chlorothiazide)
SK-Dexamethasone
  (dexamethasone)
skein
skelalgia
Skelaxin (metaxalone)
skeletal
skeletal fixation
skeletal muscle
skeletal survey
skeletal traction
skeletization
skeletogenous
skeletology
skeleton
skeleton, appendicular
skeleton, axial
skeleton, cartilaginous
Skene's gland
skenitis
skeocytosis
SK-Erythromycin
  (erythromycin stearate)
skew
skew deviation
skiascopy

skin
skin, alligator
skin, deciduous
skin, elastic
skin, glossy
skin graft (SG)
skin, hidebound
skin, loose
skin, parchment
skin, piebald
skin, scarf
skin rash
skin test
skin, true
skin cancer
skin end point titration
skinfold thickness
skin-marking
Skinner box
Skin-Prep (protective
  dressing)
SK-Lygen
  (chlordiazepoxide HCl)
skodaic
Skoda's rales
Skoda's resonance
SK-Penicillin VK
  (penicillin V
  potassium)
SK-Phenobarbital
  (phenobarbital)
SK-Potassium Chloride
  (potassium chloride)
SK-Pramine (imipramine
  HCl)
SK-Prednisone
  (prednisone)
SK-Probenecid
  (probenecid)
SK-Quinidine Sulfate
  (quinidine sulfate)
SK-Tetracycline
  (tetracycline HCl)
SK-Tolbutamide
  (tolbutamide)
skull
skull, fracture of
skullcap

slant
slave
sleep
sleep, disorders of
sleep drunkenness
sleep, hypnotic
sleep, NREM (nonrapid eye
  movement)
sleep, pathological
sleep, REM (rapid eye
  movement)
sleep, twilight
sleep deprivation
sleeping sickness
sleepwalking
slide
slime mold
slimy
sling
sling, clove-hitch
sling, counterbalanced
sling, cravat
sling, folded cravat
sling, mouth
sling, open
sling, orbicularis
sling, rectum
  (puborectalis)
sling, St. John's
sling, simple figure-of-
  eight roller arm
sling, swathe arm or
  cravat
sling, tongue
sling, triangular
sling, triangular,
  reversed
sling, trigeminal nerve
  paralysis
slinting, prepuce
slit
slit lamp
slitting, lens
slitting, removal of
  streptothrix
Slo-Bid (anhydrous
  theophylline)

Slo-Phyllin (anhydrous
  theophylline)
Slo-Phyllin GG
  (theophylline-
  guaifenesin)
Slocum operation
slope
slope, lower ridge
slough
sloughing
slow
Slow FE (iron tablets)
Slow-K (potassium
  chloride)
slow-reacting substance
  of anaphylaxis (SRS-A)
slows
slow virus infection
Sluder operation
sludge
sludged blood
slurry
SMA (iron fortified
  infant formula)
SMA-12 (blood chemistry
  tests)
small (sm)
small bowel biopsy
small bowel series
small-for-gestational age
smallpox
smallpox vaccine
smear
smear, blood
smear, Pap
smear, Papanicolaou
smegma
smegma clitordis
smegma embryonum
smegma praeputii
smegmatic
smegmolith
smell
Smith's fracture
Smith-Petersen nail
Smith-Strang disease
Smithwick operation
smog

smoke inhalation
smoke poisoning
smokeless tobacco
smoker's cancer
smoking, passive
smooth, muscle
smudging
Smurf (chewable vitamins)
snail
snake
snake, poisonous
snake bite
snap
snap, closing
snap, opening
snapping finger
snapping hip
snare
snaring rale
sneeze
sneeze reflex, solar
Snellen's chart
Snellen's reflex
Snellen's test
snip, punctum
snore
snoring rale
snow blindness
snuff
snuffbox, anatomical
snuffles
soap
soap, green
soap liniment
soap, soft medicinal
soap solution (SS)
soapsuds enema
Soave proctectomy
sob
social phobias
socialization
socioacusis
sociobiology
socioeconomic status
sociology
sociomedical
sociometry
sociopath

sociopathic personality
sociopathy
socket
socket, alveolar
socket, dry
socket, tooth
soda
soda, baking
soda, caustic
soda, lime
Soda Mint (sodium
  bicarbonate)
soda water
Sodestrin (estrogens,
  conjugated)
sodic
sodium (Na)
sodium acetate
sodium alginate
sodium amobarbital
sodium ascorbate
sodium benzoate
sodium bicarbonate
  ($NaHCO_3$)
sodium carbonate ($NaCO_3$)
sodium,
carboxymethylcellulose
sodium chloride (NaCl)
sodium citrate
Sodium Edecrin
  (ethacrynate sodium)
sodium fluoride
sodium hydroxide (NaOH)
sodium hypochlorite
sodium iodide
sodium lactate
sodium lauryl sulfate
sodium
  monofluorophosphate
sodium morrhuate
sodium nitrite ($NaNO_2$)
sodium nitroprusside
sodium phosphate, dibasic
sodium phosphate P 32
sodium polystyrene
  sulfonate
sodium propionate

sodium salicylate
  ($C_7H_5NaO_3$)
Sodium Sulamyd
  (sulfacetamide sodium)
sodium sulfate
sodium thiosulfate
Sodium Versenate (edetate
  disodium)
sodokosis
sodoku
sodomist
sodomite
sodomy
Soemmering's bone
Soemmering's foramen
Soemmering's ring
Soemmering's spot
Sofarin (warfarin sodium)
Sofield osteotomies
soft
soft diet
Soft Guard XL
soft palate
soft sore
softening
softening, anemic
softening, colliquative
softening, gray
softening, mucoid
softening, of bones
softening, of brain
softening, of heart
softening, of stomach
softening, red
softening, white
sol
solace
Solanaceae
solanaceous
solanine
Solaquin Forte
  (hydroquinone)
solar
solarium
solar plexus
solar therapy
Solatene (beta-carotene)
solation

Solbar PF 15 Cream
Solbar PF Liquid
Solbar Plus 15 Cream
solder
solder, building
solder, gold
solder, hard
solder, soft
soldering
sole
sole reflex
solenoid
soleus
Solfoton (phenobarbital)
Solganal
  (aurothioglucose)
solid
solipsism
solitary
solitary lymph nodules
solo practitioner
solubility
soluble
Solu-Cortef
  (hydrocortisone sodium
  succinate)
Solu-Medrol
  (methylprednisolone
  sodium succinate)
solum tympani
solute
solutio
solution
solution, aqueous
solution, buffer
solution, colloidal
solution, contrast
solution, hyperbaric
solution, hypertonic
solution, hypotonic
solution, iodine
solution, isobaric
solution, isohydric
solution, isosmotic
solution, isotonic
solution, Locke-Ringer's
solution, molar
solution, normal

solution, normal saline
solution, ophthalmic
solution, physiological
  saline
solution, repair
solution, Ringer's
solution, saline
solution, saturated
solution, sclerosing
solution, seminormal
solution, standard
solution, supersaturation
solution, test
solution, Tyrode's
solution, volumetric
solv
solvate
solvation
solvent
solvolysis
soma
Soma (carisoprodol)
Soma Compound
  (carisoprodol and
  aspirin)
Soma Compound with
  Codeine (carisoprodol,
  aspirin, and codeine)
soman
somasthenia
somatasthenia
somatesthesia
somatic
somatic nerves
somaticosplanchnic
somaticovisceral
somatist
somatization
somatization disorder
somatoceptors
somatochrome
somatocrinin
somatoform disorders
somatogenic
somatology
somatomammotropin,
  chorionic
somatome

somatomedin (SM)
somatomegaly
somatometry
somatopagus
somatopathic
somatoplasm
somatopleure
somatoplural
somatopsychic
somatopsychosis
somatoschisis
somatoscopy
somatosensory testing
somatosexual
somatostatin
somatotherapy,
  psychiatric
somatotonia
somatotopic
somatotrophic
somatotrophin
somatotropic
somatotype
Sombulex (hexobarbital)
somesthesia
somesthetic
somesthetic area
somesthetic path
somite
somnambulance
somnambule
somnambulism
somnambulist
somniferous
somnific
somniloquence
somniloquism
somniloquist
somnipathist
somnipathy
somnocinematograph
somnolence
somnolent
somnolentia
somnolism
Somogyi phenomenon
Somophyllin-CRT
  (theophylline)

Somophylline
  (aminophylline)
sone
sonicate
sonication
sonic boom
sonitus
Sonneberg operation
sonogram
sonographer
sonographer, diagnostic
  medical
sonography
sonolucent
sonometer
sonorous
sonorous rale
sophistication
sophomania
sopor
soporiferous
soporific
soporose
soporous
Soques' phenomenon
sorbefacient
sorbitol
Sorbitrate (isosorbide
  dinitrate)
sorcery
sordes
sore
sore, bed
sore, canker
sore, cold
sore, Delhi
sore, desert
sore, hard
sore, Oriental
sore, pressure
sore, soft venereal
sore, tropical
sore, venereal
sore throat
sore throat, diphtheritic
sore throat, quinsy
sore throat, septic
soroche

Sorondo-Ferre operation
sororiation
sorption
s.o.s (if necessary or
  required)
sotalol hydrochloride
Sotradecol (sodium
  tetradecyl sulfate)
souffle
souffle, cardiac
souffle, fetal
souffle, funic
souffle, placental
souffle, splenic
souffle, uterine
sound
sound, anasarcous
sound, blowing
sound, bottle
sound, breath
sound, bronchial
sound, bronchovesicular
sound, cracked-pot
sound, ejection
sound, fetal heart
sound, friction
sound, heart
sound, Kortfkoff's
sound, percussion
sound, physiological
sound, respiratory
sound, succussion
sound, to-and-fro
sound, tracheal
sound, tubular
sound, urethral
sound, vesicular
source-skin distance
Soutter fasciotomy
soybean oil
spa
space
space, anatomical dead
space, axillary
space, circumlental
space, dead
space, epidural
space, of Fontana

space, intercostal
space, interfascial
space, interpleural
space, interproximal
space, interradicular
space, intervillous
space, lymph
space maintainer
space, Meckel's
space, mediastinal
space medicine
space, Nuel's
space, palmar
space, parasinoidal
space, perforated
space, perivascular
space, physiological dead
space, plantar
space, pneumatic
space, popliteal
space, prezonular
space, Prussak's
space, retroperitoneal
space, retropharyngeal
space sickness
space, subarachnoid
space, subdural
space, subphrenic
space, suprasternal
space, Tenon's
space, zonular
spallation
span
Span R/D (phentermine
  HCl)
Span-FF (ferrous
  fumarate)
Spanish fly
sparer
sparer, protein
sparganosis
Sparganum
Sparganum mansoni
Sparganum mansonoides
Sparganum proliferum
sparge
spargosis
Sparine (promazine HCl)

spark coil
spark gap
spark gap, quenched
spasm
spasm, Bell's
spasm, bronchial
spasm, choreiform
spasm, clonic
spasm of esophagus
spasm, habit
spasm, nodding
spasm, saltatory
spasm, tetanic
spasm, tonic
spasm, torsion
spasm, toxic
spasm, winking
spasmatic
spasmatic asthma
spasmatic croup
spasmatic stricture
spasmodic
spasmogen
spasmology
spasmolygmus
spasmolysin
spasmolytic
spasmophemia
spasmophilia
spasmous
spasmus
spasmus agitans
spasmus bronchialis
spasmus caninus
spasmus coordinatus
spasmus cynicus
spasmus Dubini
spasmus glottidis
spasmus nictitans
spasmus nutans
spastic
spastic colon
spastic gait
spastic hemiplegia
spasticity
spastic paralysis
spastic paraplegia
spatial

spatial discrimination
spatium
spatula
spatula, eye
spatula, nasal
spatulate
Spaulding-Richardson
  operation
spay
spaying
specialist
specialization
specialty
speciation
species
species-specific
species type
specific
specific dynamic action
  (SDA)
specific gravity (SG, Sp
  gr)
specificity
specificity, diagnostic
specillum
specimen
spectacle fitting
spectacles
Spectazole (econazole
  nitrate)
spectinomycin
  hydrochloride, sterile
spectral
Spectrobid (bacampicillin
  HCl)
spectrocolorimeter
spectrofluorometer
spectrograph
spectrograph, mass
spectrometer
spectrometry
spectrophotometer
spectrophotometric
  amniotic fluid scan
spectrophotometry
spectropolarimeter
spectropyrheliometer
spectroscope

spectroscopic
spectroscopy
spectrum
spectrum, absorption
spectrum, broad
spectrum, chromatic
spectrum emission
spectrum, invisible
spectrum, visible
spectrum, visible
  electromagnetic
speculum
speculum, ear
speculum, eye
speculum, vaginal
speech
speech abnormalities
speech, aphonic
speech, ataxic
speech, clipped
speech, echo
speech, esophageal
speech, explosive
speech, interjectional
speech, mirror
speech pathologist
speech, scamping
speech, scanning
speech, slurring
speech, staccato
speech synthesizer
speech therapy
sperm
sperma
spermacrasia
spermagglutination
spermatemphraxis
spermatic
spermatic arteries
spermatic cord
spermatic duct
spermaticidal
spermatic vein
spermatid
spermatin
spermatitis
spermatoblast
spermatocele

spermatocelectomy
spermatocidal
spermatocyst
spermatocystectomy
spermatocystitis
spermatocystotomy
spermatocytal
spermatocyte
spermatocyte, primary
spermatocyte, secondary
spermatocytogenesis
spermatogenesis
spermatogenic
spermatogenous
spermatogeny
spermatogonium
spermatoid
spermatology
spermatolysin
spermatolysis
spermatolytic
spermatopathia
spermatopathy
spermatophobia
spermatopoietic
spermatorrhea
spermatoschesis
spermatospore
spermatotoxin
spermatovum
spermatoxin
spermatozoa
spermatozoal
spermatozoon
spermaturia
spermectomy
spermic
spermicidal
spermicide
spermidine
spermiduct
spermine
spermiogenesis
spermiogram
spermoblast
spermolith
spermolysin
spermolytic

spermoneuralgia
spermophlebectasia
spermoplasm
spermosphere
spermospore
spermotoxin
sphacelate
sphacelation
sphacelism
sphaceloderma
sphacelotoxin
sphacelous
sphacelus
sphagiasmus
sphagitis
sphenethmoid
sphenobasilar
sphenoccipital
sphenocephalus
sphenoethmois
sphenoethmoid recess
sphenofrontal
sphenoid
sphenoidal
sphenoid bone
sphenoid fissure
sphenoiditis
sphenoidostomy
sphenoidotomy
sphenomalar
sphenomaxillary
spheno-occipital
sphenopalatine
sphenoparietal
sphenorbital
sphenosis
sphenosquamosal
sphenotemporal
sphenotic
sphenotresia
sphenotribe
sphenoturbinal
sphenovomerine
sphenozygomatic
sphere
sphere, attraction
sphere, segmentation
spheresthesia

spherical
spherocylinder
spherocyte
spherocytosis
spherocytosis, hereditary
spheroid
spheroidal
spherolith
spheroma
spherometer
spheroplast
spherospermia
spherule
sphincter
sphincter, ampullae
sphincter, ani
sphincter, bladder
sphincter, cardiac
sphincter choledochus
sphincter, ileocecal
sphincter of Oddi
sphincter, pancreaticus
sphincter, pyloric
sphincteral
sphincteralgia
sphincterectomy
sphincteric
sphincterismus
sphincteritis
sphincterolysis
sphincteroplasty
sphincterorrhaphy, anal
sphincteroscope
sphincteroscopy
sphincterotome
sphincterotomy
sphingolipid
sphingolipidosis
sphingolipodystrophy
sphingomyelins
sphingosine ($C_{18}H_{37}O_2N$)
sphygmic
sphygmobolometer
sphygmocardiogram
sphygmocardiograph
sphygmocardioscope
sphygmochronograph

sphygmogram
sphygmograph
sphygmography
sphygmoid
sphygmology
sphygmomanometer
sphygmomanometer, random-
   zero
sphygmometer
sphygmopalpation
sphygmophone
sphygmoplethysmograph
sphygmoscope
sphygmosystole
sphygmotonograph
sphygmotonometer
sphygmus
sphyrectomy
sphyrotomy
spica
spica hip cast
spicular
spicule
spicule, bony
spiculed red cell
spiculum
spider
spider bites or poisoning
spider, black widow
spider, brown recluse
spider cells
spider fingers
spider nevus
spider-burst
Spielmeyer-Vogt disease
spigelian line
spigelian lobe
spike
spikeboard
spill
spill, cellular
spill, radioactive
spillway
spiloma
spilus
spiloplania
spiloplaxia
spina

spina bifida
spina bifida occulta
spina ventosa
spinal
spinal accessory nerve
spinal anesthesia
spinal canal
spinal column
spinal cord
spinal curvature
spinal curvature, angular
spinal curvature, lateral
spinal fluid (SF)
spinal fusion
spinal ganglion
spinal instrumentation
spinal nerves
spinal puncture
spinal reflex
spinal shock
spinal vessels
spinalgia
spinalis
spinate
spindle
spindle, aortic
spindle, enamel
spindle, muscle
spindle, neuromuscular
spindle, neurotendinous
spindle, sleep
spine
spine, alar
spine, anterior nasal
spine, fracture of
spine, frontal
spine, hemal
spine, Henle's
spine, iliac
spine, ischial
spine, mental
spine, nasal
spine, pharyngeal
spine, posterior nasal
spine of pubis
spine of scapula
spine, sciatic
spine of sphenoid

spine, suprameatal
spine, typhoid
Spinelli operation
spinifugal
spinipetal
spinnbarkeit (SBK)
spinobulbar
spinocellular
spinocerebellar
spinocortical
spinocostalis
spinoglenoid
spinoglenoid ligament
spinose
spinotectal
spinous
spinous point
spinous process
spintherism
spintheropia
spiradenitis
spiradenoma
spiral
spiral, Curschmann's
spiral bandage
spiral canal of cochlea
spiral canal of modiolus
spiral lamina
spiral organ of Corti
spirilla
spirillicidal
spirillicide
spirillolysis
spirillosis
spirillotropic
spirillotropism
Spirillum
Spirillum minus
spirillum
spirit
spirit of ammonia
spirit of bitter almond
spirit of camphor
spirit of juniper
spirit of lavender
spirit of mustard
spirit of peppermint
spiritual therapy

spirituous
spiritus
spiritus frumenti
  (whiskey)
spiritus juniperi (gin)
spiritus myrciae (bay
  rum)
spiritus vini gallici
  (brandy)
Spirochaeta
*Spirochaeta
  icterohaemorrhagiae*
Spirochaeta pallida
Spirochaetales
spirochetal
spirochetalytic
spirochete
spirochetemia
spirocheticidal
spirocheticide
spirochetolysis
spirochetosis
spirochetotic
spirocheturia
spirogram
spirograph
spiroid
spirokinesis
spiroma
spirometer
spirometry
spironolactone
spissated
spissitude
spit
spittle
Spivack operation
splanchna
splanchnapophysis
splanchnectopia
splanchnesthesia
splanchnesthetic
splanchnic
splanchnicectomy
splanchnic nerves
splanchnicotomy
splanchnoblast
splanchnocele

splanchnocoele
splanchnocranium
splanchnodiastasis
splanchnodynia
splanchnography
splanchnolith
splanchnology
splanchnomegaly
splanchnomicria
splanchnopathia
splanchnopleural
splanchnopleure
splanchnoptosia
splanchnoptosis
splanchnosclerosis
splanchnoscopy
splanchnoskeleton
splanchnosomatic
splanchnotomy
splanchnotribe
splayfoot
spleen
spleen, accessory
spleen, floating
spleen, lardaceous
spleen, sago
splenadenoma
splenalgia
splenceratosis
splenectasia
splenectasis
splenectomy
splenectomy, infections
  following
splenectopia
splenectopy
splenelcosis
splenemia
splenemphraxis
spleneolus
splenetic
splenetic cords
splenetic nodule
splenetic sinus
splenetic vein
splenial
splenic
splenic artery

splenic flexure
splenic sequestration
splenicterus
splenification
spleniform
splenitis
splenium
splenium corporis callosi
splenius
splenization
splenocele
splenoceratosis
splenocleisis
splenocolic
splenocyte
splenodynia
splenogenic
splenogenous
splenogram
splenography
splenohemia
splenohepatomegaly
splenoid
splenokeratosis
splenolaparotomy
splenology
splenolymphatic
splenolysin
splenolysis
splenoma
splenomalacia
splenomedullary
splenomegalia
splenomegaly
splenomegaly, congestive
splenomegaly, hemolytic
splenometry
splenomyelogenous
splenomyelomalacia
splenoncus
splenonephric
splenonephroptosis
splenopancreatic
splenopathy
splenopexy
splenophrenic
splenoplasty
splenopneumonia

splenoportogram
splenoportography
splenoptosis
splenorenal
splenorenal anastomosis
splenorenal bypass graft
splenorenal shunt
splenorrhagia
splenorrhaphy
splenotomy
splenotoxin
splenulus
splenunculus
splint
splint, acrylic resin
  bite-guard
splint, Agnew's
splint, airplane
splint, anchor
splint, Ashhurst's
splint, Balkan
splint, banjo traction
splint, Bavarian
splint, blow-up
splint, Bond's
splint, Bowlby's
splint, bracketed
splint, Cabot's
splint, Carter's
  intranasal
splint, coaptation
splint, Denis Browne
splint, dental
splint, Dupuytren's
splint, dynamic
splint, Fox's
splint, functional
splint, Gibson walking
splint, Gordon's
splint, inflatable
splint, Jones' nasal
splint, Kanavel
splint, Levis'
splint, McIntire's
splint, permanent fixed
splint, Sayre's
splint, Stromeyer's

splint, temporary
  removable
splint, Thomas
splint, Thomas' knee
splint, Thomas' posterior
splint, Volkmann's
splinter
splinter hemorrhage
splinter skill
splinting
splinting, dental
splinting,
  musculoskeletal
splinting, orthodontic
splinting, ureteral
split
split foot
split hand
split pelvis
split thickness skin
  graft (STSG)
splitting
splitting, canaliculus
splitting, hand
splitting, lacrimal
  papilla
splitting, percutaneous
splitting, spinal cord
  tracts
splitting, tendon sheath
split tongue
spodogenous
spodophagous
spondee
spondylalgia
spondylarthritis
spondylarthrocace
spondylexarthrosis
spondylitic
spondylitis
spondylitis, ankylosing
spondylitis deformans
spondylitis, hypertrophic
spondylitis, Kümmell's
spondylitis, Marie-
  Strümpell
spondylitis, rheumatoid

spondylitis, tuberculous
spondylizema
spondylocace
spondylodiagnosis
spondylodymus
spondylodynia
spondylolisthesis
spondylolysis
spondylomalacia
spondylopathy
spondyloptosis
spondylopyosis
spondyloschisis
spondylosis
spondylosis, cervical or
  lumbar
spondylosis, rhizomelic
spondylosyndesis
spondylotherapy
spondylotomy
spondylous
sponge
sponge, abdominal
sponge, contraceptive
sponge, gauze
sponge, gelatin
sponge graft
spongiform
spongioblast
spongioblastoma
spongiocyte
spongioid
spongioplasm
spongiosis
spongiositis
spongy
spongy bone
spontaneous
spontaneous delivery (SD)
spontaneous fracture
spontaneous nystagmus
  test
spontaneous vaginal
  delivery (SVD)
spontaneous version
spoon
spoon nail
sporadic

sporangiophore
sporangium
spore
sporicidal
sporicide
sporiferous
spork
sporoblast
sporocyst
sporogenesis
sporogenic
sporogenous
sporgeny
sporogony
sporophore
sporophyte
sporoplasm
Sporothrix
Sporothrix schenckii
sporotrichin
sporotrichosis
Sporotrichum
Sporotrichum schenckii
Sporozoa
sporozoan
sporozoite
sporozoon
sport
sports medicine
sporular
sporulation
spot
spot, blind
spot, blue
spot, cherry-red
spot, cold
spot, corneal
spot, genital
spot, hot
spot, hypnogenic
spot, milk
spot, mongolian
spot, ruby
spot, temperature
spot, yellow
spots, Fordyce's
spots, Koplik's
spots, liver

spots, rose
spots, warm
spots, white
spotted fever
spotting
sprain
sprain of ankle or foot
sprain of back
sprain fracture
sprain, riders'
spray
spray tube
spreader
spreader, bladder-neck
spreader, root canal
spreading
spreading factor
Sprengel's deformity
spring
spring conjunctivitis
spring fever
spring finger
spring ligament
S.P. Rogers operation
sprue
S-P-T (pork thyroid "liquid" capsules)
spud
spur
spur, calcaneal
spur, femoral
spur, scleral
spurious
sputum
sputum, bloody
sputum, nummular
sputum, prune juice
sputum, rusty
sputum, septicemia
sputum specimen
squalene
squama
squamate
squamatization
squame
squamocellular
squamofrontal
squamomastoid

squamo-occipital
squaomoparietal
squamopetrosal
squamosa
squamosal
squamosphenoid
squamous
squamous bone
squamous cell
squamous cell carcinoma (SCC)
squamous epithelium
squamous suture
squamozygomatic
square centimeter (cm^2)
square knot
square lobe
squarrose
squarrous
squatting position
squeeze-bottle
squill
squint
squint, convergent
squint, divergent
squint, external
squint, internal
SSKI (potassium iodide)
stab
stab culture
stabile
stabilization
stabilization, joint
stable
staccato speech
stachyose
Stacke operation
stactometer
stadium
stadium acmes
stadium augmenti
stadium caloris
stadium decrementi
stadium fluorescentiae
stadium frigoris
stadium incrementi
stadium invasionis
stadium sudoris

Stadol (butorphanol
  tartrate)
staff
staff, attending
staff, consulting
staff, house
staff of Wrisberg
stage
stage, algid
stage, amphibolic
stage, asphyxial
stage, cold
stage, defervescent
stage, eruptive
stage, expulsive, of
  labor
stage, first, of labor
stage, fourth, of labor
stage, hot
stage of invasion
stage of latency
stage, placental, of
  labor
stage, preeruptive
stage, pyrogenetic
stage, resting
stage, second, of labor
stage, sweating
stage, third, of labor
staggers
staghorn calculus
staging
staging celiotomy
stagnation
stain
stain, acid
stain, acid-fast
stain, basic
stain, Commission
  Certified
stain, contrast
stain, counter
stain, dental
stain, differential
stain, double
stain, Giemsa
stain, Gram's
stain, hematoxylin-eosin

stain, intravital
stain, inversion
stain, metachromatic
stain, neutral
stain, nuclear
stain, port-wine
stain, substantive
stain, supravital
stain, tumor
stain, vital
stain, Wright's
staining
staircase breaths
staircase phenomenon
stalagmometer
stalk
stalk, belly
stalk, body
stalk, cerebellar
stalk, infundibular
stalk, optic
stalk, yolk
Stallard operation
Stamey vesical neck
  suspension
stamina
stammering
stammering of bladder
Stamm operation
standard
standard, biological
standard deviation (SD)
standard deviation of the
  mean (SDM)
standard error (SE)
standard operating
  procedure (SOP)
Standard Vivonex
  (nutritionally complete
  elemental diet formula)
standardization
standards of practice
standing orders
standstill
standstill, atrial
standstill, cardiac
standstill, inspiratory
standstill, ventricular

Stanford-Binet test
stannic
stannous
stannous fluoride
stannum
stanolone
stanozolol
Stanton's disease
stapedectomy
stapedial
stapediolysis
stapediotenotomy
stapediovestibular
stapedius
stapes
Staphage Lysate (SPL)
  (staphylococcus
  antigen)
Staphcillin (methicillin
  sodium)
staphylagra
staphyle
staphylectomy
staphyledema
staphyline
staphylion
staphylitis
staphyloangina
staphylococcal
staphylococcal
  actinophytosis
staphylococcal food
  poisoning
staphylococcemia
staphylococci
Staphylococcus
Staphylococcus aureus
Staphylococcus
  epidermidis
Staphylococcus
  saprophytricus
staphylococcus (staph)
staphyloderma
staphylodermatitis
staphylodialysis
staphylohemia
staphylokinase
staphylolysin

staphyloma
staphyloma, anterior
staphyloma, ciliary
staphyloma, corneae
staphyloma, equatorial
staphyloma, intercalary
staphyloma, partial
staphyloma, posterior
staphyloma, total
staphyloma uveal
staphylomatous
staphyloncus
staphylopharyngeus
staphylopharyngorrhaphy
staphyloplasty
staphyloptosia
staphyloptosis
staphylorrhaphy
staphyloschisis
staphylotome
staphylotomy
staphylotoxin
staple food
stapling
stapling, artery
stapling, blebs, lung
stapling, diaphysis
stapling, epiphyseal
  plate
stapling, femur
stapling, fibula
stapling, gastric varices
stapling, graft
stapling, humerus
stapling, radius
stapling, tibia
stapling, ulna
stapling, vein
star
star, lens
stars of Verheyen
starch
starch, animal
starch, corn
starch glycerite
stare
Stark esophageal dilation
Starling's law of heart

Starling's law of
  intestine
starter
startle syndrome
starvation
stasibasiphobia
stasimorphia
stasimorphy
stasiphobia
stasis
stasis, diffusion
stasis, intestinal
stasis, venous
state
state, anxiety
state, central excitatory
  (CES)
state, central inhibitory
  (CIS)
state, dream
state, excited
state, fatigue
state, ground
state, refractory
state, steady
static
static electricity
static equilibrium
static pressure
static reflex
statics
static splint
statim (stat)
station
station, aid
station, dressing
station, rest
stationary
statistical
statistical significance
statistics
statistics, medical
statistics, morbidity
statistics, vital
statoacoustic
statoconia
statokinetic
statokinetic reflexes

statolith
statometer
statosphere
stature
stature, short
status
status anginosus
status arthriticus
status asthmaticus
status dysgraphicus
status epilepticus
status parathyreoprivus
status praesens
status raptus
status sternuens
status verrucosus
status vertiginosus
staunch
staurion
stauroplegia
steal
steal, subclavian
steam
steam tent
steapsin
stearate
stearic acid
steariform
stearin
stearoderma
stearopten
stearoptene
stearrhea
stearrhea flavescens
stearrhea nigricans
stearrhea simplex
steatadenoma
steatite
steatitis
steatocele
steatocryptosis
steatocystoma multiplex
steatogenous
steatolysis
steatolytic
steatoma
steatomatous
steatonecrosis

steatopathy
steatopygia
steatopygous
steatorrhea
steatorrhea, idiopathic
steatorrhea simplex
steatosis
stege
stegnosis
stegnotic
Stegomyia
Steinberg operation
Steindler flexor-plasty
Steindler stripping
Steinert's disease
Stein-Leventhal syndrome
Steinmann's extension
Steinmann pin
Stelazine
  (trifluoperazine HCl)
stella
stella lentis hyaloidea
stella lentis iridica
stellate
stellate bandage
stellate cell
stellate fracture
stellate ganglion
stellate ligament
stellate veins
stellectomy
Stellwag's sign
stem
stem, brain
stem cell
Stenger test
stenion
stenobregmatic
stenocardia
stenocephaly
stenochoria
stenocompressor
stenocoriasis
stenocrotaphia
stenopaic
stenopeic
stenosal
stenosed

stenosis
stenosis, aortic
stenosis, cardiac
stenosis, cicatricial
stenosis, mitral
stenosis, pulmonary
stenosis, pyloric
stenosis, subaortic
stenosis, tricuspid
stenostomia
stenothermal
stenothorax
stenotic
Stensen's duct
Stensen's foramina
stent
step, Rönne's
stephanion
steppage gait
stepping reflex
steradian
Sterane (prednisolone)
Sterapred DS Unipak
  (prednisone)
Sterapred Unipak
  (prednisone)
stercobilin
stercobilinogen
stercolith
stercoraceous
stercoral
stercorin
stercorolith
stercoroma
stercorous
stercus
stere
stereoagnosis
stereoanesthesia
stereoarthrolysis
stereoauscultation
stereocampimeter
stereochemical
stereochemistry
stereocilia
stereocinefluorography
stereoencephalotomy
stereognosis

stereogram
stereoisomer
stereoisomerism
stereology
stereometer
stereometry
stereo-ophthalmoscope
stereo-orthopter
stereophantoscope
stereophorometer
stereophotography
stereophotomicrograph
stereopsis
stereoradiography
stereo radiologic exam
stereoroentgenography
stereoscope
stereoscopic
stereoscopic vision
stereoscopical
stereospecific
stereotactic
stereotaxis
stereotropic
stereotropism
stereotypy
sterile
sterile supply unit (SSU)
sterility
sterility, absolute
sterility, acquired
sterility, female
sterility, male
sterility, primary
sterility, relative
sterilization
sterilization, dry heat
sterilization, fractional
sterilization, gas
sterilization,
   intermittent
sterilization,
   laparoscopic
sterilization, steam
sterilize
sterilizer
sterilizer, steam
sternad

sternal
sternalgia
sternal puncture
Sternberg-Reed cell
sternebra
sternen
sternoclavicular
sternoclavicular joint
sternocleidal
sternocleidomastoid
sternocostal
sternodymia
sternodynia
sternohyoid
sternoid
sternomastoid
sternomastoid region
sternopagia
sternopericardial
sternoschisis
sternothyroid
sternotomy
sternotracheal
sternotrypesis
sternovertebral
sternum
sternum, cleft
sternutament
sternutatio
sternutatio convulsiva
sternutation
sternutation, convulsive
sternutator
sternutatory
steroid
steroidal withdrawal
   syndrome
steroid hormones
steroid hormone therapy
steroidogenesis
sterol
sterotactic frame
stertor
stertorous
stethalgia
stethocyrtograph
stethogoniometer
stethogram

stethograph
stethokyrtograph
stethometer
stethomyitis
stethomyositis
stethoparalysis
stethophonometer
stethoscope
stethoscope, binaural
stethoscope, compound
stethoscope, double
stethoscope, single
stethoscopic
stethoscopy
stethospasm
Stevens-Johnson syndrome
Stewart operation
S-T Forte
sthenia
sthenic
sthenometer
sthenometry
stibialism
stibiated
stibium
stibophen
stichochrome
stiff
stiff joint
stiff man syndrome
stiff neck
stiff-neck fever
stigma
stigma of degeneration
stigma, hysterical
stigma, psychic
stigmatic
stigmatism
stigmatization
stigmatometer
stilbestrol
stilet
stilette
stillbirth (SB)
stillborn
Still's disease
stillicidium
stillicidium lacrimarum

stillicidium narium
stillicidium urinae
Stilphostrol
  (diethylstilbestrol
  diphosphate)
Stimate (desmopressin
  acetate)
stimulant
stimulate
stimulation
stimulator
stimulator, long-acting
  thyroid
stimulus
stimulus, adequate
stimulus, chemical
stimulus, conditioned
stimulus, electric
stimulus, homologous
stimulus, iatrotropic
stimulus, liminal
stimulus, mechanical
stimulus, minimal
stimulus, nociceptive
stimulus, subliminal
stimulus, thermal
stimulus, threshold
stimulus, unconditioned
sting
stingray
S-T interval
stippling
stippling, gingival
stir (agit)
stirrup
stirrup bone
stitch
stitch abscess
stitch, Kelly-Stöeckel
stochastic model
stock
stock culture
stockinet
stocking
stoichiology
stoichiometry
stoke
Stokes-Adams syndrome

Stokes' disease
Stokes' law
Stokes' lens
stoma
stomach
stomach ache
stomach, bilocular
stomach cancer
stomach, cardiac
stomach, cascade
stomach, cow horn
stomach, foreign bodies
  in
stomach, hourglass
stomach intubation
stomach, leather-bottle
stomach pump
stomach, thoracic
stomach tooth
stomach tube
stomach, water-trap
stomachal
stomachalgia
stomachic
stomachoscopy
stomal
stomata
stomatal
stomatalgia
stomatic
stomatitis
stomatitis, aphthous
stomatitis, catarrhal
stomatitis, corrosive
stomatitis, diphtheritic
stomatitis, follicular
stomatitis, herpetic
stomatitis, membranous
stomatitis, mercurial
stomatitis, mycotic
stomatitis parasitica
stomatitis, simple
stomatitis, traumatic
stomatitis, ulcerative
stomatitis, vesicular
stomatitis, Vincent's
stomatodynia
stomatogastric

stomatognathic
stomatologist
stomatology
stomatomalacia
stomatomenia
stomatomy
stomatomycosis
stomatonecrosis
stomatonoma
stomatopathy
stomatoplasty
stomatorrhagia
stomatorrhaphy
stomatoscope
stomatotomy
stomion
stomocephalus
stomodeal
stomodeum
stone
stone, dental
stone, red
stone, salivary
Stone operation
stool
stool, bilious
stool, fatty
stool, lienteric
stool, pea soup
stool, rice water
stool softeners
stopcock
stop needle
stoppage
storax
storm
storm, renal
storm, thyroid
stout
Stoxil (idoxuridine)
strabismal
strabismic
strabismometer
strabismus
strabismus, accommodative
strabismus, alternating
strabismus, concomitant
strabismus, convergent

strabismus, deorsum
  vergens
strabismus, divergent
strabismus, horizontal
strabismus, intermittent
strabismus, monocular
strabismus, monolateral
strabismus,
  nonconcomitant
strabismus, paralytic
strabismus, spastic
strabismus, sursum
  vergens
strabismus, vertical
strabometer
strabotome
strabotomy
strain
strainer
strain x-ray
strait
strait, inferior
straits of pelvis
strait, superior
straitjacket
stramonium
stramonium poisoning
strand
strangalesthesia
strangle
strangulated
strangulation
strangulation, internal
strangury
strap
strap, Montgomery
strapping
Strassman hysterectomy
stratification
stratified
stratified epithelium
stratiform
stratum
stratum basale
stratum compactum
stratum corneum
stratum disjunction
stratum germinativum

stratum granulosum
stratum lucidum
stratum malpighii
stratum mucosum
stratum papillare
stratum reticulare
stratum spinosum
stratum spongiosum
stratum submucosum
stratum subserosum
stratum supravasculare
stratum vasculare
strawberry mark
strawberry tongue
Strayer operation
streak
streak, angioid
streak, medullary
streak, meningitic
streak, Moore's lightning
streak, primitive
stream
strength
strength, breaking
strength, compression
strength, ego
strength, impact
strength, sheer
strephosymbolia
strepitus
strep quick test
Streptase (streptokinase)
strepticemia
streptoangina
streptobacillus
streptococcal
streptococcemia
streptococci
streptococcic
streptococcicosis
streptococcolysin
Streptococcus
Streptococcus pneumoniae
Streptococcus pyogenes
*Streptococcus
  thermophilus*
Streptococcus viridans
streptococcus (strep)

streptococcus ß-hemolytic
streptocolysin
streptodermatitis
streptodornase
streptokinase (STK)
streptokinase-
  streptodornase
streptoleukocidin
streptolysin
streptolysin O
streptolysin S
streptomycin sulfate
streptomycosis
streptosepticemia
streptothricin
streptothricosis
stress
stress-breaker
stress fracture
stress radiography
stress test
stress ulcer
stress urinary
  incontinence (SUI)
Stresscaps (stress
  formula B+C vitamins)
stressor
stressor, systemic
stressor, topical
Stresstabs 600 with Iron
  (stress formula
  vitamins with iron)
Stresstabs 600 with Zinc
  (stress formula
  vitamins with zinc)
stretch
stretch marks
stretch receptor
stretch reflex
stretcher
stretching
stretching, eyelid
stretching, fascia
stretching, foreskin
stretching, iris
stretching, muscle
stretching, nerve

stretching of
  contractures
stretching, tendon
stria
striae acusticae
striae atrophica
striae cerebellares
striae distensae
striae gravidarum
striae longitudinalis
  lateralis
striae medullares
striae of Retzius
striae terminalis
striatal
striate
striated
striated arteries
striated body
striated muscle
striated veins, inferior
striation
striatum
stricture
stricture, annular
stricture, anorectal
stricture, bridle
stricture, cicatricial
stricture, functional
stricture, impermeable
stricture, irritable
stricture, spasmodic
stricture of urethra
stricturotome
stricturotomy
stride length
strident
stridor
stridor, congenital
  laryngeal
stridor dentium
stridor serraticus
stridulous
string-of-pearls
  deformity
string sign
striocerebellar

strip
stripping, bone
stripping, carotid sinus
stripping, cranial suture
stripping, fascia
stripping, hand
stripping, membranes-
  induction of labor
stripping, meninges
stripping, saphenous
  veins
stripping, subdural
  membrane
stripping, varicose veins
stripping, vocal cords
strobila
strobiloid
stroboscope
stroke
stroke, heat
stroke, paralytic
stroke volume
stroking
stroma
stromal
stromatic
stromatolysis
stromatosis
Stromeyer-Little
operation
Stromeyer's splint
stromuhr
Strong operation
Strongyloides
Strongyloides stercoralis
strongyloidosis
strongylosis
Strongylus
strontium (Sr)
Strophanthus
strophocephaly
structural
structure
structure, denture
  supporting
struma aberranta
struma, cast iron
struma congenita

struma lingualis
struma lymphomatosa
struma maligna
struma ovarii
struma, Riedel's
strumectomy
strumiprivous
strumitis
strumous
Strümpell's disease
Strümpell-Marie disease
Strümpell's sign
struvite
strychnine
strychnine poisoning
strychninism
strychnism
Stryker frame
Stuart factor
Stuart Prenatal
  (multivitamin/multi-
  mineral supplement)
Stuartinic (hematinic)
study, case-control
stump
stump hallucination
stun
stupe
stupefacient
stupefactive
stupemania
stupor
stupor, anergic
stupor, delusional
stupor, epileptic
stupor, lethargic
stupor melancholicus
stuporous
stuporous depression
Sturge-Weber syndrome
sturine
Sturmdorf operation
stutter
stuttering
stuttering, urinary
sty(e)
stye
sty, meibomian

sty, zeisian
style
stylet
styliform
styliscus
styloglossus
stylohyal
stylohyoid
stylohyoideus
styloid
styloidectomy
styloiditis
styloid process
stylomandibular
stylomastoid
stylopharyngeus
stylostaphyline
stylosteophyte
stylus
stype
stypsis
styptic
subabdominal
subabdominoperitoneal
subacetate
subacid
subacromial
subacromial bursa
subacute
subacute bacterial
  endocarditis (SBE)
subacute myelo-optic
  neuropathy (SMON)
subacute sclerosing
  panencephalitis (SSPE)
subalimentation
subanal
subanconeus
subapical
subaponeurotic
subarachnoid
subarachnoid cisternae
subarachnoid injection
subarachnoid shunt
subarachnoid space
subarcuate
subarcuate fossa
subareolar

subastragalar
subastringent
subatomic
subaural
subauricular
subaxial
subaxillary
subbrachycephalic
subcalcarine
subcapsular
subcarbonate
subcartilaginous
subception
subchondral
subchronic
subclass
subclavian
subclavian artery
subclavian-axillary
  bypass graft
subclavian-carotid bypass
  graft
subclavian shunt
subclavian steal syndrome
subclavian triangle
subclavian vein
subclavian-vertebral
  bypass graft
subclavicular
subclavius
subclinical
subcollateral
subconjunctival
subconjunctival foreign
  body
subconsciousness
subcontinuous
subcontinuous fever
subcoracoid
subcortex
subcortical
subcortical electrodes
subcortical structure
subcostal
subcostalgia
subcranial
subcrepitant
subcrureus

subculture
subcutaneous
subcutaneous fasciotomy
subcutaneous fistulectomy
subcutaneous fistulotomy
subcutaneous injection
subcutaneous mastectomy
subcutaneous
  musculoaponeurotic
  system flap
subcutaneous placement of
  neurostimulator
subcutaneous surgery
subcutaneous tenotomy
subcutaneous tissue
subcutaneous vulvectomy
subcutaneous wound
subcuticular
subcutis
subdelirium
subdeltoid
subdeltoid calcareous
  deposits
subdental
subdermal
subdiaphragmatic abscess
  drainage
subdorsal
subduct
subdural
subdural burr holes
subdural catheter
subdural injection
subdural laminectomy
subdural puncture
subdural shunt
subdural space
subdural tap
subendothelial
subendothelium
subependymal
subepidermal
subepithelial
suberosis
subfamily
subfascial
subfascial benign tumor
  excision

subfascial ligation of
  perforators
subfebrile
subfertility
subflavous
subflavous ligament
subfolium
subfrontal
subgenus
subgingival
subglenoid
subglossal
subglossitis
subglottic
subgranular
subgrondation
subgrundation
subhepatic
subhyaloid
subicteric
subicular
subiliac
subilium
subincision
subinfection
subinflammation
subintimal
subintrant
subintrant fever
subinvolution
subjacent
subject
subjective
subjective, objective,
  assessment, plan (SOAP)
subjective sensation
subjective symptoms
subjugal
sublatio
sublatio retinae
sublation
sublesional
sublethal
sublethal dose
sublimate
sublimation
Sublimaze (fentanyl
  citrate)

sublime
subliminal
subliminal self
sublimis
sublimis transfer
sublingual
sublingual abscess
  drainage
sublingual gland
sublingual salivary cyst
sublingual sialolithotomy
sublinguitis
sublobular
sublumbar
subluxation
submammary
submandibular
submandibular gland
submandibularitis
submarginal
submaxilla
submaxillary
submaxillary abscess
  drainage
submaxillary gland
  excision
submaxillary
  sialolithotomy
submedial
submedian
submembranous
submental
submerge
submetacentric
submicron
submicroscopic
submorphous
submucosa
submucous
submucous resection (SMR)
submucous resection and
  rhinoplasty (SMRR)
subnarcotic
subnasal
subnasal pint
subnasale
subnasion
subneural

subnormal
subnormality
subnucleus
suboccipital
suboccipital craniectomy
suboperculum
suboptimal
suborder
suboxides
subpapular
subparietal
subpectoral
subpeduncular
subpeduncular lobe
subpericardial
subperiosteal
subperitoneal
subperitoneoabdominal
subpharyngeal
subphrenic
subphrenic abscess
subphrenic abscess
  drainage
subphylum
subpial
subplacenta
subpleural
subpontine
subpreputial
subpubic
subpulmonary
subpyramidal
subretinal
subcapular
subscleral
subsclerotic
subscription
subserous
subsibilant
subsidence
subsistence
subspecies
subspinous
subspinous dislocation
substage
substance
substance, anterior
  perforated

substance, anterior
  pituitary-like
substance, black
substance, chromophilic
substance, colloid
substance, gray
substance, ground
substance, ketogenic
substance, medullary
substance, Nissl
substance P
substance, posterior
  perforated
substance, pressor
substance, reticular
substance, slow-reacting
substance, specific
  soluble (SSS)
substance, threshold,
  high
substance, threshold, low
substance, transmitter
substance, white
substance, white, of
  Schwann
substandard
substantia
substantia alba
substantia, cinerea
substantia ferruginea
substantia gelatinosa
substantia griesea
substantia nigra
substantia propria
  membranae tympani
substernal
substernomastoid
substituent
substitute
substitute, blood
substitution
substitution products
substitution therapy
substitutive
substitutive therapy
substrate
substratum
substructure

subsultus
subsultus tendinum
subsylvian
subtarsal
subtentorial
subterminal
subtetanic
subthalamic
subthalamic nucleus
subthalamus
subtile
subtilin
subtle
subtotal
subtraction
subtraction contrast
  studies
subtrapezial
subtribe
subtrochanteric
subtrochanteric femoral
  fracture treatment
subtrochlear
subtuberal
subtympanic
subumbilical
subumbilical space
subungual
subungual hematoma
subunguial
subunit
suburethral
subvaginal
subvalvular stenosis
  resection, aortic valve
subvertebral
subvirile
subvitrinal
subvolution
subwaking
subzonal
subzygomatic
succagogue
succedaneous
succedaneum
succenturiate
succi
succinate

succinic acid
succinylcholine chloride
succinylsulfathiazole
succorrhea
succubus
succus
succus entericus
succus gastricus
succus pyloricus
succussion
suck
sucking pad
suckle
Sucostrin Chloride
  (succinylcholine
  chloride)
sucrase
sucrose
sucrose polyester
sucrosemia
sucrosuria
suction
suction, post-tussive
suction abortion
suction biopsy
suction lipectomy
suctorial
Sudafed (pseudephedrine
  HCl)
sudamen
sudamina
sudaminal
Sudan
sudanophil
sudanophilia
sudanophilic
sudation
sudatoria
sudatorium
sudden death (SD)
sudden death syndrome
  (SDS)
sudden infant death (SID)
sudden infant death
  syndrome (SIDS)
Sudeck's disease or
  atrophy
sudokeratosis

sudomotor
sudor
sudor cruentus
sudoral
sudoresis
sudoriferous
sudoriferous glands
sudorific
sudoriparous
suet
Sufenta (sufentanil
  citrate)
suffocate
suffocation
suffusion
sugar
sugar and acetone (S&A)
sugar, beet (sucrose)
sugar, blood (glucose)
sugar, brain (galactose)
sugar, cane (sucrose)
sugar, diabetic (glucose)
sugar, fruit (levulose or
  fructose)
sugar, grape (glucose)
sugar, invert (glucose
  and fructose)
sugar, liver (glycogen)
sugar, malt (maltose)
sugar, milk (lactose)
sugar, muscle (inositol)
sugar, starch (dextrin)
sugar, wood (xylose)
suggestibility
suggestible
suggestion
suggestion, auto-
suggestion, hypnotic
suggestion, posthypnotic
suggestive
suggestive medicine
suggestive therapeutics
suggillation
suicide
suicidology
suint
suit
suit, anti-G

sulcal
sulcal artery
sulcate
sulcated
sulci cutis
sulciform
sulculus
sulcus
sulcus, alveololingual
sulcus centralis
sulcus, collateral
sulcus, gingival
sulcus, hippocampal
sulcus, intraparietal
sulcus precentralis
sulcus pulmonalis
sulcus spiralis cochleae
Sulf-10 (sulfacetamide
  sodium)
sulfa drugs
Sulfacet-R (sodium
  sulfacetamide and
  sulfur)
sulfacetamide
sulfacetamide, sodium
sulfadiazine
sulfamerazine
sulfameter
sulfamethazine
sulfamethizole
sulfamethoxazole
Sulfamylon (mafenide
  acetate)
sulfanilamide
sulfapyridine
sulfapyridine, sodium
  monohydrate
sulfarsphenamine
sulfasalazine
sulfatase
sulfate
sulfate, cupric
sulfate, ferrous
sulfate, iron
sulfate, magnesium
sulfathiazole
sulfatide
sulfhemoglobin

sulfhemoglobinemia
sulfhydryl
sulfide
sulfinpyrazone
sulfisoxazole
sulfmethemoglobin
sulfobromophthalein
sulfonamides
sulfone
sulfourea
sulfoxide
sulfoxone sodium
sulfur (S)
sulfur dioxide
sulfur, precipitated
sulfur, sublimed
sulfurated
sulfurated hydrogen
sulfuric acid
sulfuric acid, dilute
sulfuric acid poisoning
Sultrin (triple sulfa
  cream and vaginal
  tablets)
sumac
sumac, poison
summation
summer
**Summer's Eve Medicated
  Douche** (povidone-iodine)
Summerskill operation
Sumycin '250' Tablets
  (tetracycline HCl)
Sumycin Syrup
  (tetracycline HCl)
sunburn
Sunday morning paralysis
sunflower eyes
sunglasses
sunscreen
sunscreen protective
  factor index
sunstroke
Supac (analgesic
  compound)
superabduction
superacidity
superacromial

superactivity
superacute
superalimentation
superalkalinity
superciliary
supercilium
superclass
superduct
superego
SuperEPA 1200 (fish oil
  omega-3 fatty acid
  concentrate)
superexcitation
superextension
superfamily
superfecundation
superfemale
superfetation
superficial
superficialis
superficial reflex
superficies
superflexion
supergenual
superimpregnation
superinduce
superinfection
superinvolution
superior
superior temporal-middle
  cerebral artery
  anastomosis (ST-MCA)
superiority complex
superjacent
superlactation
superlethal
supermedial
supermoron
supermotility
supernatant
supernate
supernumerary
supernumerary teeth
supernutrition
superolateral
superovulation
superoxide
superoxide dismutase

superparasite
superparasitism
superphosphate
supersaturate
superscription
supersecretion
supersensitiveness
supersoft
supersonic
superstructure
supertension
supervenosity
supervention
supervirulent
supervisor
supervitaminosis
supervoltage
supinate
supination
supinator
supinator longus reflex
supine
suppedania
supplemental
supplemental air
support
suppository
suppression
suppression of menses
suppurant
suppurate
suppuration
suppurative
suppurative fever
supra-acromial
supra-anal
suprabuccal
suprabulge
supracerebellar
supracervical
  hysterectomy
suprachoroid
suprachoroidea
suprachoroid lamina
supraciliary
supraclavicular
supraclavicular fossa
supraclavicular point

supracondylar
supracondylar fracture
supracondylar osteotomy
supracostal
supracotyloid
supradiaphragmatic
supraduction
supraepicondylar
supraglenoid
supraglenoid tuberosity
supraglottic
supraglottic laryngectomy
suprahepatic
suprahyoid
suprahyoid
  lymphadenectomy
suprahyoid muscles
suprainguinal
supraintestinal
supralevator abscess I&D
supraliminal
supralumbar
supramalleolar
supramammary
supramandibular
supramarginal
supramarginal convolution
supramastoid
supramastoid crest
supramaxilla
supramaxillary
suprameatal
suprameatal spine
suprameatal triangle
supramental
supranasal
supranuclear
supraoccipital
supraocclusion
supraorbital
supraorbital nerve
  destruction
supraorbital neuralgia
supraorbital notch
suprapatellar
suprapelvic
suprapontine
suprapubic

suprapubic aspiration of
  urine
suprapubic catheter
suprapubic catheter
  aspiration of bladder
suprapubic cystotomy
suprapubic prostatectomy
  (SPP)
suprapubic reflex
suprarenal
suprarenalectomy
sprarenal gland
suprarenalopathy
suprascapular
suprascapular nerve
  injection
suprascleral
suprasegmental
suprasegmental brain
suprasellar
suprasonic
supraspinal
supraspinatus tendon
  repair
supraspinous
supraspinous fossa
suprastapedial
suprasternal
suprasterol
suprasylvian
supratemporal
supratentorial
supratentorial burr holes
supratentorial
  craniectomy
supratentorial craniotomy
supratentorial
  decompression
suprathoracic
supratonsillar
supratrochlear
supratympanic
supravaginal
supravalvular stenosis
  aortoplasty
supraventricular
supravergence
supraversion

Suprol (suprofen)
sura
sural
suralimentation
suramin sodium
Surbex (vitamin B
  complex)
surditas
surdity
surdomute
surefooted
Surfacaine
  (cyclomethycaine
  sulfate)
surface
surface, body
surface tension
surfactant
surfactant, pulmonary
Surfak (docusate calcium)
surfer's knots
surgeon
surgeon, dental
surgeon general
surgery (surg)
surgery, aseptic
surgery, aural
surgery, conservative
surgery, cosmetic
surgery, major
surgery, maxillofacial
surgery, minor
surgery, mucogingival
surgery, oral
surgery, orthopedic
surgery, plastic
surgery, radical
surgical
surgical collapse therapy
surgical consultation
surgical diathermy
surgical dressing
surgical fever
surgical intensive care
  unit (SICU)
surgical neck
surgical pathology
surgical resident

surgical suture,
  absorbable
surgical suture,
  nonabsorbable
Surgicel (oxidized
  cellulose)
Surgicel Nu-Knit
  (absorable hemostat)
Surital (thiamylal
  sodium)
Surmay operation
Surmontil (trimipramine
  maleate)
surrogate
surrogate parenting
sursumduction
sursumvergence
sursumversion
surveillance
surveillance,
  immunological
survivor guilt
susceptibility
susceptible
suscitate
suscitation
sushi
suspended
suspension
suspension, cephalic
suspension, colloid
suspension, tendon
suspensoid
suspensory
suspensory bandage
suspensory ligament
Sus-Phrine (epinephrine)
suspiration
suspirious
Sustacal (nutritionally
  complete food)
Sustagen (nutritional
  supplement)
Sustaire (anhydrous
  theophylline)
sustentacular
sustentacular cell

sustentacular fibers of
  Müller
sustentaculum
sustentaculum hepatis
sustentaculum lienis
sustentaculum tali
susurrus
sutilains
Sutton's disease
Sutton's law
sutura
sutura dentata
sutura, harmonia
sutura limbosa
sutura notha
sutura serrata
sutura squamosa
sutura vera
sutural
sutural joint
sutural ligament
suturation
suture
suture, absorbable
  surgical
suture, Acutrol
suture, Albert's
suture, Alcon's
suture, Allison's
suture, alternating
suture, angle
suture, Appolito's
suture, apposition
suture, approximation
suture, Argyll-Robertson
suture, Arlt's
suture, Atroloc
suture, Axedfeld's
suture, Babcock's
suture, back-and-forth
suture, Barraquer's
suture, baseball
suture, basilar
suture, Beclard's
suture, Bell's
suture, bifrontal
suture, biparietal
suture, black silk

suture, black-braided
suture, blanket
suture, bolster
suture, Bozeman's
suture, braided
suture, bridle
suture, bunching
suture, Bunnell's
suture, buried
suture, button
suture, cable wire
suture, capitonnage
suture, cardiovascular
suture, catgut
suture, celluloid
suture, chain
suture, chromic catgut
suture, circular
suture, circumcision
suture, clavate
suture, Coakley's
suture, coaptation
suture, cobbler's
suture, collagen
suture, compound
suture, Connell's
suture, continuous
suture, corneoscleral
suture, coronal
suture, cranial
suture, Cushing's
suture, cutaneous
suture, Czerny's
suture, Czerny-Lembert
suture, dacron
suture, dekalon
suture, deknatel
suture, delayed
suture, dentate
suture, dermal
suture, Dermalene
suture, Dexon
suture, double-armed
suture, double-button
suture, dulox
suture, Dupuytren's
suture, Duvergier's
suture, edge-to-edge

suture, elastic
suture, Emmet's
suture, Equisetene
suture, Ethibond
suture, Ethicon
suture, Ethiflex
suture, Ethilon
suture, ethmoidofrontal
suture, ethmoidolacrimal
suture, ethmoidomaxillary
suture, ethmoidosphenoid
suture, everting
suture, false
suture, far and near
suture, figure-of-eight
suture, fixation
suture, Flaxedil
suture, Flexiton
suture, Flexon
suture, free ligature
suture, frontal
suture, frontolacrimal
suture, frontomalar
suture, frontomaxillary
suture, frontonasal
suture, frontoparietal
suture, frontotemporal
suture, Frost's
suture, furrier's
suture, Gaillard-Arlt
suture, Gambee's
suture, Gely's
suture, Gibson's
suture, glover's
suture, Gould's
suture, groove
suture, Gussenbauer's
suture, gut chromic
suture, Guyton-
  Friedenwald
suture, Halsted's
suture, harmonic
suture, Harris
suture, helical
suture, hemostatic
suture, horizontal
  mattress
suture, horsehair

suture, implanted
suture, interlocking
suture, intermaxillary
suture, internasal
suture, interparietal
suture, interrupted
suture, intradermal
suture, inverted
suture, Ivalon's
suture, Jobert's
suture, Kalt's
suture, kangaroo tendon
suture, Kelly's
suture, Kirby's
suture, Kirschner's
suture, lace
suture, lambdoid
suture, Le Drar's
suture, LeFort's
suture, Lembert's
suture, ligatiot
suture, limbal
suture, Littre's
suture, living
suture, lock-stitch
suture, locking
suture, Loffler's
suture, longitudinal
suture, loop
suture, Marlex
suture, mattress
suture, Maunsell's
suture, maxillolacrimal
suture, Mayo-linen
suture, mediofrontal
suture, Medrafil's wire
suture, Meigs'
suture, monofilament
suture, metopic
suture, multifilament
suture, multistrand
suture, nasomaxillary
suture, near-and-far
suture, Neurolon
suture, nonabsorbable
suture, nonabsorbable
  surgical
suture, noose

suture, nylon
  monofilament
suture, occipital
suture, occipitomastoid
suture, occipitoparietal
suture, over-and-over
suture, overlapping
suture, palatine
suture, palatine
  transverse
suture, Palfyn's
suture, Pancoast's
suture, Pare's
suture, parietal
suture, parietomastoid
suture, Parker-Kerr
suture, pericostal
suture, Petit's
suture, petro-occipital
suture, petrosphenoidal
suture, pin
suture, plain catgut
suture, plastic
suture, plicating
suture, Polydek
suture, polyester
suture, polyethylene
suture, polyfilament
suture, polypropylene
suture, presection
suture, primary
suture, prolene
suture, pull-out wire
suture, pulley
suture, purse-string
suture, quilled
suture, quilted
suture, Ramdohr's
suture, reinforcing
suture, relaxation
suture, relief
suture, retention
suture, ribbon gut
suture, Richardson's
suture, Richter's
suture, Rigal's
suture, right-angled
suture, rubber

suture, running
  continuous
suture, Saenger's
suture, sagittal
suture, secondary
suture, seminal
suture, seromuscular
suture, serrated
suture, shotted
suture, silk
suture, silk-braided
suture, silkworm gut
suture, silver wire
suture, Simon's
suture, Sims'
suture, single-armed
suture, sling
suture, sphenosquamous
suture, sphenotemporal
suture, spiral
suture, squamoparietal
suture, squamosphenoidal
suture, squamous
suture, stainless steel
suture, staple
suture, steel mesh
suture, stick-tie
suture, Sturmdorf's
suture, subcuticular
suture, superficial
suture, support
suture, Supramid
suture, surgical
suture, Surgilene
suture, Surgilon
suture, Surgilope
suture, tantalum-wire
suture, Taylor's
suture, temporo-occipital
suture, temporoparietal
suture, tendon
suture, tension
suture, Tevdek
suture, Thermo-flex
suture, Thiersch's
suture, through-and-
  through
suture, tiger gut

suture, Tom-Jones
suture, tongue-and-groove
suture, traction
suture, transfixing
suture, twisted
suture, Tycron
suture, unabsorbable
suture, uninterrupted
suture, Verhoeff's
suture, vertical mattress
suture, Vicryl
suture, Viro-Tec
suture, visceroparietal
suture, whipstitch
suture, white braided
suture, white silk
suture, wire
suture, Wolfler's
suture, Wysler's
suture, Y
suture, Z
suture, Zytor's
suxamethonium chloride
SV-40 virus
swab
swab, test tube
swab, urethral
swab, uterine
swaddling
swage
swallow
swallowing
swallowing, air
swallowing function test
swallowing, tongue
swallow's nest
Swan-Ganz catheter
swan neck deformity
Swanson osteotomy
swarming
sway-back
sweat
sweat, bloody
sweat centers
sweat collection by
  iontophoresis
sweat, colliquative
sweat, colored

sweat, fetid
sweat glands
sweat, night
sweat, profuse
sweat, scanty
sweating
sweating, deficiency of
sweating, excessive
sweating, insensible
sweating, sensible
sweating, urinous
Swedish gymnastics
Swedish massage
Sween Cream (protective
  cream)
Sween Prep (protective
  skin barrier film)
Sween-A-Peel (wafer skin
  protectant)
sweep, anterior iris
sweet
Sweet's syndrome
swelling
swelling, albuminous
swelling, Calabar
swelling, cloudy
swelling, fugitive
swelling, glassy
swelling, white
Swenson proctectomy
Swift's disease
swimmer's ear
swimmer's itch
Swinney operation
switch
switch, foot
switch, pole-changing
swoon
sycoma
sycophant
sycosiform
sycosis
sycosis, barbae
sycosis, lupoid
sycosis, vulgaris
Sydenham's chorea
syllabic utterance
syllable stumbling

syllabus
syllepsis
sylvatic plague
sylvian aqueduct
sylvian artery
sylvian fissure
sylvian line
symballophone
symbion
symbiont
symbiosis
symbiote
symbiotic
symblepharon
symblepharopterygium
symbol
symbol, phallic
symbolia
symbolism
symbolization
symbolophobia
symbrachydactyly
symdesmotomy
Syme's amputation
symmelia
symmelus
Symmetrel (amantadine HCl)
symmetromania
symmetry
symmetry, bilateral
symmetry, radial
sympathectomize
sympathectomy
sympathectomy, chemical
sympathectomy, periarterial
sympatheoneuritis
sympathetic
sympatheticalgia
sympathetic nervous system
sympatheticoparalytic
sympatheticopathy
sympathetic ophthalmia
sympatheticotonia
sympatheticotonic
sympatheticotripsy

sympathetic plexuses
sympathetoblast
sympathic
sympathicectomy
sympathicoblast
sympathicoblastoma
sympathicolytic
sympathicomimetic
sympathiconeuritis
sympathicopathy
sympathicotonia
sympathicotripsy
sympathicotropic
sympathicus
sympathism
sympathist
sympathoadrenal
sympathoblast
sympathoblastoma
sympathoglioblastoma
sympathogonia
sympathogonioma
sympatholytic
sympathoma
sympathomimetic
sympathy
sympexion
sympexis
symphalangism
symphyogenetic
symphyseal
symphyseotomy
symphysiectomy
symphysion
symphysiorrhaphy
symphysiotomy
symphysis
symphysis cartilaginosa
symphysis ligamentosa
symphysis mandibulae
symphysis menti
symphysis of jaw
symphysis pubis
symphysodactyly
symplasm
sympodia
symporter
symptom (Sx)

symptom, accessory
symptom, accidental
symptom, assident
symptom, cardinal
symptom complex
symptom, concomitant
symptom, constitutional
symptom, delayed
symptom, direct
symptom, dissociation
symptom, equivocal
symptom, focal
symptom, general
symptom, indirect
symptom, labyrinthine
symptom, local
symptom, negative
  pathognomonic
symptom, objective
symptom, passive
symptom, pathognomonic
symptom, presenting
symptom's, prodromal
symptom, rational
symptom, signal
symptom, static
symptom, subjective
symptom, sympathetic
symptom's, withdrawal
symptomatic
symptomatology
symptomatolytic
symptomolytic
symptosis
sympus
synache
Synacort (hydrocortisone)
synactosis
synadelphus
Synalar (fluocinolone
  acetonide)
Synalar-HP (fluocinolone
  acetonide)
synalgia
synalgic

Synalgos-DC
  (dihydrocodeine
  bitartrate, aspirin and
  caffeine)
synapse
synapse, axodendritic
synapse, axodendrosomatic
synapse, axosomatic
synapsis
synaptic cleft
synaptic field
synaptolemma
synaptology
synarthrodia
synarthrodial
synarthrophysis
synarthrosis
syncanthus
syncaryon
syncephalus
synchilia
synchiria
synchondroseotomy
synchondrosis
synchondrotomy
synchorial
synchronism
synchronous
synchrotron
synchysis
synchysis scintillans
syncinesis
syncinesis, imitative
syncinesis, spasmodic
synciput
synclinical
synclitism
synclonus
synclonus ballismus
synclonus tremens
syncopal
syncope
syncope anginosa
syncope, cardiac
syncope, carotid sinus

syncope, cough
syncope, defecation
syncope, hysterical
syncope, laryngeal
syncope, local
syncope, micturition
syncope, swallow
syncope, vasovagal
syncopic
syncretio
syncytial
syncytiolysin
syncytioma
syncytioma benignum
syncytioma malignum
syncytiotrophoblast
syncytium
syndactylism
syndactylous
syndectomy
syndesis
syndesmectomy
syndesmectopia
syndesmitis
syndesmochorial
syndesmography
syndesmologia
syndesmology
syndesmoma
syndesmopexy
syndesmophyte
syndesmoplasty
syndesmorrhaphy
syndesmosis
syndesmotomy
syndrome
syndrome, Adair-Dighton
syndrome, adiposogenital
syndrome, adrenogenital
syndrome, angelucci's
syndrome, dumping
syndrome, Fröhlich's
syndrome, Gilles de la
  Tourette's
syndrome, Gradenigo's
syndrome, Horner's
syndrome, Korsakoff's
syndrome, Marfan's

syndrome, sick-sinus
syndrome, skin-eye
syndrome, Stokes-Adams
syndrome, toxic shock
syndrome, Weber's
syndromic
synechia
synechia, annular
synechia, anterior
synechia, posterior
synechia, total
synechia, vulvae
synechotome
synechotomy
synechtenterotomy
synecology
Synemol (fluocinolone
  acetonide)
synencephalocele
syneresis
synergetic
synergia
synergic
synergism
synergist
synergistic
synergy
synesthesia
synesthesia algica
synesthesialgia
synezesis
Syngamus
Syngamus laryngeus
syngamy
syngeneic
syngenesioplasty
syngenesious
syngenesis
syngnathia
synhidrosis
synizesis
synizesis pupillae
synkaryon
Synkayvite (menadiol
  sodium diphosphate)
synkinesis
synkinesis, imitative
synnecrosis

synonym (syn)
synophrys
synophthalmus
synopsia
synopsis
synoptophore
synoptoscope
synorchidism
synorchism
synoscheos
synosteology
synosteosis
synosteotomy
synostosis
synostotic
synotia
synotus
synovectomy
synovia
synovial
synovial biopsy
synovial bursa
synovial crypt
synovial cyst
synovial fluid
synovial folds
synovial hernia
synovialis
synovial membrane
synovialoma
synovial tendon sheaths
synovial villi
synovioma
synoviparous
synovitis
synovitis, chronic
synovitis, dendritic
synovitis, dry
synovitis, purulent
synovitis, serous
synovitis, sicca
synovitis, simple
synovitis, tendinous
synovitis, vaginal
synovitis, vibration
synovium
syntactic
syntasis

syntaxis
syntectic
syntexis
synthase
synthermal
synthesis
synthesize
synthetase
synthetic
synthetic sentence
   identification test
synthorax
Synthroid (levothyroxine
   sodium)
Syntocinon (oxytocin)
Syntocinon Nasal Spray
   (oxytocin nasal
   solution)
syntone
syntonic
syntonin
syntoxoid
syntripsis
syntrophism
syntrophoblast
syntropic
syntropy
synulosis
synulotic
syphilelcosis
syphilelcus
syphilid
syphilide
syphilionthus
syphiliphobia
syphilis
syphilis, cardiovascular
syphilis, congenital
syphilis, extragenital
syphilis insontium
syphilis, latent
syphilis, meningovascular
syphilis, neuro-
syphilis, nonvenereal
syphilis, prenatal
syphilis, visceral
syphilitic
syphilitic fever

syphilitic macules
syphiloderm
syphiloderma
syphilogenesis
syphilogeny
syphilographer
syphilography
syphiloid
syphilology
syphiloma
syphilomania
syphilopathy
syphilophobia
syhphilophobic
syphilophyma
syphilosis
syphilotherapy
syphilotropic
syphilous
syphionthus
syrigmophonia
syrigmus
syringadenoma
syringe
syringe, hypodermic
syringe, oral
syringectomy
syringing, lacrimal duct
  or sac
syringing, nasolacrimal
  duct
syringitis
syringoadenoma
syringobulbia
syringocarcinoma
syringocele
syringocystadenoma
syringocystoma
syringoencephalomyelia
syringoid
syringoma
syringomeningocele
syringomyelia
syringomyelitis
syringomyelocele
syringomyelus
syringopontia
syringosystrophy

syringotome
syringotomy
syrinx
syrup (syr)
syssarcosis
systaltic
system
system, alimentary
system, autonomic nervous
system, cardiovascular
system, centimeter-gram-
  second
system, central nervous
system, chromaffin
system, circulatory
system, conduction, of
  the heart
system, cytochrome
system, digestive
system, endocrine
system, extrapyramidal
  motor
system, genital
system, genitourinary
system, haversian
system, hematopoietic
system, homogeneous
system, hypophyseoportal
system, impulse-
  conducting
system, integumentary
system, lymphatic
system, metric
system, muscular
system, nervous
system, osseous
system, parasympathetic
  nervous
system, peripheral
  nervous
system, portal
system, reproductive
system, respiratory
system,
  reticuloendothelial
  (RES)
system review (SR)
system, skeletal

system, skeletal
system, sympathetic
  nervous
System of Units,
  International (SI)
system, urinary
system, urogenital
system, vascular
system, vasomotor
system, vegetative
  nervous
system, visceral
  efferent
systema
systematic
systematization
systemic
systemic circulation
systemic lupus
  erythematosus (SLE)
systemic remedies
systemoid
systems theory
systole
systole, aborted
systole, anticipated
systole, arterial
systole, atrial
systole, electrical
systole, extra-
systole, premature
systole, ventricular
systolic
systolic discharge
systolic murmur
systolic pressure
systremma
Sytobex (cyanocobalamin)
syzygial
syzygiology
syzygium
syzygy

T

T-Diet (phentermine HCl)
T-Dry (pseudoephedrine
  HCl)
T fracture
T-group
T-lymphocytes
T-Stat (erythromycin)
T-tube biliary duct stone
  extraction
tabacism
tabacosis
tabacum
tabagism
tabanid
Tabanidae
Tabanus
tabardillo
tabatière anatomique
tabella
tabes
tabes, diabetic
tabes dorsalis
tabes ergotica
tabes mesenterica
tabescent
tabetic
tabetic crisis
tabetic foot
tabetiform
tabic
tabid
tablature
table
table, periodic
table, tilt
table, vitreous
table, water
tables, of skull
tablespoon (T, Tbs)
tablet, buccal
tablet, coated
tablet, compressed

tablet, dispensing
tablet, enteric-coated
tablet, fluoride
tablet, hypodermic
tablet, sublingual
tablet triturate
tablier
Tabloid (thioguanine)
taboo
taboparalysis
taboparesis
tabophobia
Tabron Filmseal
tabular
tabular bone
tabun
Tacaryl (methdilazine HCl)
TACE (chlorotrianisene)
tache
tache blanche
tache bleuatre
tache cérébrale
tache motrice
tache noire
tachetic
tachistoscope
tachogram
tachography
tachyarrhythmia
tachyauxesis
tachycardia
tachycardia, atrial
tachycardia, ectopic
tachycardia, essential
tachycardia, nodal
tachycardia, paroxysmal atrial
tachycardia, paroxysmal nodal
tachycardia, paroxysmal ventricular
tachycardia, polymorphic ventricular
tachycardia, reflex
tachycardia, sinus
tachycardia strumosa exophthalmica

tachycardia, ventricular
tachycardiac
tachylalia
tachymeter
tachyphagia
tachyphasia
tachyphemia
tachyphrasia
tachyphrenia
tachyphylaxis
tachypnea
tachypnea, nervous
tachyrhythmia
tachysterol
tachysystole
tachytrophism
Tack operation
tactile
tactile corpuscles
tactile defensiveness
tactile discrimination
tactile disk
tactile localization
tactile system
taction
tactometer
tactor
tactual
tactus
tactus eruditus
taedium vitae
taenia
taenia coli
taenia fimbriae
taenia pontis
taenia semicircularis
taenia thalami
taenia ventriculi tertii
Taenia
Taenia echinococcus
Taenia saginata
Taenia solium
taeniacide
taeniafuge
taeniasis
taeniform
taenifuge
taeniophobia

tag
tag, anus papillectomy
tag, hemorrhoidal
tag, radioactive
tag, skin
Tagamet (cimetidine HCl)
tagging
tagliacotian operation
tags, hemorrhoid excision
tail
tailgut
tailor's cramp
taint
Takayasu's arteritis
take
Talacen (pentazocine HCl
  and acetaminophen)
talalgia
talar
talbutal
talc
talcosis
talcum
talectomy
tali
talipedic
talipes
talipes arcuatus
talipes calcaneus
talipes cavus
talipes equinus
talipes percavus
talipes valgus
talipes varus
talipomanus
tallow
Talma-Morison operation
talocalcaneal
talocrural
talocrural articulation
talofibular
talon
talon noir
talonavicular
talonid
taloscaphoid
talotibial
talotibial capsulotomy

talus
Talwin (pentazocine
  lactate)
Talwin Compound
  (pentazocine HCl and
  aspirin)
Talwin Nx (pentazocine
  and naloxone HCl)
Tambocor (flecainide
  acetate)
tambour
Tamm-Horsfall mucoprotein
tamoxifen citrate
tampon
tampon, menstrual
tampon, Mikulicz's
tampon, nasal
tamponade
tamponade, balloon
tamponade, cardiac
tamponage
tamponing
tamponment
Tandearil
  (oxyphenbutazone)
tang
Tangier disease
tank, Hubbard
tannase
tannate
Tanner operation
tannic acid
tannin
tantalum (TA)
tantrum
TAO (troleandomycin)
tap
tap water (TW)
Tapar (acetaminophen)
Tapazole (methimazole)
tape
tape, adhesive
tapeinocephalic
tapeinocephaly
tapetum
tapetum choroideae
tapetum lucidum
tapeworm

tapeworm, armed (*Taenia solium*)
tapeworm, beef (*Taenia saginata*)
tapeworm, broad (*Diphyllobothrium latum*)
tapeworm, dog (*Dipylidium caninum*)
tapeworm, dwarf (*Hymenolepis nana*)
tapeworm, fish (*Diphyllobothrium latum*)
tapeworm, hydatid (*Echinococcccus granulosus*)
tapeworm, mouse (*Hymenolepis nana*)
tapeworm, pork (*Taenia solium*)
tapeworm, rat (*Hymenolepis nana*)
tapeworm, unarmed (*Taenia saginata*)
taphephobia
taphophilia
Tapia syndrome
tapinocephalic
tapinocephaly
tapiroid
tapotement
tapping
tar
tar, coal
tar, juniper
tar, pine
Taractan Ampuls (chlorprothixene HCl)
Taractan Concentrate (chlorprothixene lactate and HCl)
Taractan Tablet (chlorprothixene)
tarantism
tarantula
Tardieu's spots
tardive

tare
tared
tarentism
target
target cell
target organ
tarichatoxin
Tarnier's sign
tarnish
tarsadenitis
tarsal
tarsal arches
tarsal bones
tarsal cartilages
tarsal coalition osteotomy
tarsalgia
tarsal glands
tarsalis
tarsal lacrimal glands
tarsal plate transposition
tarsal tunnel
tarsal tunnel release
tarsal tunnel syndrome
tarsal wedge osteotomy
tarsectomy
tarsectopia
tarsi
tarsitis
tarsocheiloplasty
tarsoclasia
tarsoclasis
tarsolevator resection
tarsomalacia
tarsomegaly
tarsometatarsal
tarsometatarsal joint arthrodesis
tarsometatarsal joint arthrotomy
tarsometatarsal joint dislocation
tarsometatarsal joint synovectomy
tarso-orbital
tarsophalangeal

tarsophyma
tarsoplasia
tarsoplasty
tarsoptosis
tarsorrhaphy
tarsotarsal
tarsotibial
tarsotomy
tarsus
tarsus inferior palpebrae
tarsus superior palpebrae
tartar
tartar, cream of
tartar emetic
tartaric acid
tart cells
tartrate
tartrazine
taste
taste, after
taste area
taste blindness
taste buds
taste cells
taster
tattoo
tattooing
tattooing, traumatic
Tatum-T (intrauterine
  copper contraceptive)
taurine
taurocholate
taurocholemia
taurocholic acid
taurodontism
Taussig-Bing syndrome
tautomenial
tautomer
tautomeral
tautomeric
tautomerase
tautomerism
tautorotation
Tavist (clemastine
  fumarate)
Tavist-1 (clemastine
  fumarate)

Tavist-D (clemastine
  fumarate,
  phenylpropanolamine
  HCl)
taxis
taxis, bipolar
taxon
taxonomic
taxonomy
Taylor brace
Tay-Sachs disease (TSD)
Tazicef (ceftazidime)
Tazidime (ceftazidime)
T bandage
T-bar
T cells
tea
tea, black
tea, green
tea, Paraguay copper
tear
tear duct, test of
  patency of
tears
tears, artificial
tears, crocodile
tease
teaspoon (tsp)
teat
teatulation
technetium (Tc)
technetium-99m
technetium Tc 99m albumin
  aggregated injection
technic
technical
technician
technician, biomedical
  engineering
technician, dental
technician, dialysis
technician, dietetic
technician,
  electrocardiographic
technician,
  electromyographic
technician, emergency
  medical

technician, emergency-
   paramedic
technician, environmental
   health
technician, histologic
technician, medical
   laboratory
technician, medical
   record
technician, orthopedic
technician, pharmacy
technician, psychiatric
technician, respiratory
   therapy
technique
technologist
technologist, blood bank
technologist,
   cardiovascular
technologist, cyto-
technologist,
   electroencephalographic
technologist, histologic
technologist, medical
technologist, nuclear
   medicine
technologist, radiation
   therapy
technologist, radiologic
technologist, surgical
technology
tectocephalic
tectocephaly
tectorial
tectorium
tectospinal
tectospinal tract
tectum
tectum mesencephali
Tedral (theophylline,
   ephedrine, and
   phenobarbital)
Tedral SA
teenage
teeth
teeth, anterior
teeth, auditory

teeth, charting and
   numbering
teeth, deciduous
teeth, Hutchinson's
teeth, malacotic
teeth, milk
teeth, permanent
teeth, reimplantation or
   repair of
teeth, sclerotic
teeth, secondary
teeth, stained
teeth, temporary
teeth, wisdom
teething
Tegison (etretinate)
tegmen
tegmen mastoideum
tegmen tympani
tegmen ventriculi quarti
tegmental
tegmental nuclei
tegmentum
Tegopen (cloxacillin
   sodium)
Tegretol (carbamazepine)
tegument
tegumental
tegumentary
teichopsia
teinodynia
tela
tela choroidea
tela conjunctiva
tela elastica
tela subcutanea
tela submucosa
telalgia
telangiectasia
telangiectasia,
   hereditary hemorrhagic
telangiectasia,
   lymphatica
telangiectasia, spider
telangiectasis
telangiectatic
telangiectodes

telangiitis
telangioma
telangion
telangiosis
telarche
Teldrin (chlorpheniramine maleate)
telecanthus
telecardiogram
telecardiography
telecardiophone
teleceptive
teleceptor
telecinesia
telecurietherapy
teledendrite
teledendron
telediagnosis
telediastolic
Tel-E-Dose (Bactrim)
Tel-E-Dose (Bumex)
Tel-E-Dose (Dalmane)
Tel-E-Dose (Gantanol)
Tel-E-Dose (Gantrisin)
Tel-E-Dose (Librax)
Tel-E-Dose (Librium)
Tel-E-Dose (Limbitrol)
Tel-E-Dose (Trimpex)
Tel-E-Dose (Valium)
telefluoroscopy
telekinesis
telelectrocardiogram
telemeter
telemetry
telemnemonic
telencephalic
telencephalization
telencephalon
teleneurite
teleneuron
telelogical
teleology
teleomitosis
teleonomic
teleonomy
teleopsia
teleorganic
teleotherapeutics

Telepaque (iopanoic acid)
telepathist
telepathy
telephonic analysis
teleradiography
teleradium
telergy
teleroentgenogram
teleroentgenography
telesthesia
telesystolic
teletactor
teletherapy
teletypewriter (TTY)
telluric
tellurism
tellurium (Te)
tellurium poisoning
telocentric
teloceptor
telodendron
telogen
teloglia
telolecithal
telolemma
telomere
telophase
telophragma
telosynapsis
telotism
Temaril (trimeprazine tartrate)
Temovate (clobetasol propionate)
tempeh
temper
temperament
temperament assessment
temperate
temperature (T, temp)
temperature, absolute
temperature, ambient
temperature, axillary
temperature, body
temperature, core
temperature, critical
temperature gradient studies

temperature, inverse
temperature, maximum
temperature, mean
temperature, minimum
temperature, normal
temperature, optimum
temperature, oral
temperature, pulse,
  respiration (TPR)
temperature, rectal
temperature, room
temperature senses
temperature, subnormal
temper tantrums
template
template, occlusal
template, wax
temple
tempolabile
tempora
temporal
temporal bone
temporalis
temporal line
temporal lobe
temporoauricular
temporohyoid
temporomalar
temporomandibular (TM)
temporomandibular joint
  (TMJ)
temporomandibular joint
  syndrome
temporomaxillary
temporo-occipital
temporoparietal
temporopontine
temporosphenoid
temporozygomatic
tempostabile
Tempra (acetaminophen)
tenacious
tenacity
tenaculum
tenalgia
tenalgia crepitans

Tencet (acetaminophen,
  butalbital, and
  caffeine)
Tenckhoff peritoneal
catheter
tender loving care (TLC)
tenderizers
tenderness
tenderness, rebound
tendinitis
tendinoplasty
tendinosuture
tendinous
tendinous synovitis
tendolysis
tendon
tendon, Achilles
tendon, calcaneal
tendon cells
tendon, central
tendon, superior, of
  Lockwood
tendon of Zinn
tendonitis
tendon reflex
tendon reflex, patellar
tendon release (patellar
  retinacula)
tendon sheath dissection
tendon spindle
tendon transfer (biceps
  femoris tendon)
tendoplasty
tendosynovitis
tendosynovitis crepitans
tendotome
tendotomy
tendovaginal
tendovaginitis
Tenebrio
tenectomy
tenectomy, graduated
tenesmic
tenesmus
Tenex (guanfacine HCl)
tenia

teniasis
tenicide
tenifuge
Ten-K (potassium
  chloride)
tennis elbow
tenodesis
tenodesis splint
tenodynia
tenofibril
tenolysis
tenomyoplasty
tenomyotomy
Tenon's capsule
tenonectomy
tenonitis
tenonometer
Tenon's space
tenontitis
tenontodynia
tenontography
tenontolemmitis
tenontology
tenontomyoplasty
tenontomyotomy
tenontoplasty
tenontothecitis
tenontothecitis stenosans
tenophyte
tenoplastic
tenoplasty
tenoreceptor
Tenoretic (atenolol and
  chlorthalidone)
Tenormin (atenolol)
tenorrhaphy
tenositis
tenostosis
tenosuspension
tenosuture
tenosynovectomy
tenosynovitis
tenosynovitis crepitans
tenosynovitis
  hyperplastica
tenotome
tenotomist
tenotomy

tenovaginitis
tenovaginotomy
tense
Tensilon (edrophonium
  chloride)
Tensilon test for
  myasthenia gravis
tensing, orbicularis
  oculi
tensiometer
tension
tension, arterial
tension of gases
tension headache
tension, intraocular
tension, intravenous
tension, muscular
tension pneumothorax
tension, premenstrual
tension, surface
tension suture
tension, tissue
tensometer
tensor
tensor tympani muscle
tent
tent, oxygen
tent, sponge
tentacle
tentative
tenth cranial nerve
tentorial
tentorial notch
tentorial pressure cone
tentorium
tentorium cerebelli
Tenuate (diethylpropion
  HCl)
Tepanil (diethylpropion
  HCl)
Tepanil Ten-Tab
  (diethylpropion HCl)
tephromalacia
tephromyelitis
tephrosis
tephrylometer
tepid
tepidarium

tepor
ter in die (t.i.d.)
teracurie
teramorphous
teras
teratic
teratism
teratism, acquired
teratism, atresic
teratism, ceasmic
teratism, ectogenic
teratism, ectopic
teratism, hypergenic
teratism, symphysic
teratoblastoma
teratocarcinoma
teratogen
teratogenesis
teratogenetic
teratogenous
teratogeny
teratoid
teratoid tumor
teratologic
teratology
teratoma
teratomatous
teratophobia
teratosis
teratospermia
terbium (Tb)
terbutaline sulfate
terchloride
terebrant
terebration
teres
tergal
tergum
term
term, normal delivery
  (TND)
terminal
terminal bars
terminal cancer
terminal device
terminal ganglia
terminal illness
terminal infection

terminal veins
terminatio
termination
termination of pregnancy
terminology
terminus
ternary
teroxide
terpene
terpin hydrate
terra
terra alba
terra fullonica
terracing
Terra-Cortril
  (oxytetracycline HCl
  and hydrocortisone
  acetate)
Terramycin
  (oxytetracycline HCl)
Terramycin Ointment
  (oxytetracycline
  HCl/polymyxin B
  sulfate)
territoriality
terror
terror, night
tertian
tertiary
tertiary alcohol
tertiary care
tertiary syphilis
tertigravida
tertipara
tervone
Teslac (testolactone)
Tessalon (benzonatate)
tessellated
test
test, acetic acid
test, acetone
test, agglutination
test, alkali denaturation
test, Allen-Doisy
test, aptitude
test, Aschheim-Zondek
test, association
test, autohemolysis

test, biuret
test, challenge
test, chromatin
test, coin
test, complement-fixation
test, concentration
test, conjunctival
test, creatinine
  clearance
test, double-blind
test, finger-nose
test, Friedman
test, galactose tolerance
test, Gelle's
test, glucose tolerance
test, guaiac
test, hardness
test, histamine
test, Huhner
test, human repeated
  patch insult
test, intracutaneous
test, Kahn
test, McMurray
test, meal
test, multiple-puncture
test, neutralization
test, patch
test, precipitin
test, pregnancy
test, prothrombin
  consumption
test, pulp vitality
test, Rubin
test, Schiller's
test, Schwabach
test, scratch
test, serial sevens
test, serologic
test, sickling
test, standardized
test, thematic
  apperception
test, three-glass
test, tine
test, tolerance
test, tourniquet
test, tuberculin

test, urea balance
test, Wassermann
testa
testalgia
testectomy
testes
testicle
testicond
testicular
testis
testis, descent of
testis, displaced
testis, femoral
testis, inverted
testis, perineal
testis, rete
testis, undescended
testis compression reflex
testitis
testitoxicosis
testoid
testolactone
testopathy
testosterone
testosterone toxicology
  test
Testred
  (methyltestosterone)
test tube baby
test type
tetanic
tetanic convulsion
tetaniform
tetanigenous
tetanilla
tetanism
tetanization
tetanize
tetanode
testanoid
tetanoid paraplegia
tetanolysin
tetanomotor
tetanophil
tetanophilic
telanospasmin
tetanus
tetanus anticus

tetanus antitoxin
tetanus, artificial
tetanus, ascending
tetanus, cephalic
tetanus, cerebral
tetanus, chronic
tetanus, cryptogenic
tetanus, descending
tetanus dorsalis
tetanus, extensor
tetanus, hydrophobic
tetanus, idiopathic
tetanus, imitative
tetanus immune globulin
tetanus, infantum
tetanus lateralis
tetanus, local
tetanus neonatorum
tetanus paradoxus
tetanus, postoperative
tetanus, puerperal
tetanus, toxic
tetanus toxoid
**Tetanus and Diphtheria
Toxoids Absorbed
  Purogenated**
**Tetanus Toxoid, Absorbed
  Purogenated**
tetany
tetany, alkalotic
tetany, duration
tetany, epidemic
tetany, gastric
tetany, hyperventilation
tetany, hypocalcemic
tetany, latent
tetany, manifest
tetany, parathyroid
tetany, rachitic
tetany, thyreoprival
tetarcone
tetartanopia
tetartanopsia
tetartocone
tetrabasic
tetrablastic
tetrabrachius
tetrabromofluorescein

tetracaine hydrochloride
tetrachirus
tetrachlorethylene
tetrachloride
  2,3,7,8-
  tetrachlorodibenzo-p
  dioxin (TCDD)
tetracid
Tetracoccus
tetracrotic
tetracycline
tetrad
tetradactyly
tetraethylammonium
  chloride (TEAC)
tetraethylpyrophosphate
  (TEPP)
tetragenous
tetrahydrocannabinol THC
  (marijuana)
tetraiodothyronine (T_4)
tetralogy
tetralogy of Fallot
tetramastia
tetramastigote
tetramazia
tetrameric
tetramerous
tetranopsia
tetraotus
tetraparesis
tetrapeptide
tetraplegia
tetraploid
tetrapus
tetrasaccharide
tetrascelus
tetrasomic
tetraster
tetrastichiasis
tetratomic
tetravalent
Tetrex (tetracycline
  phosphate complex)
tetrodotoxin
tetrotus
tetroxide
Texacort (hydrocortisone)

texis
textiform
textoblastic
textural
texture
textus
Thal operation
Thal-Nissen procedure
thalamencephalon
thalamic
thalamic syndrome
thalamocele
thalamocoele
thalamocortical
thalamolenticular
thalamotomy
thalamus
thalassemia
thalassophobia
thalassoposia
thalassotherapy
thalidomide
Thalitone
  (chlorthalidone)
thallinization
thallitoxicosis
thallium (Tl)
thallium poisoning
thallium sulfate
THAM (tromethamine)
thamuria
thanatobiological
thanatognomonic
thanatoid
thanatology
thanatomania
thanatophidia
thanatophobia
thanatophoric
thanatophoric dwarfism
thaumaturgic
Thayer-Martin medium
The Stuart Formula
  (multivitamin/
  multimineral
  supplement)
theaism

thebaic
thebaine
thebesian foramina
thebesian valve
thebesian veins
theca
theca cordis
theca folliculi
thecal
thecitis
thecodont
thecoma
thecomatosis
thecostegnosia
thecostegnosis
Theelin (estrone)
theine
theinism
thelalgia
thelarche
thelasis
Thelazia
thelaziasis
theleplasty
thelerethism
thelitis
thelium
theloncus
thelophlebostemma
thelorrhagia
thelothism
thelygenic
thenad
thenal
thenal aspect
thenar
thenar cleft
thenar eminence
thenar fascia
thenar muscles
Theo-24 (theophylline,
  anhydrous)
Theobid (theophylline,
  anhydrous)
theobromine
Theochron (theophylline,
  anhydrous)

Theoclear (theophylline anhydrous)
Theo-Dur (theophylline, anhydrous)
Theolair (anhydrous theophylline)
Theolair Plus (anhydrous theophylline and guaifenesin)
theomania
Theo-Organidin (bronchodilator/ mucolytic-expectorant)
Theon Syrup (theophylline and alcohol)
theophobia
theophylline
theophylline ethylenediamine
theophylline olamine
theoplylline sodium glycinate
theophylline (Theodur) toxicology test
theorem
theorem, Bayes
theory
theory, cell
theory, clonal selection, of immunity
theory, germ
theory, quantum
theory, recapitulation
Theospan-SR (theophylline, anhydrous)
Theostat (theophylline, anhydrous)
theotherapy
Theovent (theophylline, anhydrous)
thèque
Thera-Flur (acidulated phosphate fluoride)
Thera-Flur-N (neutral sodium fluoride)
Therabid (multivitamin)

Theragran Hematinic (vitamin tablets with hematinics)
Theragran Jr. (children's chewable vitamin formula)
Theragran Liquid (high potency vitamin supplement)
Theragran Stress Formula (multivitamin with iron and biotin)
Theragran Tablets (high potency multivitamin formula)
Theragran-M Tablets (high potency multivitamin formula, minerals)
Theralax (bisacodyl)
therapeusis
therapeutic
therapeutic abortion (TA)
therapeutic exercise
therapeutic recreation
therapeutics
therapia sterilisans magna
therapist
therapist, occupational
therapist, physical
therapist, radiation
therapist, respiratory
therapist, speech
therapy (Rx)
therapy, anticoagulant
therapy, aversion
therapy, behavior
therapy, collapse
therapy, electroconvulsive
therapy, fever
therapy, group
therapy, immunosuppressive
therapy, inhalation
therapy, insulin shock
therapy, light
therapy, milieu

therapy, nonspecific
therapy, occupational
therapy, opsonic
therapy, photodynamic
therapy, physical
therapy, play
therapy, radiation
therapy, replacement
therapy, serum
therapy, shock
therapy, specific
therapy, speech
therapy, spiritual
therapy, substitution
therapy, vaccine
Therevac S.B. (docusate sodium and glycerine)
thermacogenesis
thermaerotherapy
thermal
thermal death point
thermal destruction
thermalgesia
thermalgia
thermal radiation
thermal sense
thermanalgesia
thermanesthesia
thermatology
thermelometer
thermesthesia
thermesthesiometer
thermhyperesthesia
thermhypesthesia
thermic
thermic sense
thermistor
thermoalgesia
thermoanalgesia
thermoanesthesia
thermobiosis
thermobiotic
thermocauterectomy
thermocauterization
thermocautery
thermochemistry
thermochroic
thermochroism

thermocoagulation
thermocouple
thermocurrent
thermode
thermodiffusion
thermodilution
thermoduric
thermodynamics
thermoelectric
thermoelectricity
thermoesthesia
thermoexcitatory
thermogenesis
thermogenics
thermogram
thermograph
thermography
thermohyperalgesia
thermohyperesthesia
thermohypesthesia
thermohypoesthesia
thermoinhibitory
thermokeratoplasty
thermolabile
thermolamp
thermology
thermoluminescent dosimeter
thermolysis
thermolytic
thermomassage
thermometer
thermometer, air
thermometer, alcohol
thermometer, Celsius
thermometer, centigrade
thermometer, clinical
thermometer, differential
thermometer, disinfection of
thermometer, Fahrenheit
thermometer, gas
thermometer, Kelvin
thermometer, mercury
thermometer, recording
thermometer, rectal
thermometer, self-registering

thermometer, spirit
thermometer, surface
thermometer, wet-and-dry-
   bulb
thermometric
thermometry
thermometry, clinical
thermoneurosis
thermonuclear
thermopenetration
thermoperiodicity
thermophagy
thermophilic
thermophils
thermophobia
thermophore
thermophylic
thermopile
thermoplacentography
thermoplastic
thermoplegia
thermopolypnea
thermoradiotherapy
thermoreceptor
thermoregulation
thermoregulatory
thermoregulatory centers
thermoresistant
thermosclerectomy
thermostabile
thermostasis
thermostat
thermosteresis
thermosterilization
thermosystaltic
thermotactic
thermotaxic
thermotaxis
thermotherapeutics
thermotherapy
thermotics
thermotolerant
thermotonometer
thermotoxin
thermotropism
theroid
thesaurismosis
thesaurosis

thiabendazole
thiaminase
thiamine hydrochloride
   (vitamin B_1)
thiamine mononitrate
thiamine pyrophosphate
thiamylal sodium
thiemia
Thiersch's graft
Thiersch operation
Thiersch wire or suture
   removal
thiethylperazine malate
thigh
thigmesthesia
thigmotaxis
thigmotropism
thimerosal
thinking
thin-layer chromatography
   (TLC)
thiocyanate
thiogenic
thioglucosidase
thioguanine
thioneine
thionic
thiopectic
thiopental sodium
thiopexic
thiopexy
thiophil
thiophilic
thioridazine
   hydrochloride
thiosulfate
Thiosulfil Forte
   (sulfamethizole)
Thiosulfil-A Forte
   (sulfamethizole with
   phenazopyridine HCl)
thiotepa
thiothixene
thiouracil
thiourea
thiram
thiram poisoning
third cranial nerve

third intention
third ventricle
thirst
Thiry's fistula
Thiuretic
  (hydrochlorothiazide)
Thixokon (sodium
  acetrizoate)
thixolabile
thixotropy
thlipsencephalus
Thomas shunt
Thomas splint
Thomas-White hypothesis
Thompson operation
Thompson quadriceps palsy
Thomsen's disease
thoracalgia
thoracectomy
thoracentesis
thoracic
thoracic aorta aneurysm
thoracic aorta
  aortography
thoracic aorta graft
thoracic cage
thoracic cavity
thoracic duct
thoracic duct cannulation
thoracic gas volume
thoracic limbs
thoracic outlet
  compression syndrome
thoracic spine
  arthrodesis
thoracic squeeze
thoracic surgery
thoracicoabdominal
thoracicohumeral
thoracoacromial
thoracobronchotomy
thoracocautery
thoracoceloschisis
thoracocentesis
thoracocyllosis
thoracocyrtosis
thoracodelphus
thoracodidymus

thoracodynia
thoracogastroschisis
thoracograph
thoracolaparotomy
thoracolumbar
thoracolysis
thoracomelus
thoracometer
thoracometry
thoracomyodynia
thoracopagus
thoracoparacephalus
thoracopathy
thoracoplasty
thoracopneumoplasty
thoracoschisis
thoracoscope
thoracoscopy
thoracostenosis
thoracostomy
thoracotomy
thoracotomy, barrel-
  shaped
thoracotomy, bony
thoracotomy paralyticus
thoracotomy, Peyrot's
thorax
Thorazine
  (chlorpromazine)
Thorek operation
Thorel's bundle
thorium (Th)
Thorn test
thoron (Tn)
thread
threadworm
three-day fever
thremmatology
threonine
threshold
threshold, absolute
threshold, auditory
threshold of
  consciousness
threshold, differential
threshold dose
threshold, erythema
threshold, ketosis

threshold, renal
threshold, sensory
threshold stimulus
threshold substance
thrill
thrill, aneurysmal
thrill, aortic
thrill, arterial
thrill, diastolic
thrill, hydatid
thrill, presystolic
thrill, systolic
thrix
thrix annulata
throat
Throat Discs (throat
  lozenges)
throb
throbbing
Throckmorton's reflex
throe
thrombase
thrombasthenia
thrombectomy
thrombi
thrombin
Thrombinar (thrombin,
  topical [bovine])
thrombinogen
thromboangiitis
thromboangiitis
  obliterans (TAO)
thromboarteritis
thromboclasis
thromboclastic
thrombocyst
thrombocyte
thrombocythemia
thrombocytocrit
thrombocytolysis
thrombocytopathy
thrombocytopenia
thrombocytopoiesis
thrombocytosis
thromboembolism
thromboendarterectomy
thromboendarteritis

thromboendocarditis
Thrombogen (thrombin
  [bovine origin])
thrombogenesis
thrombogenic
thromboid
thrombokinase
thrombokinesis
thrombolymphangitis
thrombolysis
thrombolysis and
  angioplasty in
  myocardial infarction
  (TAMI)
thrombolytic
thrombon
thrombopathy
thrombopenia
thrombophilia
thrombophlebitis
thrombophlebitis migrans
thrombophlebitis,
  postpartum, iliofemoral
thromboplastic
thromboplastid
thromboplastin
thromboplastinogen
thrombopoiesis
thrombosed
thrombosinusitis
thrombosis
thrombosis, cardiac
thrombosis, coagulation
thrombosis, coronary
thrombosis, embolic
thrombosis, infective
thrombosis, marasmic
thrombosis, placental
thrombosis, plate
thrombosis, puerperal
thrombosis, sinus
thrombosis, traumatic
thrombosis, venous
thrombostasis
Thrombostat (thrombin)
thrombosthenin
thrombotic

thrombotic thrombocyto-
  penia purpura
  (TTP)
thrombus
thrombus, annular
thrombus, antemortem
thrombus, ball
thrombus, hyaline
thrombus, Laennec's
thrombus, lateral
thrombus, milk
thrombus, mural
thrombus, obstructing
thrombus, occluding
thrombus, parietal
thrombus, progressive
thrombus, stratified
thrombus, white
through-and-through
  drainage
through illumination
thrush
thrust
thrypsis
thulium (Tm)
thumb
thumb sign
thumb sucking
thumb, tennis
thus
thylacitis
thylakoid
thymectomize
thymectomy
thymelcosis
thymic
thymicolymphatic
thymidine
thymine
thymion
thymitis
thymocyte
thymokesis
thymokinetic
thymol
thymol iodide
thymolysis
thymolytic

thymoma
thymopathy
thymopexy
thymopoietin
thymoprivic
thymotoxic
thymus
thymus, accessory
thymus persistens
  hyperplastica
thymusectomy
thyreoplasia
thyroadenitis
thyroaplasia
thyroarytenoid
thyrocalcitonin
thyrocardiac
thyrocele
thyrochondrotomy
thyrocolloid
thyrocricoidectomy
thyrocricotomy
thyroepiglottic
thyroepiglottic muscle
thyroepiglottideus
thyrofissure
thyrogenic
thyrogenous
thyroglobulin
thyroglossal
thyroglossal cyst I&D
thyroglossal duct
thyrohyal
thyrohyoid
thyroid
thyroid autoantibodies
thyroid cachexia
thyroid cartilage
thyroid crisis
thyroid function tests
thyroid gland
thyroid microsomal
  antibody
thyroid panel
thyroid storm
Thyroid Strong
thyroid-stimulating
  hormone (TSH)

thyroidea accessoria
thyroidea ima
thyroidectomized
thyroidectomy
thyroidism
thyroiditis
thyroiditis, giant cell
thyroiditis, Hashimoto's
thyroidomania
thyroidorrhaphy
thyroidotomy
thyroidotoxin
Thyrolar (T_3/T_4 liotrix)
thyrolysin
thyrolytic
thyromegaly
thyromimetic
thyroparathyroidectomy
thyropathy
thyroprival
thyroprivia
thyroptosis
thyrosis
thyrotherapy
thyrotome
thyrotomy
thyrotoxic
thyrotoxicosis
thyrotoxin
thyrotrophic
thyrotropic
thyrotropic hormone
thyrotropin
thyrotropism
thyroxine (T_4)
thyroxine-binding
  globulin (TBG)
Thytropar (thyrotropin)
tibia
tibia, saber-shaped
tibia valga
tibia vara
tibiad
tibial
tibial bypass graft
tibial vein
tibialgia
tibialis

tibioadductor reflex
tibiocalcanean
tibiofemoral
tibiofibular
tibiofibular joint
tibionavicular
tibioperoneal
tibioperoneal artery
tibioscaphoid
tibiotarsal
tic
tic, convulsive
tic douloureux
tic, facial
tic, habit
tic rotatoire
tic, spasmodic
Ticar (ticarcillin
  disodium)
ticarcillin disodium,
  sterile
tick
tick bite
tick-borne rickettsiosis
tickle
tickling
tidal
tidal air
tidal drainage
tidal volume (TV)
tide
tide, acid
tide, alkaline
tide, fat
Tietze's syndrome
Tigan (trimethobenzamide
  HCl)
tigering
tigretier
tigroid
tigroid bodies
tigrolysis
tilmus
tiltometer
timbre
time
time, bleeding
time, clot retraction

time, coagulation
time, doubling
time frame
time inventory
time, median lethal
time, prothrombin
time, reaction
time, setting
time, thermal death
timer
times (x)
Timolide (timolol maleate-hydrochlorothiazide)
Timoptic (timolol maleate)
tin (Sn)
tin poisoning
Tinactin (tolnaftate)
tinctable
tinction
tinctorial
tinctura
tincturation
tincture
tincture of iodine
tincture of iodine poisoning
Tindal (acetophenazine maleate)
tine test
tinea
tinea amiantacea
tinea barbae
tinea capitis
tinea corporis
tinea cruris
tinea imbricata
tinea kerion
tinea nigra
tinea nodosa
tinea pedis
tinea profunda
tinea sycosis
tinea unguium
tinea versicolor
Tinel's sign
tingibility

tingible
tingle
tinnitus
tinnitus aurium
tintometer
tintometric
tintometry
tip
tipped uterus
tipping
tiqueur
tire
tirefond
tires
tiring
tissue
tissue, adenoid
tissue, adipose
tissue, areolar
tissue bank
tissue, bony, bone
tissue, brown adipose
tissue, brown fat
tissue, cancellous
tissue, cartilage
tissue, chondral
tissue, chordal
tissue, cicatricial
tissue, connective
tissue culture
tissue, elastic
tissue, embryonic
tissue, endothelial
tissue, epithelial
tissue, erectile
tissue, extracellular
tissue factor
tissue, fatty
tissue, fibrous
tissue, gelatiginous
tissue, glandular
tissue, granulation
tissue, hard
tissue immunoperoxidase histochemistry
tissue, indifferent
tissue, interstitial
tissue, lymphadenoid

tissue, lymphoid
tissue macrophage
tissue, mesenchymal
tissue, mucous
tissue, muscular
tissue, myeloid
tissue, nerve
tissue, nervous
tissue, osseous
tissue plasminogen
  activator (t-PA)
tissue, reticular
tissue, scar
tissue, sclerous
tissue, skeletal
tissue, splenic
tissue, subcutaneous
tissue, subcutaneous
  adipose
tissue typing
tissue, white fibrous
tissue, white nervous
tissues, chromaffin
tissues, chromophil
tissular
titanium (Ti)
titanium dioxide
titer
titer, agglutination
titillation
titrate
titration
titre
titrimetric
titrimetry
titubation
titubation, lingual
toadskin
toadstool
toadstool poisoning
tobacco
tobramycin
Tobrex (tobramycin)
tocainide
tocodynagraph
tocodynamometer
tocograph
tocography

tocology
tocolysis
tocometer
tocopherol, alpha
  (vitamin E)
tocophobia
tocus
toe
toe, claw
toe clonus
toe, dislocations of
toe drop
toe, hammer-
toe, Morton's
toe, pigeon
toe reflex
toes, fanning of
toes, webbed
toenail
Tofranil (imipramine HCl)
Tofranil-PM (imipramine
  pamoate)
Togaviridae
toilet
toilet training
toilette
to keep open (TKO)
toko
tokodynagraph
tolazamide
tolazoline hydrochloride
tolbutamide
Tolectin 200 (tolmetin
  sodium)
tolerance
tolerance, drug
tolerance, exercise
tolerance, glucose
tolerance, immunologic
tolerant
tolerogen
tolerogenic
Toleron (ferrous
  fumarate)
Tolfrinic (ferrous
  fumarate, vitamin B_{12}
  and ascorbic acid)
Tolinase (tolazamide)

tollwut (rabies)
tolnaftate
tolu balsam
toluene
toluene poisoning
toluidine
tomaculous neuropathy
tomatine
Tomkins operation
tomogram
tomograph
tomography
tomography, computerized
  axial (CAT)
tomography, computerized-
  body
tomography, computerized-
  head
tonaphasia
tone
tone deafness
tone decay test
tone, muscular
tongs
tongs, Crutchfield
tongue
tongue, bifid
tongue, black hairy
tongue, burning
tongue, cleft
tongue, coated
tongue, deviation of
tongue, dry
tongue, fern-leaf
tongue, filmy
tongue, fissured
tongue, forked
tongue, geographic
tongue, magenta
tongue, parrot
tongue, raspberry
tongue, scrotal
tongue, smoker's
tongue, smooth
tongue, strawberry
tongue, trifid
tongue, trombone
tongue-swallowing

tongue-tie
tongue-tie operation
tonic
tonic labyrinthine reflex
tonic neck reflex
tonic spasm
tonicity
tonicoclonic
Tonocard (tocainide HCl)
tonoclonic
tonofibril
tonofilament
tonogram
tonograph
tonography
tonometer
tonometry
tonometry, digital
tonometry, non-contact
tonoplast
tonsil
tonsil, cerebellar
tonsil, faucial
tonsil, lingual
tonsil, Luschka's
tonsil, nasal
tonsil, palatine
tonsil, pharyngeal
tonsil, tubal
tonsilla
tonsillar
tonsillar area
tonsillar crypt
tonsillar fossa
tonsillar ring
tonsillar sinus
tonsillectomy
tonsillectomy and
  adenoidectomy (T&A)
tonsillitis
tonsillitis, acute
tonsillitis, follicular
tonsillitis,
  parenchymatous, acute
tonsilloadenoidectomy
tonsillolith
tonsillopathy
tonsillotome

tonsillotomy
tonus
too numerous to count
   (TNTC)
tooth
toothache
toothbrush
topagnosis
topalgia
topectomy
topesthesia
tophaceous
tophus
tophyperidrosis
topical
topically
Topicort (desoximetasone)
Topicycline (tetracycline
   HCl)
topoalgia
topoanesthesia
topognosia
topognosis
topographic
topographic anatomy
topography
topology
toponarcosis
toponym
toponymy
topophobia
topothermesthesiometer
TOPS (Take Off Pounds
   Sensibly)
Topsyn (fluocinonide)
TOPV (trivalent oral
   polio vaccine)
torcular Herophili
Torecan (thiethylperazine
   maleate)
Torek orchiopexy
toric
toric lens
Torkildsen operation
tormina
Tornalate (bitolterol
   mesylate)
Torpin operation

torose
torous
torpent
torpid
torpidity
torpor
torpor intestinorum
torpor peristalticus
torpor retinae
torque
torr
torrefaction
torrefy
Torsade de pointes
torsiometer
torsion
torsion swing test
torsionometer
torsive
torsiversion
torso
torsoclusion
torticollar
torticollis
torticollis, fixed
torticollis, intermittent
torticollis, ocular
torticollis, rheumatic
torticollis, spasmodic
torticollis, spurious
torticollis, symptomatic
tortipelvis
tortuous
torture
Torula
toruloid
toruloma
Torulopsis glabrata
torulosis
torulus
torulus tactiles
torus
torus mandibularis
torus palatinus
Totacillin (ampicillin)
total abdominal
   hysterectomy (TAH)
total allergy syndrome

total body density (TBD)
total body fat (TBF)
total body weight (TBW)
total disability (TD)
Total Formula (high
  potency multivitamin/
  multimineral)
total hip replacement
total lymphocyte count
  (TLC)
total parenteral
  nutrition (TPN)
total pulmonary blood
  flow (TPBF)
total vaginal
  hysterectomy (TVH)
total serum protein (TSP)
Toti operation
totipotency
totipotent
touch
touch, abdominal
touch, after-
touch, double
touch, rectal
touch, vaginal
touch, vesical
Touchas operation
tour de maître
Tourette's syndrome
Tournay's sign
tourniquet
tourniquet paralysis
tourniquet, rotating
tourniquet test
Touroff operation
Touton cells
towelette
toxanemia
toxemia
toxemia, alimentary
toxemia, eclamptogenic
toxemia of pregnancy
toxenzyme
toxic
toxic-allergic syndrome
toxicant
toxicemic

toxic erythema
toxicide
toxicity
Toxicodendron
toxicoderma
toxicodermatitis
toxicodermatosis
toxicogenic
toxicoid
toxicologist
toxicology
toxicomania
toxicopathic
toxicopathy
toxicopexy
toxicophidia
toxicophobia
toxicosis
toxicosis, endogenic
toxicosis, exogenic
toxicosis, retention
toxic shock syndrome
  (TSS)
toxic substance
toxidermitis
toxiferous
toxigenic
toxigenicity
toxignomic
toxin
toxin, bacterial
toxin, botulinus
toxin, dermonecrotic
toxin, Dick
toxin, diphtheria
toxin, dysentery
toxin, erythrogenic
toxin, extracellular
toxin, fatigue
toxin, intracellular
toxin, plant
toxin-antitoxin (TAT)
toxinicide
toxinology
toxinosis
toxipathic
toxipathy
toxiphobia

toxisterol
toxitabellae
toxitherapy
toxituberculid
toxoalexin
toxocariasis
toxogenin
toxoid
toxoid, alum-precipitated
toxoid, diphtheria
toxoid, tetanus
toxolecithin
toxolyxin
toxomucin
toxonosis
toxopeptone
toxophil
toxophile
toxophilic
toxophore
toxophorous
toxophylaxin
Toxoplasma
Toxoplasma gondii
toxoplasmosis
toxoplasmosis skin test
trabecula
trabeculae carneae cordis
trabecular
trabecularism
trabeculate
trabeculectomy
trabeculodialysis
trabeculoplasty
trabeculotomy
trabs
trabs cerebri
trace
trace elements
trace, primitive
tracer
trachea
tracheaectasy
tracheal
tracheal fistula
tracheal tugging
trachealis
tracheitis

trachelagra
trachelectomopexy
trachelectomy
trachelematoma
trachelism
trachelismus
trachelitis
trachelobregmatic
trachelocele
trachelocyrtosis
trachelocystitis
trachelodynia
trachelokyphosis
trachelology
trachelomastoid
trachelomyitis
trachelopexy
tracheloplasty
trachelorrhaphy
tracheloschisis
trachelotomy
tracheoaerocele
tracheobronchial
tracheobronchial tree
tracheobronchomegaly
tracheobronchoscopy
tracheocele
tracheocricotomy
tracheoesophageal
tracheoesophageal fistula
tracheofissure
tracheography
tracheolaryngeal
tracheolaryngotomy
tracheomalacia
tracheopathia
tracheopathy
tracheopharyngeal
tracheophonesia
tracheophony
tracheoplasty
tracheorrhagia
tracheoschisis
tracheoscopy
tracheostenosis
tracheostoma
tracheostomize
tracheostomy

tracheostomy care
tracheotome
tracheotomy
trachitis
trachoma
trachoma, brawny
trachoma deformans
trachoma, diffuse
trachomatous
trachychromatic
trachyphonia
tracing
Tracrium (atracurium besylate)
tract
tract, afferent
tract, alimentary
tract, ascending
tract, biliary
tract, descending
tract, digestive
tract, dorsolateral
tract, extrapyramidal
tract, gastrointestinal
tract, genitourinary
tract, iliotibial
tract, intestinal
tract, motor
tract, olfactory
tract, optic
tract, pyramidal
tract, respiratory
tract, rubrospinal
tract, supraoptico-hypophyseal
tract, urinary
tract, uveal
tractellum
traction (Tx)
traction, adhesive tape
traction, axis
traction, boot
traction, Bryant's skeletal
traction, Buck's
traction, caliper tongs
traction, Crutchfield tongs

traction, Dunlop's skeletal
traction, elastic
traction, gallows
traction, Gardner Wells
traction, halo device, skull
traction, head
traction, Lyman Smith skeletal
traction, manual, intermittent
traction, mechanical, intermittent
traction, Russell's skeletal
traction, skeletal
traction, skin, limbs
traction, spinal
traction, Thomas' splint
traction, Vinke tongs
traction, weight
tractor
tractotomy
tractus
tragacanth
tragal
tragi
tragicus
tragion
tragomaschalia
tragophonia
tragophony
tragopodia
tragus
train
trainable
training
training, assertiveness
trait
trait, acquired
trait, inherited
trajector
Tral (hexocyclium methylsulfate)
tramazoline hydrochloride
trance
trance, death

trance, induced
Trancopal (chlormezanone)
Trandate (labetalol HCl)
Trandate HCT (labetalol HCl/hydrochloro-thiazide)
tranquilizer
transabdominal
transacetylation
transactional analysis
transamidination
transaminase
transaminase, glutamic-oxaloacetic (GOT or S[serum]GOT)
transaminase, glutamic-pyruvic (GPT or S[serum]GPT)
transamination
transaortic
transatrial
transaudient
transaxial
transbronchial biopsy
transcalent
transcapillary
transcapillary exchange
transcatheter therapy
transcervical
transcortical
transcortin
transcriptase
transcription
transcutaneous electrical nerve stimulation (TENS)
transcutaneous pacing
transdermal infusion system
Transderm-Nitro (nitroglycerin [transdermal])
Transderm Scop (scopolamine [transdermal])
transducer
transduction
transection

transfection
transfer
transfer board
transfer factor
transfer factor test (TFT)
transferase
transference
transferrin
transferring
transfix
transfixion
transforation
transforator
transformation
transformer
transformer, step-down
transformer, step-up
transfusion
transfusion, cadaver blood
transfusion, direct
transfusion, exchange
transfusion, indirect
transfusion reactions
transfusion, replacement
transfusion, single unit
transfusion syndrome, multiple
Transgrow
transient ischemic arrhythmia (TIA)
transient ischemic attack (TIA)
transiliac
transilient
transillumination
transinsular
transischiac
transisthmian
transistor
transition
transitional
translation
translocation
translucent
translumbar aortogram
transmethylation

transmigration
transmigration, external
transmigration, internal
transmissible
transmission
transmission, biological
transmission, duplex
transmission, mechanical
transmission, neuromyal
transmission, placental
transmission, synaptic
transmission, transovarial
transmural
transmutation
transocular
transonance
transorbital
transovarial passage
transparent
transparietal
transpeptidase
transperitoneal
transphosphorylase
transphosphorylation
transpirable
transpiration
transpiration, cutaneous
transpiration, pulmonary
transplacental
transplant
transplantar
transplantation
transplantation, autoplastic
transplantation, heteroplastic
transplantation, heterotopic
transplantation, homoplastic
transplantation, homotopic
transplantation, tenoplastic
transpleural
transport
transport, active

transportation of the injured
transposition
transposition of great vessels
transposon
transsection
transsegmental
transseptal
transsexual
transsexual surgery
transsexualism
transsphenoidal
transtemporal
transthalamic
transthermia
transthoracic
transthoracotomy
transtracheal
transtracheal injection
transtracheal neurectomy
transubstantiation
transudate
transudation
transureteroureterostomy
transurethral
transurethral resection (TUR)
transvaginal
transvector
transvenous electrodes
transversalis
transversalis fascia
transverse
transversectomy
transverse foramen
transverse plane
transversion
transversocostal
transversospinalis
transversourethralis
transversus
transvesical
transvestism
transvestitism
transvestite
Tranxene (clorazepate dipotassium)

tranylcypromine
trapeze bar
trapezial
trapeziform
trapeziometacarpal
trapezium
trapezius
trapezoid
trapezoid body
trapezoid bone
trapezoid ligament
trapping, aneurysm
trauma
trauma, birth
trauma, occlusal
trauma, psychic
trauma, toothbrush
Traumacal (nutritionally
  complete liquid)
traumatic
traumatic psychosis
traumatism
traumatology
traumatonesis
traumatopathy
traumatophilia
traumatopnea
traumatopyra
traumatotherapy
Trauner operation
travail
Travase (sutilains
  ointment)
travelers' diarrhea
tray
tray, impression
Treacher Collins syndrome
treacle
tread
treadmill exercise
treatment
treatment, active
treatment, causal
treatment, conservative
treatment, dental
treatment, dietetic
treatment, electric shock
treatment, empiric

treatment, expectant
treatment, Kenny
treatment, palliative
treatment plan
treatment, preventive
treatment, rational
treatment, shock
treatment, specific
treatment, starvation
treatment, supportive
treatment, surgical
treatment, symptomatic
Trecator-SC (ethionamide)
tree
tree, bronchial
tree, tracheobronchial
trehala
trehalase
trehalose
Trematoda
trematode
trematodiasis
tremble
trembles
tremelloid
tremellose
tremetol
Tremin (trihexyphenidyl
  HCl)
tremogram
tremograph
tremolabile
tremophobia
tremor
tremor, coarse
tremor, continuous
tremor, enhanced
physiologic
tremor, essential
tremor, fibrillary
tremor, fine
tremor, flapping
tremor, forced
tremor, Hunt's
tremor, hysterical
tremor, intention
tremor, intermittent
tremor, muscular

tremor, parkinsonian
tremor, physiologic
tremor, rest
tremor, senile
tremor, static
tremor, volitional
tremorgram
tremulor
tremulous
trench fever
trench foot
trench mouth
trend
Trendelenburg position
trepan
trepanation
trepanation, corneal
trephination
trephine
trephine exploratory
trephining
trephocyte
trepidant
trepidatio
trepidatio cordis
Treponema
Treponema carateum
Treponema pallidum
Treponema pallidum
  agglutination (TPA)
Treponema pertenue
Treponemataceae
treponematosis
treponeme
treponemiasis
treponemicidal
trepopnea
tresis
tretinoin
Trexan (naltrexone HCl)
triacetate
triacetin
triacetyloleandomycin
triacylglycerols
triad
triad, Hutchinson's

Triad (butalbital,
  acetaminophen, and
  caffeine)
triage
triakaidekaphobia
Tri-Immunol (diphtheria,
  tetanus toxoid, and
  pertussis)
Tri-Levlen 21
  (levonorgestrel and
  ethinyl estradiol-
  triphasic)
Tri-Levlen 28
  (levonorgestrel and
  ethinyl estradiol-
  triphasic)
Tri-Norinyl
  (norethindrone and
  ethinyl estradiol)
Tri-Vi-Flor (vitamins
  A,D,C, and fluoride)
triamcinolone acetonide
triamcinolone acetonide
  inhaler
triamcinolone diacetate
triamcinolone
  hexacetonide
Triaminic Cold Tablets
Triaminic Expectorant
Triaminic Expectorant
  with Codeine
Triaminic Expectorant DH
Triaminic Multi-Symptom
  Cold Syrup
Triaminic Multi-Symptom
  Cold Tablets
Triaminic Oral Infant
  Drops
Triaminic Tablets
Triaminic TR Tablets
Triaminic-12 Tablets
Triaminic-DM Cough
  Formula
triamterene
triangle
triangle, anal
triangle, anterior, of
  neck

triangle, carotid,
  inferior
triangle, carotid,
  superior
triangle, cephalic
triangle, digastric
triangle of elbow
triangle, facial
triangle, femoral
triangle, frontal
triangle, Hesselbach's
triangle, interior
  occipital
triangle, inguinal
triangle, Lesser's
triangle,
  lumbocostoabdominal
triangle, muscular
triangle, mylohyoid
triangle of necessity
triangle, occipital, of
  the neck
triangle, omoclavicular
triangle, omohyoid
triangle of Petit
triangle, posterior
  cervical
triangle, pubourethral
triangle, Scarpa's
triangle, subclavian
triangle, submandibular
triangle, suboccipital
triangle, supraclavicular
triangle, suprameatal
triangle, urogenital
triangle, vesical
triangular
triangular bandage
triangular ligament
triangular nucleus of
  Schwalbe
Triatoma
triatomic
Triavil (perphenazine-
  amitriptyline HCl)
tribadism
tribasic
tribasilar

tribasilar synostosis
tribe
tribology
triboluminescence
tribrachia
tribrachius
tribromide
tribromoethanol
TRIC agents
tricarboxylic acid cycle
tricellular
tricephalus
triceps
triceps reflex
triceps skin-fold (TSF)
Tricercomonas
trichangiectasia
trichangiectasis
trichatrophia
trichauxe
trichauxis
trichiasis
trichilemmoma
Trichina
trichina
Trichinella
Trichinella spiralis
trichinelliasis
trichinellosis
trichiniasis
trichiniferous
trichinization
trichinophobia
trichinosis
trichinosis skin test
trichinous
trichinous myositis
trichion
trichitis
trichloride
trichlormethiazide
trichloroacetic acid
trichloroethanol
trichloroethylene
2,4,5-trichlorophenoxy-
  acetic acid (2,4,5-T)
trichoanesthesia
trichobacteria

trichobezoar
trichocardia
trichoclasia
trichoclasis
trichocryptosis
trichocyst
Trichodectes
trichoepithelioma
trichoesthesia
trichoesthesiometer
trichogen
trichogenous
trichoglossia
trichohyalin
trichoid
trichokryptomania
tricholith
trichologia
trichology
trichoma
trichomadesis
trichomatosis
trichomatous
trichome
trichomegaly
trichomonacide
trichomonad
Trichomonas
Trichomonas hominis
Trichomonas tenax
Trichomonas vaginalis
trichomoniasis
trichomycosis
trichomycosis axillaris
trichomycosis nodosa
trichonodosis
trichonosis
trichonosus
trichopathic
trichopathophobia
trichopathy
trichophagia
trichophagy
trichophobia
trichophytic
trichophytic granulosa
trichophytid
trichophytin

trichophytobezoar
Trichophyton
Trichophyton
  mentagrophytes
Trichophyton
  schoenleinii
Trichophyton tonsurans
Trichophyton violaceum
trichophytosis
trichoptilosis
trichorrhea
trichorrhexis
trichorrhexis nodosa
trichorrhexomania
trichoschisis
trichoscopy
trichosiderin
trichosis
trichosis decolor
trichosis setosa
Trichosporon
Trichosporon beigelii
trichosporosis
trichostasis spinulosa
trichostrongyliasis
trichostrongylosis
Trichostrongylus
Trichothecium
Trichothecium roseum
trichotillomania
trichotomous
trichotomy
trichotoxin
trichotrophy
trichroic
trichroism
trichromatic
trichromatism
trichromatopsia
trichromic
trichterbrust
trichuriasis
Trichuris
Trichuris trichiura
tricipital
tricitrates oral solution
triclofos sodium
tricornic

tricornute
tricrotic
tricrotism
tricuspid
tricuspid area
tricuspid atresia
tricuspid murmur
tricuspid orifice
tricuspid tooth
tricuspid valve
trident
tridentate
tridermic
tridermoma
Tridesilon (desonide)
tridihexethyl chloride
Tridil (nitroglycerin)
Tridione (trimethadione)
tridymite
trielcon
triencephalus
triethanolamine
triethylenemelamine (TEM)
triethylene-
  thiophosphoramide
trifacial
trifacial neuralgia
trifid
trifluoperazine
  hydrochloride
triflupromazine
trifocal
trifurcation
trigastric
trigeminal
trigeminal cough
trigeminal nerve (V)
trigeminal neuralgia
trigeminal pulse
trigeminus
trigeminy
trigenic
trigger
trigger action
trigger finger
trigger finger tendon
  sheath incision
trigger point

trigger substance
trigger zone
triglycerides
trigone
trigone of bladder
trigone, carotid
trigone, olfactory
trigone, vesical
trigonectomy
trigonid
trigonitis
trigonocephalic
trigonocephalus
trigonum
trigonum lumbale
TriHEMIC 600 (hematinic)
trihexyphenidyl
  hydrochloride
trihybrid
tri-iniodymus
triiodothyronine (T_3)
triiodothyronine resin
  uptake test (T_3 RU)
trikates
trilabe
Trilafon (perphenazine)
trilaminar
trilateral
Trilisate (choline
  magnesium
  trisalicylate)
trill
trilobate
trilocular
trilogy
trimalleolar ankle
  fracture
trimanual
trimeprazine tartrate
trimester
trimester, first
trimester, second
trimester, third
trimethadione
trimethaphan camsylate
trimethidinium
  methosulfate

trimethobenzamide
  hydrochloride
trimethoprim
trimethylene
trimmer
trimmer, gingival margin
trimmer, model
trimming, amputation
  stump
trimorphous
**Trimox '125' For Oral
  Suspension**
  (amoxicillin)
Trimox '250' Capsules
  (amoxicillin)
**Trimox '250' For Oral
  Suspension**
  (amoxicillin)
Trimox '500' Capsules
  (amoxicillin)
Trimpex (trimethoprim)
Trimstat (phendimetrazine
  tartrate)
Trinalin (azatadine
  maleate and
  pseudoephedrine
  sulfate)
Trind (decongestant/
  antihistamine)
Trind-DM (antitussive,
  decongestant,
  antihistamine)
Trinitroglycerol
  (nitroglycerin)
trinitrophenol
trinitrotoluene
Trinsicon (hematinic with
  intrinsic factor)
Trinsicon M (hematinic
  concentrate modified)
triocephalus
triolein
triolism
triophthalmos
triopodymus
triorchid
triorchis
triorchidism

triose
triotus
trioxsalen
trip
tripara
tripelennamine citrate
tripeptide
triphalangia
triphasic
Triphasil-21
  (levonorgestrel and
  ethinyl estradiol)
Triphasil-28
  (levonorgestrel and
  ethinyl estradiol)
triphenylmethane
Tripier's amputation
triple
triple arthrodesis
triplet
triplex
triploblastic
triploid
triploidy
triplokoria
triplopia
tripod
tripod, Haller's
tripod, vital
tripodia
tripoding
triprolidine
  hydrochloride
triprosopus
tripsis
triquetral
triquetral bone
triquetrous
triquetrum
triradial
triradiate
triradius
trisaccharide
triskaidekaphobia
trismic
trismoid
trismus
trismus nascentium

trisomic
trisomy
trisomy 13
trisomy 18
trisomy 21
trisplanchnic
Trisoralen (trioxsalen)
tristichia
tristimania
trisulcate
trisulfapyrimidines oral
  suspension
trisulfate
trisulfide
tritanomalopia
tritanomaly
tritanopia
Triten (dimethindene
maleate)
tritiate
triticeous
triticeous cartilage
tritium
triturable
trituration
trivalence
trivalent
trivalve
trivial name
trizonal
Trobicin (spectinomycin
  HCl)
trocar
trochanter
trochanter, greater
trochanter, lesser
trochanter major
trochanter minor
trochanter tertius
trochanter, third
trochanterian
trochanteric
trochanterplasty
trochantin
trochantinian
troche
trochiscus
trochlea

trochlea of the elbow
trochlear fovea
trochleariform
trochlearis
trochlear nerve (IV)
trochocardia
trochocephalia
trochocephaly
trochoid
trochoides
Trofan (L-tryptophan)
Troglotrematidae
Troisier's node
trolamine
troland
troleandomycin
trolnitrate phosphate
Trombicula
Trombicula akamushi
trombiculiasis
Trombiculidae
tromethamine
tromomania
Tronothane Hydrochloride
  (pramoxine HCl)
Tropamine (amino acid,
  mineral and vitamin
  combination)
trophectoderm
trophedema
trophic
trophism
trophoblast
trophoblastic
trophoblastoma
trophocyte
trophoderm
trophodynamics
trophology
trophoneurosis
trophoneurosis,
  disseminated
trophoneurosis, facial
trophoneurosis, muscular
trophoneurotic
trophonosis
trophonucleus
trophopathia

trophopathy
trophotaxis
trophotherapy
trophotonus
trophotropism
trophozoite
tropia
tropical
tropical immersion foot
tropical lichen
tropicamide
tropine ($C_8H_{15}NO$)
tropism
tropocollagen
tropometer
tropomyosin
troponin
trough
trough, gingival
trough, synaptic
Trousseau's sign
Trousseau's spots
Trousseau's symptom
troxidone
troy weight
true
true conjugate diameter
  of pelvic inlet
true pelvis
true ribs
truncal
truncate
truncus
truncus arteriosus
truncus brachiocephalicus
truncus celiacus
truncus pulmonalis
trunk
trunk, celiac
trunk, lumbosacral
trunk, sympathetic
trusion
truss
truth serum
try-in
Trymex (triamcinolone
  acetonide)
Trypanoplasma

Trypanosoma
Trypanosoma brucei
Trypanosoma cruzi
Trypanosoma gambiense
Trypanosoma
  rhodesiense
trypanosomal
trypanosome
trypanosomiasis
trypanosomiasis, African
trypanosomiasis, American
trypanosomic
trypanosomicide
trypanosomid
tryparsamide
trypsin
trypsin, crystallized
trypsinogen
Tryptacin (L-tryptophan)
tryptic
tryptolysis
tryptone
tryptophan
tryptophanase
tryptophanuria
Tryptoplex
  (serotoninergic
  precursor)
Trysul (triple sulfa
  vaginal cream)
tsetse fly
tsutsugamushi disease
T-tube
tuaminoheptane sulfate
tub
tuba
tubal
tubal nephritis
tubal pregnancy
tubatorsion
tubba
tubboe
tube
tube, auditory
tube, Cantor
tube, cathode-ray
tube, Coolidge
tube, Crookes'

tube, drainage
tube, endobronchial
tube, endotracheal
tube, esophageal
tube, eustachian
tube, fallopian
tube feeding
tube, fermentation
tube, hot-cathode
tube, hot cathode
  roentgen-ray
tube, intestinal
  decompression
tube, intubation
tube, Levin
tube, Miller-Abbott
tube, nasogastric
tube, neural
tube, otopharyngeal
tube, Sengstaken-
Blakemore
tube, Southey's
tube, stomach
tube, test
tube, thoracostomy
tube, tracheotomy
tube, uterine
tube, ventilation
tube, Wangensteen
tubectomy
tuber
tuber cinereum
tubercle
tubercle, adductor
tubercle, articular
tubercle, bacillus
tubercle, condyloid
tubercle, dental
tubercle, deltoid
tubercle, fibrous
tubercle, genial
tubercle, genital
tubercle, lacrimal
tubercle, laminated
tubercle, Lisfranc's
tubercle, mental
tubercle, miliary
tubercle, pharyngeal

tubercle, pubic
tubercle, supraglenoid
tubercle, of the upper
  lip
tubercle, zygomatic
tubercula
tubercular
tuberculate
tuberculated
tuberculation
tuberculid(e)
tuberculid(e), follicular
tuberculid(e),
  papulonecrotic
tuberculigenous
tuberculin
tuberculin, new
tuberculin, old
tuberculin, purified
  protein derivative
tuberculin test
tuberculin tine test
tuberculitis
tuberculocele
tuberculocidal
tuberculoderma
tuberculofibroid
tuberculofibrosis
tuberculoid
tuberculoma
tuberculophobia
tuberculoprotein
tuberculosilicosis
tuberculosis (TB)
tuberculosis, avian
tuberculosis, bovine
tuberculosis, exogenous
tuberculosis,
  hematogenous
tuberculosis, open
tuberculosis skin test
  (patch, Mantoux, and
  Tine/Mono-Vacc)
tuberculosis, verrucosa
tuberculostatic
tuberculotic
tuberculous
tuberculum

tuberculum acusticum
tuberculum majus humeri
tuberculum minus humeri
tuberin
tuberosis
tuberositas
tuberosity
tuberosity, ischial
tuberosity, maxillary
tuberous
tuberous sclerosis
Tubersol (tuberculin
  purified protein
  derivative)
**Tubex Closed Injection
  System**
tuboabdominal
tuboabdominal pregnancy
tubocurarine chloride
tuboligamentous
tubo-ovarian
tubo-ovariotomy
tubo-ovaritis
tuboperitoneal
tuboplasty
tuborrhea
tubotorsion
tubotympanal
tubouterine
tubouterine implantation
tubovaginal
tubular
tubule
tubule, collecting
tubule, Henle's
tubule, junctional
tubules, convoluted, of
  kidney
tubules, convoluted
  seminiferous
tubules, dentinal
tubules, excretory
tubules, galactophorous
tubules, lactiferous
tubules, mesonephric
tubules, metanephritic
tubules, renal
tubules, seminiferous

tubules, uriniferous
tubulin
tubulization
tubuloalveolar
tubulocyst
tubulodermoid
tubuloracemose
tubulorrhexis
tubulous
tubulus
tubus
tucking
Tudor "rabbit ear"
  operation
Tuffier operation
tuft
tuft, enamel
tuft, malpighian
tugging
tugging, tracheal
tularemia
tumbu fly
tumefacient
tumefaction
tumentia
tumentia, vasomotor
tumescence
tumid
tumor
tumor angiogenesis factor
  (TAF)
tumor, carotid body
tumor, connective tissue
tumor, desmoid
tumor, erectile
tumor, Ewing's
tumor, false
tumor, fibroid
tumor, giant cell, of
  bone
tumor, giant cell, of
  tendon sheath
tumor, granulosa
tumor, granulosa cell
tumor, granulosa-theca
  cell
tumor, heterologous
tumor, homoiotypic

tumor, homologous
tumor, Hürthle cell
tumor, islet cell
tumor, Krukenberg's
tumor, lipoid cell, of the ovary
tumor, mast cell
tumor, melanotic neuroectodermal
tumor, mesenchymal mixed
tumor, phantom
tumor of pregnancy
tumor, sand
tumor, turban
tumor viruses
tumor, Wilms'
tumoraffin
tumoricidal
tumorigenesis
tumorigenic
tumor markers, serum
tumor necrosis factor (TNF)
tumorous
Tums
tumultus
tumultus cordis
tumultus sermonis
Tunga
Tunga penetrans
tungiasis
tungsten (W)
tunic
tunic, Bichat's
tunica
tunica adventitia
tunica albuginea
tunica conjunctiva
tunica dartos
tunica externa
tunica interna
tunica intima
tunica media
tunica mucosa
tunica muscularis
tunica propria
tunica serosa
tunica vaginalis

tunica vaginalis surgery
tunica vasculosa
tunicin
tuning fork
tunnel
tunnel, carpal
tunnel, flexor
tunnel, inner
tunnel, tarsal
tunnel vision
turbid
turbidimeter
turbidimetry
turbidity
turbinal
turbinate
turbinate cauterization
turbinate cryosurgery
turbinate excision
turbinate injection
turbinate submucous resection
turbinated
turbinectomy
turbinotome
turbinotomy
Turco operation
turgescence
turgescent
turgid
turgometer
turgor
turgor, skin
turgor vitalis
Turing test
turista
Turner's syndrome
turning
turpentine
turpentine poisoning
turricephaly
turunda
Tussagesic
tussal
Tussar DM
Tussar-2
Tussend (antitussive-decongestant)

Tussend Expectorant
  (antitussive-
  decongestant-
  expectorant)
tussicular
tussiculation
Tussi-Organidin
  (antitussive/mucolytic-
  expectorant)
Tussionex (hydrocodone
  and phenyltoloxamine)
tussis
tussis convulsiva
tussis stomachalis
tussive
tussive syncope
Tuss-Ornade
tutin
T wave
twelfth
twice a day (b.i.d.)
twig
twilight sleep
twilight state
twin
twins, biovular
twins, conjoined
twins, dizygotic
twins, enzygotic
twins, fraternal
twins, identical
twins, impacted
twins, interlocked
twins, monozygotic
twins, parasitic
twins, Siamese
twins, true
twins, unequal
twinge
Twin-K (potassium)
Twin-K-Cl (potassium and
  chloride)
twinning
twitch
twitching
TwoCal HN (high nitrogen
  liquid nutrition)

two-point discrimination
  test
tybamate
tylectomy
Tylenol (acetaminophen)
**Tylenol with codeine
  phosphate**
  (acetaminophen, codeine
  phosphate)
Tylenol Sinus Medication
  (acetaminophen and
  pseudoephedrine HCl)
tylion
tyloma
tylosis
Tylox (oxycodone and
  acetaminophen)
tyloxapol
Tympagesic (analgesic-
  decongestant ear drops)
tympanectomy
tympania
tympanic
tympanic membrane
tympanicity
tympanism
tympanites
tympanitic
tympanitic resonance
tympanitis
tympanoeustachian
tympanography
tympanohyal
tympanolysis
tympanomandibular
tympanomastoidectomy
tympanomastoiditis
tympanometry
tympanoplasty
tympanosclerosis
tympanosis
tympanosquamosal
tympanostapedial
tympanostomy tubes
tympanosympathectomy
tympanotemporal
tympanotomy

tympanous
tympanum
tympany
type
type, asthenic
type, athletic
type, blood
type, phage
type, pyknic
typhlectasis
typhlectomy
typhlenteritis
typhlitis
typhlodicliditis
typhloempyema
typhloenteritis
typhlolexia
typhlolithiasis
typhlology
typhlon
typhlopexy
typhlorrhaphy
typhlosis
typhlospasm
typhlostenosis
typhlostomy
typhlotomy
typhloureterostomy
typhohemia
typhoid
typhoid agglutinin
typhoid carrier
typhoid fever
typhoid immunization
typhoid vaccine
typhoidal
typholysin
typhomalarial
typhomania
typhopneumonia
typhous
typhus
typhus, classic
typhus, endemic
typhus, epidemic
typhus, flea-borne
typhus, Mexican
typhus, mite-borne

typhus, murine
typhus, recrudescent
typhus, rural
typhus, scrub
typhus, shop
typhus, urban
typhus vaccine
typical
typing
typing, bacteriophage
typing, blood
typing, tissue
typoscope
typus
tyramine
tyrannism
tyrogenous
Tyroglyphus
tyroid
tyroma
tyromatosis
tyrosinase
tyrosine
tyrosinemia
tyrosinosis
tyrosinuria
tyrosis
tyrosyluria
tyrothricin
tyrotoxism
Tyrrell's fascia
Tyson's glands
tysonitis
tyvelose
Tyzine (tetrahydrozoline
  HCl)
Tzanck test
tzetze

U

uberous
uberty
ubiquinol
ubiquinone
Uchida operation

udder
Uffelmann's test
U-Gencin (gentamicin
  sulfate)
Uhthoff's sign
ulaganactesis
ulalgia
ulatrophia
ulcer
ulcer, amputating
ulcer, atonic
ulcer, callous
ulcer, chronic leg
ulcer, Curling's
ulcer, decubitus
ulcer, duodenal
ulcer, follicular
ulcer, fungus
ulcer, gastric
ulcer, Hunner's
ulcer, indolent
ulcer, peptic
ulcer, perforating
ulcer, phagedenic
ulcer, rodent
ulcer, serpiginous
ulcer, simple
ulcer, specific
ulcer, stasis
ulcer, stercoral
ulcer, stress
ulcer, trophic
ulcer, tropical
ulcer, varicose
ulcer, venereal
ulcera
ulcerate
ulcerated
ulceration
ulcerative
ulcerative colitis (UC)
ulcerogangrenous
ulcerogenic drugs
ulceromembranous
ulceromembranous
  tonsillitis
ulcerous
ulcus

ulcus cancrosum
ulcus induratum
ulcus vulvae acutum
ulectomy
ulna
ulnad
ulnar
ulnar artery
ulnar motor nerve
ulnar nerve neurolysis
ulnar nerve transposition
ulnar resection
ulnocarpal
ulnoradial
Ulo (chlophedianol HCl)
ulocace
ulocarcinoma
ulodermatitis
uloglossitis
uloid
uloncus
ulorrhagia
ulorrhea
ulosis
ulotic
ulotomy
ulotrichous
ulotripsis
ultimate
ultimobranchial bodies
ultrabrachycephalic
Ultracef (cefadroxil)
Ultracholine
  (phosphatidylcholine
  and phospholipid)
Ultralente Iletin I
  (extended insulin zinc
  suspension)
Ultralente Insulin
  (extended insulin zinc)
ultrasonic (US)
ultrasonic fragmentation
  of calculus
ultrasonic removal of
  lens
ultrasonogram
ultrasonography

ultrasonography, abdominal aorta
ultrasonography, arteries and veins
ultrasonography, brain
ultrasonography, gallbladder
ultrasonography, heart
ultrasonography, kidneys
ultrasonography, liver
ultrasonography, pancreas
ultrasonography, pelvic and uterus (pregnant)
ultrasonography, spleen
ultrasonography, thyroid
ultrasound, A-mode
ultrasound diagnostic
ultrasound therapeutic
ultrastructure
ultraviolet (UV)
ultraviolet light actinotherapy
ultraviolet rays
ultraviolet therapy
ululation
umbilectomy
umbilical
umbilical artery catheter
umbilical cord
umbilical fissure
umbilical hernia
umbilical souffle
umbilical vein catheterization, newborn
umbilical vesicle
umbilicate
umbilication
umbilicus (umb)
umbilicus excision
umbo
umbo of tympanic membrane
umbra
umbrella filter
umbrella interruption, inferior vena cava

Unasyn (ampicillin sodium/sulbactam sodium)
unbridling
uncal
uncal herniation
unciform
unciform bone
unciform fasciculus
unciform process
unciforme
uncinariasis
uncinate
uncinate bundle of Russell
uncinate convolution
uncinate epilepsy
uncinate fasciculus
uncinate fits
uncinate gyrus
uncinatum
uncipressure
uncomplemented
unconditioned reflex
unconscious
unconscious, collective
unconsciousness
unco-ossified
uncovertebral
unction
unctuous
uncus
undecylenic acid
underachiever
undercut
undernutrition
undertoe
underweight
undifferentiation
undine
undinism
undulant
undulant fever
undulate
undulation
undulation, jugular
undulation, respiratory
unemployment

ungual
ungual phalanx
ungual tuberosity
unguent
unguentum
unguiculate
unguinal
unguis
ungus incarnatus
ungula
uniarticular
uniaxial
unibasal
unicameral
Unicare (skin care lotion)
unicellular
unicentral
uniceps
Unicontin (anhydrous theophylline)
unicorn
unicornous
unicuspid
Uni Derm (protective moisturizer)
uniflagellate
Uniflex
uniforate
unigerminal
uniglandular
unigravida
unilaminar
unilateral
unilobar
unilocular
uninuclear
uninucleated
uniocular
union
union, non-
union, secondary
union, vicious
unioval
uniovular
unipara
uniparous
Unipen (nafcillin sodium)

Uniphyl (anhydrous theophylline)
unipolar
unipotent
unipotential
Uni Salve (protective ointment)
uniseptate
unisex
Unisom Dual Relief (diphenhydramine/ acetaminophen)
Unisom Night Time Sleep Aid (doxylamine succinate)
unit (u)
unit, amboceptor
unit, angström (A, AU)
unit, antigen
unit, antitoxin
unit, atomic mass (AMU)
unit, Bodansky
unit, British thermal (BTU)
unit of capacity
unit, cat
unit, complement
unit, dental
unit dose
unit, electrostatic (ESU, ESE)
unit, hemolytic
unit, international
unit, light
unit, Mache (Mu)
unit, motor
unit, mouse
unit, rat
unit, SI
unit, Todd
unit, USP
unitarian
unitary
Unites States Adopted Names (USAN)
United States Pharmacopeia (USP)
uniterminal

univalence
univalent
universal
universal antidote
universal cuff
universal donor
universal dressing
universal recipient
Uni Wash (skin cleanser)
unknown (UK)
unmedullated
unmyelinated
Unna's boot
Unna's (paste) boot
unofficial
unorganized
unphysiological
unrest
unroofing
unsaturated
unsaturated compound
unsex
unstriated
Unverricht's disease,
  syndrome
unwell
upper airway obstruction
  (UAO)
upper extremity (UE)
upper gastrointestinal
  (UGI)
upper left quadrant (ULQ)
upper lobe (UL)
upper motor neuron lesion
upper outer quadrant
  (UOQ)
upper respiratory
  infection (URI)
upper right quadrant
  (URQ)
upsiloid
uptake
urachal
urachal cyst or sinus
urachal, patent
urachus
uracil ($C_4H_4N_2O_2$)
uracil mustard

uracrasia
uracratia
uragogue
uranisconitis
uraniscoplasty
uraniscorrhaphy
uraniscus
uranium (U)
uranoplasty
uranoplegia
uranorrhaphy
uranoschisis
uranostaphyloplasty
uranostaphylorrhaphy
uranostaphyloschisis
uranyl (UO^{++})
urapostema
uraroma
urarthritis
urase
urate
uratemia
uratic
uratoma
uratosis
uraturia
Urban mastectomy
urceiform
urceolate
ur-defense(s)
urea (CH_4N_2O)
urea cycle
urea frost
urea nitrogen (blood-BUN)
Ureacin-10 Lotion (urea)
Ureacin-20 Creme (urea)
Ureacin-40 Creme (urea)
ureagenetic
ureal
ureameter
ureametry
Ureaphil (urea)
Ureaplasma urealyticum
ureapoiesis
urease
urecchysis
Urecholine (bethanechol
  chloride)

uredema
ureide
urelcosis
uremia
uremia, extrarenal
uremia, prerenal
uremic
uremigenic
ureogenesis
ureometer
ureometry
ureotelic
uresiesthesia
uresiesthesis
uresis
ureter
ureteral
ureteral endoscopy
ureteralgia
ureteral reflux study
uretercystoscope
ureterectasis
ureterectomy
ureteric
ureteritis
ureterocalycostomy
ureterocele
ureterocecostomy
ureterocele repair
ureterocervical
ureterocolostomy
ureterocutaneous fistula
ureterocutaneous
    transplantation
ureterocystanastomosis
ureterocystoneostomy
ureterocystoscope
ureterocystostomy
ureterodialysis
ureteroenterostomy
ureterography
ureteroheminephrectomy
ureterohydronephrosis
ureteroileostomy
ureterolith
ureterolithiasis
ureterolithotomy

ureterolysis
ureteroneocystostomy
ureteroneopyelostomy
ureteronephrectomy
ureteropathy
ureteropelvioplasty
ureterophlegma
ureteroplasty
ureteroplication
ureteroproctostomy
ureteropyelitis
ureteropyelography
ureteropyeloneostomy
ureteropyeloplasty
ureteropyelostomy
ureteropyosis
ureterorectostomy
ureterorrhagia
ureterorrhaphy
ureteroscopy
ureterosigmoidostomy
ureterostegnosis
ureterostenosis
ureterostoma
ureterostomy
ureterostomy, cutaneous
ureterotomy
ureterotrigonoenterostomy
ureteroureteral
ureteroureterostomy
ureterouterine
ureterovaginal
ureterovesical
ureterovesical junction
    (UVJ)
ureterovesicostomy
ureterovisceral fistula
ureters
urethra
urethra, muliebris
urethra, virilis
urethral
urethral catheterization
urethral fistula
urethral pressure profile
    (UPP)
urethral syndrome

urethralgia
urethrascope
urethratresia
urethrectomy
urethremphraxis
urethreurynter
urethrism
urethrismus
urethritis
urethritis, anterior
urethritis, gonococcal
urethritis, nongonococcal
urethritis, nonspecific
urethritis, posterior
urethritis, specific
urethrobulbar
urethrocele
urethrocele repair
urethrocystitis
urethrocystography
urethrocystopexy
urethrodynia
urethrograph
urethrography
urethrography, voiding
urethrometer
urethropenile
urethroperineal
urethroperineoscrotal
urethropexy
urethrophraxis
urethrophyma
urethroplasty
urethroprostatic
urethrorectal
urethrorrhagia
urethrorrhaphy
urethrorrhea
urethrorrhea ex libidine
urethroscope
urethroscopy
urethrospasm
urethrostaxis
urethrostenosis
urethrostomy
urethrotome
urethrotomy
urethrotrigonitis

urethrovaginal
urethrovaginal fistula
urethrovesical
urethrovesical junction
Urex (methenamine
  hippurate)
urhydrosis
uric
uric acid ($C_5H_4N_4O_3$)
uric acid, endogenous
uric acid, exogenous
uricacidemia
uricaciduria
uricase
uricemia
uricocholia
uricolysis
uricolytic
uricometer
uricopoiesis
uricosuria
uricosuric
uricosuric agent
uricotelic
uricoxidase
uridine
uridine diphosphate
uridrosis
uridrosis crystallina
uridyl transferase
uriesthesis
urina
urina cibi
urina galactodes
urina hysterica
urina jumentosa
urinaccelerator
urinal
urinalysis
urinary
urinary bladder
urinary calculi
urinary casts
urinary chorionic
  gonadotropin (UCG)
urinary director
  appliance
urinary diversion

urinary extravasation
  drainage
urinary incontinence
urinary infection
urinary meatus
urinary organs
urinary pigments
urinary reflex
urinary sediment
urinary stammering
urinary system
urinary tract
urinary tract infection
  (UTI)
urinate
urination
urine
urine assay test
urine, residual
urinemia
uriniferous
urinific
uriniparous
urinogenital
urinogenous
urinology
urinoma
urinometer
urinometry
urinophil
urinoscopy
urinose
urinosexual
uriposia
Urised (antiseptics and
  parasympatholytics
  combination)
urisolvent
Urispas (flavoxate HCl)
uroammoniac
uroanthelone
urobilin
urobilinemia
urobilinicterus
urobilinogen
urobilinogenemia
urobilinuria
Urobiotic-250

urocele
urocheras
urochesia
urochrome
Urocit-K (potassium
  citrate)
uroclepsia
urocrisia
urocyanin
urocyanogen
urocyanosis
urocyst
urocystic
urocystis
urocystitis
urodynamics
urodynia
uroedema
uroenterone
uroerythrin
uroflavin
uroflowmetry (UFR)
urofuscin
urofuscohematin
urogastrone
urogenital (UG)
urogenital fold
urogenous
uroglaucin
urogram
urography
urography, ascending
urography, cystoscopic
urography, descending
urography, excretion
urography, excretory
urography, intravenous
urography, retrograde
urohematin
urohematonephrosis
urohematoporphyrin
urokinase
urokinase pulmonary
  embolism trials (UPET)
urokinase-streptokinase
  pulmonary embolism
  trials (USPET)
urokinetic

urolagnia
urolith
urolithiasis
urolitic
urolithology
urologic
urologist
urology
urolutein
Uro-Mag (magnesium oxide)
uromancy
uromelanin
uromelus
urometer
uroncus
uronephrosis
uronology
uronophile
uropathogen
uropathy
uropathy, obstructive
uropenia
uropepsin
urophanic
urophein
Uro-Phosphate Tablets
urophosphometer
uroplania
uropoiesis
uropoietic
uroporphyria
uroporphyrin (UP)
uroporphyrinogen
uropsammus
uropyonephrosis
uropyoureter
Uroqid-Acid (methenamine
  mandelate and sodium
  acid phosphate)
urorosein
urorrhagia
urorrhea
urorrhodin
urorrhodinogen
urorubin
urorubrohematin
urosacin
uroscheocele

uroschesis
uroscopy
urosepsis
Ursinus Inlay-Tabs
urospectrin
urostealith
urotoxia
urotoxicity
urotoxin
uroureter
urous
uroxanthin
uroxin
urtica
urticant
urticaria
urticaria, aquagenic
urticaria bullosa
urticaria, cold
urticaria factitia
urticaria gigantea
urticaria haemorrhagica
urticaria maculosa
urticaria maritima
urticaria medicamentosa
urticaria papulosa
urticaria pigmentosa
urticaria pigmentosa
  juvenilis
urticaria solaris
urticarial
urticate
urtication
urushiol
Usher's syndrome
Ustilago
ustion
ustulation
ustus
usual and customary (U&C)
usual childhood diseases
  (UCHD)
ut dict (as directed)
uta
utend
uteralgia
uterectomy
uterine

uterine adnexa
uterine bleeding
uterine cervix
uterine glands
uterine ligament
uterine milk
uterine souffle
uterine subinvolution
uterine tube
uteroabdominal
uterocele
uterocervical
uterocystostomy
uterofixation
uterogenic
uterogestation
uterography
uterolith
uterometer
uteroovarian
uteropexia
uteropexy
uteroplacental
uteroplasty
uterorectal
uterosacral
uterosacral ligament
uterosalpingography
uteroscope
uterotome
uterotomy
uterotonic
uterotractor
uterotubal
uterotubography
uterovaginal
uteroventral
uterovesical
uterus
uterus acollis
uterus arcuatus
uterus bicornis
uterus biforis
uterus bilocularis
uterus bipartite
uterus, cancer of
uterus cordiformis
uterus, Couvelaire

uterus didelphys
uterus duplex
uterus, fetal
uterus, gravid
uterus masculinus
uterus parvicollis
uterus, prolapse of
uterus, pubescent
uterus, rupture of, in
  pregnancy
uterus septus
uterus, subinvolution of
uterus, tipped
uterus, tumors of
uterus unicornis
Uticillin VK (penicillin
  V potassium)
Uticort (betamethasone
  benzoate)
utilization review
Utimox (amoxicillin)
utricle
utricle, prostatic
utricle of urethra
utricle of vestibule
utricular
utriculitis
utriculoplasty
utriculosaccular
utriculosaccular duct
utriculus
utriculus masculinus
utriculus prostaticus
uva
uvea
uveal
uveitic
uveitis
uveitis, heterochromic
uveitis, sympathetic
uveoparotitis
uveoplasty
uveoscleritis
uviform
uviofast
uviol
uviolize
uviometer

uvioresistant
uviosensitive
uvula
uvula of cerebellum
uvula fissa
uvula vermis
uvula vesicae
uvulaptosis
uvular
uvularis
uvulatome
uvulatomy
uvulectomy
uvulitis
uvulopalatopharyngoplasty
 (UPPP)
uvulopharyngoplasty
uvuloptosis
uvulotome
uvulotomy
U wave

V

vaccigenous
vaccina
vaccinable
vaccinal
vaccinate
vaccination
vaccination, aqueous
vaccination, anthrax
vaccination, autogenous
vaccination, bacterial
vaccination, BCG
vaccination, brucellosis
vaccination, cholera
vaccination, DTP
vaccination, encephalitis
vaccination, epidemic
 typhus fever
vaccination, German
 measles
vaccination, hepatitis B
vaccination, heterologous

vaccination, homologous
vaccination, human
 diploid cell rabies
 (HDCV)
vaccination, hydrophobia
vaccination, infectious
 parotitis
vaccination, influenza
vaccination, killed
vaccination, measles
 virus, inactivated
vaccination, measles
 virus, live attenuated
vaccination, mixed
vaccination, multivalent
vaccination, mumps
vaccination, paratyphoid
 fever
vaccination, pertussis
vaccination, plague
vaccination,
 pneumococcal,
 polyvalent
vaccination,
 poliomyelitis
vaccination, poliovirus,
 inactivated
vaccination, poliovirus,
 live oral
vaccination, polyvalent
vaccination, rabies
vaccination, Rocky
 Mountain Spotted Fever
vaccination, rubella
vaccination, rubeola
vaccination, Sabin
vaccination, Salk
vaccination, sensitized
vaccination, smallpox
vaccination,
 staphylococcus
vaccination,
 streptococcus
vaccination, triple
vaccination, tuberculosis
vaccination, tularemia
vaccination, typhoid

vaccination, typhus
vaccination, undulant
    fever
vaccination, viral
    hepatitis
vaccination, yellow fever
vaccinator
vaccine
vaccine, aqueous
vaccine, autogenous
vaccine, bacterial
vaccine, BCG
vaccine, cholera
vaccine, DTP
vaccine, epidemic typhus
    fever
vaccine, heterologous
vaccine, homologous
vaccine, human diploid
    cell rabies
vaccine, humanized
vaccine, influenza
vaccine, killed
vaccine, measles virus,
    inactivated
vaccine, measles virus,
    live attenuated
vaccine, mixed
vaccine, multivalent
vaccine, mumps
vaccine, plague
vaccine, pneumococcal,
    polyvalent
vaccine, poliovirus,
    inactivated
vaccine, poliovirus, live
    oral
vaccine, polyvalent
vaccine, rabies
vaccine, Sabin
vaccine, Salk
vaccine, sensitized
vaccine, smallpox
vaccine, triple
vaccine, typhoid
vaccine, yellow fever
vaccinia
vaccinia necrosum

vaccinia immune globulin
vaccinial
vacciniform
vacciniola
vaccinogen
vaccinogenous
vaccinoid
vaccinostyle
vaccinotherapeutics
vaccinum
vacuolar
vacuolar degeneration
vacuolated
vacuolation
vacuole
vacuole, autophagic
vacuole, contractile
vacuole, heterophagous
vacuole, plasmocrine
vacuole, rhagiocrine
vacuolization
vacuome
vacuum
vacuum aspiration (VA)
vacuum extraction, fetal
    head
vacuum extractor
vacuum tube
vade mecum
vagabond's disease
vagal
vagal attack
vagal escape
vagal tone
**Vagesic Medicated Douche
    Liquid Concentrate**
vagi
vagina
vagina, bulb of
vagina fibrosa tendinis
vagina masculina
vagina mucosa tendinis
vagina, septate
vaginal
vaginal cytopathology
vaginal delivery
vaginal douche
vaginal episiotomy

vaginal hysterectomy (VH)
vaginal mucosa
vaginal septum
vaginal specimen
vaginal vibrator
vaginalectomy
vaginalitis
vaginapexy
vaginate
vaginectomy
vaginismus
vaginismus, deep
vaginismus, mental
vaginismus, posterior
vaginitis
vaginitis adhaesiva
vaginitis, atrophic
vaginitis, diphtheritic
vaginitis, emphysematous
vaginitis, *Gardnerella vaginalis*
vaginitis, granular
vaginitis, nonspecific
vaginitis, postmenopausal
vaginitis, senile
vaginitis testis
vaginitis, *Trichomonas vaginalis*
vaginoabdominal
vaginocele
vaginodynia
vaginofixation
vaginogenic
vaginogram
vaginography
vaginolabial
vaginometer
vaginomycosis
vaginopathy
vaginoperineal
vaginoperineorrhaphy
vaginoperineotomy
vaginoperitoneal
vaginopexy
vaginoplasty
vaginorrhaphy
vaginoscope
vaginoscopy

vaginosis, bacterial
vaginotome
vaginotomy
vaginovesical
vaginovulvar
Vagisec Plus Suppositories
vagitis
vagitus
vagitus uterinus
vagitus vaginalis
vagolysis
vagolytic
vagomimetic
vagosympathetic
vagotomy
vagotomy and pyloroplasty (V&P)
vagotomy, medical
vagotonia
vagotonic
vagotropic
vagotropism
vagovagal
vagrant
vagus
vagus pulse
vagus nerve (X)
Valadol (acetaminophen)
valence
valency
Valentin's ganglion
valethamate bromide
valetudinarian
valgus
valgus, cubitus hemiepiphyseal arrest
valgus, genu osteotomy
valgus, hallux exostectomy
valgus, hallux osteotomy
validity
valine ($C_5H_{11}NO_2$)
valinemia
Valisone (betamethasone valerate)
Valium (diazepam)
vallate

vallate papilla
vallecula
vallecula cerebelli
vallecula epiglottica
vallecula ovata
vallecula sylvii
vallecula unguis
Valleix's points
valley fever
valley of cerebellum
vallis
vallum unguis
Valmid (ethinamate)
Valpin 50 (anisotropine
  methylbromide)
Valrelease (diazepam)
Valsalva's maneuver
Valsalva's sinuses
value
valva
valvate
valve
valve, aortic
valve, atrioventricular,
  left
valve, atrioventricular,
  right
valve, bicuspid
valve, coronary
valve, ileocecal
valve, mitral
valve, pulmonary
valve, pyloric
valve, semilunar
valve, thebesian
valve, tricuspid
valve, of Varolius
valves, cardiac
valves, Houston's
valvectomy
valvoplasty
valvotomy
valvula
valvula bicuspidalis
valvula coli
valvula pylori
valvula semilunaris
valvula tricuspidalis

valvulae
valvulae conniventes
valvular
valvular disease of the
  heart (VDH)
valvulitis
valvuloplasty
valvulotome
valvulotomy
vanadium (V)
vanadiumism
van Buren's disease
Vancenase (beclomethasone
  dipropionate)
Vanceril (beclomethasone
  dipropionate)
Vancocin HCl (vancomycin
  HCl)
van den Bergh's test
van der Hoeve's syndrome
van der Waals forceps
vanilla
vanillin
vanillism
vanillylmandelic acid
  (VMA)
Vanoxide-HC (acne lotion)
Vanquish
Vansil (oxamniquine)
van't Hoff's rule
Vapo-Iso (isoproterenol
  HCl)
vapor
vapor permeable membrane
vaporium
vaporization
vaporize
vaporizer
vaporous
vapotherapy
Vaquez's disease
variability
variable
variance
variant
variate
variation
variation, continuous

variation, meristic
varication
variced
varicella
varicella gangrenosa
varicella-zoster immune
  globulin
varicelliform
varicelloid
varices
varices esophageal
variciform
varicoblepharon
varicocele
varicocele, ovarian
varicocele, utero-ovarian
varicocelectomy
varicocelectomy,
  spermatic cord
varicography
varicoid
varicole
varicomphalus
varicophlebitis
varicose
varicose ulcers
varicose veins
varicosis
varicosity
varicotomy
varicula
variety
Vari-Flavors
variola
variola minor
variolar
variolate
variolation
variolic
varioliform
variolization
varioloid
variolous
varix
varix, aneurysmal
varix, arterial
varix, chyle
varix, lymphaticus

varix, turbinal
varnish
varolian
varolian bend
varus
vas
vas aberrans
vas afferens
vas afferens glomeruli
vas capillare
vas deferens
vas lymphaticum
vas prominens
vas spirale
vasa
vasa afferentia
vasa brevia
vasa efferentia
vasa praevia
vasa recta
vasa vasorum
vasa vorticosa
vasal
vascular
vascular ring
vascular system
vascular tuft
vascular tumor
vascularity
vascularization
vascularize
vasculature
vasculitis
vasculogenesis
vasculomotor
vasculopathy
vasculum
vasectomy
Vaseline (petrolatum)
Vaseretic (enalapril
  maleate-
  hydrochlorothiazide)
vasifactive
vasiform
vasitis
vasoactive
vasoactive intestinal
  polypeptide (VIP)

vasoconstriction
vasoconstrictive
vasoconstrictor
vasodentin
vasodepression
vasodepressor
Vasodilan (isoxsuprine HCl)
vasodilatation
vasodilatation, antidromic
vasodilatation, reflex
vasodilation
vasodilative
vasodilator
vasoepididymostomy
vasofactive
vasoformative
vasoganglion
vasography
vasohypertonic
vasohypotonic
vasoinhibitor
vasoinhibitory
vasoligation
vasomotion
vasomotor
vasomotor epilepsy
vasomotor reflex
vasomotor spasm
vasoneuropathy
vasoneurosis
vaso-orchidostomy
vasoparesis
vasopressin
vasopressin injection
vasopressor
vasopuncture
vasoreflex
vasorelaction
vasorrhaphy
vasosection
vasosensory
vasospasm
vasospastic
vasostimulant
vasostomy

Vasotec (enalapril maleate)
vasotomy
vasotonia
vasotonic
vasotribe
vasotripsy
vasotrophic
vasotropic
vasovagal
vasovagal syncope
vasovasostomy
vasovesiculectomy
vasovesiculitis
Vasoxyl (methoxamine HCl)
vastus
Vater's ampulla
Vater's corpuscles
Vater's papilla
vault
V-Cillin (penicillin V)
V-Cillin K (penicillin V potassium)
vection
vectis
vector
vector, biological
vector, mechanical
vectorcardiogram
vectorcardiography
vectorial
Veetids '125' For Oral Solution (penicillin V potassium)
Veetids '250' For Oral Solution (penicillin V potassium)
Veetids '250' Tablets (penicillin V potassium)
Veetids '500' Tablets (penicillin V potassium)
vegan
veganism
vegetable
vegetal

vegetarian
vegetarianism
vegetate
vegetation
vegetation, adenoid
vegative
vegetoanimal
vehicle
veil
vein
velamen
velamen nativum
velamen vulvae
velamentous
velamentum
velar
Velban (vinblastine
  sulfate)
Velcro
veliform
vellication
vellus
velopharyngeal
**Velosef '125' for Oral
  Suspension** (cephradine)
Velosef '250' Capsules
  (cephradine)
**Velosef '250' for Oral
  Suspension** (cephradine)
Velosef '500' Capsules
  (cephradine)
Velosef for Injection
  (cephradine)
Velosulin (U-100 purified
  pork insulin)
Velosulin Human (U-100
  human insulin)
velosynthesis
Velpeau's deformity
velum
velum palatinum
vena
vena cava inferior
vena cava superior
venacavography
venae comitantes
venation
venectasia

venectomy
veneer
venenation
venene
veneniferous
venenific
venenosalivary
venenosity
venenous
venepuncture
venereal
venereal bubo
venereal collar
venereal disease (VD)
venereal sore
venereal urethritis
venereal wart
venereologist
venereology
venereophobia
venery
venesection
venin
venine
venipuncture
venisection
venisuture
venoatrial
venoauricular
venoclysis
venofibrosis
venogram
venography
venom
venom, Russell's viper
venom, snake
venomization
venomosalivary
venomotor
venomous
venomous snake
veno-occlusive
venoperitoneostomy
venopressor
venosclerosis
venose
venosinal
venosity

venospasm
venostasis
venostat
venothrombotic
venotomy
venous
venous blood
venous hum
venous hyperemia
venous return
venous sinus
venous sinus of sclera
venos thrombosis
venovenostomy
vent
vent, alveolar
venter
ventilation
ventilation coefficient
ventilation, continuous
  positive-pressure
ventilation, intermittent
  postive-pressure
ventilation, pulmonary
ventilation rate (VR)
ventilation tube
ventilator
Ventolin (albuterol)
ventouse
ventrad
ventral
ventral hernia
ventralis
ventricle
ventricle, aortic
ventricle of Arantius
ventricle, fifth
ventricle, fourth
ventricle of larynx
ventricle, lateral
ventricle, left
ventricle, Morgagni's
ventricle, pineal
ventricle, right
ventricle, third
ventricornu
ventricose
ventricular

ventricular assist
  pumping
ventricular compliance
ventricular folds
ventricular ligament
ventricular septal defect
ventriculitis
ventriculoatriostomy
ventriculocisternostomy
ventriculocordectomy
ventriculogram
ventriculography
ventriculometry
ventriculonector
ventriculopuncture
ventriculoscopy
ventriculostomy
ventriculosubarachnoid
ventriculotomy
ventriculus
ventriculus tertius
ventricumbent
ventriduct
ventriduction
ventrimeson
ventripyramid
ventrocystorrhaphy
ventrodorsal
ventrofixation
ventrohysteropexy
ventroinguinal
ventrolateral
ventromedial
ventroptosia
ventroptosis
ventroscopy
ventrose
ventrosity
ventrosuspension
ventrotomy
ventrovesicofixation
Venturi mask
venturimeter
venula
venule
Venus, crown of
Venus, mount of
Venus's collar

Vepesid (etoposide [VP
  16-213])
verbigeration
verbomania
Vercyte (pipobroman)
verdigris
verdigris poisoning
verdohemoglobin
Verga's ventricle
verge
verge, anal
vergence
Verheyen's stars
vermicidal
vermicide
vermicular
vermicular movements
vermicular pulse
vermiculation
vermicule
vermiculose
vermiculous
vermiform
vermiform appendix
vermifugal
vermifuge
vermilion border
vermilionectomy
vermin
verminal
vermination
verminosis
verminous
vermiphobia
vermis
vermis cerebelli
vermis, inferior
vermis, superior
Vermox (mebendazole)
vernal
Vernet's syndrome
vernix
vernix caseosa
Verr-Canth-C&M
Verrex-C&M
verruca
verruca acuminata
verruca digitata

verruca filiformis
verruca gyri hippocampi
verruca plana
verruca plantaris
verruca vulgaris
verruciform
verrucose
verrucosis
verrucous
verruga peruana
Verrusol-C&M
Versapen (hetacillin)
Versapen K (hetacillin
  potassium)
Versed (midazolam HCl)
Versene
  (ethylene-
  diaminetetraacetic
  acid)
versicolor
version
version, bipolar
version, cephalic
version, combined
version, external
version, internal
version, pelvic
version, podalic
version, spontaneous
vertebra
vertebra, basilar
vertebra, cervical
vertebra, coccygeal
vertebra dentata
vertebra, false
vertebra, fixed
vertebra, flexion
vertebra, lumbar
vertebra magnum
vertebra, odontoid
vertebra prominens
vertebra, rotation
vertebra, sacral
vertebra, sternal
vertebra, thoracic
vertebra, true
vertebral
vertebral body fracture

vertebral canal
vertebral-carotid
  transposition
vertebral column
vertebral corpectomy
vertebral foramen
vertebral groove
vertebral notch
vertebral ribs
vertebrarium
Vertebrata
vertebrate
vertebrated
vertebrectomy
vertebroarterial
vertebrobasilar
vertebrochondral
vertebrocostal
vertebrofemoral
vertebroiliac
vertebromammary
vertebrosacral
vertebrosternal
vertex
vertex cordis
vertical
verticalis
verticality
verticillate
verticomental
vertiginous
vertigo
vertigo, auditory
vertigo, central
vertigo, cerebral
vertigo, epileptic
vertigo, essential
vertigo, gastric
vertigo, hysterical
vertigo, labyrinthine
vertigo, laryngeal
vertigo, objective
vertigo, ocular
vertigo, organic
vertigo, peripheral
vertigo, positional
vertigo, postural
vertigo, subjective

vertigo, toxic
vertigo, vestibular
verumontanitis
verumontanum
very low density
  lipoproteins (VLDL)
vesalianum
Vesalius, foramen of
Vesalius, veins of
vesica
vesica fellea
vesica prostatica
vesica urinaria
vesical
vesical neck dilation
vesical neck excision
vesical neck repair
vesical reflex
vesicant
vesication
vesicatory
vesicle
vesicle, allantoic
vesicle, auditory
vesicle, blastodermic
vesicle, chorionic
vesicle, compound
vesicle, lens
vesicle, otic
vesicle, seminal
vesicle, umbilical
vesicles, brain
vesicles, brain, primary
vesicles, cerebral
vesicles, encephalic
vesicles, multilocular
vesicles, optic
vesicoabdominal
vesicocele
vesicocervical
vesicoclysis
vesicoenteric
vesicofixation
vesicointestinal
vesicolithotomy
vesicoprostatic
vesicopubic
vesicopustule

vesicosigmoid
vesicosigmoidostomy
vesicospinal
vesicostomy
vesicotomy
vesicoumbilical
vesicoureteral
vesicourethropexy
vesicouterine
vesicouterine fistula
vesicouterine pouch
vesicouterovaginal
vesicovaginal
vesicovaginal fistula
vesicovaginorectal
vesicula
vesicula seminalis
vesicular
vesicular breathing
vesicular eczema
vesicular murmur
vesicular rale
vesicular resonance
vesiculase
vesiculated
vesiculation
vesiculectomy
vesiculiform
vesiculitis
vesiculobronchial
vesiculocavernous
vesiculogram
vesiculogram, seminal
vesiculography
vesiculopapular
vesiculopustular
vesiculotomy
vesiculotubular
vesiculotympanic
Vespidae
Vesprin (triflupromazine
  HCl)
vessel
vessel, blood
vessel, collateral
vessel, lacteal
vessel, radicular
vessels, absorbent

vessels, chyliferous
vessels, great
vessels, lymphatic
vessels, nutrient
vestibular
vestibular bulbs
vestibular caloric test
vestibular membrane
vestibular nerve
vestibular nerve section
vestibule
vestibule of aorta
vestibule, aortic
vestibule of ear
vestibule of larynx
vestibule of mouth
vestibule of vagina
vestibulocochlear nerve
  (VIII)
vestibuloplasty
vestibulotomy
vestibulourethral
vestibulum
vestige
vestigial
vestigium
veta
veterinarian
veterinary
veterinary medicine
via
viability
viable
viable birth (VB)
vial
vibex
Vibramycin (doxycycline
  hyclate)
vibrapuncture
Vibra-Tabs (doxycycline
  hyclate)
vibratile
vibration
vibrative
vibrator
vibrator, vaginal
vibrator, whole body
vibratory

vibratory sense
Vibrio
Vibrio cholerae
Vibrio fetus
vibriocidal
vibrion
vibriosis
vibrissae
vibromassage
vibromasseur
vibrometer
vibrotherapeutics
vicarious
vicarious learning
vicarious menstruation
vicarious respiration
Vicks Children Cough Syrup
Vicks Cough Silencers
Vicks Daycare
Vicks Formula 44
Vicks Formula 44D
Vicks Formula 44M
Vicks Inhaler
Vicks Nyquil
Vicks Sinex
Vicks Throat Lozenges
Vicks Vaporub
Vicks Vaposteam
Vicks Vatronol
Vicodin (hydrocodone bitartrate and acetaminophen)
Vicon Forte (therapeutic vitamins and minerals)
Vicon Plus (therapeutic vitamins and minerals)
Vicon-C (therapeutic vitamins and minerals)
Vicq d'Azyr's tract
Vidal operation
vidarabine
Vi-Daylin ADC Vitamin Drops
Vi-Daylin/F ADC Vitamin Drops with Fluoride
Vi-Daylin Multivitamin + Iron Chewable Tablets
Vi-Daylin Multivitamin + Iron Drops
Vi-Daylin Multivitamin + Iron Liquid
Vi-Daylin Multivitamin Chewable Tablets
Vi-Daylin Multivitamin Drops
Vi-Daylin Multivitamin Liquid
video display terminal (VDT)
videognosis
vidian artery
vidian canal
vidian nerve
vidianectomy
vigil
vigil, coma
vigilambulism
vigilance
vigintinormal
vigor
Villaret's syndrome
villi
villi, chorionic
villiferous
villoma
villose
villous
villositis
villosity
villus
villus, arachnoid
villus, chorionic
villus, intestinal
villus, synovial
villusectomy
vinblastine sulfate
vinca
vinca alkaloids
Vincasar PFS (vincristine sulfate)
Vincent's angina
vincristine sulfate
vinculum
vinculum tendinum
Vineberg operation

vinegar
vinic
vinous
vinum
vinyl
vinyl chloride
vinyl cyanide
vinyl ether
Vioform (clioquinol)
Vioform-Hydrocortisone
  (clioquinol and
  hydrocortisone)
Viokase (pancrelipase)
violaceous
violate
violence
violet
violet blindness
violet, gentian
viomycin
viosterol
viper
viper venom prothrombin
  time
Vira-A (vidarabine
  concentrate)
viraginity
viral
viral hemagglutination
  inhibition tests (HAI)
viral interference
viral neutralization test
Viranol (salicylic acid
  and lactic acid)
Virazole (ribavirin)
Virchow's node
viremia
vires
virgin
virginal
virginal membrane
virginity
viricidal
viricide
virile
virile reflex
virilescence
virilia

virilism
virility
virilization
virion
viripotent
viroids
virology
viropexis
Viroptic (trifluridine)
virose
virous
virtual
virucidal
virucide
virulence
virulent
viruliferous
viruria
virus
virus, arbor
virus, attenuated
virus, bacterial
virus, chikungunya
virus, coxsackie
virus, cytomegalic (CMV)
virus, defective
virus, enteric
  cytopathogenic human
  orphan (ECHO)
virus, enteric
virus, Epstein-Barr (EB)
virus, filtrable
virus, fixé
virus, fixed
virus, helper
virus, hepadna-
virus, herpes
virus, human
  immunodeficiency (HIV)
virus identification
virus, latent
virus, lytic
virus, masked
virus, parainfluenza
virus, plant
virus, pox
virus, respiratory
  syncytial

virus, slow
virus, street
virus, tumor
virusemia
viruses, neurotropic
viruses, orphan
virustatic
vis
vis afronte
vis formativa
vis medicatrix naturae
viscera
viscerad
visceral
visceral angiography
visceral angioplasty
visceral arches
visceral cavity
visceral clefts
visceralgia
viscereal skeleton
viscerimotor
viscerocranium
viscerogenic
visceroinhibitory
visceromegaly
visceromotor
visceromotor reflex
visceroparietal
visceroperitoneal
visceropleural
visceroptosis
visceroreceptors
viscerosensory
viscerosensory reflex
visceroskeletal
viscerosomatic
viscerosomatic reaction
viscerotome
viscerotonia
viscerotrophic
viscerotropic
viscerovisceral reaction
viscid
viscidity
viscometer
viscosimeter
viscosimetry

viscosity
viscosity, specific
viscous
viscus
visibility
visible
visile
vision
vision, achromatic
vision, artificial
vision, binocular
vision, central
vision, day
vision, dichromatic
vision, double
vision, field of
vision, half
vision, indirect
vision, monocular
vision, multiple
vision, night
vision, oscillating
vision, peripheral
vision, phantom
vision, tunnel
visit
Visiting Nurse
  Association
Visken (pindolol)
Vistaril (hydroxyzine
  HCl)
Vistaril Pamoate
  (hydroxyzine pamoate)
visual acuity (VA)
visual angle
visual cone
visual evoke potential
  (VEP)
visual field
visual field examination
visual function
visual plane
visual point
visual yellow
visualization
visualize
visually evoked response
visuoauditory

visuognosis
visuopsychic
visuosensory
vita glass
Vita-Plus H
vital
vital capacity (VC, vit
  cap)
vital center
Vital High Nitrogen
Vitaline's 8X Pancreatin
  (lipase, protease and
  amylase)
vitalism
vitalist
vitalistic
vitality
vitalize
vital signs (VS)
vital statistics
vitamer
vitamin A
vitamin A_1
vitamin A_2
vitamin B_1 (thiamine)
vitamin B_2 (riboflavin)
vitamin B_6 (pyridoxine)
vitamin B_{12}
  (cyanocobalamin)
vitamin C (ascorbic acid)
vitamin D
vitamin E (tocopherol,
  alpha)
vitamin, folacin
vitamin K
vitamin loss
vitamin, niacin
vitaminoid
vitaminology
vitellary
vitellin
vitelline
vitelline circulation
vitelline duct
vitelline membrane
vitelline veins
vitellogenesis
vitellointestinal

vitellolutein
vitellorubin
vitellose
vitellus
vitiation
vitiligines
vitiliginous
vitiligo
vitiligo capitis
vitiligo perinevic
vitiligoidea
vitium
vitium cordis
vitrectomy
vitreocapsulitis
vitreodentin
vitreoretinal
vitreous
vitreous body
vitreous chamber
vitreous degeneration
vitreous humor
vitreous membrane
vitreous table
vitrescence
vitreum
vitriol
vitriol, blue
vitriol, green
vitriol, oil of
vitriol, white
vitropression
vitrum
Vivactil (protriptyline
  HCl)
vividialysis
vividiffusion
vivification
viviparity
viviparous
vivisect
vivisection
vivisectionist
vivisector
vivisepulture
Vivonex Acutrol (enteral
  feeding system)

Vivonex Delivery System
(tube feeding system)
Vivonex Jejunostomy Kit
(needle catheter
jejunostomy kit)
Vivonex T.E.N. (elemental
diet for total enteral
nutrition)
Vivonex Tungsten Tip Tube
(nasogastric/
nasointestinal feeding)
Vi-Zac (therapeutic
vitamin-mineral)
Vlemasque (sulfurated
lime)
Vleminckx's solution
vocal
vocal cords
vocal folds
vocal fremitus
vocal ligament
vocal lips
vocal muscle
vocal process
vocal resonance
vocal signs
voces
voice
voice, amphoric
voice, cavernous
voice, eunuchoid
voice training
voiceprint
voices
void
voiding
urethrocystography
vola
vola manus
vola pedis
volaris
volatile
volatilization
volatilize
vole
volition
volitional
Volkmann's canals

Volkmann's contracture
volley
volsella
volt
voltage
voltaic
voltaism
voltammeter
voltampere
volubility
volume
volume, airway closing
volume, blood or plasma
volume, expiratory rate
volume, expiratory
reserve
volume index (VI)
volume, inspiratory
reserve
volume, mean corpuscular
volume, minute
volume of packed red
cells (VPRC)
volume preset ventilators
volume, residual lung
volume, respiratory flow
loop
volume, screen
volume, stroke
volume, thoracic gas
volume, tidal
volume, urine
voluntary
voluntary health agency
voluntary muscle
voluptuous
volupty
volute
volvulosis
volvulus
volvulus decompression
volvulus imaging
volvulus reduction
vomer
vomerine
vomerobasilar
vomeronasal
vomeronasal cartilages

vomeronasal organ
vomica
vomicose
vomit
vomit, bilious
vomit, black
vomit, coffee-ground
vomiting
vomiting, cyclic
vomiting, dry
vomiting, epidemic
vomiting, incoercible
vomiting, induced
vomiting, pernicious
vomiting of pregnancy
vomiting, projectile
vomiting, stercoraceous
vomitive
vomitory
vomiturition
vomitus
vomitus, coffee-ground
vomitus cruentus
vomitus marinus
vomitus matutinus
von Gierke disease
von Graefe's sign
von Hippel's disease
von Jaksch's disease
von Kraske operation
von Pirquet's test
von Recklinghausen's
  canals
von Recklinghausen's
  disease
von Recklinghausen's
  tumor
Vontrol (diphenidol)
von Willebrand's disease
voodoo
Voorhees' bag
voracious
vortex
vortex, coccygeal
vortex of heart
vortex lentis
vortices
vortices pilorum

vorticose
vorticose veins
VoSol (acetic acid
  nonaqueous)
Voss operation
vox
vox abscissa
vox capitus
vox cholerica
vox rauca
voyeur
voyeurism
vuerometer
vulgaris
vulnerable
vulnerant
vulnerary
vulnerate
vulnus
Vulpian-Heidenhain-
  Sherrington phenomenon
vulsella
vulsellum
vulva
vulva abscess, I&D
vulva benign lesion
  cryosurgery
vulva biopsy
vulva connivens
vulva cryosurgery
vulva destruction of
  lesion
vulva hians
vulva laser surgery
vulva, velamen
vulval
vulvar
vulvar leukoplakia
vulvar vestibulitis
  syndrome
vulvectomy
vulvismus
vulvitis
vulvitis, acute
  nongonorrheal
vulvitis, follicular
vulvitis, gangrenous
vulvitis, leukoplakic

vulvitis, mycotic
vulvocrural
vulvopathy
vulvouterine
vulvovaginal
vulvovaginal glands
vulvovaginitis
vulvovaginitis, diabetic
V-Y operation, bladder
V-Y operation, lip
V-Y operation, skin
V-Y operation,
  subcutaneous tissue
V-Y operation, tongue
Vytone (hydrocortisone
  iodoquinol)

W

Waardenburg syndrome
Wachendorf's membrane
Wada activation test
wafer
Wagstaffe's fracture
waist
wakeful
Walcher's position
Wald cycle
Wald, Lillian
Waldenström's disease
Waldeyer's gland
Waldeyer's neuron
Waldeyer's ring
walk
walker
walking
walking cast
walking, sleep
walking well
walking wounded
wall
Wallenberg's syndrome
wallerian degeneration
walleye

Walthard's islets or
  inclusions
wandering
wandering abcess
wandering kidney
wandering mind
wandering spleen
Wangesteen tube
Warburg apparatus
ward
ward, accident
ward, psychiatric
Wardrop's disease
Wardrop's operation
warehousemen's itch
warfarin poisoning
warfarin potassium
warfarin sodium
war gases
wart
wart, fig
wart, genital
wart, plantar
wart, seborrheic
wart, senile
wart, venereal
Wart-Off (salicylic acid,
  alcohol, ether)
wash
wash, eye
washerwoman's itch
washout, nitrogen
wasp
wasp sting
Wassermann reaction
Wassermann-fast
waste
waste products
waste products, metabolic
wasting
wasting palsy
water
water bed
water, bound
water brash
water cure
water, deionized

water, distilled
water, hard
water, heavy
water intoxication
water, lime
water on brain
water, purified
water, pryogen-free
water, soft
waterhammer pulse
Waterhouse-Friderichsen
  syndrome
waters
Watson-Crick helix
Watson-Schwartz test
watt
wattage
wave
wave, alpha
wave, beta
wave, brain
wave, delta
wave, electromagnetic
wave, excitation
wave, pulse
wave, ultrashort
wave, ultrasonic
waves, hertzian
waves, light
waves, radio
waves, sound
waves, theta
wavelength
wax
wax, dental
waxing-up
waxy
waxy cast
waxy degeneration
weak
wean
weanling
weanling diarrhea
web
web, esophageal
web, terminal
webbed
Weber's glands

Weber's paralysis
Weber test
Weber-Christian disease
Wechsler Intelligence
  Scale for Children
  (WISC)
wedge pressure
weeping
weeping eczema
weeping sinew
Wegener's granulomatosis
  or syndrome
Weidel reaction
Weigert's law
weight
weight, apothecaries'
weight, atomic
weight, avoirdupois
weight, equivalent
weight, molecular
weight, set point
weightlessness
weights and measures
Weil-Felix reaction, test
Weil's disease
Weir Mitchell's treatment
weismannism
Weitbrecht's foramen
Weitbrecht's ligament
Welch's bacillus
welding
Wellcovorin (leucovorin)
welt
wen
Wenckebach's period,
  pauses, or phenomenon
Werdnig-Hoffmann disease
Werdnig-Hoffmann
  paralysis
Werdnig-Hoffmann syndrome
Werlhof's disease
Wermer's syndrome
Wernicke's encephalopathy
Wernicke's syndrome
Westcort (hydrocortisone
  valerate)
western blotting
Westphal-Edinger nucleus

Westphal-Stûmpell
  pseudosclerosis
wet
wet brain
wet cup
wet dream
wet nurse
wet pack
wet-dry dressing or pack
Wetzel grid
Wharton's duct
Wharton's jelly
wheal
wheat
wheatstone bridge
wheel
wheel, carborundum
wheel, diamond
wheel, polishing
wheel, wire
wheelchair
wheeze
wheezing
whelk
whiff
whinolalia
whiplash injury
Whipple's disease
whipworm
whirl
whirlbone
whirlpool bath
whiskey, whisky
whisper
whisper, cavernous
whistle
whistling face syndrome
white
white cell
white of egg
white of eye
white gangrene
white leg
white line
white lotion
white matter
white ointment
white precipitate

white softening
whitehead
whitepox
whitlow
Whitman acetabuloplasty
Whitmore's disease
whole blood (WB)
whole body bone imaging
whole body bone marrow
  imaging
whole body counter
whole body tumor
  localization
wholism
wholistic health
whoop
whooping cough
whorl
Widal's reaction or test
Wigand-Martin maneuver
wild cherry
Wilke parotid duct
  diversion
will
Willebrand factor assay
Williams-Richardson
  operation
Willis' circle
Willis' cords
Wilms' tumor
Wilson acetabular
  augmentation
Wilson's disease
Wilson-Mikity syndrome
Winckel's disease
windburn
windchill
windchill factor
windchill index
winding sheet
window
window, aortic
window, aortopulmonary
window, cochlear
window, oval, repair
window, pericardial
window, round, repair
window, vestibular

windowing of cast
windpipe
wine (vin)
wine sores
wing
WinGel (aluminum-
  magnesium hydroxide)
Winiwarter operation
wink
winking
winking, jaw
Winslow, foramen of
Winslow, ligament of
Winslow, pancreas of
Winstrol (stanozolol)
wintergreen oil
winter itch
Winter procedure
Wintrobe sedimentation
  rate
wire
wire, arch
wire, Kirschner
wire, ligature
wire, separating
wiring, aneurysm
wiring, circumferential
wiring, continuous loop
wiring, craniofacial
  suspension
wiring, dental
wiring, Gilmer
wiring, Ivy Loop
wiring, perialveolar
wiring, pyriform
wiring, Stout's
Wirsung, duct of
wisdom tooth
Wiskott-Aldrich syndrome
witches' milk
withdrawal
withdrawal syndrome
within normal limits
  (WNL)
witkop
Witzel operation
witzelsucht

witzelsucht, primary
  affective
Wohlfahrtia
Wohlfahrtia magnifica
Wohlfahrtia opaca
Wohlfahrtia vigil
wolffian body
wolffian cyst
wolffian duct
wolffian tubules
Wolff-Parkinson-White
  syndrome
Wolfina 100 (rauwolfia
  serpentina)
wolfram
wolfsbane
Wolhynia fever
Wolman's disease
womb
wood alcohol
Wood's ray
wood tick
Woodward operation
Wookey esophagectomy
wool fat
woolsorter's disease
word blindness
word salad
work
work-up
worm
wormian bones
wormseed
wormseed, American
wormwood
worried well
wound
wound, abdominal
wound, bullet
wound, cellulitis of
wound, contused
wound, crushing
wound dehiscence
wound, fishhook
wound, incised
wound infection
wound, lacerated

wound, nonpenetrating
wound, open
wound, penetrating
wound, perforating
wound, puncture
wound repair
wound, subcutaneous
wound, tunnel
W-plasty
wrapping, aneurysm
wreath
Wright's stain
Wright's technique
wrinkle
Wrisberg's cardiac
  ganglion
Wrisberg's cartilages
Wrisberg's ganglion
Wrisberg's nerve
wrist
wrist bones
wrist drop
wrist unit
writer's cramp
writing
writing, dextrad
writing hand
writing, mirror
wrongful birth
wrongful life
wryneck
Wuchereria
Wuchereria bancrofti
Wuchereria malayi
wuchereriasis
Wyamine Sulfate
  (mephentermine sulfate)
Wyamycin Liquid
  (erythromycin
  ethylsuccinate)
Wyamycin S (erythromycin
  stearate)
Wyanoids (hemorrhoidal
  suppositories)
Wycillin (penicillin G
  procaine)

Wycillin and Probenecid
  (penicillin G procaine
  and probenecid)
Wydase (hyaluronidase)
Wygesic (propoxyphene HCL
  and acetaminophen)
Wymox (amoxicillin)
Wytensin (guanabenz
  acetate)

X

Xanax (alprazolam)
xanchromatic
xanthelasma
xanthelasmoidea
xanthematin
xanthemia
xanthene
xanthic
xanthic calculus
xanthine
xanthine base
xanthinuria
xanthiuria
xanthochroia
xanthochromatic
xanthochromia
xanthochromic
xanthochroous
xanthocyanopia
xanthocyanopsia
xanthocyte
xanthoderma
xanthodont
xanthoerythrodermia
  perstans
xanthogranuloma
xanthogranuloma, juvenile
xanthokyanopy
xanthoma
xanthoma, diabetic
xanthoma disseminatum

xanthoma multiplex
xanthoma palpebrarum
xanthoma tuberosum
xanthomatosis
xanthomatous
xanthophose
xanthophyll
xanthoprotein
xanthopsia
xanthopsin
xanthopsis
xanthorrhea
xanthosine
xanthosis
xanthous
xanthurenic acid
xanthuria
xenobiotic
xenogeneic
xenogenesis
xenogenous
xenograft
xenography, breast
xenology
xenomenia
xenon (Xe)
xenon-133
xenon arc
   photocoagulation
xenoparasite
xenophobia
xenophonia
xenophthalmia
Xenopsylla
Xenopsylla cheopsis
xenorexia
Xerac (alcohol gel)
Xerac AC (aluminum
   chloride hexahydrate in
   anhydrous ethanol)
Xerac BP10
Xerac BP5 (benzoyl
   peroxide water gel)
xerantic
xerasia
xerocheilia
xeroderma

xeroderma pigmentosum
   (XDP)
xerography
xeroma
xeromammography
xeromenia
xeromycteria
xeronosus
xerophagia
xerophagy
xerophthalmia
xerophthalmus
xeroradiography
xerosis
xerostomia
xerotes
xerotic
xerotocia
xerotripsis
xiphisternum
xiphocostal
xiphocostal ligament
xiphodynia
xiphoid
xiphoid process
xiphoidectomy
xiphoiditis
xiphopagotomy
xiphopagus
X-linked
X-Prep (extract of senna
   fruit)
x-radiation
x-ray (XR)
x-ray, abdomen
x-ray, bite-wing
x-ray, chest
x-ray diffraction,
   calculus
x-ray dermatitis
x-ray, heart
x-ray, skull
x-ray, strain
x-ray, uterus, bladder
xylene
xylene poisoning
xylenin
xylenol

Xylocaine (lidocaine HCl)
xylol
xylometazoline
  hydrochloride
xylose
xylose absorption test
xylose excretion test
xylulose
xylyl
xyrospasm
xysma
xyster

Y

Y cartilage
Y chromosome
yard
yaw
yaw, mother
yawn
yawning
yaws
year (yr)
year of birth (YOB)
yeast
yeast, brewer's
yeast, dried
yellow
yellow body
yellow fever
yellow ointment
yellow spot
yellow vision
yerba
yerba maté
Yersin's serum
Yersinia
Yersinia enterocolitica
Yersinia pestis
Yersinia
  pseudotuberculosis
yersiniosis

YF-VAX (live, 17D virus,
  Avian Leukosis-free,
  stablilized)
yin-yang
Yocon (yohimbine HCl)
Yodoxin (iodoquinol)
yoga
yoghurt
yogurt
yohimbine
Yohimex (yohimbine HCl)
yoke
yolk
yolk sac
yolk stalk
Young-Helmholtz theory
Young's operation
Young's rule
youth
Yount operation
Y-plasty, bladder
ypsiliform
Y-pyeloplasty (Yb)
ytterbium (Y)
yttrium
yttrium aluminum garnet
  (Yag)
yushi
Yutopar (ritodrine HCl)

Z

Z disk
Zaglas' ligament
Zahn's lines
Zancolli operation
Zang's space
Zantac (ranitidine HCl)
Zarontin (ethosuximide)
Zaroxolyn (metolazone)
zeatin
zeaxanthin
zein

Zeis' glands
zeisian
zelotypia
Zenate Prenatal Tablets
  (iron)
Zenker, Friedrich Albert
  von
Zenker's degeneration
Zenker's diverticulum
zenkerism
Zephiran chloride
  (benzalkonium chloride)
Zephrex-LA
  (pseudoephedrine HCl
  and guaifenesin)
zero (Z; 0)
zero, absolute
zero, limes (L0)
zero population growth
  (ZPG)
zestocausis
Zetar Emulsion (coal tar)
Zetar Shampoo (coal tar)
Zide
  (hydrochlorothiazide)
Ziegler discission,
  membranous cataract
Ziegler operation
Ziehl-Neelsen method
Zieve's syndrome
Zim jar opener
Zinacef (cefuroxime
  sodium, Glaxo)
zinc (Zn)
zinc acetate
zinc bacitracin
zinc cadmium sulfide
zinc carbonate
zinc chloride
zinc gelatin
zinc ointment
zinc oxide
zinc oxide and eugenol
zinc peroxide
zinc salts
zinc salts poisoning
zinc stearate
zinc sulfate

zinc undecylenate
zinc white
Zinc-220 (zinc sulfate)
zinciferous
zincoid
Zincon (dandruff shampoo)
zinconium (Zr)
Zinctrace (zinc chloride)
Zinn's ligament
zipper pull
zoacanthosis
zoanthropy
zoescope
zoetic
zoic
Zollinger-Ellison
secretin test
Zollinger-Ellison
  syndrome
Zolyse (chymotripsin)
Zomax (zomepirac sodium)
zona
zona ciliaris
zona facialis
zona fasciculata
zona glomerulosa
zona pellucida
zona radiata
zona reticularis
zona striata
zonae
zonal
zonary
zonary placenta
Zondek-Aschheim test
zone
zone, cell-free
zone, cell-rich
zone, ciliary
zone, comfort
zone, epileptogenic
zone, erogenous
zone, hypnogenic
zone, hypnogenous
zone, transitional
Zone-A Cream 1% (topical
  corticosteroid)
zonesthesia

zonifugal
zoning
zonipetal
zonoskeleton
zonula
zonula adherens
zonula ciliaris
zonula occludens
zonular
zonular cataract
zonular fibers
zonular spaces
zonule
zonule of Zinn
zonulitis
zonulolysis
zonulotomy
zonulysis
zoobiology
zooblast
zoochemistry
zoodermic
zoodynamics
zooerasty
zoofulvin
zoogenesis
zoogenous
zoogeny
zoogeography
zooglea
zoogonous
zoogony
zoograft
zoografting
zooid
zoolagnia
zoologist
zoology
zoomania
zoonoses
zoonotic
zooparasite
zoopathology
zoophagous
zoophile
zoophilism
zoophobia
zoophyte

zooplankton
zooplasty
zoopsia
zoopsychology
zoosadism
zooscopy
zoosmosis
zoospore
zoosterol
zootechnics
zootic
zootomy
zootoxin
zootrophic
ZORprin (aspirin)
zoster
zoster auricularis
zoster ophthalmicus
zosteriform
zosteroid
Zostrix (capsaicin)
Zovirax Capsules
  (acyclovir)
Zovirax Ointment
  (acyclovir)
Zovirax Sterile Powder
  (acyclovir)
Z-plasty epicanthus
Z-plasty eyelid
Z-plasty hypopharynx
Z-plasty skin
Z-track
zwitterions
Zydone (acetaminophen and
  hydrocodone bitartrate)
zygal
zygapophyseal
zygapophysis
zygion
zygocyte
zygodactyly
zygoma
zygoma fracture
zygomatic
zygomatic arch
zygomatic bone
zygomatic process
zygomatic reflex

zygomaticoauricularis
zygomaticofacial
zygomaticofrontal
zygomaticomaxillary
zygomatico-orbital
zygomaticosphenoid
zygomaticotemporal
zygomaticum
zygomaticus
zygomaxillary
zygomaxillary point
zygomycosis
zygon
zygopodium
zygosis
zygosity
zygosperm
zygopore
zygote
zygotene
zygotic
zygotoblast
zygotomere
Zyloprim (allopurinol)
zymase
zyme
zymic
zymogen
zymogen granules
zymogene
zymogenic
zymogenous
zymogram
zymohexase
zymohydrolysis
zymoid
zymologic
zymologist
zymology
zymolysis
zymolyte
zymolytic
zymometer
Zymonema
zymophore
zymophoric
zymophorous
zymophyte

zymoplastic
zymoprotein
zymosan
zymoscope
zymose
zymose secretion,
  pancreas
zymosis
zymosis gastrica
zymosterol
zymosthenic
zymotic

Medical Abbreviations

A

A	assessment; artery; ambulatory; apical; alive; anterior; acetum; accommodation; age; allergy; ampere; anode; atropine; axial; mass number; aqua; total acidity; absorbance; start of anesthesia
A$_2$	aortic second heart sound
A250	5% albumin 250 ml
A1000	5% albumin 1000 ml
A II	angiotensin II
AA	Alcoholics Anonymous; amino acid; achievement age; authorized absence; auto accident; active assistive; arm ankle (pulse ratio); acetic acid; ascending aorta; aminoacetone; alveolar-arterial
AAA	abdominal aortic aneurysmectomy; acute anxiety attack; androgenic anabolic agent; American Academy of Allergists; American Association of Anatomists
AAAS	American Association for the Advancement of Science
AAC	antimicrobial agent-associated colitis
AACCN	American Association of Critical Care Nurses
AAD	acid-ash diet
AAE	active assistive exercise; acute allergic encephalitis
AAFP	American Association of Family Practice
AAG	alpha-1-acid glycoprotein
AAGP	American Academy of General Practice
A:AGT	antiglobulin test
AAIN	American Association of Industrial Nurses; acute allergic intestinal nephritis
AAL	anterior axillary line
AAMA	American Association of Medical Assistants
AAMRL	American Association of Medical Record Librarians
AAMS	acute aseptic meningitis syndrome
AAMT	American Association for Medical Transcription
AAN	analgesic-associated nephropathy; attending's admission notes; analgesic abuse nephropathy
AANA	American Association of Nurse Anesthetists
AAO	alert, awake, and oriented
AAOx3	awake and oriented to time, place, and person

AAP	assessment adjustment pass; American Academy of Pediatrics
AAPA	American Academy of Physicians' Assistants
AAPC	antibiotic-associated pseudomembranous colitis
AAPMC	antibiotic-associated pseudomembranous colitis
AAR	antigen-antiglobulin reaction
AAROM	active assistive range of motion
AART	American Association for Respiratory Therapy
AAS	atlantoaxis subluxation; atypical absence seizure; aortic arch syndrome
AAV	adeno-associated virus
AAVV	accumulated alveolar ventilatory volume
AB	abortion; antibody; Ace bandage; antibiotic; abnormal; alcian blue; asbestos body; asthmatic bronchitis; axiobuccal
A/B	acid-base ratio
A>B	air greater than bone (conduction)
A&B	apnea and bradycardia
ABC	artificial beta cells; absolute band count; absolute basophil count; apnea, bradycardia, cyanosis; axiobuccocervical
ABCDE	botulism toxoid pentavalent
ABCs	Airway, Breathing, and Circulation
ABCDs of melanoma	asymmetry, border, color, and diameter
abd	abdomen
Abd	abdomen; abdominal; abductor
ABDCT	atrial bolus dynamic computer tomography
ABE	acute bacterial endocarditis
ABG	arterial blood gases; axiobuccogingival
ABI	atherothrombotic brain infarction
ABID	antibody identification
ABL	allograft bound lymphocytes; abetalipoproteinemia; axiobuccolingual
ABLB	alternate binaural loudness balance
ABMT	autologous bone marrow transplantation
ABN	abnormality(ies); abnormal
ABNM	American Board of Nuclear Medicine
abnor	abnormal
ABO	blood group system (A, AB, B, and O)
ABP	arterial blood pressure
ABR	absolute bed rest; auditory brain responses

ABS	at bedside; admitting blood sugar; absorption; absorbed; acute brain syndrome; absent
abs feb	absente febre (while the fever is absent)
ABT	aminopyrine breath test
ABW	actual body weight
ABx	antibiotics
ac	acute; ante cibum (before meals)
AC	antecubital; acetate; acromioclavicular; abdominal circumference; anchored catheter; air conduction; assist control; adrenal cortex; alternating current; anodal closure; anterior chamber; anticoagulant; anticomplementary; antiinflammatory corticoid; aortic closure; atriocarotid; auriculocarotid; axiocervical
A/C	anterior chamber of the eye
ACA	anterior cerebral artery; adenocarcinoma; anterior communicating artery
AC/A	accommodation convergence-accommodation
ACAD	academy
ACB	antibody-coated bacteria; alveolar-capillary block
AC&BC	air and bone conduction
ACBE	air contrast barium enema
ACC	accommodation; administrative control center; adenoid cystic carcinoma; accident; ambulatory care center; anodal closure contraction
Acc	accommodation
AcCoA	acetyl-coenzyme A
ACCL	anodal-closure clonus
accom	accommodation
ACCR	amylase creatinine clearance ratio
ACD	acid, citrate, dextrose; anterior chest diameter; absolute cardiac dullness; anterior chamber diameter
ACDs	anticonvulsant drugs
ACE	angiotensin-converting enzyme; adrenocortical extract
ACF	accessory clinical findings; acute care facility
ACG	angiocardiography; apex cardiogram
AcG	accelerator globulin
ACH	adrenal cortical hormone
ACh	acetylcholine
AChE	acetylcholinesterase
ac&hs	before meals and at bedtime

ACI	aftercare instructions; adrenal cortical insufficiency
ACIP	Advisory Committee Immunization Practices
ACL	anterior cruciate ligament
ACLS	advanced cardiac life support
ACM	albumin-calcium-magnesium
ACMV	assist-controlled mechanical ventilation
ACN	acute conditioned neurosis
ACO	anodal-closing odor
ACP	acid phosphatase; acyl-carrier protein; anodal-closing picture; aspirin, caffeine, phenacetin
AC-PH	acid phosphatase
ACPP	adrenocorticopolypeptide
ACPP PF	acid phosphatase prostatic fluid
ACR	adenomatosis of the colon and rectum; anticonstipation regimen
ACS	American Cancer Society; anodal-closing sound; antireticular cytotoxic serum
ACSV	aortocoronary saphenous vein
ACSVBG	aortocoronary saphenous vein bypass graft
ACSW	Academy of Certified Social Workers
ACT	activated clotting time; allergen challenge test; anticoagulant therapy
ACTe	anodal-closure tetanus
Act Ex	active exercise
ACTH	adrenocorticotropic hormone
ACTP	adrenocorticotropic polypeptide
ACTSEB	anterior chamber tube shunt encircling band
ACV	atrial/carotid/ventricular
ACVD	acute cardiovascular disease
AD	right ear; Alzheimer's disease; alternating days; admitting diagnosis; Aleutian disease; anodal duration; average deviation; axis deviation
A&D	ascending and descending; vitamins A & D
ad	add; let there be added
ADA	American Diabetes Association; adenosine deaminase; anterior descending artery
ADAU	adolescent drug abuse unit
ADC	Aid to Dependent Children; anxiety disorder clinic; anodal-duration contraction; average daily census; axiodistocervical
ADCC	antibody-dependent cellular cytotoxicity
ADD	attention deficit disorder; adduction; average daily dose

ADDH	attention deficit disorder with hyperactivity
ADDU	alcohol and drug dependence unit
ADE	acute disseminated encephalitis
ADEM	acute disseminated encephalomyelitis
ADFU	agar diffusion for fungus
ADG	atrial diastolic gallop; axiodistogingival
ADH	antidiuretic hormone; alcohol dehydrogenase
adhib	to be administered
ADI	allowable daily intake; axiodistoincisal
ADL	activities of daily living
ad lib	as desired; at liberty
ADM	admission; administrative medicine; administrator
adm	admission
admov	let there be added
ADO	axiodisto-occlusal
adol	adolescent
ADP	arterial demand pacing; adenosine diphosphate; automatic data processing
ADPKD	autosomal dominant polycystic kidney disease
ADPL	average daily patient load
ADR	adverse drug reaction; acute dystonic reaction
ADS	anonymous donor's sperm; anatomical dead space; antibody deficiency syndrome; antidiuretic substance
ADT	anticipate discharge tomorrow; alternate-day therapy; Auditory Discrimination Test; adenosine triphosphate; anything desired (placebo)
adv	against
ad 2 vic	ad duas vices (for two doses)
A5D5W	alcohol 5%, dextrose 5% in water for injection
AE	above elbow; air entry; accident and emergency;
A&E	accident and emergency
AEA	above elbow amputation
AEC	at earliest convenience; Atomic Energy Commission
AED	automated external defibrillator; antiepileptic drug
AEDP	automated external defibrillator pacemaker
AEG	air encephalogram
AEM	ambulatory electrogram monitor
AEP	average evoked potential
AEq	age equivalent

AER	acoustic evoked response; auditory evoked response; average evoked response; aldosterone excretion rate
Aer M	aerosol mask
Aer T	aerosol tent
AES	antiembolic stockings
AET	absorption-equivalent thickness
aet	age
aetat	aged; of age
AF	atrial fibrillation; acid-fast; anterior fontanel; amniotic fluid; antifibrinogen; aldehyde fuchsin; antibody-forming; aortic flow; atrial flutter
AFB	acid-fast bacilli; aortofemoral bypass
AFC	air filled cushions; antibody-forming cells
AFDC	Aid to Family and Dependent Children
AFE	amniotic fluid embolization
AFI	amniotic fluid index; amaurotic familial idiocy
A fib	atrial fibrillation
AFIP	Armed Forces Institute of Pathology
AFL	atrial flutter
AFLP	acute fatty liver of pregnancy
AFO	ankle-foot orthosis
AFP	alpha-fetoprotein; anterior faucial pillar
AFRD	acute febrile respiratory disease
AFV	amniotic fluid volume
AFVSS	afebrile, vital signs stable
Ag	antigen
AG	antigravity; aminoglycoside; anion gap; atrial gallop; antiglobulin; axiogingival
A/G	albumin-globulin ratio
AGA	appropriate for gestational age; acute gonococcal arthritis
AGD	agar gel diffusion
AGE	angle of greatest extension; acute gastroenteritis
AGF	angle of greatest flexion
AGG	agammaglobulinemia
agg	aggravated
agit	shake
aggl	agglutination
AGL	acute granulocytic leukemia; aminoglutethimide
A GALACTO-LK	alpha galactoside-leukocytes
AGN	acute glomerulonephritis
AgNO$_3$	silver nitrate

AGPT	agar-gel precipitation test
AGS	adrenogenital syndrome
AGT	antiglobulin test
AGTT	abnormal glucose tolerance test
AGV	aniline gentian violet
AH	amenorrhea hyperprolactinemia; abdominal hysterectomy; acetohexamide; amenorrhea and hirsutism; aminohippurate; antihyaluronidase; arterial hypertension; hypermetropic astigmatism
A&H	accident and health
AHA	autoimmune hemolytic anemia; acetohydroxamic acid; acquired hemolytic anemia; American Hospital Association
AHC	acute hemorrhagic conjunctivitis; acute hemorrhagic cystitis
AHD	autoimmune hemolytic disease; arteriosclerotic heart disease; atherosclerotic heart disease
AHE	acute hemorrhagic encephalomyelitis
AHEC	Area Health Education Center
AHF	antihemophilic factor
AHFS	American Hospital Formulary Service
AHG	antihemophilic globulin; antihuman globulin
AHGS	acute herpetic gingival stomatitis
AHH	alpha-hydrazine analogue of histidine; arylhydrocarbon hydroxylase
AHL	apparent half-life
AHLE	acute hemorrhagic leukoencephalitis
AHLS	antihuman lymphocyte serum
AHM	ambulatory Holter monitoring
AHP	acute hemorrhagic pancreatitis; air at high pressure
AHT	autoantibodies to human thyroglobulin; augmented histamine test
AI	aortic insufficiency; artificial insemination; allergy index; aortic incompetence; accidentally incurred; apical impulse; axioincisal
A&I	allergy and immunology
AIA	antiinsulin antibody; aspirin-induced asthma
AI-Ab	antiinsulin antibody
AIBA	aminoisobutyric acid
AIC	aminoimidazole carboxamide
AICA	anterior inferior communicating artery; anterior inferior cerebellar artery
AICD	automatic implantable cardioverter/defibrillator

AID	artificial insemination donor; automatic implantable defibrillator; acute infectious disease
AIDKS	acquired immunodeficiency syndrome with Kaposi's sarcoma
AIDS	acquired immunodeficiency syndrome
AIE	acute inclusion body encephalitis
AIEP	amount of insulin extracted from the pancreas
AIF	aortic-iliac-femoral
AIH	artificial insemination, homologous
AIHA	autoimmune hemolytic anemia
AIHD	acquired immune hemolytic disease
AIIS	anterior inferior iliac spine
AILD	angioimmunoblastic lymphadenopathy
AIMS	abnormal involuntary movement scale
AIN	anal intraepithelial neoplasia; acute interstitial nephritis
AINS	antiinflammatory nonsteroidal
AION	anterior ischemic optic neuropathy
AIP	acute intermittent porphyria; acute infectious polyneuritis; average intravascular pressure
AIR	accelerated idioventricular rhythm
AIS	Abbreviated Injury Score; antiinsulin serum
AITT	arginine insulin intolerance test
AIU	absolute iodine uptake
AIVR	accelerated idioventricular rhythm
AJ	ankle jerk
AJN	American Journal of Nursing
A/K,AK	above knee; artificial kidney
AKA	above-knee amputation; alcoholic ketoacidosis; all known allergies
AL	acute leukemia; axial length; albumin; axiolingual
ALA	aminolevulinic acid; axiolabial
ALAD	abnormal left axis deviation; aminolevulinic acid dehydrase
ALAG	axiolabiogingival
ALAL	axiolabiolingual
ALARA	as low as reasonably achievable
ALAT	alanine transaminase
alb	albumin
Alb	albumin
ALC	acute lethal catatonia; alcohol; alternate lifestyle checklist; approximate lethal concentration; axiolinguocervical
ALC R	alcohol rub

ALD	alcoholic liver disease; aldolase; adrenoleukodystrophy
ALDOST	aldosterone
ALFT	abnormal liver function test
ALG	antilymphocyte globulin; axiolinguogingival
ALH	anterior lobe hormone; anterior lobe, hypophysis
alk	alkaline
ALK ISO	alkaline phosphatase isoenzymes
ALK-P	alkaline phosphatase
alk phos	alkaline phosphatase
ALL	acute lymphoblastic leukemia; allergy
ALM	acral lentiginous melanoma
ALME	acetyl-lysine methyl ester
ALMI	anterolateral myocardial infarction
ALN	anterior lymph node
ALO	axiolinguoocclusal
Al(OH)$_3$	aluminum hydroxide
ALP	argon laser photocoagulation; alkaline phosphatase; antilymphocyte plasma
ALS	amyotrophic lateral sclerosis; acute lateral sclerosis; advanced life support; antilymphatic serum; antilymphocyte serum
ALT	alanine transaminase; argon laser trabeculoplasty
ALTB	acute laryngotracheobronchitis
ALTEE	acetyl-L-tyrosine ethyl ester
ALVAD	abdominal left ventricular assist device
ALW	arch-loop-whorl
ALWMI	anterolateral wall myocardial infarction
AM	morning; myopic astigmatism; amalgam; adult male; alveolar macrophage; ametropia; amperemeter; anovular menstruation; arithmetic mean; aviation medicine; axiomesial
AMA	American Medical Association; against medical advice; antimitochondrial antibody
AMAG	adrenal medullary autograft
AMAP	as much as possible
AMAT	antimalignant antibody test
A-MAT	amorphous material
AMB	ambulate; ambulatory
AMC	arm muscle circumference; axiomesiocervical
AM/CR	amylase to creatinine ratio
AMD	age-related macular degeneration; alpha methyldopa; axiomesiodistal
AMegL	acute megakaryoblastic leukemia
AMESLAN	American sign language

AMG	acoustic myography; aminoglycoside; antimacrophage globulin; axiomesiogingival
AMH	automated medical history
Amh	mixed astigmatism with myopia predominating
AMI	acute myocardial infarction; amitriptyline; axiomesioincisal
AML	acute myelocytic leukemia; acute monocytic leukemia
AMLS	antimouse lymphocyte serum
AMM	agnogenic myeloid metaplasia; ammonia
AMML	acute myelomonocytic leukemia
AMMOL	acute myelomonoblastic leukemia
AMN	adrenomyeloneuropathy
amnio	amniocentesis
AMO	axiomesioocclusal
A-mode	amplitude modulation
AMOL	acute monoblastic leukemia; acute monocytic leukemia
amp	ampere
AMP	amputation; ampul; ampule; ampicillin; adenosine monophosphate; average mean pressure; acid mucopolysaccharide
A-M pr	Austin-Moore prosthesis
AMPS	abnormal mucopolysacchariduria; acid mucopolysaccharides
AMR	alternating motor rates
AMS	amylase; acute mountain sickness; aggravated in military service; auditory memory span; antimacrophage serum; automated multiphasic screening
AMSIT	portion of the mental status examination: A-appearance, M-mood, S-sensorium, I-intelligence, T-thought process
amt	amount
amu	atomic mass unit
AMV	assisted mechanical ventilation
AMY	amylase
AN	anisometropia; anodal; anode
ANA	antinuclear antibody; American Nurses' Association; acetylneuraminic acid
ANAD	anorexia nervosa and associated disorders
anal	analysis; analyst
anat	anatomical; anatomy
ANC	absolute neutrophil count
AnCC	anodal-closure contraction
AND	anterior nasal discharge
ANDA	Abbreviated New Drug Application
AnDTe	anodal-duration tetanus

anes	anesthesia; anesthesiology
ANF	antinuclear factor; atrial natriuretic factor
ang	angiogram
ANG	angiogram
ANISO	anisocytosis
ank	ankle
ANLL	acute nonlymphoblastic leukemia
AnOC	anodal-opening contraction
ANOV	analysis of variance
ANP	atrial natriuretic peptide
ANS	autonomic nervous system; answer; antineutrophilic serum; arteriolonephrosclerosis
ant	anterior
ANT	anterior
ANTI	anti blood group A
Anti bx	antibiotic
ant sag D	anterior sagittal diamaeter
ANTR	apparent net transfer rate
ANUG	acute necrotizing ulcerative gingivitis
ANX	anxiety; anxious
AO	anodal opening; aorta; anterior oblique; aortic opening; axioocclusal
A&O	alert and oriented
A&O X3	awake and oriented to person, place, and time
A&O X4	awake and oriented to person, place, time, and date
AOAP	as often as possible
AOB	alcohol on breath
AOC	area of concern; anodal-opening contraction
AOCl	anodal-opening clonus
AOD	arterial occlusive disease
AODM	adult onset diabetes mellitus
ao-il	aorta-iliac
AOM	acute otitis media
AOO	anodal-opening odor
AOP	aortic pressure; anodal-opening picture
AOS	anodal-opening sound
AOSD	adult-onset Still's disease
AOTe	anodal-opening tetanus
AP	anterior posterior; antepartum; apical pulse; appendicitis; alkaline phosphatase; atrial pacing; acid phosphatase; action potential; angina pectoris; acute proliferative; appendix; anterior pituitary; arterial pressure; association period; axiopulpal

A&P	anterior and posterior; auscultation and percussion; assessment and plan; active and present; anatomy and physiology
A/P	ascites/plasma ratio
A$_2$>P$_2$	second aortic sound greater than second pulmonic sound
APA	aldosterone-producing adenoma; antipernicious anemia factor
APAP	acetaminophen
APB	atrial premature beat; abductor pollicis brevis; auricular premature beat
APC	aspirin, phenacetin, and caffeine; atrial premature contraction; adenoidal-pharyngeal-conjunctival; adenomatous polyposis of the colon (and rectum)
APC-C	aspirin, phenacetin, and caffeine with codeine
APCD	adult polycystic disease
APD	automated peritoneal dialysis; atrial premature depolarization; anterior-posterior diameter; action-potential duration
APDC	Anxiety and Panic Disorder Clinic
APE	acute psychotic episode; anterior pituitary extract
APF	animal protein factor
APGL	alkaline phosphatase activity of the granular leukocytes
APH	antepartum hemorrhage
APHP	anti-*Pseudomonas* human plasma
APIVR	artificial pacemaker-induced ventricular rhythm
APKD	adult polycystic kidney disease; adult-onset polycystic kidney disease
APL	acute promyelocytic leukemia; abductor pollicis longus; accelerated painless labor; anterior pituitary-like
APN	acute pyelonephritis; average peak noise
apo E	apolipoprotein E
app	appendix
appr	approximate
appt	appointment
appy	appendectomy
APR	abdominoperineal resection; amebic prevalence rate
APTT	activated partial thromboplastin time
AQ	achievement quotient
aq	water (aqua)
aq dest	distilled water

AQS	additional qualifying symptoms
AR	aortic regurgitation; active resistance; airway resistance; alcohol related; alarm reaction; at risk; Argyll Robertson; artificial respiration
Ar	argon
A&R	advised and released
A-R	apical-radial (pulses)
ARB	any reliable brand
ARC	AIDS related complex; anomalous retinal correspondence; American Red Cross
ARCBS	American Red Cross Blood Services
ARD	adult respiratory distress; acute respiratory disease; antibiotic removal device; anorectal dressing
ARDS	adult respiratory distress syndrome
ARE	active-resistive exercise
ARF	acute renal failure; acute rheumatic fever; acute respiratory failure
arg	silver (argentum)
ARG	arginine
ARI	aldose reductase inhibitor
ARL	average remaining lifetime
ARLD	alcohol related liver disease
ARM	artificial rupture of membranes; anxiety reaction, mild
AROM	active range of motion; artificial rupture of membranes
ARP	at risk period
arr	arrive
ARRT	American Registry of Radiologic Technologists
ARS	antirabies serum
art	artery
ART	automated reagin test; arterial; Achilles reflex test
ARV	AIDS related virus
AS	aortic stenosis; activated sleep; anal sphincter; left ear; ankylosing spondylitis; Adams-Stokes (disease); astigmatism; arteriosclerosis; antistreptolysin; androsterone sulfate
ASA	acetylsalicyclic acid; American Society of Anesthesiologists; Adams-Stokes attack
ASA I	Healthy patient with localized pathological process
ASA II	A patient with mild to moderate systemic disease

ASA III	A patient with severe systemic disease limiting activity but not incapacitating
ASA IV	A patient with incapacitating systemic disease
ASA V	Moribund patient not expected to live
ASAA	acquired severe aplastic anemia
ASAP	as soon as possible
ASAT	aspartate transaminase
ASB	anesthesia standby; asymptomatic bacteriuria
ASC	ambulatory surgery center; altered state of consciousness; antimony sulfur colloid; ascorbic acid
ASCVD	arteriosclerotic cardiovascular disease; atherosclerotic cardiovascular disease
ASD	atrial septal defect; aldosterone secretion defect
ASDH	acute subdural hematoma
ASE	acute stress erosion
ASH	asymmetric septal hypertrophy
AsH	hypermetropic astigmatism
ASHD	arteriosclerotic heart disease
ASI	Anxiety Status Inventory
ASIS	anterior superior iliac spine
ASK	antistreptokinase
ASL	antistreptolysin
ASLO	antistreptolysin-O
AsM	myopic astigmatism
ASMA	antismooth muscle antibody
ASMI	anteroseptal myocardial infarction
ASN	alkali-soluble nitrogen
ASO	antistreptolysin-O; arteriosclerosis obliterans; aldicarb sulfoxide; automatic stop order
ASOT	antistreptolysin-O titer
ASP	acute suppurative parotitis; aspartic acid; area systolic pressure
ASPVD	arteriosclerotic peripheral vascular disease
ASR	aldosterone secretion rate
ASRT	American Society of Radiologic Technologists
ASS	anterior superior supine
asst	assistant
Ast	astigmatism
AST	aspartate transaminase; astigmatism
ASTO	antistreptolysin-O
AS TOL	as tolerated
ASTZ	antistreptozyme test
ASU	acute stroke unit; ambulatory surgical unit
ASV	antisnake venom

ASVD	arteriosclerotic vessel disease
AT	atraumatic; antithrombin
ATA	anti-*Toxoplasma* antibodies; atmosphere absolute
ATB	antibiotic
ATC	around the clock
ATD	antithyroid drug(s); autoimmune thyroid disease; asphyxiating thoracic dystrophy
ATE	adipose tissue extract
At Fib	atrial fibrillation
AT III FUN	antithrombin III functional
ATG	antithymocyte globulin; antithyroglobulin
ATHR	angina threshold heart rate
ATL	Achilles tendon lengthening; atypical lymphocytes; adult T-cell leukemia
ATLS	advanced trauma life support
ATM	acute transverse myelitis; atmosphere
ATN	acute tubular necrosis
ATNC	atraumatic normocephalic
aTNM	autopsy staging of cancer
ATNR	asymmetrical tonic neck reflex
ATP	adenosine triphosphate; addiction treatment program
ATPase	adenosine triphosphatase
ATPS	ambient temperature and pressure, saturated (with water vapor)
ATR	atrial; Achilles tendon reflex
ATS	antitetanic serum; anxiety tension state; arteriosclerosis
ATT	arginine tolerance test; aspirin tolerance test
at wt	atomic weight
au	both ears; each ear
Au	gold
Au 198	radioactive gold
AU	both ears; allergenic units; Angstrom unit; antitoxin unit; arbitrary units; azauridine
AUB	abnormal uterine bleeding
AUC	area under the curve
AUGIB	acute upper gastrointestinal bleeding
AUL	acute undifferentiated leukemia
AUR	acute urinary retention
aus	auscultation
av	average
AV	arteriovenous; auditory-visual; atrioventricular
AVA	American Vocational Association

AV/AF	anteverted, anteflexed
AVCS	atrioventricular conduction system
AVD	aortic valve disease; apparent volume of distribution
AVDO$_2$	arteriovenous oxygen difference
avdp	avoirdupois
AVF	arteriovenous fistula
avg	average
AVGs	ambulatory visit groups
AVH	acute viral hepatitis
AVI	air velocity index
AVJR	atrioventricular junctional rhythm
AVM	atriovenous malformation
AVN	atrioventricular node; arteriovenous nicking; avascular necrosis
AVR	aortic valve replacement
AVRP	atrioventricular refractory period
AVS	atriovenous shunt
AVSS	afebrile, vital signs stable
AVT	atypical ventricular tachycardia; atrioventricular tachycardia; Allen vision test
AW	anterior wall
A/W	able to work
A&W	alive and well
AWA	as well as
A waves	atrial contraction waves
AWDW	assault with a deadly weapon
AWI	anterior wall infarction
AWMI	anterior wall myocardial infarction
AWO	airway obstruction
AWOL	absent without leave
ax	axillary; axis
AXT	alternating exotropia
Az	azote
AZT	zidovudine (azidothymidine)
A-Z test	Ascheim-Zondek test

B

B	*Bacillus;* bands; black; bloody; both; buccal; bilateral; base; bath; Baume's scale; behavior; *Balantidium;* bicuspid; boron; Bucky; barometric
B$_1$	thiamine HCl

B_2	riboflavin
B_6	pyridoxine HCl
B_7	biotin
B_8	adenosine phosphate
B_{12}	cyanocobalamin
Ba	barium
BA	blood alcohol; buccoaxial; backache; bile acid; Bachelor of Arts; bacterial agglutination; betamethasone acetate; blocking antibody; bone age; bovine albumin; brachial artery; bronchial asthma; benzyl alcohol
B>A	bone greater than air
B&A	brisk and active
Bab	Babinski
BAC	blood alcohol concentration; buccoaxiocervical
bact	bacterium
BAD	bipolar affective disorder
BaE	barium enema
BAE	bronchial artery embolization
BAEP	brain (stem) auditory evoked potential
BAERs	brain (stem) auditory evoked responses
BAG	buccoaxiogingival
BAL	blood alcohol level; bronchoalveolar lavage
BALB	binaural alternate loudness balance
bals	balsam
BaM	barium meal
BANS	back, arm, neck, and scalp
BAO	basal acid output
BAP	blood agar plate
Barb	barbiturate
BARN	bilateral acute retinal necrosis
BAS	boric acid solution
BASH	body acceleration given synchronously with the heartbeat
baso	basophil
batt	battery
BAVP	balloon aortic valvuloplasty
BAW	bronchoalveolar washing
BB	blow bottle; bed bath; buffer base; bowel or bladder; blood bank; bad breath; beta blocker; blanket bath; bed board; breast biopsy; baby boy; body belts; both bones; breakthrough bleeding
BBA	born before arrival
BBB	bundle branch block; blood-brain barrier
BBBB	bilateral bundle branch block

BBD	benign breast disease
BBM	banked breast milk
BBS	bilateral breath sounds; (electronic) bulletin board system
BBT	basal body temperature
BB to MM	belly button to medial malleolus
B Bx	breast biopsy
BC	bone conduction; blood culture; birth control; Bourn control; bed and chair; Blue Cross; back care; battle casualty; buccocervical; bactericidal concentration
B/C	because
B&C	board and care; breathed and cried; bed and chair; biopsy and curettage
BCA	balloon catheter angioplasty; basal cell atypia; brachiocephalic artery
BCAA	branched-chain amino acids
BC/BS	Blue Cross/Blue Shield
BCC	basal cell carcinoma; birth control clinic
BCCa	basal cell carcinoma
BCD	basal cell dysplasia
BCE	basal cell epithelioma
B cell	large lymphocyte
BCG	bacillus Calmette-Guérin vaccine; bicolor guaiac; ballistocardiogram
BCL	basic cycle length
BCM	birth control medication
BCNP	Board of Certified Nuclear Pharmacists
BCP	birth control pills
BCS	battered child syndrome; Budd-Chiari syndrome
BCW	biological and chemical warfare
BD	bronchial drainage; birth defect; brain dead; base deficit; bile duct; buccodistal
BDAE	Boston Diagnostic Aphasia Examination
BDBS	Bonnet-Dechaume-Blanc Syndrome
BDC	burn-dressing change
BDE	bile duct exploration
BDI SF	Beck's Depression Index-Short Form
BDL	below detectable limits; bile duct ligation
BDR	background diabetic retinopathy
BE	barium enema; below elbow; bread equivalent; bacterial endocarditis; base excess; breast examination; Bacillen Emulsion; bovine enteritis
B&E	brisk and equal
BEA	below elbow amputation
BEAM	brain electrical activity mapping
BEC	bacterial endocarditis

BEE	basal energy expenditure
BEF	bronchoesophageal fistula
BEI	butanol-extractable iodine
BEP	brain stem evoked potentials
BEV	bleeding esophageal varices; billion electron volts
BF	black female; breakfast fed; blood flow
B/F	bound-free ratio
BFC	benign febrile convulsion
BFP	biologic false positive
BFR	biologic false-positive reactor; blood flow rate; bone formation rate
B frag	*Bacillus fragilis*
BFT	bentonite flocculation test
BG	blood glucose; baby girl; bone graft; buccogingival
B-GALACTO	beta galactosidase
BGC	basal-ganglion calcification
BGDC	Bartholin gland duct cyst
BGH	bovine growth hormone
BGP	beta-glycerophosphatase
BGSA	blood granulocyte-specific activity
BGTT	borderline glucose tolerance test
BHI	biosynthetic human insulin; brain-heart infusion
BHN	bridging hepatic necrosis
BHS	beta-hemolytic streptococci
BHT	breath hydrogen test
BH/VH	body hematocrit-venous hematocrit ratio
BI	bowel impaction; burn index; bacteriological index
bib	drink (bıbe)
BIB	brought in by
BIC	brain injury center
bid	twice a day
BID	twice daily; brought in dead
BIG 6	analysis of 6 serum components
BIH	benign intracranial hypertension; bilateral inguinal hernia
bil	bilateral
BIL	bilateral; brother-in-law; bilirubin
BILAT SLC	bilateral short leg cast
BILAT SXO	bilateral salpingo-oophorectomy
Bili	bilirubin
BILI-C	conjugated bilirubin
BIMA	bilateral internal mammary arteries
bin	twice a night
BIP	bismuth iodoform paraffin

BiPD	biparietal diameter
BIW	twice a week
BJ	bone and joint; Bence-Jones; biceps jerk
BJE	bone and joint examination
BJM	bones, joints, and muscles
BJP	Bence-Jones protein
BK	below knee; bradykinin
BKA	below knee amputation
BKC	blepharokeratoconjunctivitis
bkft	breakfast
Bkg	background
BKWP	below-knee walking plaster
BL	blood loss; bronchial lavage; Burkitt's lymphoma; baseline; Bessey-Lowry; bleeding; buccolingual
BLBK	blood bank
BL=BS	bilateral equal breath sounds
bl cult	blood culture
bld tm	bleeding time
BLE	both lower extremities
BLESS	bath, laxative, enema, shampoo, and shower
BLG	beta-lactoglobulin
BLL	bilateral lower lobe
BLN	bronchial lymph nodes
BLOBS	bladder obstruction
BLQ	both lower quadrants
BLS	basic life support
BLT	bloodclot lysis time
BL unit	Bessey-Lowry unit
BM	bowel movement; bone marrow; black male; breast milk; basement membrane; body mass; buccomesial
BMA	bone marrow aspiration
BMC	bone marrow cells
BMD	bone marrow depression; bone mineral density
BME	brief maximal effort
BMI	body mass index
BMJ	bones, muscles, joints
BMK	birthmark
BMR	basal metabolic rate
BMT	bone marrow transplant; bilateral myringotomy and tubes
BMTU	bone marrow transplant unit
BNC	bladder neck contracture
BNCT	boron neutron capture therapy
BNO	bladder neck obstruction
BNR	bladder neck retraction

BO	behavior objective; body odor; bowel obstruction
B&O	belladonna and opium
BOA	born on arrival; born out of asepsis
BOB	ball on back
Bod Units	Bodansky units
BOE	bilateral otitis externa
BOM	bilateral otitis media
BOMA	bilateral otitis media, acute
BOO	bladder outlet obstruction
BOT	base of tongue
BOW	bag of water
BP	blood pressure; benzoyl peroxide; bed pan; bypass; British Pharmacopeia; bathroom privileges; birthplace; back pressure; behavior pattern; boiling point; bronchopleural; buccopulpal
BPD	biparietal diameter; bronchopulmonary dysplasia; borderline personality disorder
BPd	blood pressure (diastolic)
BPF	bronchopleural fistula
BPH	benign prostatic hypertrophy
BPG	bypass graft
BPLA	blood pressure, left arm
BPM	breaths per minute; beats per minute
BPR	blood per rectum; blood pressure recorder
BPRS	Brief Psychiatric Rating Scale
BPs	blood pressure (systolic)
BPSD	bronchopulmonary segmental drainage
BPV	benign paroxysmal vertigo; bovine papilloma virus
BR	bedrest; bridge; bathroom; Benzing retrograde
BRA	brain
BRAO	branch retinal artery occlusion
BRAT	bananas, rice, applesauce, and toast
BRATT	bananas, rice, applesauce, tea, and toast
BRB	blood-retinal barrier; bright red blood
BRBPR	bright red blood per rectum
BRBR	bright red blood (rectum)
BRCM	below right costal margin
BRJ	brachial radialis jerk
BRM	biological response modifiers
BRP	bathroom privileges
BR RAO	branch retinal artery occlusion
BR RVO	branch retinal vein occlusion
BS	blood sugar; breath sounds; bowel sounds; before sleep; bedside; Blue Shield
B&S	Bartholin and Skene

BSA	body surface area; bovine serum albumin
BSB	body surface burned
BSC	bedside commode; burn scar contracture; bedside care
BSE	breast self-examination; bilateral, symmetrical, and equal
BSER	brain stem evoked responses
BSF	back scatter factor
BSGA	beta *Streptococcus* group A
BSI	bound serum iron
BSL	blood sugar level
BSN	bowel sounds normal
BSNA	bowel sounds normal and active
BSO	bilateral salpingo-oophorectomy
BSOM	bilateral serous otitis media
BSP	bromsulphalein
BSPM	body surface potential mapping
BSR	basal skin resistance
BSSS	benign sporadic sleep spikes
BSU	Bartholin, Skene's urethra
BSW	Bachelor of Social Work
BT	breast tumor; brain tumor; bedtime; bladder tumor; blood transfusion; blood type
BTB	breakthrough bleeding
BTBV	beat to beat variability
BTC	by the clock
BTFS	breast tumor frozen section
BTL	bilateral tubal ligation
BTPS	body temperature pressure saturated
BTR	bladder tumor recheck
BTU	British thermal unit
BU	burn unit; base up
BUE	both upper extremities
BUI	boating under influence
BUN	blood urea nitrogen; bunion
BUR	back-up rate
BUS	Bartholin, urethral, and Skene's glands
bv	vapor bath
BV	biological value; blood volume; blood vessel; bronchovesicular
BVE	blood volume expander
BVH	biventricular hypertrophy
BVI	blood vessel invasion
BVL	bilateral vas ligation
BVO	branch vein occlusion
BVV	bovine vaginitis virus
BW	body weight; birth weight; body water; biological warfare

B&W	Black and White (milk of magnesia and aromatic cascara fluid extract)
BWA	bed wetter admission
BWCS	bagged white cell study
BWFI	bacteriostatic water for injection
BWS	battered woman syndrome
Bx	biopsy
BX BS	Blue Cross and Blue Shield

C

c	clubbing; cyanosis; carbohydrate; Celsius; centigrade; hundred; Catholic; Caucasian; cup
C1	first cervical vertebra
C1 to C9	precursor molecules of the complement system
CII	controlled substance, class 2
CA	cancer; chronologic age; cardiac arrest; carotid artery; coronary artery
Ca	calcium
C&A	Clinitest and Acetest
CAA	crystalline amino acids
CAB	coronary artery bypass
CABG	coronary artery bypass graft
CaBI	calcium bone index
CABS	coronary artery bypass surgery
CACI	computer-assisted continuous infusion
CaCO₃	calcium carbonate
CAD	coronary artery disease; computer-assisted design
CAE	cellulose acetate electrophoresis
CaG	calcium gluconate
CAH	chronic active hepatitis; chronic aggressive hepatitis; congenital adrenal hyperplasia
CAHEA	Committee on Allied Health Education and Accreditation
CAL	calorie; callus; chronic airflow limitation
cal ct	calorie count
CALD	chronic active liver disease
CALGB	Cancer and Leukemia Group B
CALLA	common acute lymphoblastic leukemia antigen
CAM	Caucasian adult male
CAN	cord around neck
CA/N	child abuse and neglect
CANC	cancelled
CAO	chronic airway obstruction

CAP	capsule; compound action potentials; community-acquired pneumonia
CaP	carcinoma of the prostate
Ca/P	calcium to phosphorus ratio
CAPD	chronic ambulatory peritoneal dialysis
CAR	cardiac ambulation routine
CARB	carbohydrate
CAS	carotid artery stenosis
CASS	computer aided sleep system
CAST	cardiac arrhythmia suppression trial
CAT	computed axial tomography; cataract
cath	catheter; catheterization
CAVB	complete atrioventricular block
CAVC	common artrioventricular canal
CAVH	continuous arteriovenous hemofiltration
CB	code blue; chronic bronchitis; cesarean birth; chair and bed
C&B	crown and bridge; chair and bed
CBA	chronic bronchitis and asthma
CBC	complete blood count
CBD	common bile duct; closed bladder drainage
CBF	cerebral blood flow
CBFS	cerebral blood flow studies
CBFV	cerebral blood flow velocity
CBG	capillary blood glucose
CBI	continuous bladder irrigation
CBN	chronic benign neutropenia
CBPS	coronary bypass surgery
CBR	complete bedrest; chronic bedrest; carotid bodies resected
CBRAM	controlled partial rebreathing-anesthesia method
CBS	chronic brain syndrome
CC	chief complaint; chronic complainer; clean catch; cardiac cycle; critical condition; cord compression; creatinine clearance; cerebral concussion; circulatory collapse; corpus callosum; clinical course; commission certified; compound cathartic; costochondral
cc	cubic centimeter
C&C	cold and clammy
CCA	common carotid artery; circumflex coronary artery
CCAP	capsule cartilage articular preservation
CCB	calcium channel blocker(s)
CCC	child care clinic
CC&C	colony count and culture

CCE	clubbing, cyanosis, and edema; countercurrent electrophoresis
CCF	crystal-induced chemotactic factor; compound comminuted fracture; congestive cardiac failure; cephalin-cholesterol flocculation
CCHD	cyanotic congenital heart disease
CCI	chronic coronary insufficiency
CCK	cholecystokinin
CCK-OP	cholecystokinin octapeptide
CCK-PZ	cholecystokinin-pancreozymin
CCL	critical condition list
CCl_4	carbon tetrachloride
CCMSU	clean catch midstream urine
CCMU	critical care medicine unit
C-collar	cervical collar
CCPD	continuous cycle peritoneal dialysis
CCR	continuous complete remission
CCRN	certified critical care registered nurse
CCRU	critical care recovery unit
CCT	congenitally corrected transposition; crude coal tar
CCTGA	congenitally corrected transposition of the great arteries
CCT in PET	crude coal tar in petroleum
CCTV	closed circuit television
CCU	coronary care unit; critical care unit; cardiac care unit; Cherry-Crandall units; community care unit
CCUA	clean catch urinalysis
CCUP	colpocystourethropexy
CCX	complications
CD	Crohn's Disease; common duct; continuous drainage; cesarean delivery; cadaver donor; cardiac disease; cardiac dullness; caudal; cardiovascular disease; conjugata diagonalis; consanguineous donor; curative dose; cystic duct
C/D	cup-to-disc ratio; cigarettes per day
C&D	curettage and desiccation; cystoscopy and dilatation
CDA	congenital dyserythropoietic anemia
CDAI	Crohn's Disease Activity Index
CDB	cough and deep breath
CDC	Centers for Disease Control; cancer detection center; calculated day of confinement; Communicable Disease Center
CDD	certificate of disability for discharge

CDE	common duct exploration; canine distemper encephalitis
CDGD	constitutional delay in growth and development
CDH	congenital dysplasia of hip; congenital dislocation of hip; chronic daily headache
CDK	climatic droplet keratopathy
CDLE	chronic discoid lupus erythematosus
CDP	coronary drug project
CDQ	corrected development quotient
CDSS	clinical decision support system
CDU	chemical dependency unit
CDV	canine distemper virus
cdyn	dynamic compliance
CE	central episiotomy; continuing education; cardiac enlargement; contrast echocardiology; California encephalitis; chick embryo; cholesterol esters; contractile element
C&E	curettage and electrodesiccation; cough and exercise; consultation and examination
CEA	carcinoembryonic antigen; carotid endarterectomy
CECT	contrast enhancement computed tomography
CEI	continuous extravascular infusion
CEO	chief executive officer
CEP	congenital erythropoietic porphyria; countercurrent electrophoresis; cognitive evoked potential
CEPH	cephalic
CEPH FLOC	cephalin flocculation
CE&R	central episiotomy and repair
CERA	cortical evoked response audiometry
CERV	cervical
CES	computerized educational system; cognitive environmental stimulation
CF	cystic fibrosis; Caucasian female; complement fixation; cardiac failure; cancer-free; count fingers; Christmas factor; contractile force
CFA	common femoral artery; complete Freund's adjuvant
CFAC	complement-fixing antibody consumption
CFM	close fitting mask
CFNS	chills, fever, and night sweats
CFP	cystic fibrosis protein
CFS	cancer family syndrome
CFT	complement fixation test
CF test	complement fixation test

CFU	colony forming units
CFU-S	colony forming unit-spleen
CG	cholecystogram
CGB	chronic gastrointestinal bleeding
CGD	chronic granulomatous disease
CGFNS	Commission on Graduates of Foreign Nursing Schools
CGI	Clinical Global Impression (scale)
CGL	chronic granulocytic leukemia
CGN	chronic glomerulonephritis
CGTT	cortisol glucose tolerance test
Ch	cholesterol
CH	child; chronic; chest; chief; crown-heal; convalescent hospital; cluster headache; congenital hypothyroidism
CHAI	continuous hepatic artery infusion
CHAP	child health associate practitioner
CHB	complete heart block
CHD	congenital heart disease; childhood diseases; chronic hemodialysis; center for hemodialysis
CHF	congestive heart failure
CHFV	combined high frequency ventilation
CHG	change
CHI	closed head injury; creatinine-height index
CHO	carbohydrate
chol	cholesterol
chr	chronic
CHRS	congenital hereditary retinoschisis
CHS	Chédiak-Higashi syndrome
CHU	closed head unit
CI	cesium implant; cardiac index; complete iridectomy
Ci	curie
CIA	chronic idiopathic anhidrosis
CIAED	collagen-induced autoimmune ear disease
cib	cibus (food)
CIB	cytomegalic inclusion bodies; Carnation Instant Breakfast
CIBD	chronic inflammatory bowel disease
CIC	circulating immune complexes
CICE	combined intracapsular cataract extraction
CICU	cardiac intensive care unit
CID	cytomegalic inclusion disease
CIDP	chronic inflammatory demyelinating polyradiculoneuropathy
CIDS	continuous insulin delivery system; cellular immunodeficiency syndrome

CIE	counterimmunoelectrophoresis; crossed immunoelectrophoresis
CIN	chronic interstitial nephritis; cervical intraepithelial neoplasia
CINE	chemotherapy-induced nausea and emesis
Circ	circumcision; circumference; circulation
circ&sen	circulation and sensation
CIS	carcinoma in situ
CIU	chronic idiopathic urticaria
CK	check; creatine kinase
CK-BB	creatine kinase BB band
CKC	cold knife conization
CK-ISO	creatine kinase isoenzyme
CK-MB	creatine kinase MB band
CK-MM	creatine kinase MM band
cl	cloudy
Cl	chloride
CL	critical list; clear liquid
CLA	community living arrangements
Clav	clavicle
CLBBB	complete left bundle branch block
CL/CP	cleft lip and cleft palate
CLD	chronic lung disease; chronic liver disease
CLE	continuous lumbar epidural
CLF	cholesterol-lecithin flocculation
CLH	chronic lobular hepatitis
CLL	chronic lymphocytic leukemia
CLLE	columnar-lined lower esophagus
cl liq	clear liquid
CLO	cod liver oil; close
CL&P	cleft lip and palate
CLT	chronic lymphocytic thyroiditis
CL VOID	clean voided specimen
clysis	hypodermoclysis
cm	centimeter
CM	costal margin; continuous murmur; contrast media; Caucasian male; cochlear microphonics; culture media; common migraine; cow's milk; chondromalacia
CMA	compound myopic astigmatism; certified medical assistant
CMBBT	cervical mucous basal body temperature
CMC	chronic mucocutaneous moniliasis
CME	cystoid macular edema; continuing medical education
CMG	cystometrogram
CMGN	chronic membranous glomerulonephritis
CMHC	community mental health center

CMHN	community mental health nurse
CMI	cell-mediated immunity; Cornell Medical Index
CMJ	carpometacarpal joint
CMK	congenital multicystic kidney
CML	chronic myelogenous leukemia; cell-mediated lympholysis
CMM	cutaneous malignant melanoma
CMML	chronic myelomacrocytic leukemia
CMO	cardiac minute output; card made out
CMP	cardiomyopathy; chondromalacia patella
CMRNG	chromosomally mediated resistant *Neisseria gonorrhoeae*
$CMRO_2$	cerebral metabolic rate for oxygen
CMS	circulation motion sensation
CMSUA	clean midstream urinalysis
CMT	certified medical transcriptionist
CMV	cytomegalovirus; cool mist vaporizer; controlled mechanical ventilation
CMVIG	cytomegalovirus immune globulin
CN	cranial nerve; clinical nursing
cn	cras nocte (tomorrow night)
Cn	cyanide
CNA	chart not available
CNAG	chronic narrow angle glaucoma
CND	cannot determine
CNDC	chronic nonspecific diarrhea of childhood
CNH	central neurogenic hyperpnea; community nursing home
CNM	certified nurse midwife
CNN	congenital nevocytic nevus
CNS	central nervous system; clinical nurse specialist
CO	cardiac output; carbon monoxide; castor oil; cervical orthosis; cervicoaxial; corneal opacity; compound
Co	cobalt
C/O	complains of; complaints; under care of; check out
CO_2	carbon dioxide
CoA	coarctation of aorta; coenzyme A
COAD	chronic obstructive airway disease; chronic obstructive arterial disease
COAG	chronic open angle glaucoma
COBT	chronic obstruction of biliary tract
COD	cause of death; codeine; condition on discharge
COD-MD	cerebro-ocular-dysplasia-muscular dystrophy

COEPS	cortically originating extrapyramidal symptoms
COG	cognitive function tests; Central Oncology Group
COH	carbohydrate
COHB	carboxyhemoglobin
Coke	cocaine
COLD	chronic obstructive lung disease
COLD A	cold agglutin titer
col/ml	colonies per milliliter
colp	colporrhaphy
COM	chronic otitis media
COMP	complications; compound
conc	concentrated
CONG	congenital; congius (gallon)
cont	contusions; continuous
COP	cicatricial ocular pemphigoid; colloid osmotic pressure
COPD	chronic obstructive pulmonary disease
COPE	chronic obstructive pulmonary emphysema
cor	coronary
COS	clinically observed seizure
COT	content of thought
COTA	certified occupational therapy assistant
COTX	cast off, to x-ray
COU	cardiac observation unit
COX	Coxsackie virus
CP	cerebral palsy; cleft palate; creatine phosphokinase; chest pain; chronic pain; candle power; chemically pure; combining power; combination product; chloropurine; cochlear potential; chondromalacia patella; chronic pyelonephritis; closing pressure; creatine phosphate
C&P	cystoscopy and pyelography; complete and pushing
CPA	costophrenic angle; cerebellar pontile angle; cardiopulmonary arrest; carotid phonoangiography
CPAP	continuous positive airway pressure
CPB	cardiopulmonary bypass
CPBA	competitive protein-binding assay
CPC	cerebral palsy clinic
CPCR	cardiopulmonary-cerebral resuscitation
CPCS	clinical pharmacokinetics consulting service
CPD	chorioretinopathy and pituitary dysfunction; cephalopelvic disproportion

CPE	chronic pulmonary emphysema; cardiogenic pulmonary edema; complete physical examination
CPGN	chronic progressive glomerulonephritis
CPH	chronic persistent hepatitis
CPI	constitutional psychopathic inferiority
CPID	chronic pelvic inflammatory disease
CPIP	chronic pulmonary insufficiency of prematurity
CPK	creatine phosphokinase; creatinine phosphokinase
CPKD	childhood polycystic kidney disease
CPL	criminal procedure law
CPM	central pontine myelinolysis; continuous passive motion; continue present management; counts per minute
CPN	chronic pyelonephritis
CPP	cerebral perfusion pressure; chronic pelvic pain
CPPB	continuous positive pressure breathing
CPPV	continuous positive pressure ventilation
CPR	cardiopulmonary resuscitation
CPS	complex partial seizures; clinical pharmacokinetic service; coagulase-positive staphylococci; clinical performance score; cumulative probability of success
CPT	chest physiotherapy; child protection team; Current Procedural Terminology
CPTH	chronic post-traumatic headache
CPUE	chest pain of unknown etiology
CPX	complete physical examination
CPZ	chlorpromazine
CR	cardiorespiratory; controlled release; cardiac rehabilitation; colon resection; closed reduction; complete remission; calculus removed; chest and right arm; clinical research; conditioned reflex; crown-rump
CR1	first cranial nerve
CRA	central retinal artery; chronic rheumatoid arthritis
CRAG	cerebral radionuclide angiography
CRAO	central retinal artery occlusion
CRBBB	complete right bundle branch block
CRC	colorectal cancer; child resistant container
CR&C	closed reduction and cast
CrCl	creatinine clearance
CRD	chronic renal disease

creat	creatinine
CREST	calcinosis, Raynaud's phenomenon, esophageal dysmotility, sclerodactylia, and telangiectasia
CRF	chronic renal failure; corticotropin-releasing factor
CRI	chronic renal insufficiency
CRIE	crossed radioimmunoelectrophoresis
CRIS	controlled release infusion system
crit	hematocrit
CRL	crown-rump length
CRM+	cross-reacting material positive
CRNA	certified registered nurse anesthetist
CRNP	certified registered nurse practitioner
CRO	cathode ray oscilloscope
CRP	C-reactive protein
CRS	catheter-related sepsis; Chinese restaurant syndrome; colon-rectal surgery
CRST	calcification, Raynaud's phenomenon, scleroderma, and telangiectasia
CRT	copper reduction test; cathode ray tube; central reaction time
Cr Tr	crutch training
CRTT	certified respiratory therapy technician
CRTX	cast removed, take x-ray
CRU	clinical research unit
CRV	central retinal vein
CRVO	central retinal vein occlusion
CS	clinical stage; consciousness; cat scratch; conjunctiva and sclera; cervical spine; cigarette smoker; consultation; consultation service; central service; central supply; cesarean section; conditioned stimulus; coronary sinus; corticosteroid; current strength
C&S	culture and sensitivity; conjunctiva and sclera
C/S	cesarean section; culture and sensitivity
CSA	controlled substance analogue
CSB I & II	Chemistry Screening Batteries I and II
CSBF	coronary sinus blood flow
CSC	cornea, sclera, conjunctiva
CSD	cat scratch disease
CSE	cross-section echocardiography
C sect	cesarean section
CSF	cerebrospinal fluid; colony-stimulating factor

CSFP	cerebrospinal fluid pressure
C-sh	chair shower
CSH	carotid sinus hypersensitivity; chronic subdural hematoma
CSICU	cardiac surgery intensive care unit
CSII	continuous subcutaneous insulin infusion
CS IV	clinical stage 4
CSLU	chronic status leg ulcer
CSM	circulation, sensation, movement; cerebrospinal meningitis; carotid sinus massage
CSNS	carotid sinus nerve stimulation
CSOM	chronic serous otitis media; chronic suppurative otitis media
CSP	cellulose sodium phosphate
CSR	central supply room; Cheyne-Stokes respiration; corrected sedimentation rate; cortisol secretion rate; corrected septorhinoplasty
CSS	carotid sinus stimulation; chewing, sucking, and swallowing
CST	convulsive shock therapy; contraction stress test; cardiac stress test
CSU	cardiac surveillance unit; cardiovascular surgery unit; catheter specimen of urine
CT	computed tomography; clotting time; circulation time; corneal thickness; coagulation time; cervical traction; Coombs' test; cardiothoracic; calcitonin; chest tube; coated tablet; compressed tablet; corneal transplant; carotid tracing; carpal tunnel; cerebral thrombosis; classic technique; collecting tubule; connective tissue; contraction time; coronary thrombosis; corrected transposition; corrective therapy; crest time; cytotechnologist
Cta	catamenia
CTB	ceased to breathe
CTD	chest tube drainage
CT&DB	cough, turn, and deep breathe
CTF	Colorado tick fever
CTH	clot to hold
CTL	cytotoxic T lymphocytes; cervical, thoracic, and lumbar
CT/MPR	computed tomography with multiplanar reconstruction
CTN	calcitonin

C&T N,	color and temperature normal, both lower
BLE	extremities
cTNM	clinical-diagnostic staging of cancer
CTP	comprehensive treatment plan
CTR	carpal tunnel release
CTS	carpal tunnel syndrome
CTSP	called to see patient
CTW	central terminal of Wilson
CTXN	contraction
CTZ	chemoreceptor trigger zone
Cu	copper
CU	cause unknown
CUC	chronic ulcerative colitis
CUD	cause undetermined
CUG	cystourethrogram
CUPS	carcinoma of unknown primary site
CUS	chronic undifferentiated schizophrenia
CUSA	Cavitron ultrasonic aspirator
CV	cardiovascular; cell volume
CVA	cerebrovascular accident; costovertebral angle
CVAT	costovertebral angle tenderness
CVC	central venous catheter
CVD	collagen vascular disease
CVF	cardiovascular failure; central visual field; cervicovaginal fluid
CVHD	chronic valvular heart disease
CVI	cerebrovascular insufficiency; continuous venous infusion
CVID	common variable immunodeficiency
CVO	central vein occlusion
CVP	central venous pressure
CVR	cerebral vascular resistance
CVRI	coronary vascular resistance index
CVS	clean voided specimen; chorionic villi sampling; cardiovascular surgery
CVUG	cysto-void urethrogram
CW	compare with
C/W	consistent with; crutch walking
CWD	cell wall defective
CWE	cottonwool exudate
CWMS	color, warmth, movement, sensation
CWP	coal worker's pneumoconiosis; childbirth without pain
CWS	cotton wool spots
Cx	cervix; culture; cancel; cylinder axis

CxMT	cervical motion tenderness
CXR	chest x-ray
CYTO	cytotechnology

D

D	diarrhea; day; divorced; distal; dead; diopter; dextrose; diastole; dorsal; daughter; deciduous; density; died; duration
d	dose (dosis); give (da); right (dexter)
D1,D2	dorsal vertebrae 1, 2
DA	dopamine; direct admission; drug aerosol; drug addict; direct agglutination; dental assistant; degenerative arthritis; ductus arteriosus
D/A	discharge and advise
DAB	days after birth
DACL	Depression Adjective Checklists
DAD	drug administration device; dispense as directed
DAH	disordered action of the heart
DAL	drug analysis laboratory
DAM	degraded amyloid
DANA	drug-induced antinuclear antibodies
DAP	diabetes-associated peptide; direct agglutination pregnancy
DAPT	direct agglutination pregnancy test
DAT	direct agglutination test; direct antiglobulin test; diet as tolerated; dementia of the Alzheimer type; diphtheria antitoxin; differential agglutination titer
DAW	dispense as written
dB	decibel
DB	date of birth; disability; distobuccal; dextran blue
DBC	dye-binding capacity
DB&C	deep breathing and coughing
DBCL	dilute blood clot lysis
DBE	deep breathing exercise
DBI	development-at-birth index
DBIL	direct bilirubin
DBO	distobucco-occlusal
DBP	diastolic blood pressure; distobuccopulpal
DBS	diminished breath sounds

DC	discharged; discontinue; decrease; diagonal conjugate; direct Coombs'; daily census; diagnostic code; distocervical; direct current
D&C	dilatation and curettage; dilation and curettage
DCBE	double contrast barium enema
DCC	day care center; double concave
DCCF	dural carotid-cavernous fistula
DCF	direct centrifugal flotation
DCH	delayed cutaneous hypersensitivity
DCO	diffusing capacity of carbon monoxide
DCPN	direction-changing positional nystagmus
DCR	delayed cutaneous reaction; dacryocytorhinostomy
DCSA	double contrast shoulder arthrography
DCT	direct Coombs' test; deep chest therapy
DCTM	delay computed-tomographic myelography
DCYS	Department of Children and Youth Services
DCx	double convex
dd	let it be given to (detur ad)
DD	differential diagnosis; down drain; dependent drainage; dry dressing; Duchenne's dystrophy; discharge diagnosis; died of the disease; disk diameter
D&D	diarrhea and dehydration
DDC	direct display console
DDD	degenerative disc disease; defined daily doses
DDGB	double-dose gallbladder
DDS	dialysis disequilibrium syndrome; Doctor of Dental Surgery; dystrophy-dystocia syndrome
DDST	Denver Development Screening Test
DDx	differential diagnosis
DE	dream elements; duration of ejection
D&E	dilation and evacuation
DEA	Drug Enforcement Administration
dec	deceased; decrease
DEC	decrease
decub	decubitus
DEF	decayed, extracted, or filled; defecation; deficiency
deg	degree
degen	degenerative
deglut	deglutire (to swallow)
del	delivery
dep	dependents

DEP ST SEG	depressed ST segment
DeR	reaction of degeneration
DES	disequilibrium syndrome; diffuse esophageal spasm
dest	destilla (distilled)
det	detur (give)
DEV	duck embryo vaccine; deviation
DEVR	dominant exudative vitreoretinopathy
dex	dexter (right)
DF	decayed and filled; deficiency factor; degree of freedom; diabetic father
DFA	direct fluorescent antibody; difficulty falling asleep
DFD	defined formula diet
DFE	distal femoral epiphysis
DFM	decreased fetal movement
DFMC	daily fetal movement count
DFMR	daily fetal movement record
DFP	diastolic filling period
DFR	diabetic floor routine
DFU	dead fetus in uterus
dg	decigram
DG	diagnosis; diastolic gallop; diglyceride; distogingival
DGI	disseminated gonococcal infection
DGM	ductal glandular mastectomy
DH	developmental history; delayed hypersensitivity; diaphragmatic hernia
DHBV	duck hepatitis B virus
DHF	dengue hemorrhagic fever
DHL	diffuse histocytic lymphoma
DHS	duration of hospital stay; Department of Human Services
DI	diabetes insipidus; date of injury; detrusor instability; drug interaction; diagnostic imaging; Depression Inventory
D&I	dry and intact
diag	diagnosis
Diath SW	diathermy short wave
DIB	disability insurance benefits
DIC	disseminated intravascular coagulation; drug information center; diffuse intravascular coagulation
DID	dead of intercurrent disease
DIE	died in emergency department; died in emergency room
diff	differential

DIFF	differential (blood count)
dig	digeratur (let it be digested)
DIJOA	dominantly inherited juvenile optic atrophy
dil	dilute
DILD	diffuse infiltrative lung disease; drug-induced lupus erythematous
DIM	diminish; divalent ion metabolism
DIMOAD	diabetes insipidus, diabetes mellitus, optic atrophy, and deafness
DIP	distal interphalangeal; desquamative interstitial pneumonia; drip infusion pyelogram
DIPJ	distal interphalangeal joint
dis	disease; dislocation
DIS	Diagnostic Interview Schedule
disch	discharge
DISH	diffuse idiopathic skeletal hyperostosis
disp	dispensatory; dispense
dist	distill; distilled
div	divide
DIV	double inlet ventricle
DIVA	digital intravenous angiography
DJD	degenerative joint disease
DK	diabetic ketoacidosis; dark; decay; diseased kidney; dog kidney
DKA	diabetic ketoacidosis; didn't keep appointment
dl	deciliter
DL	direct laryngoscopy; danger list; diagnostic laparoscopy; distolingual; Donath-Landsteiner
DLA	distolabial
DLAI	distolabioincisal
DLB	direct laryngoscopy and bronchoscopy
DLCO	diffusing capacity of lung for carbon monoxide
DLE	discoid lupus erythematosus; disseminated lupus erythematosus
DLF	digitalis-like factor
DLI	distolinguoincisal
DLIF	digoxin-like immunoreactive factor
DLIS	digoxin-like immunoreactive substance
DLMP	date of last menstrual period
DLNMP	date of last normal menstrual period
DLO	distolinguo-occlusal
DLP	distolinguopulpal
D_5LR	dextrose 5% in lactated Ringer's
DM	diabetes mellitus; diastolic murmur; dermatomyositis; diabetic mother; dopamine

DMD	Doctor of Dental Medicine; Duchenne's muscular dystrophy
DME	durable medical equipment
DMF	decayed, missing, or filled
DMKA	diabetes mellitus ketoacidosis
DMOOC	diabetes mellitus out of control
DMS	diagnostic medical sonography
DMV	Doctor of Veterinary Medicine
DMX	diathermy, massage, and exercise
DN	dextrose-nitrogen; down; diabetic nephropathy
D&N	distance and near
DNA	deoxyribonucleic acid; did not answer; does not apply
DNC	did not come
DND	died a natural death
DNI	do not intubate
DNKA	did not keep appointment
DNR	do not resuscitate; do not report; did not respond
DNS	did not show; deviated nasal septum; dysplastic nevus syndrome
DNT	did not test
DO	Doctor of Osteopathy; diet order; distoocclusal
D/O	disorder
DOA	dead on arrival; date of admission
DOA-DRA	dead on arrival despite resuscitative attempts
DOB	date of birth; doctor's order book
DOC	died of other causes; diabetes out of control; drug of choice
DOE	dyspnea on exertion
DOH	Department of Health
DOI	date of injury
DOL #2	second day of life
DOLV	double-outlet left ventricle
DON	Director of Nursing
DORV	double-outlet right ventricle
DORx	date of treatment
DOSS	dioctyl sodium sulfosuccinate (docusate sodium)
DOT	Doppler ophthalmic test; died on table; date of transcription; date of transfer
doz	dozen
DP	dorsalis pedis; diastolic pressure
DPA	Department of Public Assistance
DPB	days postburn

DPC	discharge planning coordinator; delayed primary closure
DPDL	diffuse poorly differentiated lymphocytic lymphoma
DPH	Department of Public Health; Doctor of Public Health
DPM	Doctor of Podiatric Medicine; disintegrations per minute
DPT	diphtheria, pertussis, and tetanus
DPU	delayed pressure urticaria
DQ	developmental quotient
DR	doctor; diabetic retinopathy; reaction of degeneration; delivery room
Dr	doctor
dr	drachm; dram
DRA	drug-related admission
DREZ	dorsal root entry zone
DRGs	diagnosis-related groups
DRI	Discharge Readiness Index
DRS	Duane's retraction syndrome
DRSG	dressing
D/S	dextrose and sodium chloride
DS	double strength; dead space; disoriented; dextrose stick; discharge summary; Down's syndrome; dry swallow
D&S	diagnostic and surgical
DSA	digital subtraction angiography
DSD	dry sterile dressing; discharge summary dictated
dsg	dressing
DSI	Depression Status Inventory; deep shock insulin
DSM	drink skim milk
DSM III	Diagnostic and Statistical Manual, 3rd Edition
DSS	dengue shock syndrome; Disability Status Scale
DST	donor specific transfusion
DSWI	deep surgical wound infection
DT	discharge tomorrow; diphtheria, tetanus; diphtheria toxoid; dietetic technician; distance test; duration tetany
DTD	detur talis dosis (let such a dose be given)
DTH	delayed-type hypersensitivity
DTP	diphtheria, tetanus, and pertussis; distal tingling on percussion
DTR	deep tendon reflex
DTs	delirium tremens

DTS	donor specific transfusion
DTT	diphtheria-tetanus toxoid
DTUS	diathermy, traction, and ultrasound
DTV	due to void
DTX	detoxification
DU	duodenal ulcer; diagnosis undetermined; diabetic urine
DUB	dysfunctional uterine bleeding; Dubowitz (score)
DUI	driving under influence
DUNHL	diffuse undifferentiated non-Hodgkins lymphoma
duod	duodenum
dur	duration
D&V	diarrhea and vomiting
DVA	distance visual acuity
DVD	dissociated vertical deviation
DVI	digital vascular imaging
DVIU	direct vision internal urethrotomy
DVM	Doctor of Veterinary Medicine
DVR	double valve replacement
DVT	deep vein thrombosis
D_5W	5% dextrose in water
$D\overline{W}$	distilled water; dry weight
D/W	dextrose in water
DWDL	diffuse well differentiated lymphocytic lymphoma
DWI	driving while intoxicated
Dx	diagnosis
DXT	deep x-ray therapy
Dz	disease; dozen

E

E	edema; eye; electron; energy; epinephrine; experimenter
E2	estradiol
E3	estriol
ea	each
EAA	electrothermal atomic absorption; essential amino acids
EAC	external auditory canal; Ehrlich ascites carcinoma
EAE	experimental allergic encephalomyelitis
EAHF	eczema, allergy, hay fever

EAHLG	equine antihuman lymphoblast globulin
EAHLS	equine antihuman lymphoblast serum
EAM	external auditory meatus
EAST	external rotation abduction stress test
EAT	ectopic atrial tachycardia
EAU	experimental autoimmune uveitis
EB	epidermolysis bullosa; elementary body
EBA	epidermolysis bullosa acquisita
EBF	erythroblastosis fetalis
EBL	estimated blood loss
EBV	Epstein-Barr virus
EC	enteric coated; eyes closed; extracellular; electron capture; excitation-contraction
E-CABG	endarterectomy and coronary artery bypass grafting
ECBD	exploration of common bile duct
ECC	emergency cardiac care; endocervical curettage; extracorporeal circulation
ECCE	extracapsular cataract extraction
ECD	endocardial cushion defect
ECEMG	evoked compound electromyography
ECF	extracellular fluid; extended care facility; effective capillary flow
ECG	electrocardiogram
EcHO	enterocytopathogenic human orphan (virus); echocardiogram
ECL	extent of cerebral lesion; extracapillary lesions
ECM	extracellular material
ECMO	extracorporeal membrane oxygenation
ECN	extended care nursery
ECOG	Eastern Cooperative Oncology Group
E. coli	*Escherichia coli*
ECR	emergency chemical restraint
ECS	electrocerebral silence
ECT	electroconvulsive therapy; enhanced computed tomography; emission computed tomography
ECV	extracellular volume
ECW	extracellular water
ED	emergency department; epidural; end-diastolic; effective dose; erythema dose
EDAP	Emergency Department Approved for Pediatrics
EDAX	energy-dispersive analysis of x-rays
EDC	estimated date of confinement; estimated date of conception; extensor digitorium communis; end-diastolic count; electrodesiccation and curettage
EDD	expected date of delivery

EDM	early diastolic murmur
EDS	Ehlers-Danlos syndrome
EDV	end-diastolic volume
EE	equine encephalitis; end to end
EEE	eastern equine encephalomyelitis; edema, erythema, and exudate; external eye examination
EEG	electroencephalogram
EENT	eyes, ears, nose, throat
EF	extended-field; endurance factor; ejection fraction
EFAD	essential fatty acid deficiency
EFHBM	eosinophilic fibrohistiocytic lesion of bone marrow
EFM	external fetal monitoring; electronic fetal monitor(ing)
EFVC	expiratory flow-volume curve
EFW	estimated fetal weight
e.g.	for example
EG	esophagogastrectomy
EGA	estimated gestational age
EGBUS	external genitalia, Bartholin, urethral, Skene's glands
EGD	esophagogastroduodenoscopy
EGG	electrogastrography; electrogastrogram
EGL	eosinophilic granuloma of the lung
EGM	electrogram
EGOT	erythrocyte glutamic oxaloacetic transaminase
EGTA	esophageal gastric tube airway
EH	enlarged heart; essential hypertension; educationally handicapped; extramedullary hematopoiesis
EHB	elevate head of bed
EHF	epidemic hemorrhagic fever
E&I	endocrine and infertility
EIA	exercise-induced asthma; enzyme immunoassay
EIAB	extracranial-intracranial arterial bypass
EIB	exercise-induced bronchospasm
EID	electronic infusion device; electroimmunodiffusion
EIP	end-inspiratory pressure
EIS	endoscopic injection scleropathy
EJ	external jugular; elbow jerk
EKC	epidemic keratoconjunctivitis
EKG	electrocardiogram
EKY	electrokymogram
E-L	external lids
ELF	elective low forceps

ELH	endolymphatic hydrops
ELISA	enzyme-linked immunosorbent assay
Elix	elixir
ELOS	estimated length of stay
ELP	electrophoresis
ELS	Eaton-Lambert syndrome
EM	electron microscope; ejection murmur; erythema multiforme; emmetropia; extensive metabolizers
EMB	endomyocardial biopsy; endometrial biopsy
EMC	encephalomyocarditis
EMD	electromechanical dissociation
EMF	erythrocyte maturation factor; evaporated milk formula
EMG	electromyography; essential monoclonal gammopathy; exophthalmos, macroglossia, gigantism
EMIC	emergency maternity and infant care
E-MICR	electron microscopy
EMIT	enzyme-multiplied immunoassay technique
EMMW	extended mandatory minute ventilation
EMR	emergency mechanical restraint; empty, measure, and record; educable mentally retarded
EMS	emergency medical services; early morning stiffness; eosinophilia-myalgia syndrome
EMT	emergency medical technician
EMT-P	emergency medical technician-paramedic
EMV	eye, motor, verbal
EMVC	early mitral valve closure
EMW	electromagnetic waves
EN	enteral nutrition; erythema nodosum
ENA	extractable nuclear antigen
ENG	electronystagmogram
ENL	erythema nodosum leprosum
ENP	extractable nucleoprotein
ENT	ears, nose, throat
EO	eyes open; elbow orthosis; eosinophilia; ethylene oxide
EOA	examine, opinion, and advice; esophageal obturator airway
EOD	every other day
EOG	electrooculogram
EOM	extraocular movement; extraocular muscles; external otitis media
EOMI	extraocular muscles intact
EORA	elderly onset rheumatoid arthritis
eos	eosinophil

EP	endogenous pyrogen; ectopic pregnancy; evoked potentials; electrophysiologic
EPB	extensor pollicis brevis
EPI	epinephrine; exocrine pancreatic insufficiency; epithelioid cells
EPIS	episiotomy
epith	epithelial
EPL	extensor pollicis longus
EPM	electronic pacemaker
EPO	erythropoietin
EPP	erythropoietic protoporphyria
EPR	electrophrenic respiration; emergency physical restraint; electron paramagnetic resonance
EPS	electrophysiologic study; extrapyramidal symptoms
EPTS	existed prior to service
ER	emergency room; estrogen receptors; endoplasmic reticulum; external rotation
E&R	equal and reactive; examination and report
ER+	estrogen receptor-positive
ERA	estrogen receptor assay; evoked response audiometry
ERCP	endoscopic retrograde cholangiopancreatography
ERE	external rotation in extension
ERF	external rotation in flexion
ERFC	erythrocyte rosette-forming cells
ERG	electroretinogram
ERL	effective refractory length
ERP	estrogen receptor protein; emergency room physician; endoscopic retrograde pancreatography
ERPF	effective renal plasma flow
ERT	estrogen replacement therapy
ERV	expiratory reserve volume
ES	emergency services; end-systolic; end-to-side; Environmental Stimulation
ESAP	evoked sensory action potential
ESC	end-systolic counts
ESD	esophagus, stomach, and duodenum
ESLD	end-stage liver disease
ESM	ejection systolic murmur
ESP	especially; end-systolic pressure; extrasensory perception
ESR	erythrocyte sedimentation rate
ESRD	end-stage renal disease
ess	essential

EST	electroshock therapy
ESWL	extracorporeal shockwave lithotripsy
ET	endotracheal; esotropia; eustachian tube; exercise treadmill; ejection time; exchange transfusion; etiology; effective temperature; electroneurodiagnostic technologist
et	and
et al	and others
ETC	estimated time of conception
ETCO$_2$	end tidal carbon dioxide
ETF	eustachian tubal function
ETKTM	every test known to man
ETO	estimated time of ovulation
ETOP	elective termination of pregnancy
ETT	endotracheal tube; exercise tolerance test
ETU	emergency and trauma unit; emergency treatment unit
EU	excretory urography; etiology unknown; enzyme units; Ehrlich units
EUA	examine under anesthesia
EUM	external urethral meatus
EUP	extrauterine pregnancy
EUS	external urethral sphincter
EVAC	evacuation
eval	evaluate
ew	elsewhere
EWB	estrogen withdrawal bleeding
EWSCLs	extended-wear soft contact lens
ex	examined; excision; exercise
exam	examination
exp	expiration
EXP	experienced; expose; exploration
expect	expectorant
exp lap	exploratory laparotomy
ext	extract; external
extrav	extravasation
ext rot	external rotation
EX U	excretory urogram

F

F	Fahrenheit; female; firm; flow; facial; French; finger; father; fat; fellow; foramen; formula
F$_1$	offspring from first generation

F$_2$	offspring from second generation
F II	factor two
F VIII	factor eight
FA	folic acid; femoral artery; foramen; far advanced; fatty acid; first aid; free acid; fluorescent antibody
FAAP	family assessment adjustment pass
FAB	French-American-British Cooperative group; functional arm brace
FABER	full abduction and external rotation
FACA	Fellow of the American College of Anesthetists
FACAG	Fellow of the American College of Angiology
FACAL	Fellow of the American College of Allergy
FACAN	Fellow of the American College of Anesthesiologists
FACAS	Fellow of the American College of Abdominal Surgeons
FACC	Fellow of the American College of Cardiology
FACCP	Fellow of the American College of Chest Physicians
FACCPC	Fellow of the American College of Clinical Pharmacology and Chemotherapy
FACD	Fellow of the American College of Dentists
FACEM	Fellow of the American College of Emergency Medicine
FACGE	Fellow of the American College of Gastroenterology
FACH	forceps-after-coming of head
FACLM	Fellow of the American College of Legal Medicine
FACN	Fellow of the American College of Nutrition
FACNP	Fellow of the American College of Neuropsychopharmacology
FACOG	Fellow of the American College of Obstetricians and Gynecologists
FACOS	Fellow of the American College of Orthopedic Surgeons
FACP	Fellow of the American College of Physicians
FACPRM	Fellow of the American College of Preventive Medicine
FACR	Fellow of the American College of Radiology
FACS	Fellow of the American College of Surgeons
FACSM	Fellow of the American College of Sports Medicine
FAGA	full-term appropriate for gestational age
FAI	functional assessment inventory
FALL	fallopian

FAM	family
FAMA	fluorescent antibody to membrane antigen
FANA	fluorescent antinuclear antibody
FAP	fibrillating action potential; familial amyloid polyneuropathy; familial adenomatous polyposis; femoral artery pressure
FAS	fetal alcohol syndrome
FAST	fluoro-allergo sorbent test
FAT	fluorescent antibody test
FB	fingerbreadth; foreign body
FBD	fibrocystic breast disease; functional bowel disease
FBG	foreign-body-type granuloma
FBRCM	fingerbreadth below right costal margin
FBS	fasting blood sugar; fetal bovine serum
FBU	fingers below umbilicus
FBW	fasting blood work
FC	Foley catheter; finger counting; fever and chills; finger clubbing; function capacity; functional class
F+C	flare and cells
F&C	foam and condom
F cath	Foley catheter
FCC	follicular center cells; familial colonic cancer; fracture compound comminuted
FCCL	follicular center cell lymphoma
FCDB	fibrocystic disease of the breast
FCH	familial combined hyperlipidemia
FCMC	family-centered maternity care
FCMN	family-centered maternity nursing
FCR	flexor carpi radialis
FCRB	flexor carpi radialis brevis
FCSNVD	fever, chills, sweating, nausea, vomiting, diarrhea
FCU	flexor carpi ulnaris
FD	focal distance; familial dysautonomia; forceps delivery; full denture; fatal dose; focal disease; foot drape; freeze-dried
F&D	fixed and dilated
FDA	Food and Drug Administration; fronto-dextra anterior
FDBL	fecal daily blood loss
FDIU	fetal death in utero
FDLMP	first day of last menstrual period
FDM	fetus of diabetic mother
FDP	fibrin-degradation products; flexor digitorum profundus

FDS	flexor digitorum superficialis; for duration of stay
Fe	iron
FEC	forced expiratory capacity
FECG	fetal electrocardiogram
FEF	forced expiratory flow
FEL	familial erythrophagocytic lymphohistiocytosis
FEM	femoral
Fem-pop	femoral popliteal (bypass)
FEN	fluid, electrolytes, nutrition
FENa	fractional extraction of sodium
FEP	free erythrocyte protoporphyrin
FES	fat embolism syndrome; forced expiratory spirogram
FeSO$_4$	ferrous sulfate
FET	forced expiratory time
FETS	forced expiratory time, in seconds
FEUO	for external use only
FEV	forced expiratory volume
FF	filtration fraction; fat free; fundus firm; flat feet; force fluids; father factor; finger-to-finger; fecal frequency; foster father
FFA	free fatty acid
FFM	fat-free mass
FFP	fresh frozen plasma
FGP	fundic gland polyps
FH	family history; fetal heart; fundal height; fetal head
FHF	fulminant hepatic failure
FHH	familial hypocalciuria hypercalcemia; fetal heart heard
FHNH	fetal heart not heard
FHP	family history positive
FHR	fetal heart rate
FHS	fetal heart sounds
FHT	fetal heart tone
FiCO$_2$	fraction of inspired carbon dioxide
FIGO	International Federation of Gynecology and Obstetrics
FIL	father-in-law
FiO$_2$	fraction of inspired oxygen
FJROM	full joint range of motion
FJS	finger joint size
FL	fluid; fetal length; fatty liver
fl	fluid
FLASH	fast low-angle shot

fl dr	fluid dram
fl oz	fluid ounce
FLP	left frontoposterior
FLS	flashing lights and/or scotoma
FLSA	follicular lymphosarcoma
FLT	left frontotransverse
FLU A	influenza A virus
FLZ	flurazepam
FM	fetal movements; face mask; flowmeter
F&M	firm and midline (uterus)
FMC	fetal movement count
FMD	foot and mouth disease; family medical doctor; fibromuscular dysplasia
FME	full mouth extraction
FMF	familial Mediterranean fever; forced midexpiratory flow; fetal movement felt
FMG	foreign medical graduate; fine mesh gauze
FMH	fibromuscular hyperplasia; family medical history
FMP	fasting metabolic panel; first menstrual period
FMR	fetal movement record
FMX	full mouth x-ray
FN	finger-to-nose; false negative
F to N	finger-to-nose
FNAB	fine-needle aspiration biopsy
FNAC	fine-needle aspiration cytology
FNCJ	fine-needle catheter jejunostomy
FNH	focal nodular hyperplasia
FNR	false negative rate
FNS	functional neuromuscular stimulation
FO	foot orthosis; frontooccipital; foramen ovale
FOB	foot of bed; fiberoptic bronchoscope; father of baby; fecal occult blood; feet out of bed;
FOBT	fecal occult blood test
FOC	father of child; fluid of choice
FOD	free of disease
FOI	flight of ideas
FOM	floor of mouth
FOOB	fell out of bed
FP	family practice; family planning; false positive; flat plate; frozen plasma; food poisoning; freezing point; frontoparietal
F-P	femoral-popliteal
fpA	fibrinopeptide A
FPAL	fullterm, premature, abortion, living
FPB	flexor pollicis brevis

FPD	feto-pelvic disproportion; fixed partial denture
FPG	fasting plasma glucose
FPIA	fluorescence-polarization immunoassay
FPL	flexor pollicis longus
FPM	full passive movements
FPNA	first-pass nuclear angiocardiography
FR	flow rate; fluid restriction
F&R	force and rhythm
FRC	functional residual capacity
FRJM	full range of joint motion
FROM	full range of motion
FS	frozen section; flexible sigmoidoscopy; full strength
F&S	full and soft
FSB	fetal scalp blood
FSBM	full strength breast milk
FSC	fracture, simple, complete
FSD	fracture, simple, depressed
FSE	fetal scalp electrode
FSG	focal and segmental glomerulosclerosis
FSH	follicle stimulating hormone; facioscapulohumeral
FSHMD	facioscapulohumeral muscular dystrophy
FSIQ	Full-Scale Intelligence Quotient
FSP	fibrin split products
FSS	French steel sound; Familiar Sensory Stimulation
FSW	field service worker
ft	foot
FT	full term; finger tip; follow through; family therapy; fibrous tissue; false transmitter; free thyroxine
FT$_3$	free triiodothyronine
FT$_4$	free thyroxine
FTA	fluorescent titer antibody; fluorescent treponemal antibody
FTA-ABS	fluorescent treponeal antibody-absorption test for syphilis
FTB	fingertip blood
FTBD	full-term born dead
FTD	failure to descend
FTE	full-time equivalent
FTFTN	finger-to-finger-to-nose
FTI	free thyroxine index
FTKA	failed to keep appointment
FTLB	full-term living birth
FTLFC	full-term living female child

FTLMC	full-term living male child
FTN	finger to nose; full-term nursery
FTNB	full-term newborn
FTND	full-term normal delivery
FTNSD	full-term, normal, spontaneous delivery
FTP	failure to progress
FTR	for the record
FTSG	full-thickness skin graft
FTT	failure to thrive
F&U	flanks and upper quadrant
F/U	follow-up; fundus at umbilicus
FUB	functional uterine bleeding
FUN	follow-up note
FUO	fever of undetermined origin; fever of unknown origin
FUOV	follow-up office visit
FUS	fusion
FVC	forced vital capacity
FVH	focal vascular headache
FVL	flow volume loop
FWB	full weight bearing
FWW	front wheel walker
Fx	fracture
Fx-dis	fracture-dislocation
FXN	function
FXR	fracture
FY	fiscal year
FYI	for your information
FZ	focal zone

G

G	gauge; gravida; gram; gallop; glucose; good; gingival; gonidial; Greek
G+	gram-positive
G-	gram-negative
G1-4	grade 1-4
GA	gastric analysis; glucose/acetone; general anesthesia; gestational age; ginger ale; general appearance; gut-associated; gingivoaxial; Gamblers Anonymous
Ga	gallium
GABA	gamma-aminobutyric acid
GABHS	group A beta hemolytic streptococci
gal	gallon

G'ale	ginger ale
GALT	gut-associated lymphoid tissue
galv	galvanic
garg	gargle
GAS	general adaption syndrome; Global Assessment Scale; group A streptococci
Ga scan	gallium scan
GAT	group adjustment therapy
GATB	General Aptitude Test Battery
GAU	geriatric assessment unit
GB	gallbladder
G&B	good and bad
GBA	ganglionic-blocking agent; gingivobuccoaxial
GBM	glomerular basement membrane
GBP	gastric bypass
GBS	gallbladder series; Guillain-Barré syndrome; group B streptococci; gastric bypass surgery
GC	gonococci; gonorrhea; geriatric chair; graham crackers; good condition; gas chromatography; ganglion cells; glucocorticoid; granular casts
G-C	gram-negative cocci
G+C	gram-positive cocci
GCDFP	gross cystic disease fluid protein
GCIIS	glucose control insulin infusion system
GCS	Glasgow coma scale; general clinical service
GCSF	granulocyte cell-stimulating factor
GCT	giant cell tumor; general care and treatment
GCU	gonococcal urethritis
GD	Graves' disease
G and D	growth and development
GDF	gel diffusion precipitin
GDM	gestational diabetes mellitus
GE	gastroenteritis; gainfully employed
gen	general
GEN/ ENDO	general anesthesia with endotracheal intubation
GENT	gentamicin
GEP	gastroenteropancreatic
GER	gastroesophageal reflux
GERD	gastroesophageal reflux disease
GET	gastric emptying time; graded exercise test
GETA	general endotracheal anesthesia
GF	grandfather; gastric fistula; gluten-free; germ-free
GFAP	glial fibrillary acid protein
GFD	gluten-free diet
GFM	good fetal movement

GFR	glomerular filtration rate
GG	gamma globulin; guaifenesin
GGE	generalized glandular enlargement
GGT	gamma-glutamyl transpeptidase
GGTP	gamma-glutamyl transpeptidase
GH	growth hormone
GHB	gamma hydroxybutyric
GHb	glycosylated hemoglobin
GHD	growth hormone deficiency
GHQ	General Health Questionnaire
GI	gastrointestinal; granuloma inguinale
GIB	gastric ileal bypass
GIC	general immunocompetence
GIFT	gamete intrafallopian transfer
GIK	glucose-insulin-potassium
ging	gingiva
GIP	giant cell interstitial pneumonia; gastric inhibitory peptide
GIS	gastrointestinal series; gas in stomach
GIT	gastrointestinal tract
GITS	gastrointestinal therapeutic system
GITSG	Gastrointestinal Tumor Study Group
giv	give; given
GJ	gastrojejunostomy
GL	greatest length; gastric lavage
GLA	gingivolinguoaxial
GLC	gas-liquid chromatography
glob	globulin
GLP	group-living program
glu	glucose
GLU 5	five-hour glucose tolerance test
gluc	glucose
GLYCOS Hb	glycosylated hemoglobin
GM	grandmother; grand mal; granulocyte-monocyte; gastric mucosa; general medical; geometric mean; grand multiparity; gram
GM+	gram-positive
GM-	gram-negative
Gm%	grams per 100 milliliters
GMC	general medical clinic; general medical council
GMP	guanosine monophosphate
GMS	general medical services
GM&S	general medicine and surgery
GMTs	geometric mean antibody titers
GN	graduate nurse; gram-negative; glomerulonephritis; glucose nitrogen
GNID	gram-negative intracellular diplococci

GNR	gram-negative rods
GnRH	gonadotropin-releasing hormone
GOG	Gynecologic Oncology Group
GOK	God only knows
GON	gonococcal ophthalmia neonatorum
GOR	general operating room
GOT	glutamic oxaloacetic transaminase; glucose oxidase test; goals of treatment
GP	general practice; general practitioner; glycoprotein; gutta percha; guinea pig
gp	group
G/P	gravida/para
G4P3104	four pregnancies (gravid), 3 went to term, one premature, no abortion, and 4 living (para) children
GPC	gram-positive cocci; giant papillary conjunctivitis
G6PD	glucose-6-phosphate dehydrogenase
GPMAL	gravida, para, multiple births, abortions, and live births
GPN	graduate practical nurse
GPS	Goodpasture's syndrome; guinea pig serum
GPT	glutamic pyruvic transaminase
gr	grain
G-R	gram-negative rods
G+R	gram-positive rods
GRASS	gradient recalled acquisition in a steady state
Grav	gravid (pregnant)
GRD	gastroesophageal reflux disease
GRT	gastric residence time
GS	gallstone; general surgery
GSD	glycogen storage disease
GSD-1	glycogen storage disease, type 1
GSE	grip strong and equal; gluten sensitive enteropathy
GSI	genuine stress incontinence
GSP	general survey panel
GSPN	greater superficial petrosal neurectomy
GSR	galvanic skin resistance
GST	gold sodium thiomalate
GSTM	gold sodium thiomalate
GSW	gunshot wound
GSWA	gunshot wound to abdomen
GT	gastrostomy tube; gait training; grand total
GTF	gastrostomy tube feedings
GTN	gestational trophoblastic neoplasm
GTP	glutamyl transpeptidase

GTS	Gilles de la Tourette's syndrome
GTT	glucose tolerance test; drop
GTT agar	gelatin-tellurite-taurocholate agar
GTTS	drops
GU	genitourinary
GUS	genitourinary sphincter; genitourinary system
GVF	good visual fields
GVHD	graft-versus-host disease
GWA	gunshot wound of abdomen
GWT	gunshot wound of throat
GXT	graded exercise test
GYN	gynecology

H

H	hypodermic; hour; heroin; hydrogen; husband; heart; height; *Hemophilus*; high; hot; henry; horizontal
3H's	high, hot, and a helluva lot .
HA	headache; hyperalimentation; hypothalamic amenorrhea; hearing aid; hemolytic anemia; hospital admission; high anxiety; height age
H/A	head-to-abdomen
HAA	hepatitis-associated antigen
HAE	hereditary angioedema; hepatic artery embolization; hearing aid evaluation
HAI	hepatic arterial infusion; hemagglutination inhibition
HAL	hyperalimentation
HAM	human albumin microspheres
HAMA	Hamilton Anxiety (Scale)
HAMD	Hamilton Depression (Scale)
HAN	heroin-associated nephropathy
HANE	hereditary angioneurotic edema
HAP	hospital-acquired pneumonia
HAPC	hospital-acquired penetration contact
HAPE	high altitude pulmonary edema
HAPS	hepatic arterial perfusion scintigraphy
HAQ	Headache Assessment Questionnaire
HAR	high altitude retinopathy
HARH	high altitude retinal hemorrhage
HARS	Hamilton Anxiety Rating Scale
HAS	hyperalimentation solution; Hamilton Anxiety (Rating) Scale
HASHD	hypertensive arteriosclerotic heart disease

HAT	head, arm, and trunk; hospital arrival time
HAV	hepatitis A virus; hallux abducto valgus
Hb	hemoglobin
HB	hemoglobin; heart block; hold breakfast; heel to buttock; housebound
HbA1c	glycosylated hemoglobin
HBBW	hold breakfast for blood work
HB core	hepatitis B core antigen
HBD	hydroxybutyric acid dehydrogenase; has been drinking
HBeAB	hepatitis Be antibody
HBeAg	hepatitis Be antigen
HBF	hepatic blood flow; fetal hemoglobin
HBGM	home blood glucose monitoring
HBI	hemibody irradiation
HBIG	hepatitis B immune globulin
Hb Kansas	mutant hemoglobin with a low affinity for oxygen
HBLV	human B-lymphotropic virus
HBO	hyperbaric oxygen
HbO$_2$	hyperbaric oxygen
HBOT	hyperbaric oxygen treatment
HBP	high blood pressure
HBS	Health Behavior Scale
HBsAg	hepatitis B surface antigen
HBSS	Hank's balanced salt solution
HBV	hepatitis B virus; hepatitis B vaccine; honeybee venom
HBW	high birth weight
H/BW	height-to-body weight
HC	hydrocortisone; home care; house call; head circumference; Hickman catheter; handicapped; hair cell; hepatic catalase; Huntington's chorea; hyaline casts
H&C	hot and cold
HCA	health care aide; Hospital Corporation of America
HCC	hepatocellular carcinoma
HCD	hydrocolloid dressing
HCFA	Health Care Financing Administration
HCG	human chorionic gonadotropin
HCl	hydrochloric acid; hydrochloride
HCL	hairy cell leukemia
HCLs	hard contact lens
HCM	health care maintenance; hypertropic cardiomyopathy
HCO$_3$	bicarbonate
HCP	hereditary coproporphyria

17-HCS	17-hydroxycorticosteroids
HCT	hematocrit; hydrocortisone; hydrochlorothiazide; human chorionic thyrotropin; histamine challenge test
HCTU	home cervical traction unit
HCTZ	hydrochlorothiazide
HCVD	hypertensive cardiovascular disease
HCWs	health-care workers
HD	hearing distance; heloma durum; Hodgkin's disease; hip disarticulation; high dose; Huntington's disease; heart disease; hospital day
HDARAC	high dose cytarabine (ara-C)
HDCV	human diploid cell vaccine
HDH	heart disease history
HDL	high-density lipoprotein
HDLW	hearing distance for watch in left ear
HDMTX	high-dose methotrexate
HDMTX/CF	high-dose methotrexate and citrovorum factor
HDMTX/LV	high-dose methotrexate and leucovorin
HDN	hemolytic disease of newborn
HDP	hydroxydimethylpyrimidine
HDPAA	heparin-dependent platelet-associated antibody
HDRS	Hamilton Depression Rating Scale
HDRW	hearing distance for watch in right ear
HDS	Hamilton Depression (Rating) Scale; herniated disk syndrome
HDU	hemodialysis unit
HDV	hepatitis delta virus
HE	hard exudate
H&E	hemorrhage and exudate; heredity and environment; hematoxylin and eosin
HEENT	head, eyes, ears, nose, and throat
HEK	human embryonic kidney
HEL	human embryonic lung
HELLP	hemolysis, elevated liver enzymes, and low platelet (count)
HEMI	hemiplegia
HEMOSID	hemosiderin
HEMPAS	hereditary erythrocytic multinuclearity with positive acidified serum
HEMS	helicopter emergency medical services
HEP	histamine equivalent prick; hepatic; heparin
HEPA	hamster egg penetration assay; high-efficiency particulate air
HERP	human exposure (dose)/rodent potency (dose)

HES	hypereosinophilic syndrome; hydroxyethyl starch
Hex	hexamethylmelamine
HF	heart failure; hard feces; hay fever; head of fetus; house formula; high flow; Hageman factor; high frequency; hemorrhagic fever
HFD	high forceps delivery; high fiber diet
HFHL	high-frequency hearing loss
HFI	hereditary fructose intolerance
H fl	*Hemophilus influenzae*
HFST	hearing-for-speech test
HFUPR	hourly fetal urine production rate
hg-cal	high caloric
HGH	human growth hormone
HG/Hgb	hemoglobin
hG/hGB	hemoglobin
HGPRT	hypoxanthine guanine phosphoribosyl transferase
HH	hiatal hernia; home health; hypogonadotrophic hypogonadism; hard of hearing; hydroxyhexamide
H&H	hematocrit and hemoglobin
HHA	hereditary hemolytic anemia; home health agency
HHC	home health care
HHD	hypertensive heart disease; home hemodialysis
HHFM	high humidity face mask
HHM	humoral hypercalcemia of malignancy
HHN	handheld nebulizer
HHNC	hyperosmolar hyperglycemic nonketotic coma
HHNK	hyperglycemic hyperosmolar nonketotic (coma)
HHS	Health and Human Services (US Department of)
HHT	hereditary hemorrhagic telangiectasis
HI	hemagglutination inhibition; head injury; hearing impaired; hospital insurance
HIA	hemagglutination inhibition antibody
5-HIAA	5 hydroxyindolacetic acid
HIB	*Hemophilus influenzae b* (vaccine)
HID	headache, insomnia, depression; herniated intervertebral disk
HIDA	hepato-iminodiacetic acid
HIE	hypoxic-ischemic encephalopathy
HIF	higher integrative function
HIHA	high impulsiveness, high anxiety
HIL	hypoxic-ischemic lesion
HILA	high impulsiveness, low anxiety
HIR	head injury routine
HIS	Health Intention Scale; hospital information system

HISMS	How I See Myself Scale
Histo	histoplasmin (skin test)
HIT	heparin-induced thrombocytopenia; histamine inhalation test
HIV	human immunodeficiency virus
HIV-I	human immunodeficiency virus-I
HIVD	herniated intervertebral disk
HJB	Howell-Jolly bodies
HJR	hepato-jugular reflex
H-K	hand to knee
HKAFO	hip-knee-ankle-foot orthosis
HKAO	hip-knee-ankle orthosis
HKO	hip-knee orthosis
HL	hairline; heparin lock; hearing level; hallux limitus; harelip; Hickman line; half-life; heart and lungs; hearing loss; hypermetropia, latent
H&L	heart and lungs
HLA	human lymphocyte antigen
HLA nega-tive	heart, lungs, and abdomen negative
HLD	herniated lumbar disk; haloperidol decanoate
HLHS	hypoplastic left heart syndrome
HLK	heart, liver, and kidney
HLV	hypoplastic left ventricle; herpes-like virus
HM	hand motion; heart murmur; human milk; heavily muscled; hand movement(s); hydatidiform mole
HMA	hemorrhage and microaneurysm
HMB	homatropine methylbromide
HMBA	hexamethylenebisacetamide
HMD	hyaline membrane disease
HMDP	hydroxymethyline diphosphonate
HME	heat, massage, and exercise
HMg	human menopausal gonadotropin
HMG CoA	hepatic hydroxymethylglutaryl coenzyme A
HMI	healed myocardial infarction
HMM	hexamethylmelamine
HMO	Health Maintenance Organization
HMP	hexose monophosphate; hot moist packs
HMR	histocytic medullary reticulosis
HMX	heat massage exercise
HN	high nitrogen; head nurse; head and neck
H&N	head and neck
HN$_2$	mechlorethamine HCl
HNKDS	hyperosmolar nonketotic diabetic state
HNLN	hospitalization no longer necessary
HNP	herniated nucleus pulposus

HNRNA	heterogeneous nuclear ribonucleic acid
HNS	head, neck, and shaft; head and neck surgery
HNV	has not voided
HO	house officer; hand orthosis; hip orthosis; hyperbaric oxygen
H/O	history of
H_2O	water
H_2O_2	hydrogen peroxide
HOA	hip osteoarthritis
HOB	head of bed
HOB UPSOB	head of bed up for shortness of breath
HOC	Health Officer Certificate
HOCM	hypertrophic obstructive cardiomyopathy
HOG	halothane, oxygen, and gas
HOH	hard of hearing
HOI	hospital onset infection
HONDA	hypertensive, obese, Negro, diabetic, arthritic
HOPI	history of present illness
HP	hemiplegia; hydrophilic petrolatum; hot packs; hemipelvectomy; hard palate; high protein; human pituitary
H&P	history and physical
HPA	hypothalamic-pituitary-adrenal (axis)
HPE	history and physical examination
HPF	high-power field
HPFH	hereditary persistence of fetal hemoglobin
HPG	human pituitary gonadotropin
HPI	history of present illness
HPL	human placenta lactogen; hyperplexia
HPLC	high-pressure liquid chromatography
HPM	hemiplegic migraine
HPN	home parenteral nutrition
HPO	high pressure oxygen; hypertrophic pulmonary osteoarthropathy
HPT	hyperparathyroidism; histamine provocation test
HPV	human papilloma virus; human parvovirus
HPZ	high pressure zone
HQC	hydroquinone cream
HR	heart rate; hour; hallux rigidus; Harrington rod; hospital record
H&R	hysterectomy and radiation
HRA	histamine releasing activity; high right atrium
HRC	Human Rights Committee
HRL	head rotated left
HRLA	human reovirus-like agent

HRP	horseradish peroxidase; high-risk pregnancy
HRR	head rotated right
HRS	hepatorenal syndrome
HRT	heart rate; hormone replacement therapy
hs	bedtime (hour of sleep)
HS	Hartman's solution; hereditary spherocytosis; heel spur; horse serum; heel stick; herpes simplex; half strength; heart sounds; heavy smoker; heat stable; Hurler's syndrome
H&S	hemorrhage and shock; hysterectomy and sterilization
HSA	human serum albumin; Health Systems Agency; hypersomnia-sleep apnea
HSBG	heel stick blood gas
HSCL	Hopkins Symptom Check List
HSE	herpes simplex encephalitis
HSG	hysterosalpingogram; herpes simplex genitalis
HSL	herpes simplex labialis
HSM	hepato-splenomegaly; holosystolic murmur
HSP	Henoch-Schönlein purpura
HSR	heated serum reagin
HSSE	high soap suds enema
HSV	herpes simplex virus
HSVI	herpes simplex virus type 1
Ht	height
HT	height; Hubbard tank; heart; hypertension; heart test; hypermetropia; hammertoe; hearing test; heart transplant; high temperature; histotechnology
H&T	hospitalization and treatment
5-HT	5-hydroxytryptamine
ht aer	heated aerosol
HTAT	human tetanus antitoxin
HTB	hot tub bath
HTC	hypertensive crisis
HTF	house tube feeding
HTK	heel-to-knee
HTL	human thymic leukemia; hearing threshold level
HTLV-I	human T-lymphotropic virus-I
HTLV-III	human T-lymphotropic virus-III
HTN	hypertension
HTP	House-Tree-Person-Test
5-HTP	5-hydroxytryptophan
HTS	head traumatic syndrome; heel-to-shin
HTT	hand thrust test
HTV	herpes-type virus

HTVD	hypertensive vascular disease
HU	hydroxyurea; head unit
HUIFM	human leukocyte interferon meloy
HUK	human urinary kallikrein
HUS	hemolytic uremic syndrome
husb	husband
HV	has voided; hallux valgus; hospital visit
H&V	hemigastrectomy and vagotomy
HVA	homovanillic acid
HVD	hypertensive vascular disease
HVE	high-voltage electrophoresis
HVH	herpes virus hominis
HW	heparin well; housewife
hwb	hot water bottle
HWP	hot wet pack
Hx	history; hospitalization
HXM	hexamethylmelamine
hy	hysteria
Hy	hypermetropia
hypo	hypodermic (injection)
hys	hysteria
Hz	Hertz
HZ	herpes zoster
HZO	herpes zoster ophthalmia
HZV	herpes zoster virus

I

I	iodine; independent; one; intensity of magnetism; permanent incisor; impression
I^{131}	radioactive iodine
IA	intra-aortic; intra-arterial; intra-amniotic; internal auditory
I&A	irrigation and aspiration
IAA	interrupted aortic arch
IABC	intra-aortic balloon counterpulsation
IABP	intra-aortic balloon pump
IAC	internal auditory canal; intra-arterial chemotherapy
IAC-CPR	interposed abdominal compressions-cardiopulmonary resuscitation
IACP	intra-aortic counterpulsation
IA DSA	intra-arterial subtraction arteriography
IAHA	immune adherence hemagglutination
IAI	intra-abdominal infection

IAM	internal auditory meatus
IAN	intern admission note
IAO	immediately after onset
IAP	intermittent acute porphyria
IASD	interatrial septal defect
IAT	indirect antiglobulin test
IAV	interactive video
IB	isolation bed
IBBB	intra-blood-brain barrier
IBBBB	incomplete bilateral bundle branch block
IBC	iron binding capacity
IBD	inflammatory bowel disease
IBI	intermittent bladder irrigation
ibid	at the same place
IBNR	incurred but not reported
IBOW	intact bag of waters
IBRS	Inpatient Behavior Rating Scale
IBS	irritable bowel syndrome
IBU	ibuprofen
IBW	ideal body weight
IC	individual counseling; intracranial; irritable colon; intercostal; incomplete; intensive care; intermediate care; indirect Coombs' (test)
ICB	intracranial bleeding
ICBT	intercostobronchial trunk
ICCE	intracapsular cataract extraction
ICCU	intermediate coronary care unit; intensive coronary care unit
ICD	isocitrate dehydrogenase; instantaneous cardiac death; International Classification of Diseases
ICE	ice, compression, and elevation; individual career exploration
ICF	intracellular fluid; intermediate care facility
ICG	indocyanine green
ICH	intracranial hemorrhage; intracerebral hemorrhage
ICM	intracostal margin
ICN	intensive care nursery
ICP	intracranial pressure
ICPP	intubated continuous positive pressure
ICRF-159	razoxane
ICS	intercostal space; ileocecal sphincter
ICSH	interstitial cell-stimulating hormone

ICT	intensive conventional therapy; inflammation of connective tissue; indirect Coombs' test; intermittent cervical traction; intracranial tumor; insulin coma therapy; isovolumic contraction time
ict ind	icterus index
ICU	intensive care unit; intermediate care unit
ICVH	ischemic cerebrovascular headache
ICW	intercellular water
ID	intradermal; initial dose; infectious disease; identify; initial diagnosis; infant death; identification; immunodiffusion; infective dose; inside diameter; internal diameter
I&D	incision and drainage
id	idem (the same)
IDA	iron deficiency anemia; image display and analysis
IDDM	insulin-dependent diabetes mellitus
IDDS	implantable drug delivery system
IDE	Investigational Device Exemption
IDFC	immature dead female child
IDI	induction-delivery interval
IDK	internal derangement of knee
IDM	infant of diabetic mother
IDMC	immature dead male child
IDP	initial dose period
IDR	intradermal reaction
IDS	infectious disease service; immunity deficiency state
IDU	idoxuridine; iododeoxyuridine
IDV	intermittent demand ventilation
IDVC	indwelling venous catheter
IE	international unit (European abbreviation); induced emesis; inner ear; immunizing unit; immunoelectrophoresis
i.e.	that is
I/E	inspiratory-expiratory (ratio)
I&E	internal and external
IEC	inpatient exercise center
IEF	iso-electric focusing
IEM	immune electron microscopy
IEP	individualized education program; immunoelectrophoresis
IF	intrinsic factor; involved field; interferon; internal fixation; immunofluorescence; interstitial fluid

IFA	indirect fluorescent antibody; immunofluorescent assay
IFE	immunofixation electrophoresis
IFM	internal fetal monitoring
IFN	interferon
IG	immune globulin; intragastric
Ig	immunoglobulin
IgA	immunoglobulin A
IgD	immunoglobulin D
IGDM	infant of gestational diabetic mother
IgE	immunoglobulin E
IgG	immunoglobulin G
IGIM	immune globulin intramuscular
IGIV	immune globulin intravenous
IgM	immunoglobulin M
IGR	intrauterine growth retardation
IGT	impaired glucose tolerance
IH	infectious hepatitis; indirect hemagglutination; inguinal hernia
IHA	indirect hemagglutination; immune hemolytic anemia
IHC	immobilization hypercalcemia
IHD	ischemic heart disease; intrahepatic duct(ule)
IHH	idiopathic hypogonadotropic hypogonadism
IHS	Idiopathic Headache Score
IHs	iris hamartomas
IHSA	iodinated human serum albumin
IHSS	idiopathic hypertrophic subaortic stenosis
IHT	insulin hypoglycemia test
IHW	inner heel wedge
IICP	increased intracranial pressure
IICU	infant intensive care unit
IJ	internal jugular; ileojejunal
IJD	inflammatory joint disease
IJV	internal jugular vein
IK	immobilized knee; interstitial keratitis
IL	interleukin
ILA	indicated low forceps
ILBBB	incomplete left bundle branch block
ILD	ischemic leg disease; interstitial lung disease
ILE	infantile lobar emphysema
ILFC	immature living female child
ILM	internal limiting membrane
ILMC	immature living male child
ILMI	inferolateral myocardial infarction

IM	intramuscular; infectious mononucleosis; internal medicine; intermetatarsal; intramedullary
IMA	inferior mesenteric artery; internal mammary artery
IMAG	internal mammary artery graft
IMB	intermenstrual bleeding
IMF	intermaxillary fixation
IMG	internal medicine group
IMH test	indirect microhemagglutination test
IMI	inferior myocardial infarction; imipramine
IMIG	intramuscular immunoglobulin
IMN	internal mammary node
IMP	impression; impacted; important; improved
IMV	intermittent mandatory ventilation; inferior mesenteric vein
in	inch
In	indium
INC	incontinent; incomplete; inside-the-needle catheter; increase; incision; incorporated
IND	Investigational New Drug
INDM	infant of nondiabetic mother
INDO	indomethacin
INEX	inexperienced
INF	inferior; infusion; infant; infected; infarction; information
info	information
ING	inguinal
INH	isoniazid
inj	injection
INK	injury not known
INO	internuclear ophthalmoplegia
INS	insurance; idiopathic nephrotic syndrome
inspir	inspiration
INST	instrumental (delivery)
INT	internal; intermittent needle therapy
int rot	internal rotation
int trx	intermittent traction
inver	inversion
IO	intraocular pressure; inferior oblique; initial opening
I&O	intake and output
IOC	intern on call; intraoperative cholangiogram
IOCG	intraoperative cholangiogram
IOD	interorbital distance
IOF	intraocular fluid
IOFB	intraocular foreign body
IOH	idiopathic orthostatic hypotension

IOL	intraocular lens
ION	ischemic optic neuropathy
IOP	intraocular pressure
IORT	intraoperative radiation therapy
IOS	intraoperative sonography
IOV	initial office visit
IP	intraperitoneal; incubation period; interphalangeal
IPA	isopropyl alcohol; invasive pulmonary aspergillosis
IPCD	infantile polycystic disease
IPD	immediate pigment darkening; intermittent peritoneal dialysis; inflammatory pelvic disease
IPF	idiopathic pulmonary fibrosis
IPFD	intrapartum fetal distress
IPG	individually polymerized grass; impedance plethysmography
IPJ	interphalangeal joint
IPK	intractable plantar keratosis
IPMI	inferoposterior myocardial infarction
IPN	infantile periarteritis nodosa; intern's progress note
IPOF	immediate postoperative fitting
IPOP	immediate postoperative prosthesis
IPP	inflatable penile prosthesis
IPPA	inspection, palpation, percussion, and auscultation
IPPB	intermittent positive pressure breathing
IPPI	interruption of pregnancy for psychiatric indication
IPPV	intermittent positive pressure ventilation
IPS	infundibular pulmonic stenosis
IPSF	immediate postsurgical fitting
IPV	inactivated polio vaccine
IPW	interphalangeal width
IQ	intelligence quotient
IR	infrared; internal rotation
IRB	institutional review board
IRBBB	incomplete right bundle branch block
IRBC	immature red blood cell
IRBP	interphotoreceptor retinoid-binding protein
IRCU	intensive respiratory care unit
IRDS	infant respiratory distress syndrome
IRH	intraretinal hemorrhage
IRMA	intraretinal microvascular abnormalities
IRR	intrarenal reflux
IRV	inspiratory reserve volume

IS	intercostal space; incentive spirometer; induced sputum; ipecac syrup; inventory of systems
ISB	incentive spirometry breathing
ISCs	irreversible sickle cells
ISD	inhibited sexual desire
ISDN	isosorbide dinitrate
ISG	immune serum globulin
ISH	isolated systolic hypertension
ISMA	infantile spinal muscular atrophy
ISO	isoproterenol
ISS	Injury Severity Score
IST	insulin sensitivity test; insulin shock therapy
ISW	interstitial water
ISWI	incisional surgical wound infection
IT	intrathecal; inhalation therapy; inferior-temporal; intermittent traction; intensive therapy; intertuberous; intradermal test; intratracheal tube; isomeric transition
ITC	incontinence treatment center
ITCP	idiopathic thrombocytopenia purpura
ITCU	intensive thoracic cardiovascular unit
ITE	insufficient therapeutic effect
ITP	idiopathic thrombocytopenic purpura; interim treatment plan
ITT	identical twins (raised) together; insulin tolerance test; iliotibial tract
ITVAD	indwelling transcutaneous vascular access device
IU	International Unit; immunizing unit; intrauterine
IUD	intrauterine device; intrauterine death
IUDR	iododeoxyuridine; idoxuridine
IUFD	intrauterine fetal death; intrauterine fetal distress
IUGR	intrauterine growth retardation
IUP	intrauterine pregnancy
IUPC	intrauterine pressure catheter
IUPD	intrauterine pregnancy delivered
IUP,TBCS	intrauterine pregnancy, term birth, cesarean section
IUP,TBLC	intrauterine pregnancy, term birth, living child
IUR	intrauterine retardation
IV	intravenous; four; invasive; intravascular; interventricular; intervertebral; class 4 controlled substance

IVA	Intervir-A
IVAP	implantable vascular access device
IVC	intravenous cholangiogram; inferior vena cava; intraventricular catheter
IVD	intravenous drip; intervertebral disk
IVDA	intravenous drug abuse
IVDU	intravenous drug user
IVF	in vitro fertilization; intravenous fluid(s); intravascular fluid
IVFE	intravenous fat emulsion
IVFT	intravenous fetal transfusion
IVGTT	intravenous glucose tolerance test
IVH	intravenous hyperalimentation; intraventricular hemorrhage
IVIG	intravenous immunoglobulin
IVLBW	infant of very low birth weight
IVP	intravenous pyelogram; intravenous push
IVPB	intravenous piggyback
IVR	idioventricular rhythm
IVS	intraventricular septum
IVSD	intraventricular septal defect
IVSE	intraventricular septal excursion
IVTTT	intravenous tolbutamide tolerance test
IVU	intravenous urography
IWL	insensible water loss
IWMI	inferior wall myocardial infarction

J

J	Jewish; joint; juice; Joule's equivalent; journal
JAMG	juvenile autoimmune myasthenia gravis
JBE	Japanese B encephalitis
JC	junior clinicians
JDMS	juvenile dermatomyositis
JE	Japanese encephalitis
jej	jejunum
JF	joint fluid
JFS	Jewish Family Service
JG	juxtaglomerular
JGC	juxtaglomerular cell
JGI	juxtaglomerular granulation index
JI	jejunoileal

JIB	jejunoileal bypass
JJ	jaw jerk
JLP	juvenile laryngeal papillomatosis
JMS	junior medical student
JND	just noticeable difference
jnt	joint
JODM	juvenile onset diabetes mellitus
JOMACI	judgment, orientation, memory, abstraction, and calculation intact
JPB	junctional premature beats
JPC	junctional premature contraction
JPS	joint position sense
JPTS	juvenile tropical pancreatitis syndrome
JRA	juvenile rheumatoid arthritis
JRC	joint replacement center
jt	joint
JT	joint; jejunostomy tube
JTF	jejunostomy tube feeding
juv	juvenile
JV	jugular vein; jugular venous
JVD	jugular venous distention
JVP	jugular venous pulse; jugular venous pressure
JVPT	jugular venous pulse tracing
JW	Jehovah's witness

K

K	potassium; vitamin K; thousand; kathode (cathode); Kelvin
17K	17-ketosteroids
KA	ketoacidosis; kathode; King-Armstrong (units)
KAB	knowledge, attitude, and behavior
KAFO	knee-ankle-foot orthosis
KAO	knee-ankle orthosis
KAP	knowledge, attitudes, and practice
KAS	Katz Adjustment Scale
KAU	King-Armstrong units
KB	ketone bodies
KC	keratoconjunctivitis; knees to chest; kathodal closing
kc	kilocycle
kcal	kilocalorie
KCC	kathodal-closing contraction
KCG	kinetocardiogram

kCi	kilocurie
KCl	potassium chloride
kcps	kilocycles per second
KCS	keratoconjunctivitis sicca
KCT	kathodal-closing tetanus
KD	Kawasaki's disease; knee disarticulation; kathodal duration
KDA	known drug allergies
KE	kinetic energy
keV	kiloelectron volts
KF	kidney function
KFAO	knee-foot-ankle orthosis
KFR	Kayser-Fleischer ring
KFS	Klippel-Feil syndrome
kg	kilogram
kg-cal	kilogram-calorie
kHz	kilohertz
K24H	potassium, urine 24 hour
KI	potassium iodide; karyopyknotic index
KID	keratitis, ichthyosis, and deafness
kilo	kilogram
KISS	kidney internal splint/stint; saturated solution of potassium iodide
KIT	Kahn intelligence test
KJ	knee jerk
kJ	kilojoule
KK	knee kick
Kleb	*Klebsiella*
KLS	kidneys, liver, and spleen
KMnO$_4$	potassium permanganate
KNO	keep needle open
KO	keep open
KOH	potassium hydroxide
KP	hot pack
Kr	krypton
KS	Kaposi's sarcoma
17-KS	17-ketosteroids
KSA	knowledge, skills, and abilities
KS/OI	Kaposi's sarcoma and opportunistic infection
KT	kidney treatment
KTU	kidney transplant unit
KUB	kidney, ureter, and bladder
KUS	kidney(s), ureter(s), and spleen
KVO	keep vein open
kW	kilowatt
K-wire	Kirschner's wire

L

L	liter; left; fifty; lumbar; lingual; liver; lung; Latin; length; low; lethal; ligament; lower
L2	second lumbar vertebra
LA	left atrium; long acting; local anesthesia; Latin American; left atrial; left arm; linguoaxial; low anxiety; latex agglutination
L+A	light and accommodation;living and active
Lab	laboratory
LAC	laceration; long arm cast
LAD	left anterior descending; left axis deviation
LADCA	left anterior descending coronary artery
LADD	left anterior descending diagonal
LAD-MIN	left axis deviation minimal
LAE	left atrial enlargement; long above elbow
LAF	Latin-American female; lymphocyte-activating factor; laminar air flow
LAG	lymphangiogram
LAK	lymphokine-activated killer
LAL	left axillary line
LAM	Latin-American male; laminectomy
LAN	lymphadenopathy
LANC	long arm navicular cast
LAO	left anterior oblique
LAP	laparotomy; laparoscopy; left atrial pressure; leukocyte alkaline phosphatase; lyophilized anterior pituitary
LAPMS	long arm posterior molded splint
LAPW	left atrial posterior wall
LAR	left arm, reclining; left arm, recumbent
LAS	lymphadenopathy syndrome; laxative abuse syndrome; long arm splint
LASER	Light Amplification by Stimulated Emission of Radiation
lat	lateral
LAT	lateral; left anterior thigh
lat men	lateral meniscectomy
LATS	long-acting thyroid stimulator
LAV	lymphadenopathy-associated virus
LAW	left atrial wall

LB	low back; left breast; left buttock; large bowel; live births; lung biopsy; laboratory data; lipid body; loose body
lb	pound
L&B	left and below
LBB	left breast biopsy
LBBB	left bundle branch block
LBCD	left border of cardiac dullness
LBD	left border dullness; large bile duct
LBE	long below elbow
LBH	length, breadth, and height
LBO	large bowel obstruction
LBP	low back pain; low blood pressure
LBT	low back tenderness; low back trouble
LBV	left brachial vein
LBW	low birth weight; lean body weight
LC	living children; low calorie; late clamped; lethal concentration; lipid cytosomes
LCA	left coronary artery; Leber's congenital amaurosis
LCB	left costal border
LCCA	leukocytoclastic angiitis; left common carotid artery
LCCS	low cervical cesarean section
LCD	coal tar solution; localized collagen dystrophy; low calcium diet
LCF	left circumflex
LCFA	long-chain fatty acid
LCGU	local cerebral glucose utilization
LCH	local city hospital
LCLC	large cell lung carcinoma
LCM	left costal margin; lymphocytic choriomeningitis
LCR	late cutaneous reaction
LCS	low constant suction; low continuous suction
LCSW	licensed clinical social worker
LCT	long chain triglyceride; low cervical transverse; lymphocytotoxicity
LCTD	low-calcium test diet
LCV	low cervical vertical
LD	lethal dose; liver disease; lactic dehydrogenase; loading dose; labor and delivery; learning disorder; learning disability; living donor; left deltoid; light difference; low dosage; labyrinthine defect; lymphocyte-defined
L-D	Leishman-Donovan (bodies)
L/D	light-dark (ratio)

LDA	left dorsoanterior; linear displacement analysis
LDB	Legionnaires' disease bacterium
LDD	light-dark discrimination
LDH	lactic dehydrogenase
LDIH	left direct inguinal hernia
LDL	low-density lipoprotein
LDR	labor, delivery, and recovery
LDR/P	labor, delivery, recovery, and postpartum
LDT	left dorsotransverse
LDUB	long double upright brace
LDV	laser Doppler velocimetry
LE	lupus erythematosus; lower extremities; left ear; left eye; live embryo
LED	lupus erythematosus disseminatus
LEHPZ	lower esophageal high pressure zone
LEJ	ligation of the esophagogastric junction
LEM	lateral eye movements; light electron microscope
LEP	lower esophageal pressure
LEP2	leptospirosis 2
L-ERX	leukoerythroblastic reaction
LES	lower esophageal sphincter; local excitatory state; lupus erythematosus systemic
LESP	lower esophageal sphincter pressure
LET	linear energy transfer
lf	left
LF	low forceps; left foot; Lassa fever; low fat; limit flocculation; laryngofissure
LFA	left frontoanterior; low friction arthroplasty; left femoral artery; left forearm
LFC	living female child; low fat and cholesterol
LFD	low fat diet; low forceps delivery; lactose free diet; low fiber diet; least fatal dose
LFL	left frontolateral
LFP	left frontoposterior
LFS	liver function series
LFT	liver function test; left frontotransverse; latex flocculation test
LFU	limit flocculation unit
LG	laryngectomy; left gluteal; linguogingival
lg	large
LGA	large for gestational age; left gastric artery
LGI	lower gastrointestinal (series)
LGL	lobular glomerulonephritis
LH	luteinizing hormone; left hyperphoria; left

LHA	left hepatic artery
LHF	left heart failure
LHG	left hand grip
LHL	left hemisphere lesions; left hepatic lobe
LHP	left hemiparesis
LHR	leukocyte histamine release
LHRH	luteinizing hormone-releasing hormone
LHS	left hand side
LHT	left hypertropia
LI	lactose intolerance; large intestine; learning impaired; linguoincisal; low impulsiveness
Li	lithium
LIB	left in bottle
LIC	left iliac crest; left internal carotid
LICA	left internal carotid artery
LICD	lower intestinal Crohn's disease
LICM	left intercostal margin
LICS	left intercostal space
LIF	left iliac fossa; liver inhibitory factor; left index finger
lig	ligament
LIH	left inguinal hernia
LIHA	low impulsiveness, high anxiety
LIMA	left internal mammary artery (graft)
LIO	left inferior oblique
LIP	lymphocytic interstitial pneumonia; lithium-induced polydipsia
LIQ	liquid; lower inner quadrant
liq	liquid
LIR	left iliac region; left inferior rectus
LIS	low intermittent suction; left intercostal space; lobular in situ
LISS	low ionic strength saline
LIV	left innominate vein
LIVC	left inferior vena cava
LK	left kidney
LKS	liver, kidneys, and spleen
LKSB	liver, kidneys, spleen, and bladder
LL	large lymphocyte; lumbar length; left leg; lower lip; left lower; left lung; lower lobe; lymphoblastic lymphoma
LLA	limulus lysate assay
LLB	long leg brace; left lateral border
LLC	long leg cast
LLD	left lateral decubitus; left length discrepancy

LLE	left lower extremity
LL-GXT	low-level graded exercise test
LLL	left lower lobe; left lower lid
LLLE	lower lid, left eye
LLLNR	left lower lobe, no rales
LLOD	lower lid, right eye
LLOS	lower lid, left eye
LLQ	left lower quadrant
LR	left lateral rectus
LLRE	lower lid, right eye
LLS	lazy leukocyte syndrome
LLSB	left lower sternal border
LLT	left lateral thigh
LLWC	long leg walking cast
LLX	left lower extremity
L/M	liters per minute
LMA	liver membrane autoantibody
LMB	Laurence-Moon-Biedl (syndrome)
LMC	living male child
LMCA	left main coronary artery; left middle cerebral artery
LMCAT	left middle cerebral artery thrombosis
LMCL	left midclavicular line
LME	left mediolateral episiotomy
LMEE	left middle ear exploration
LMF	left middle finger
L/min	liters per minute
LML	left medial lateral; left middle lobe
LMLE	left mediolateral episiotomy
LMM	lentigo maligna melanoma
LMP	last menstrual period; left mentoposterior
LMR	left medial rectus
LMT	left mentotransverse
LN	lymph nodes; lipoid nephrosis; lupus nephritis
L/N	letter-numerical (system)
LNCs	lymph node cells
LND	lymph node dissection
LNMP	last normal menstrual period
LO	lateral oblique; low; linguoocclusal
LOA	left occipitoanterior; leave of absence
LOC	loss of consciousness; laxative of choice; level of consciousness; level of care; local
LOD	line of duty
LOIH	left oblique inguinal hernia
LOL	left occipitolateral
LOM	limitation of motion; left otitis media; loss of motion

LOMSA	left otitis media, suppurative, acute
LOMSC	left otitis media, suppurative, chronic
LoNa	low sodium
LOP	leave on pass; left occipitoposterior
LOQ	lower outer quadrant
LORS-I	Level of Rehabilitation Scale-I
LOS	length of stay
LOT	left occipitotransverse
LOV	loss of vision
LOZ	lozenge
LP	lumbar puncture; light perception; low protein; latency period; lipoprotein; lymphoid plasma; linguopulpal; leukocyte-poor
L/P	lactate-pyruvate (ratio)
LPA	left pulmonary artery
LPC	laser photocoagulation
LPD	luteal phase defect; low protein diet
lpf	low-power field
LPF	liver plasma flow
LPH	left posterior hemiblock
LPL	lipoprotein lipase
LPM	liters per minute
LPN	licensed practical nurse
LPO	left posterior oblique; light perception only
LPS	lipopolysaccharide
LR	light reflex; labor room; left-right; lactated Ringer's
LRD	living renal donor
LREH	low resin essential hypertension
LRM	left radical mastectomy
LRMP	last regular menstrual period
LRND	left radical neck dissection
LRQ	lower right quadrant
LRS	lactated Ringer's solution
LRT	lower respiratory tract
LRTI	lower respiratory tract infection
LS	lumbosacral; left side; legally separated; low salt; liver and spleen; lymphosarcoma
L5-S1	lumbar fifth vertebra to sacral first vertebra
LSA	left sacrum anterior; lymphosarcoma
LSB	left sternal border
LS BPS	laparoscopic bilateral partial salpingectomy
LSC	late systolic click
LSCA	left scapuloanterior
LSCP	left scapuloposterior
LSD	low salt diet; lysergic acid diethylamide
LSE	local side effects

LSF	low saturated fat
LSL	left sacrolateral; left short leg (brace)
LSM	late systolic murmur
LSO	left salpingo-oophorectomy; left superior oblique; lumbosacral orthosis
LSP	left sacrum posterior; liver-specific lipoprotein
LSR	left superior rectus
LSS	liver-spleen scan
LST	left sacrum transverse
LSTL	laparoscopic tubal ligation
LSV	left subclavian vein
LSVC	left superior vena cava
LT	light; left; lumbar traction; left thigh; Levin tube; leukotrienes
LTB	laparoscopic tubal banding; laryngotracheobronchitis
LTB$_4$	leukotriene B$_4$
LTC	left to count; long-term care
LTCF	long-term care facility
LTCS	low transverse cesarean section
LTD	largest tumor dimension
LTGA	left transposition of great artery
LTL	laparoscopic tubal ligation
LTM	long-term memory
LTT	lymphocyte transformation test; lactose tolerance test
LU	left upper
L&U	lower and upper
LUA	left upper arm
LUE	left upper extremity
Lues I	primary syphilis
LUL	left upper lobe; left upper lid
LUOB	left upper outer buttock
LUOQ	left upper outer quadrant
LUQ	left upper quadrant
LUSB	left upper sternal border
LV	left ventricle; leave; leukemia virus; live virus
LVA	left ventricular aneurysm
LVAD	left ventricular assist device
LVD	left ventricular dysfunction
LVE	left ventricular enlargement
LVEDP	left ventricular end-diastolic pressure
LVEDV	left ventricular end-diastolic volume
LVEF	left ventricular ejection fraction
LVF	left ventricular failure
LVFP	left ventricular filling pressure

LVH	left ventricular hypertrophy
LVL	left vastus lateralis
LVMM	left ventricular muscle mass
LVN	licensed visiting nurse; licensed vocational nurse
LVP	left ventricular pressure; large volume parenteral
LVPW	left ventricular posterior wall
LVSEMI	left ventricular subendocardial myocardial ischemia
LVSP	left ventricular systolic pressure
LVSWI	left ventricular stroke work index
LVV	left ventricular volume; live varicella vaccine
LVW	left ventricular wall
LVWI	left ventricular work index
LVWMA	left ventricular wall motion abnormality
LVWMI	left ventricular wall motion index
L&W	living and well
LWBS	left without being seen
LWCT	Lee-White clotting time
LWP	large whirlpool
lx	larynx; lower extremity
LXT	left exotropia
lymphs	lymphocytes
LYS	lysine
lytes	electrolytes

M

M	murmur; monocytes; male; molar; married; meter; medial; thousand; myopia; million; Monday; mouth; mother; myopic; mass; meta; minim; minute; mix; multipara; muscle
M1	first mitral sound
MA	mental age; Miller-Abbott; menstrual age; Mexican American; monoclonal antibodies; medical assistant; medical authorization; medical audit; moderately advanced
ma	meter-angle; milliampere
M/A	mood and/or affect
MAB	monoclonal antibody
MABP	mean arterial blood pressure

MAC	maximal allowable concentration; midarm circumference; minimum alveolar concentration;macula
MADRS	Montgomery-Asburg Depression Rating Scale
MAE	moves all extremities
MAEEW	moves all extremities equally well
MAEW	moves all extremities well
MAFAs	movement-associated fetal (heart rate) accelerations
mag cit	magnesium citrate
mag sulf	magnesium sulfate
MAHA	macroangiopathic hemolytic anemia
MAI	maximal aggregation index; minor acute illness
MAL	midaxillary line; malignant
malig	malignant
MALT	mucosa-associated lymphoid tissue
MAMC	midarm muscle circumference
Mammo	mammography
Mand	mandibular
MAO	maximum acid output
MAOI	monoamine oxidase inhibitor
MAP	mean arterial pressure; megaloblastic anemia of pregnancy
MAR	medication administration record
MAS	meconium aspiration syndrome; mobile arm support
MAST	military antishock trousers; mastectomy
MAT	multifocal atrial tachycardia; mature; medication administration team; maternal; maternity
MAVR	mitral and aortic valve replacement
max	maximal; maxillary
MB	mesiobuccal; methylene blue
MBC	maximum breathing capacity; maximum bladder capacity; minimal bactericidal concentration;
MBD	minimal brain damage; minimal brain dysfunction
MBE	medium below elbow
MBF	myocardial blood flow
MBI	methylene blue instillation
MBL	menstrual blood loss
MBM	mothers breast milk
MBNW	multiple-breath nitrogen washout
MC	mast cell; metacarpal; maximum concentration; mineralocorticoid; mouth care; myocarditis
Mc	megacurie; megacycle

MCA	middle cerebral aneurysm; middle cerebral artery; motorcycle accident; monoclonal antibodies; multichannel analyzer
McB pt	McBurney's point
MCC	midstream clean-catch
MCCU	mobile coronary care unit
MCDT	mast cell degranulation test
mcg	microgram
MCGN	minimal-change glomerular nephritis
MCH	mean corpuscular hemoglobin; muscle contraction headache
MCHC	mean corpuscular hemoglobin concentration
mCi	millicurie
MCL	midclavicular line; midcostal line; medial collateral ligament
MCLNS	mucocutaneous lymph node syndrome
MCMI	Million Clinical Multiaxial Inventory
MCP	metacarpophalangeal (joint)
MCQ	multiple choice question
MCS	microculture and sensitivity
MCT	mean circulation time; manual cervical traction; mean corpuscular thickness; medium-chain triglyceride
MCTD	mixed connective tissue disease
MCV	mean corpuscular volume
MD	medical doctor; mental deficiency; muscular dystrophy; manic depressive; movement disorder; Mantoux diameter; Marek's disease; medium dosage; myocardial disease; mediodorsal
MDA	manual dilation of anus; motor discriminative acuity
MDC	medial dorsal cutaneous (nerve); minimum detectable concentration
MDD	manic depressive disorder; major depressive disorder; mean daily dose
MDE	major depressive episode
MDF	myocardial depressant factor; mean dominant frequency
MDI	multiple daily injection; metered dose inhaler; manic depressive illness
MDIA	Mental Development Index Adjusted
MDII	multiple daily insulin injection
MDPI	maximum daily permissible intake
MDR	minimum daily requirement
MDS	maternal deprivation syndrome; myelodysplasia syndrome
MDTP	multidisciplinary treatment plan

MDUO	myocardial disease of unknown origin
MDV	Marek's disease virus; multiple dose vial
MDY	month, date, year
ME	macula edema; medical examiner; middle ear; manic episode
Me	methyl
M/E	myeloid-erythroid (ratio)
MEA-I	multiple endocrine adenomatosis type I
MEC	meconium; middle ear canal
MECG	maternal electrocardiogram
MED	minimal effective dose; minimal erythema dose; median erythrocyte diameter; medical; medication; medium; medicine
MEDAC	multiple endocrine deficiency-autoimmune-candidiasis
MEDs	medications
MEE	middle ear effusion
MEF	maximum expiratory flow rate; middle ear fluid
MEFV	maximum expiratory flow-volume
men	meningeal; meninges; meningitis
MEN II	multiple endocrine neoplasia type II
MEO	malignant external otitis
MEOS	microsomoal ethanol oxidizing system
mEq	milliequivalent
mEq/L	milliequivalent per liter
M/E ratio	myeloid-erythroid ratio
MET	metastasis; metabolic equivalent test
META	metamyelocytes
METHb	methemoglobin
METT	maximum exercise tolerance test
MEV	million electron volts
MEX	Mexican
MF	myocardial fibrosis; mycosis fungoides; midcavity forceps; meat free
M&F	mother and father; male and female
MFAT	multifocal atrial tachycardia
MFD	mid-forceps delivery; milk-free diet
MFEM	maximal forced expiratory maneuver
MFH	malignant fibrous histiocytoma
MFR	mid-forceps rotation
MFT	muscle function test
MG	myasthenia gravis; muscle group; mesiogingival; Marcus Gunn
mg	milligram
Mg	magnesium
MGF	maternal grandfather
mg/kg	milligram per kilogram

MGM	maternal grandmother
MGN	membranous glomerulonephritis
MgO	magnesium oxide
MgSO$_4$	magnesium sulfate
MGUS	monoclonal gammopathies of undetermined significance
M-GXT	multi-stage graded exercise test
MH	marital history; mental health; menstrual history; malignant hyperthermia; moist heat; medical history
MHA	microangiopathic hemolytic anemia; mixed hemadsorption
MHB	maximum hospital benefit; mental health (assistance) benefit
MHb	methemoglobin
MHC	major histocompatibility complex; mental health center; mental health counselor
MH/MR	mental health and mental retardation
MHN	massive hepatic necrosis
MHR	maximal heart rate
MHS	major histocompatibility system; malignant hyperthermia susceptible
MHW	medial heel wedge; mental health worker
MHz	megahertz
MI	myocardial infarction; mitral insufficiency; mental institution; mental illness
MIA	medically indigent adult; missing in action
MIC	minimum inhibitory concentration; maternal and infant care; medical intensive care; microscope
MICN	mobile intensive care nurse
MICU	medical intensive care unit; mobile intensive care unit
MIF	migration inhibitory factor; Merthiolate-iodine-formalin
MIH	migraine with interparoxysmal headache
MIL	mother-in-law; military
MIN	minimum; minute; minor; mineral
MIO	minimum identifiable odor
MIP	metacarpointerphalangeal; maximum inspiratory pressure
MIRD	Medical Internal Radiation Dose
MIRP	myocardial infarction rehabilitation program
MISC	miscellaneous; miscarriage
MISS	Modified Injury Severity Score
mix mon	mixed monitor
MJ	marijuana; megajoule
MJT	Mead Johnson tube

ML	midline; middle lobe
ml	milliliter
mL	milliliter
M/L	monocyte to lymphocyte (ratio); mother-in-law
MLA	mentolaeva anterior; mesiolabial; monocytic leukemia, acute
MLC	mixed lymphocyte culture; minimal lethal concentration; mixed leukocyte culture; myelomonocytic leukemia, chronic
ML-CVP	multi-lumen central venous pressure
MLD	metachromatic leukodystrophy; minimal lethal dose
MLF	median longitudinal fasciculus
MLNS	mucocutaneous lymph node syndrome
MLR	mixed lymphocyte reaction
MLU	mean length of utterance
MM	mucous membrane; multiple myeloma; malignant melanoma; meningococci meningitis; methadone maintenance; morbidity and mortality; medial malleolus; Marshall-Marchetti; muscularis mucosa
mm	millimeter
mM	millimole
μm	micrometer (formerly micron)
M&M	milk and molasses; morbidity and mortality
MMAP	Medicare/Medicaid Assistance Program
MMECT	multiple monitor electroconvulsive therapy
MMEFR	maximal midexpiratory flow rate
MMF	mean maximum flow
MMFR	maximal midexpiratory flow rate
mmHg	millimeters of mercury
MMK	Marshall-Marchetti-Krantz
MMM	myeloid metaplasia with myelofibrosis
MMPI	Minnesota Multiphasic Personality Inventory
MMPI-D	Minnesota Multiphasic Personality Inventory Depression Scale
MMR	measles, mumps, rubella; midline malignant reticulosis; mobile mass x-ray; myocardial metabolic rate
MMT	manual muscle test; Mini Mental Test
MMTP	Methadone Maintenance Treatment Program
MMWR	Morbidity and Mortality Weekly Report
Mn	midnight; maganese
M&N	morning and night
MNA	maximum noise area
MNCV	motor nerve conduction velocity
MND	motor neuron disease; modified neck dissection
MNG	multinodular goiter

MNR	marrow neutrophil reserve
Mn SSEPS	median nerve somatosensory evoked potentials
MNTB	medial nucleus of the trapezoid body
mo	month; months old
MO	mineral oil; medial oblique; morbidly obese, mother; mesioocclusal
MOA	medical office assistant; mechanism of action
MoAb	monoclonal antibody
MOB	medical office building
MOC	mother of child
MOD	moderate; medical officer of the day; maturity onset diabetes; mesioocclusodistal
mod	moderate
MODY	maturity onset diabetes of youth
MOJAC	mood orientation, judgement, affect, and content
MOM	milk of magnesia; mucoid otitis media
mono	monocyte; mononucleosis
MOPV	monovalent oral poliovirus vaccine
mOsm	milliosmole
mOsmol	milliosmole
MOTT	mycobacteria other than tubercle
MOUS	multiple occurrences of unexplained symptoms
MP	metacarpal phalangeal (joint); menstrual period; moist pack; mean pressure; melting point; mesiopulpal; multiparous
MPB	male pattern baldness
MPH	Master of Public Health
MPJ	metacarpophalangeal joint
MPL	maximum permissible level; mesiopulpolabial
MPOA	medial preoptic area
MPS	mucopolysaccharide; multiphasic screening
MR	mental retardation; may repeat; magnetic resonance; mitral regurgitation; moderate resistance; medical record; measles-rubella; metabolic rate; methyl red; mitral reflux; mortality rate; mortality ratio; muscle relaxant
M&R	measure and record
MR X1	may repeat times one
MRA	medical record administrator; main renal artery; mid-right atrium
MRAN	medical resident admitting note
MRAP	mean right atrial pressure
MRAS	main renal artery stenosis
MRD	Medical Records Department; margin reflex distance
MRDM	malnutrition-related diabetes mellitus

MRG	murmurs, rubs, and gallops
MRI	magnetic resonance imaging
MRM	modified radical mastectomy
mRNA	messenger ribonucleic acid
MRS	magnetic resonance spectroscopy
MRSA	methicillin-resistant *Staphylococcus aureus*
MS	morphine sulfate; mitral stenosis; multiple sclerosis; musculoskeletal; medical student; minimal support; muscle strength; mental status; milk shake; mitral sounds; mucosubstance
M&S	microculture and sensitivity
MS III	third-year medical student
MSAF	meconium-stained amniotic fluid
MSAFP	maternal serum alpha fetoprotein
MSAP	mean systemic arterial pressure
MSBOS	maximum surgical blood order schedule
MSCU	medical special care unit
MSE	Mental Status Examination
MSER	mean systolic ejection rate; Mental Status Examination Record
MSF	megakaryocyte stimulating factor
MSG	monosodium glutamate
MSH	melanocyte-stimulating hormone
MSK	medullary sponge kidney
MSL	midsternal line
MSLT	multiple sleep latency test
MSO$_4$	morphine sulfate
MSPU	medical short procedure unit
MSR	muscle stretch reflexes
MSS	minor surgery suite; muscular subaortic stenosis; Marital Satisfaction Scale
MST	mean survival time
MSTI	multiple soft tissue injuries
MSU	midstream urine; maple syrup urine
MSUD	maple syrup urine disease
MSW	multiple stab wounds; Master of Social Work
MT	music therapy; malaria therapy; malignant teratoma; metatarsal; medical technologist; muscles and tendons
M/T	masses of tenderness; myringotomy with tubes
M&T	*Monilia* and *Trichomonas*; myringotomy and tubes
MTAD	membrane-tympanic, right ear
MTAS	membrane-tympanic, left ear
MTAU	membrane-tympanic, both ears
MTB	*Mycobacterium tuberculosis*
MTD	Monroe Tidal drainage

MTET	modified treadmill exercise testing
MTI	malignant teratoma intermediate; minimum time interval
MTP	metatarsal phalangeal
MTR-O	no masses, tenderness, or rebound
MTSO	medical transcription service owners
MTST	maximal treadmill stress test
MTU	malignant teratoma undifferentiated
Mu	million units
mU	milliunit
mu	mouse unit
MUAC	middle upper arm circumference
muc	mucilage
multip	pregnant woman, borne two or more children
mus-lig	musculoligamentous
MUST	medical unit, self-contained, transportable
MUU	mouse uterine units
MV	mitral valve; mechanical ventilation; mixed venous; multivesicular; minute volume
mV	millivolt
MVA	motor vehicle accident; malignant ventricular arrhythmia
MVB	mixed venous blood
MVC	maximal voluntary contraction
MVD	mitral valve disease; multivessel disease
MVE	mitral valve excursion
MVI	multiple vitamin injection
MVO$_2$	myocardial oxygen consumption
MVP	mitral valve prolapse
MVR	mitral valve replacement; mitral valve regurgitation; massive vitreous retraction
MVS	mitral valve stenosis
MVV	maximum voluntary ventilation
MW	molecular weight; microwave
mw	microwave
MWD	microwave diathermy
MWS	Mickety-Wilson syndrome
My	myopia
my	mayer
myelo	myelocytes; myelogram
MyG	myasthenia gravis
MZ	monozygotic
MZL	marginal zone lymphocyte

N

N	normal; Negro; never; no; not; negative; nodes; nasal; size of sample; neurology
Na	sodium
NA	nursing assistant; not applicable; nurse anesthetist; Native American; not admitted; nicotinic acid; Negro adult; not available; numerical aperture
N&A	normal and active
NAA	neutron activation analysis; no apparent abnormalities
NABS	normoactive bowel sounds
NaCl	sodium chloride
NAD	no acute distress; no apparent distress; no appreciable disease; normal axis deviation; nothing abnormal detected
NADSIC	no apparent disease seen in chest
NaF	sodium fluoride
NAF	Negro adult female
NAG	narrow angle glaucoma
NaHCO$_3$	sodium bicarbonate
NAI	no acute inflammation; non-accidental injury
NaI	sodium iodide
NANB	non-A, non-B (hepatitis)
NANDA	North American Nursing Diagnosis Association
NAPD	no active pulmonary disease
NARC	narcotic(s)
NAS	no added salt; neonatal abstinence syndrome; nasal
NAT	no action taken
NB	newborn; note well; needle biopsy; nail bed; nitrogen balance
NBD	neurologic bladder dysfunction; no brain damage
NBF	not breast fed
NBI	no bone injury
NBICU	newborn intensive care unit
NBM	nothing by mouth; no bowel movement; normal bowel movement; normal bone marrow
NBN	newborn nursery
NBP	needle biopsy of prostate
NBS	normal bowel sound; no bacteria seen; newborn screen

NBTE	nonbacterial thrombotic endocarditis
NBTNF	newborn, term, normal female
NBTNM	newborn, term, normal male
NC	neurologic check; no complaints; not completed; nasal cannula; no charge; Negro child; not cultured
N/C	no complaints
nc	nanocurie
NCA	neurocirculatory asthenia; no congenital abnormalities
NC/AT	normal cephalic atraumatic
NCB	no blue code
NCC	no concentrated carbohydrates
NCD	normal childhood diseases; not considered disabling
nCi	nanocurie
NCI	National Cancer Institute
NCJ	needle catheter jejunostomy
NCM	nailfold capillary microscope
NCO	no complaints offered; noncommissioned officer
NCPAP	nasal continuous positive airway pressure
NCPR	no cardiopulmonary resuscitation
NCRC	non-child resistant container
NCS	no concentrated sweets; nerve conduction studies
NCT	neutron capture therapy
NCV	nerve conduction velocity
ND	no data; normal delivery; normal development; not done; nasal deformity; not diagnosed; none detectable; nose drops; nothing done; natural death; nondisabling; no disease; neonatal death; New Drugs
N&D	nodular and diffuse
NDA	New Drug Application; no data available; no detectable activity
NDD	no dialysis days
NDI	neurogenic diabetes insipidus
NDP	net dietary protein
NDR	neurotic depressive reaction
NDT	neurodevelopmental treatment; noise detection threshold
NDV	Newcastle disease virus
NE	norepinephrine; not elevated; not examined; no effect; never exposed; no enlargement
NEC	not elsewhere classified
NED	no evidence of disease
NEEP	negative end-expiratory pressure

NEFA	nonesterified fatty acids
neg	negative
NEM	nonspecific esophageal motility disorder
NEOH	neonatal high (risk)
NEOM	neonatal medium (risk)
NEP	no evidence of pathology
NER	no evidence of recurrence
NERD	no evidence of recurrent disease
NES	nasoendotracheal tube
NEX	nose to ear to xiphoid
NF	Negro female; not found; neurofibromatosis; normal flow; National Formulary
NFD	no family doctor
NFL	nerve fiber layer
NFP	no family physician
NFTD	normal full-term delivery
NFTSD	normal full-term spontaneous delivery
NFTT	nonorganic failure to thrive
NFW	nursed fairly well
NG	nasogastric; nitroglycerin
ng	nanogram
NGF	nerve growth factor
n giv	not given
NGR	nasogastric replacement
NGT	nasogastric tube; normal glucose tolerance
NGU	nongonococcal urethritis
NH	nursing home; nonhuman
NHC	neighborhood health center; neonatal hypocalcemia; nursing home care
NH$_4$Cl	ammonium chloride
NHD	normal hair distribution
NHL	non-Hodgkin's lymphoma; nodular histiocytic lymphoma
NHP	nursing home placement
NI	neurological improvement; no information; not identified; not isolated
NIA	no information available
NICC	neonatal intensive care center
NICU	neurosurgical intensive care unit; neonatal intensive care unit
NIDD	noninsulin-dependent diabetes
NIDDM	noninsulin-dependent diabetes mellitus
NIF	negative inspiratory force
NIH	National Institutes of Health
NIHL	noise-induced hearing loss
NIL	not in labor
NIMH-DIS	National Institute for Mental Health Diagnostic Interview Schedule

NINVS	noninvasive neurovascular studies
NIP	no infection present; no inflammation present
Nitro	nitroglycerin
NJ	nasojejunal
NK	not known; natural killer (cells)
NKA	no known allergies
NKC	nonketotic coma
NKDA	no known drug allergies
NKH	nonketotic hyperosmolar
NKHA	nonketotic hyperosmolar acidosis
NKHS	nonketotic hyperosmolar syndrome
NKMA	no known medication allergies
NL	normal; nasolacrimal
NLB	needle liver biopsy
NLC&C	normal libido, coitus, and climax
NLD	nasolacrimal duct
NLF	nasolabial fold
NLP	no light perception
NLS	neonatal lupus syndrome
NLT	not later than; not less than
NM	Negro male; nodular melanoma; neuromuscular; not measured; not measurable; not mentioned; nuclear medicine; nonmalignant
N&M	nerves and muscles; night and morning
NMD	normal muscle development
NMI	no middle initial; no mental illness; normal male infant
nmol	nanomole
NMP	normal menstrual period
NMR	nuclear magnetic resonance
NMS	neuroleptic malignant syndrome
NMSIDS	near-miss sudden infant death syndrome
NMT	no more than
NMTB	neuromuscular transmission blockade
NN	neonatal; nurses' notes
NND	neonatal death
NNE	neonatal necrotizing enterocolitis
NNM	Nicolle-Novy-MacNeal
NNO	no new orders
NNP	neonatal nurse practitioner
NNS	neonatal screen
NNU	net nitrogen utilization
NO	number; nitrous oxide; nursing office; none obtained
N$_2$O	nitrous oxide
noc	night
noct	nocturnal
NOD	notify of death; nonobese diabetic

NOK	next of kin
NOMI	nonocclusive mesenteric infarction
non pal	not palpable
NOOB	not out of bed
NOR	normal
NOR-EPI	norepinephrine
norm	normal
NOS	not otherwise specified
NOSIE	Nurse's Observation Scale for Inpatient Evaluation
NOT	nocturnal oxygen therapy
NP	neuropsychiatric; newly presented; no pain; not pregnant; not present; nursed poorly; nasal prongs; nurse practitioner; nuclear pharmacy; nuclear pharmacist; near point; not performed; nonpalpable; nasopharyngeal; nasopharynx; neuropathology; normal plasma; nursing procedure; nucleoprotein; nucleoplasmic
NPA	near point of accommodation
NPC	near point of convergence; nodal premature contraction; nonpatient contact; nonprotein calorie; nonproductive cough
NPDL	nodular poorly differentiated lymphocytic
NPDR	nonproliferative diabetic retinopathy
NPE	neuropsychologic examination; no palpable enlargement
NPF	nasopharyngeal fiberscope; no predisposing factor
NPG	nonpregnant
NPH	normal pressure hydrocephalus; no previous history; neutral protamine Hagedorn (insulin)
NPhx	nasopharynx
NPI	no present illness
NPN	nonprotein nitrogen
NPO	nothing by mouth
NPPNG	nonpenicillinase-producing *Neisseria gonorrhoeae*
NPR	normal pulse rate; nothing per rectum
NPT	normal pressure and temperature; nocturnal penile tumescence
NPU	net protein utilization
NQMI	non-Q wave myocardial infarction
NR	nonreactive; no report; no response; no return; normal range; normal reaction; no refills; no radiation; non repetatur; not readable; not resolved
NRAF	nonrheumatic atrial fibrillation

NRBC	normal red blood cell; nucleated red blood cell
NRBS	nonrebreathing system
NRC	normal retinal correspondence; National Research Council; Nuclear Regulatory Commission
NREM	nonrapid eye movement
NREMS	nonrapid eye movement sleep
NRF	normal renal function
NRI	nerve root involvement; nerve root irritation
NRM	normal range of motion; normal retinal movement
NRN	no return necessary
NROM	normal range of motion
NRT	neuromuscular re-education techniques
NS	normal saline solution; nephrotic syndrome; not seen; nuclear sclerosis; nylon suture; nonsmoker; not significant; no sample; neurosurgery; nervous system; neurologic survey; no specimen; nonspecific; nonsymptomatic; not sufficient
NSA	normal serum albumin; no significant abnormality
NSABP	National Surgical Adjuvant Breast Project
NSAD	no signs of acute disease
NSAIA	nonsteroidal antiinflammatory agent
NSAID	nonsteroidal antiinflammatory drug
NSC	no significant change; not service-connected
NSD	normal spontaneous delivery; nominal standard dose; no significant disease (defect, deviation, or difference)
NSDA	nonsteroid dependent asthmatic
NSE	normal saline enema
NSFTD	normal spontaneous full-term delivery
NSG	nursing
NSI	negative self-image; no signs of infection; no signs of inflammation
NSILA	nonsuppressible insulin-like activity
NSN	nephrotoxic serum nephritis
NSPVT	nonsustained polymorphic ventricular tachycardia
NSR	normal sinus rhythm; not seen regularly; nonspecific reaction; nasoseptal repair
NSS	normal saline solution; nutritional support service; normal size and shape
NSSL	normal size, shape, and location
NSSP	normal size, shape, and position
NSSTT	nonspecific ST and T (wave)

NST	nutritional support team; nonstress test; not sooner than
NSU	nonspecific urethritis; neurosurgical unit
NSV	nonspecific vaginitis
NSVD	normal spontaneous vaginal delivery
NSX	neurosurgical examination
NT	not tested; nasotracheal; not tender; normal temperature
NTBR	not to be resuscitated
NTC	neurotrauma center
NTD	neural tube defect
NTE	not to exceed
NTF	normal throat flora
NTG	nitroglycerin; nontoxic goiter; nontreatment group
NTGO	nitroglycerin ointment
NTMB	nontuberculous mycobacteria
NTP	normal temperature and pressure
NTS	nasotracheal suction
NTT	nasotracheal tube
NU	name unknown
NUD	nonulcer dyspepsia
NUG	necrotizing ulcerative gingivitis
nullip	nullipara
NV	neurovascular; next visit; nonvaccinated; normal value; not verified; nausea and vomiting; nonveteran; negative variation
N&V	nausea and vomiting
NVA	near visual acuity
NVAF	nonvalvular atrial fibrillation
NVD	neck vein distention; nausea, vomiting, and diarrhea; no venereal disease; neurovesicle dysfunction; nonvalvular disease; neovascularization of the disc; Newcastle virus disease
NVE	neovascularization elsewhere
NVG	neovascular glaucoma
NVS	neurological vital signs
NVSS	normal variant short stature
NW	naked weight; nasal wash; not weighed
NWB	nonweight bearing; no weight bearing
NX	nephrectomy
NYD	not yet diagnosed
nyst	nystagmus
NZ	enzyme

O

O	oxygen; objective (findings); oral; open; obvious; often; other; occlusal; pint; zero; none
O$_2$	oxygen
OA	oral alimentation; Overeaters Anonymous; occiput anterior; osteoarthritis; oral airway
O&A	observation and assessment
OAD	obstructive airway disease; occlusive arterial disease
OAF	osteoclast activating factor
OAG	open angle glaucoma
OASDHI	Old Age, Survivors, Disability, and Health Insurance
OASO	overactive superior oblique
OASR	overactive superior rectus
OAW	oral airway
OB	obstetrics; occult blood
OBG	obstetrics and gynecology
OB-GYN	obstetrics and gynecology
Obj	objective
obl	oblique
OBS	organic brain syndrome; obstetrical service
OC	oral contraceptive; oral care; on call; office call; only child; original claim; obstetrical conjugate
O&C	onset and course
OCA	oculocutaneous albinism; oral contraceptive agent
OCAD	occlusive carotid artery disease
OCCC	open chest cardiac compression
occl	occlusion
OCCM	open chest cardiac massage
OCCPR	open chest cardiopulmonary resuscitation
OCC Th	occupational therapy
Occup Rx	occupational therapy
OCD	obsessive-compulsive disorder
OCG	oral cholecystogram
OCP	ova, cysts, parasites; oral contraceptive pills
OCT	oxytocin challenge test
OCU	observation care unit

OD	oculus dexter (right eye); overdose; on duty; Doctor of Optometry; optic disc; optical density; outside diameter
ODA	occipitodextra anterior
ODAT	one day at (a) time
ODP	occipitodextra posterior
OE	on examination; otitis externa; orthopedic examination
O&E	observation and examination
OER	oxygen enhancement ratio
OET	oral esophageal tube
OF	occipital-frontal; optic fundi
OFC	occipital-frontal circumference; orbitofacial cleft
OG	orogastric; obstetrics and gynecology
OGTT	oral glucose tolerance test
OH	occupational history; open heart; oral hygiene; on hand; outside hospital
OHA	oral hypoglycemic agent
OHC	outer hair cell
OHCS	hydroxycorticosteroid
OHD	organic heart disease
OHG	oral hypoglycemic
OHL	oral hairy leukoplakia
OHP	oxygen under hyperbaric pressure
OHRR	open heart recovery room
OHS	open heart surgery
OI	osteogenesis imperfecta; otitis interna; opportunistic infection
OIF	oil immersion field
OJ	orange juice; orthoplast jacket
OK	all right; approved; correct
OKAN	optokinetic after nystagmus
OKN	optokinetic nystagmus
ol	oil
OLA	occipitolaeva anterior
OLP	occipitolaeva posterior
OLR	otology, laryngology, and rhinology
OLT	occipitolaeva transverse
OL&T	owners, landlords, and tenants
OM	otitis media; osteomalacia; osteomyelitis
om	omni mane (every morning)
OMAS	otitis media, acute, suppurative
OMCA	otitis media, catarrhal, acute
OMD	ocular muscle dystrophy
OME	office of medical examiner; otitis media (with) effusion
OMI	old myocardial infarction

omn bih	omni bihora (every two hours)
omn hor	omni hora (every hour)
OMPA	otitis media, purulent, acute
OMPC	otitis media, purulent, chronic
OMR	operative mortality rate
OMSA	otitis media secretory (or suppurative), acute
OMSC	otitis media secretory (or suppurative), chronic
OMVC	open mitral valve commissurotomy
ON	overnight; oronasal; otic nerve
on	omni nocte (every night)
ONC	over-the-needle catheter
ONTR	orders not to resuscitate
o/o	on account of
OOB	out of bed
OOBBRP	out of bed with bathroom privileges
OOC	out of control; onset of contractions
OOL	onset of labor
OOLR	ophthalmology, otology, laryngology, and rhinology
OOP	out on pass; out of pelvis; out of plaster
OOR	out of room
OOT	out of town
OOW	out of wedlock
OP	outpatient; operation; opening pressure; osmotic pressure; open; oblique presentation; oropharynx; osteoporosis; oscillatory potentials
O&P	ova and parasites
OPB	outpatient basis
OPC	outpatient clinic
op cit	in the work cited
OPD	outpatient department
OPG	ocular plethysmography
ophth	ophthalmology
OPM	occult primary malignancy
OPP	opposite
OPPG	oculopneumoplethysmography
OPS	operations; outpatient service
opt	optimum
OPV	oral polio vaccine
OR	operating room; oil retention; open reduction
ORIF	open reduction internal fixation
ORL	otorhinolaryngology
ORN	operating room nurse
ORT	operating room technician
OR X1	oriented to time

OR X2	oriented to time and place
OR X3	oriented to time, place, and person
OS	oculus sinister (left eye); opening snap; mouth; oral surgery; occipitosacral
OSA	obstructive sleep apnea
OSAS	obstructive sleep apnea syndrome
OSD	overside drainage
OSFT	outstretched fingertips
OSHA	Occupational Safety and Health Administration
OSM S	osmolarity serum
OSM U	osmolarity urine
OSN	off service note
OSS	osseous; over-shoulder strap
OT	old tuberculin; occupational therapy; old term; orotracheal; occlusion time
OTC	over-the-counter
OTD	organ tolerance dose
OTH	other
oto	otology
OTR	occupational therapist, registered
OTS	orotracheal suction
OTT	orotracheal tube
OU	oculi unitas (both eyes); oculus uterque (each eye)
OV	office visit
ov	ovum (egg)
OW	out of wedlock
O/W	oil in water
oz	ounce

P

P	plan; protein; pulse; para; peripheral; phosphorus; pupil; position; postpartum; pressure; presbyopia; primipara
P$_2$	pulmonic second heart sound
PA	posterior-anterior; pulmonary artery; pernicious anemia; physician assistant; presents again; psychiatric aide; professional association; phenol alcohol
P&A	percussion and auscultation; position and alignment
PAB	premature atrial beat
PAC	premature atrial contraction

PADP	pulmonary artery diastolic pressure
PAE	progressive assistive exercise
PAEDP	pulmonary artery and end-diastolic pressure
PAF	paroxysmal atrial fibrillation; platelet activating factor
PA&F	percussion, auscultation, and fremitus
PAGA	premature appropriate for gestational age
PAI	plasminogen activator inhibitor
PAIVS	pulmonary atresia with intact ventricle septum
PAL	posterior axillary line
Pa Line	pulmonary artery line
PALN	para-aortic lymph node
PAMP	pulmonary arterial (artery) mean pressure
PAN	periodic alternating nystagmus; polyarteritis nodosa
PANESS	physical and neurological examination for soft signs
PaO$_2$	partial pressure of oxygen in arterial blood
PAOP	pulmonary artery occlusion pressure
PAP	pulmonary artery pressure; prostatic acid phosphatase; passive aggressive personality
PA/PS	pulmonary atresia/pulmonary stenosis
Pap smear	Papanicolaou smear
PAR	postanesthetic recovery; platelet aggregate ratio; paraffin; parallel
PARA	number of pregnancies
para	paraplegic
PARR	postanesthesia recovery room
PARU	postanesthesia recovery unit
PAS	pulmonary artery stenosis; periodic acid Schiff (reagent); Professional Activities Study; para-aminosalicylic (acid)
PASG	pneumatic antishock garment
PASP	pulmonary artery systolic pressure
PAT	paroxysmal atrial tachycardia; pre-admission testing; percent acceleration time; pregnancy at term; patella; patient
Path	pathology
PAWP	pulmonary artery wedge pressure
Pb	lead
PB	powder board; paraffin bath; premature beat; protein-bound; Pharmacopoeia Britannica
P&B	pain and burning
PBA	percutaneous bladder aspiration
PBC	point of basal convergence; primary biliary cirrhosis
PBD	percutaneous biliary drainage

PBF	placenta blood flow; pulmonary blood flow
PBI	protein-bound iodine
PBL	peripheral blood lymphocyte
PBMC	peripheral blood mononuclear cell
PBO	placebo
pc	after meals (post cibum)
PC	packed cells; professional corporation; platelet concentrate; poor condition; popliteal cyst; productive cough; phosphate cycle; platelet count; portacaval; pubococcygeal; pulmonic closure
PCA	patient care assistant; patient-controlled analgesia; posterior cerebral artery; passive cutaneous anaphylaxis; posterior communicating artery
PCC	pheochromocytoma; poison control center
PCCC	pediatric critical care center
PCD	postmortem cesarean delivery
PCFT	platelet complement fixation test
PCG	phonocardiogram
PCH	paroxysmal cold hemoglobinuria
pc&hs	after meals and at bedtime
PCI	prophylactic cranial irradiation
PCIOL	posterior chamber intraocular lens
PCKD	polycystic kidney disease
PCL	posterior chamber lens; posterior cruciate ligament
PCM	protein-calorie malnutrition
PCO	polycystic ovary
PCO$_2$	partial pressure of carbon dioxide
PCOD	polycystic ovarian disease
PCP	pulmonary capillary pressure; *Pneumocystis carinii*
PCS	portable cervical spine; portacaval shunt
PCT	post coital test; progestin challenge test; portacaval transposition
PCU	progressive care unit; primary care unit; protective care unit
PCXR	portable chest radiograph
PCV	packed cell volume
PD	peritoneal dialysis; postural drainage; Parkinson's disease; pupillary distance; percutaneous drain; plasma defect; poorly differentiated; prism diopter; progression of disease; psychotic depression; pulmonary disease
Pd	palladium; paid
P/D	packs per day (cigarettes)

PDA	patent ductus arteriosus; parenteral drug abuser
PDE	paroxysmal dyspnea on exertion; pulsed Doppler echocardiography
PDFC	premature dead female child
PDGF	platelet-derived growth factor
PDMC	premature dead male child
PDN	private duty nurse
PD&P	postural drainage and percussion
PDR	Physicians' Desk Reference; proliferative diabetic retinopathy; postdelivery room
PDS	pain dysfunction syndrome
PDT	photodynamic therapy
PDU	pulsed Doppler ultrasonography
PE	physical examination; physical evaluation; pulmonary embolism; pressure equalization; plural effusion; plasma exchange; physical exercise; pulmonary edema; probable error; pharyngoesophageal
PEARLA	pupils equal and react to light and accommodation
PECHO	prostatic echogram
Peds	pediatrics
PEEP	positive end-expiratory pressure
PEFR	peak expiratory flow rate
PEG	pneumoencephalogram; percutaneous endoscopic gastrostomy
PEJ	percutaneous endoscopic jejunostomy
PEM	protein-energy malnutrition
PEMF	pulsing electromagnetic field
PEN	parenteral and enteral nutrition
PENS	percutaneous epidural nerve stimulator
PEP	protein electrophoresis
PER	pediatric emergency room; protein efficiency ratio
PERC	percutaneous
perf	perforation; perfect
PERL	pupils equal, reactive to light
per os	by mouth
PERR	pattern evoked retinal response
PERRLA	pupils equal, round, reactive to light and accommodation
PET	positron-emission tomography; pre-eclamptic toxemia; pressure equalizing tubes; poor exercise tolerance
PF	power factor; peripheral fields; prostatic fluid
PF$_3$	platelet factor 3

PFR	peak flow rate; parotid flow rate
PFT	pulmonary function test
PG	pregnant; postgraduate; prostaglandins
pg	picogram; page
PGE	posterior gastroenterostomy
PGE$_2$	prostaglandin E$_2$
PGF	paternal grandfather
PGH	pituitary growth hormone
PGM	paternal grandmother
PGR	progesterone receptor
PGU	postgonococcal urethritis
PH	past history; poor health; public health; prostatic hypertrophy; pulmonary hypertension
pH	hydrogen ion concentration
Ph	phenyl
PHA	peripheral hyperalimentation; photohemagglutinin
PHAR	pharmacy; pharmacist; pharynx
Pharm	Pharmacy
PHC	primary hepatocellular carcinoma
PHN	public health nurse
PHT	portal hypertension; primary hyperthyroidism; pulmonary hypertension
PHx	past history
Phx	pharynx
PI	present illness; poison ivy; pulmonary infarction; premature infant
PIAT	Peabody Individual Achievement Test
PICA	Porch Index of Communicative Ability
PICC	peripherally inserted central catheter
PICU	pediatric intensive care unit
PID	pelvic inflammatory disease; prolapsed intervertebral disc
PIE	pulmonary interstitial emphysema
PIG	pertussis immune globulin
PIH	pregnancy-induced hypertension
PINS	persons in need of supervision
PIP	proximal interphalangeal (joint); postinspiratory pressure
PITP	pseudo-idiopathic thrombocytopenic purpura
PIV	peripheral intravenous
PIVD	protruded intervertebral disc
PJB	premature junctional beat
PJC	premature junctional contraction
PK	penetrating keratoplasty; psychokinesis
PKD	polycystic kidney disease
PKP	penetrating keratoplasty
PKU	phenylketonuria

PL	place; plantar
pl	picoliter
PLAP	placenta alkaline phosphatase
PLBO	placebo
PLFC	premature living female child
PLL	prolymphocytic leukemia
PLMC	premature living male child
PLN	pelvic lymph node; popliteal lymph node
PLR	pupillary light reflex
PLS	primary lateral sclerosis; plastic surgery
pls	please
PLT	platelet
PLT EST	platelet estimate
plts	platelets
PM	post mortem; evening; afternoon; petit mal; pretibial myxedema; presents mainly; pacemaker; primary motivation; poor metabolizers; prostatic massage; physical medicine
PMA	progressive muscular atrophy; premenstrual asthma
PMB	polymorphonuclear basophil; postmenopausal bleeding
PMC	pseudomembranous colitis
PMD	primary myocardial disease; private medical doctor
PME	postmenopausal estrogen; polymorphonuclear eosinophil
PMEC	pseudomembranous enterocolitis
PMH	past medical history
PMI	past medical illness; point of maximal impulse
PML	polymorphonuclear leukocytes
PMN	polymorphonuclear neutrophil
PMO	postmenopausal osteoporosis
PMP	previous menstrual period
PMR	perinatal mortality rate
PM&R	physical medicine and rehabilitation
PMS	premenstrual syndrome; postmenopausal syndrome
PMT	premenstrual tension
PMW	pacemaker wires
PN	practical nurse; pneumonia; percussion note; periarteritis nodosa; postnasal
PNB	premature newborn; premature nodal beat
PNC	penicillin; prenatal care; premature nodal contraction
PND	postnasal drip; paroxysmal nocturnal dyspnea

pnd	pound
PNH	paroxysmal nocturnal hemoglobinuria
PNI	peripheral nerve injury
PNMG	persistent neonatal myasthenia gravis
PNP	peak negative pressure; pediatric nurse practitioner
PNS	practical nursing student; peripheral nervous system
PNT	percutaneous nephrostomy tube
PNU	protein nitrogen units
Pnx	pneumothorax
PO	by mouth (per os); phone order; postoperative
PO$_2$	partial pressure of oxygen
PO$_4$	phosphate
POA	point of application
POAG	primary open-angle glaucoma
POB	place of birth
POC	postoperative care; product of conception
POD	place of death; polycystic ovarian disease; postoperative day
POG	products of gestation; Pediatric Oncology Group
POIK	poikilocytosis
POL	premature onset of labor
POLY	polymorphonuclear leukocyte
POM	pain on motion
POMR	problem-oriented medical record
POMS	Profile of Mood States
POP	plaster of paris; popliteal; plasma oncotic pressure
PORT	postoperative respiratory therapy
pos	positive
pos pr	positive pressure
poss	possible
post	posterior; postmortem
post op	postoperative
POU	placenta, ovaries, and uterus
PP	postprandial; pin prick; postpartum; private patient; partial pressure; proximal phalanx; pulse pressure; pedal pulse; plasmapheresis; punctum proximum (near point of accommodation)
P&P	pins and plaster
PPA	palpitation, percussion, and auscultation; postpartum amenorrhea; phenylpyruvic acid
PP&A	palpitation, percussion, and auscultation
PPAS	postpolio atrophy syndrome
PPB	positive-pressure breathing

ppb	parts per billion
PPBS	postprandial blood sugar
PPC	progressive patient care
PPD	purified protein derivative; postpartum day; packs per day
PPD-B	Purified Protein Derivative Battery
PPD-S	Purified Protein Derivative Standard
PPG	photoplethysmography
PPH	postpartum hemorrhage
PPI	patient package insert
PPLO	pleuropneumonia-like organisms
ppm	parts per million
PPM	permanent pacemaker
PPMA	postpoliomyelitis muscular atrophy
PPO	preferred provider organization
PPP	postpartum psychosis
PPROM	prolonged premature rupture of membranes
PPS	postpartum sterilization; peripheral pulmonary stenosis; postpump syndrome; post polio syndrome
PPTL	postpartum tubal ligation
PPU	perforated peptic ulcer
PPV	positive-pressure ventilation
PPVT	Peabody Picture Vocabulary Test
PQ	permeability quotient
PR	punctum remotum (far point); Puerto Rican; pulse rate; premature; peer review; pregnancy rate; public relations; protein; partial remission
P&R	pulse and respiration; pelvic and rectal
Pr	presbyopia; prism
PRA	plasma renin activity
PRAT	platelet radioactive antiglobulin test
PRBC	packed red blood cells
PRC	packed red cells; peer review committee
PRCA	pure red cell aplasia
pre	preliminary
preg	pregnancy
preop	preoperative
prep	prepare
PRERLA	pupils round, equal, react to light and accommodation
prev	prevent; previous
prim	primary
PRL	prolactin
PRLA	pupils react to light and accommodation
PRM	phosphoribomutase

prn	as the occasion requires; as necessary; when needed
PRO	prothrombin; protein
prob	probable
PROCT	proctology
PROCTO	proctoscopic
prog	prognosis; program; progressive
PROM	premature rupture of membranes; passive range of motion
PRO PAC	Prospective Payment Assessment Commission
pros	prosthesis, prostate
prot	protein
prox	proximal
PRRE	pupils round, regular, and equal
PS	plastic surgery; pulmonary stenosis; physical status; performance status; pyloric stenosis; population sample; peripheral smear
P&S	pain and suffering; paracentesis and suction
PSA	prostate-specific antigen
PSC	posterior subcapsular cataract
PSE	portal-systemic encephalopathy
PSF	posterior spinal fusion
PSG	peak systolic gradient; presystolic gallop
PSH	postspinal headache
psi	pounds per square inch
PSM	presystolic murmur
P/sore	pressure sore
PSP	phenolsulfonphthalein; periodic short pulse; progressive supranuclear palsy
PSS	progressive systemic sclerosis; physiological saline solution; painful shoulder syndrome
PST	paroxysmal supraventricular tachycardia
PSVT	paroxysmal supraventricular tachycardia
PSY	psychiatry; psychology
PSYCH	psychiatry; psychology
pt	pint; patient
PT	physical therapy; patient; permanent and total; pine tar; prothrombin time; paroxysmal tachycardia
P&T	permanent and total
PTA	physical therapy assistant; plasma thromboplastin antecedent; prior to admission; prior to arrival; percutaneous transluminal angioplasty; posttraumatic amnesia
PTB	prior to birth; patellar tendon bearing; pulmonary tuberculosis
PTBA	percutaneous transluminal balloon angioplasty

PTBS	posttraumatic brain syndrome
PTC	patient to call; prior to conception; plasma thromboplastin component; phenylthiocarbamide
PTCA	percutaneous transluminal coronary angioplasty
PTCL	peripheral T-cell lymphoma
PTD	permanent and total disability; prior to delivery
PTE	pulmonary thromboembolism; pretibial edema
PTG	parathyroid gland
PTH	prior to hospitalization; posttransfusion hepatitis; parathyroid hormone
PTL	preterm labor
PTM	posttransfusion mononucleosis
PTPM	posttraumatic progressive myelopathy
PTR	patient to return; patella tendon reflex; peripheral total resistance
PTS	prior to surgery
PTSD	posttraumatic stress disorder
PTT	partial thromboplastin time; particle transport time; platelet transfusion therapy
PTU	pain treatment unit
PTX	pelvic traction; pneumothorax; parathyroidectomy
Pu	plutonium
PU	peptic ulcer
PUBS	percutaneous umbilical blood sampling
PUE	pyrexia of unknown etiology
PUFA	polyunsaturated fatty acid
pul	pulmonary
pulv	pulvis (powder)
PUN	plasma urea nitrogen
PUO	pyrexia of unknown origin
PUPP	pruritic urticarial papules and plaque of pregnancy
PUVA	psoralen-ultraviolet A light
PV	polio vaccine; peripheral vascular; plasma volume; polycythemia vera; portal vein; pulmonary vein; per vagina; papillomavirus
P&V	pyloroplasty and vagotomy
PVA	polyvinyl alcohol
PVB	premature ventricular beat
PVC	premature ventricular contraction; polyvinyl chloride; pulmonary venous congestion; postvoiding cystogram
PVD	peripheral vascular disease; posterior vitreous detachment
PVE	premature ventricular extrasystole

PVF	peripheral visual field; portal venous flow
PVH	periventricular hemorrhage
PVM	proteins, vitamins, and minerals
PVO	peripheral vascular occlusion; pulmonary venous occlusion
PVO_2	mixed venous pressure of oxygen
PVOD	pulmonary vascular obstructive disease
PVP	portal venous pressure; peripheral venous pressure
PVR	pulmonary vascular resistance; postvoiding residual; pulse-volume recording; peripheral vascular resistance
PVS	pulmonic valve stenosis; percussion, vibration,and suction; premature ventricular systole
pvt	private
PVT	private; paroxysmal ventricular tachycardia; portal vein thrombosis
PW	posterior wall
PWB	partial weight bearing
PWC	physical work capacity
PWI	posterior wall infarct
PWP	pulmonary wedge pressure
PWS	port-wine stain
Px	physical examination; pneumothorax; prognosis
PY	pack years
PZI	protamine zinc insulin

Q

q	every
QA	quality assurance
qAM	every morning
QCA	quantitative coronary angiography
qd	every day
qh	every hour
q2h	every two hours
q3h	every three hours
q4h	every four hours
qhs	every night
qid	four times a day
QIG	quantitative immunoglobulins
QMI	Q wave myocardial infarction
QMT	quantitative muscle testing
qm	every morning

qn	every night
QNS	quantity not sufficient
qod	every other day
qoh	every other hour
qPM	every evening
QS	quantity sufficient
qt	quart; quiet
quant	quantity
qwk	once a week
qv	quantum vis (as much as you like)

R

R	respiration; right; rectal; radiology; remote; regular; rate
RA	rheumatoid arthritis; right atrium; renal artery; right arm; right atrial; repeat action; room air
RAA	renin-angiotensin-aldosterone
RABG	room air blood gas
RAC	right atrial catheter
RAD	radical; radiation absorbed dose; right axis deviation
RAE	right atrial enlargement
RAF	rheumatoid arthritis factor
RAH	right atrial hypertrophy
RAI	radioactive iodine
RAIU	radioactive iodine uptake
RAM	rapid alternating movements; radioactive material
RAO	right anterior oblique
RAP	right atrial pressure
RAPD	relative afferent pupillary defect
RAQ	right anterior quadrant
RAS	renal artery stenosis
RAST	radioallergosorbent test
RATx	radiation therapy
RB	right buttock; retinoblastoma
R&B	right and below
RBA	right brachial artery; right basilar artery; rose bengal antigen
RBB	right breast biopsy; right bundle branch
RBBB	right bundle branch block
RBC	red blood cell
RBCM	red blood cell mass

RBCV	red blood cell volume
RBF	renal blood flow
RBOW	ruptures bag of waters
RBP	retinol-binding protein
RBS	random blood sugar
RCA	right coronary artery; radionuclide cerebral angiogram
RCC	renal cell carcinoma
RCD	relative cardiac dullness
RCM	red cell mass; right costal margin; radiographic contrast media
RCS	repeat cesarean section; reticulum cell sarcoma
RCT	root canal therapy
RCV	red cell volume
RD	renal disease; right deltoid; respiratory disease; Reye's disease; ruptured disc; retinal detachment
RDA	recommended daily allowance
RDP	right dorsoposterior
RDPE	reticular degeneration of the pigment epithelium
RDS	respiratory distress syndrome
RDT	regular dialysis treatment
RDVT	recurrent deep vein thrombosis
RE	rectal examination; right eye; right ear; reflux esophagitis; reticuloendothelial; regional enteritis; concerning; resting energy
R&E	round and equal; research and education
REC	recommend; record; recovery recreation; recur
REF	referred; renal erythropoietic factor
rehab	rehabilitation
Rel	religion
REM	rapid eye movement
REMS	rapid eye movement sleep
rep	repeat
repol	repolarization
RES	reticuloendothelial system; resident; resection
RESC	resuscitation
resp	respiratory; respirations
RET	right esotropia; retention; reticulocyte; retina; retired;
RF	rheumatoid factor; renal failure; rheumatic fever
RFA	right frontoanterior; right femoral artery
RFL	right frontolateral

RFP	right frontoposterior
RFS	rapid frozen section; renal function study
RFT	right frontotransverse
RG	right gluteal
Rh	Rhesus (factor)
RHB	raise head of bed
RHC	respiration has ceased
RHD	rheumatic heart disease; relative hepatic dullness
RHF	right heart failure
rhm	roentgen (per) hour (at one) meter
Rh neg	Rhesus factor negative
Rh pos	Rhesus factor positive
RI	refractive index; regional ileitis; respiratory illness
RIA	radioimmunoassay
RIAT	radioimmune antiglobulin test
RIC	right iliac crest; right internal carotid
RICE	rest, ice, compression, and elevation
RICM	right intercostal margin
RICS	right intercostal space
RICU	respiratory intensive care unit
RIF	right iliac fossa; right index finger
RIG	rabies immune globulin
RIP	rapid infusion pump
RISA	radioactive iodinated serum albumin
RIST	radioimmunosorbent test
RK	right kidney; radial keratotomy
RL	right leg; right lung;
R-L	right to left
RLC	residual lung capacity
RLD	related living donor
RLE	right lower extremity
RLF	retrolental fibroplasia
RLL	right lower lobe
RLN	recurrent laryngeal nerve
RLQ	right lower quadrant
RM	radical mastectomy; room; respiratory movement
RMD	rapid movement disorder
RML	right middle lobe
RMR	resting metabolic rate
RMSF	Rocky Mountain spotted fever
RN	registered nurse
RNA	ribonucleic acid, radionuclide angiography
RND	radical neck dissection
RO	routine order
R/O	rule out

ROC	resident on call
ROM	range of motion; right otitis media
ROS	review of systems
ROSC	restoration of spontaneous circulation
RP	retinitis pigmentosa; refractory period; radial pulse; reactive protein; retrograde pyelogram
RPA	right pulmonary artery
RPCF	Reiter protein complement fixation
RPE	retinal pigment epithelium
RPF	renal plasma flow
RPG	retrograde pyelogram
RPGN	rapidly progressive glomerulonephritis
R Ph	registered pharmacist
rpm	revolution per minute
RPN	renal papillary necrosis
RPR	rapid plasma reagin
RPT	registered physical therapist
RR	recovery room; retinal reflex; respiratory rate; renin release; radiation response; response rate
R&R	rate and rhythm; rest and recuperation
RR&E	round, regular, and equal
RREF	resting radionuclide ejection fraction
rRNA	ribosomal ribonucleic acid
RRND	right radical neck dissection
RRP	relative refractory period
RRR	regular rhythm and rate; renin-release rate
RS	rhythm strip; Reye's syndrome; Ringer's solution; Reiter's syndrome; Raynaud's syndrome; rating schedule; right side; respiratory syncytial
R/S	rupture spontaneous
RSA	right subclavian artery; right sacrum anterior; reticulum cell sarcoma
RSB	right sternal border
RSDS	reflex-sympathetic dystrophy syndrome
RSO	right salpingo-oophorectomy; right superior oblique
RSR	relative survival rate; regular sinus rhythm; right superior rectus
RST	radiosensitivity test; right sacrotransverse
RSV	respiratory syncytial virus; right subclavian vein
rt	right

RT	right; recreational therapy; radiation therapy; renal transplant; right thigh; rectal temperature; radiotherapy; reaction time; room temperature
rt lat	right lateral
RTA	renal tubular acidosis
RTC	round the clock; return to clinic
rtd	retarded
RTD	routine test dilution
RTM	routine medical care
RTN	renal tubular necrosis
RTO	return to office
RTOG	Radiation Therapy Oncology Group
rtPA	recombinant tissue-type plasminogen activator
RTU	ready-to-use
RTW	return to work
RTx	radiation therapy
RU	routine urinalysis; retrograde urogram; right upper; roentgen unit
RUE	right upper extremity
RUG	retrograde urethrogram
RUL	right upper lobe
RUQ	right upper quadrant
RUR	resin-uptake ratio
RURTI	recurrent upper respiratory tract infection
RV	residual volume; right ventricle; retrovaginal; rubella vaccine; return visit; respiratory volume
RVA	rabies vaccine adsorbed
RVET	right ventricular ejection time
RVF	Rift Valley fever
RVG	radionuclide ventriculography
RVH	right ventricular hypertrophy
RVL	right vastus lateralis
RVO	retinal vein occlusion; relaxed vaginal outlet
RVR	rapid ventricular response; renal vascular resistance; resistance to venous return
RVS	Relative Value Schedule; Relative Value Study
RVSWI	right ventricular stroke work index
RVT	renal vein thrombosis
RV/TLC	residual volume to total lung capacity ratio
RVV	rubella vaccine virus
RVVT	Russell's viper venom time
RW	ragweed
R/W	return to work
RWM	regional wall motion
Rx	therapy; treatment; take; prescription

RXN	reaction
RXT	right exotropia

S

S	subjective findings; son; sister; sacral; second; serum; single; suction; subject; surgery; soluble
S1	first heart sound
S2	second heart sound
SA	sinoatrial; salicylic acid; sarcoma; Spanish American; sustained action; specific activity; surface area; slightly active
S/A	sugar and acetone; same as
SAB	subarachnoid bleed; serum albumin; subarachnoid block
SAC	short arm cast
SAD	seasonal affective disorder
Sag D	sagittal diameter
SAL	*Salmonella*; salicylate
SAM	self-administered medication; systolic anterior motion
SAN	sinoatrial node
SAO	small airway obstruction
SAS	statistical analysis system; sleep apnea syndrome; short arm splint; subarachnoid space
SAT	Scholastic Aptitude Test; Saturday; saturated; subacute thyroiditis; saturation
SAVD	spontaneous assisted vaginal delivery
SB	single breath; stillbirth; serum bilirubin; spina bifida; small bowel; stand-by; sternal border; Stanford-Binet
SBA	serum bactericidal activity
SBC	standard bicarbonate; strict bed confinement
SBE	subacute bacterial endocarditis; short below elbow (cast); shortness of breath on exertion
SBFT	small bowel follow through
SBGM	self blood glucose monitoring
SBI	systemic bacterial infection
SBO	small bowel obstruction
SBP	systolic blood pressure; spontaneous bacterial peritonitis
SBR	strict bed rest
SBS	shaken baby syndrome

SBT	single-breath test; serum bactericidal titer
SC	subcutaneous; sickle cell; sacrococcygeal; self-care; subclavian; Snellen's chart; semicircular; semiclosed; service connected; sick call; special care; sugar-coated
SCAN	suspected child abuse and neglect
SCAT	sheep cell agglutination test; sickle cell anemia test
SCBC	small cell bronchogenic carcinoma
SCC	squamous cell carcinoma
SCD	service-connected disability; subacute combined degeneration; sickle cell disease; sudden cardiac death; spinal cord disease
SCEP	somatosensory cortical evoked potential
sched	schedule
schiz	schizophrenia
SCI	spinal cord injury; structured clinical interview
SCID	severe combined immunodeficiency disorder
SCIU	spinal cord injury unit
SCIV	subclavian intravenous
SCL	soft contact lens
SCLC	small-cell lung cancer
SCLE	subcutaneous lupus erythematosus
SCM	sternocleidomastoid; sensation, circulation, and motion; spondylitic caudal myelopathy
SCr	serum creatinine
SCT	sickle cell trait; sugar-coated tablet
SCU	self-care unit; special care unit
SCUBA	self-contained underwater breathing apparatus
SCUT	schizophrenia chronic undifferentiated type
SCV	subcutaneous vaginal (block); subclavian vein
SD	standard deviation; septal defect; serum defect; skin dose; spontaneous delivery; sterile dressing; surgical drain; scleroderma; senile dementia; severely disabled; shoulder disarticulation; sudden death
S&D	stomach and duodenum
S/D	systolic to diastolic
SDA	Seventh-Day Adventist; specific dynamic action; steroid-dependent asthmatic
SDAT	senile dementia of Alzheimer's type
SDB	sleep disorder breathing
SDH	subdural hematoma
SDL	speech discrimination loss; serum drug level
SDP	stomach, duodenum, and pancreas

SDS	same day surgery; Self-Rating Depression Scale
SDT	speech detection threshold
SE	side effect; soft exudate; saline enema; standard error; Starr-Edwards (prosthesis)
sec	secondary; secretary; second
SED	skin erythema dose; sedimentation; spondyloepiphyseal dysplasia
sed rt	sedimentation rate
SEER	surveillance, epidemiology, and end results
SEG	segment
segs	segmented neutrophils
SEM	systolic ejection murmur; scanning electron microscope; standard error of the mean; semen
SEMI	subendocardial myocardial infarction
SENS	sensorium
SEP	systolic ejection period; separate; sensory evoked potential; somatosensory evoked potential
SEQ	sequella
SER-IV	supination external rotation, type 4 fracture
SERs	somatosensory evoked responses
SES	socioeconomic status
SF	scarlet fever; salt free; sugar free; spinal fluid; soft feces; seminal fluid; symptom free; saturated fat; seizure frequency; shell fragment
SFA	saturated fatty acids; superficial femoral artery
SFC	spinal fluid count
SFEMG	single-fiber electromyography
SFP	spinal fluid pressure
SFPT	standard fixation preference test
SFTR	sagittal, frontal, transverse, rotation
SG	Swan-Ganz; serum glucose; specific gravity; signs; surgeon general; skin graft
SGC	Swan-Ganz catheter
SGE	significant glandular enlargement
SGOT	serum glutamic oxaloacetic transaminase
SGPT	serum glutamic pyruvic transaminase
SH	social history; shower; serum hepatitis; short; shoulder; sex hormone; surgical history
S&H	speech and hearing
S/H	suicidal/homicidal (ideation)
S Hb	sickle hemoglobin (screen)
SHEENT	skin, head, eyes, ears, nose, throat
Shig	*Shigella*

SHL	supraglottic horizontal laryngectomy
SHS	student health service
SI	small intestine; self-inflicted; sacroiliac; seriously ill; stress incontinence; serum iron; stroke index
S&I	suction and irrigation
SIB	self-injurious behavior
sibs	siblings
SICU	surgical intensive care unit
SIDS	sudden infant death syndrome
Sig	signetur (let it be labeled)
SIJ	sacroiliac joint
SIMV	synchronized intermittent mandatory ventilation
SISI	short increment sensitivity index
SIT	Slossen Intelligence Test; sperm immobilization test
SIV	Simian immunodeficiency virus
SIW	self-inflicted wound
SJS	Stevens-Johnson syndrome
SK	streptokinase; senile keratosis; solar keratosis
SL	slight; short leg; sensation level; sublingual
SLA	sacrolaeva anterior; slide latex agglutination
SLB	short leg brace
SLC	short leg cast
SLE	systemic lupus erythematosus; slit lamp examination
SLGXT	symptom-limited graded exercise test
SLKC	superior limbic keratoconjunctivitis
SLR	straight leg raising
SLS	short leg splint; single limb support
SLUD	salivation, lacrimation, urination, and defecation
SLWC	short leg walking cast
SM	small; systolic murmur; skim milk; simple mastectomy; submucous; suction method; symptoms; systolic mean
SMA	sequential multiple analyzer; simultaneous multichannel auto-analyzer; superior mesenteric artery; spinal muscular atrophy
SMBG	self-monitoring blood glucose
SMC	special mouth care
SMCD	senile macular chorioretinal degeneration
SMI	severely mentally impaired; small volume infusion; sustained maximal inspiration

SMP	self-management program
SMR	submucous resection; senior medical resident; skeletal muscle relaxant; standard mortality ratio
SMRR	submucous resection and rhinoplasty
SMV	superior mesenteric vein; submentovertical
SMVT	sustained monomorphic ventricular tachycardia
SN	student nurse; suprasternal notch; serum-neutralizing
SNCV	sensory nerve conduction velocity
SNE	subacute necrotizing encephalomyelopathy
SNF	skilled nursing facility
SNOOP	Systematic Nursing Observation of Psychopathology
SNT	sinuses, nose, and throat
SO	salpingo-oophorectomy; sphincter of Oddi; sutures out; standing orders; superior oblique; supraoptic
S&O	salpingo-oophorectomy
SO_4	sulfate
SOA	supraorbital artery; swelling of ankles
SOAA	signed out against advice
SOAMA	signed out against medical advice
SOAP	subjective, objective, assessment, and plan
SOB	shortness of breath
sol	solution
SOM	serous otitis media
SOMI	sterno-occipital mandibular immobilizer
Sono	sonogram
SOP	standing operating procedure
SOR	sign own release
sos	if necessary or required
SP	suprapubic; systolic pressure; sacrum to pubis; sequential pulse; status post; symphysis pubis; shunt procedure
S/P	serum protein; suicide precautions; semiprivate; systolic pressure; status post; suprapubic
SPA	stimulation-produced analgesia; serum prothrombin activity; suprapubic aspiration
SPBI	serum protein-bound iodine
SPBT	suprapubic bladder tap
SPE	serum protein electrophoresis
SPEC	specimen
Spec Ed	special education
SPECT	single photon emission computer tomography
SPEP	serum protein electrophoresis
SPF	sun protective factor

Sp G	specific gravity
sp gr	specific gravity
SPH	spherocytes
SPIA	solid phase immunoabsorbent assay
SPIF	spontaneous peak inspiratory force
SPMA	spinal progressive muscle atrophy
SPN	student practical nurse
spont	spontaneous
SPP	suprapubic prostatectomy
SPROM	spontaneous premature rupture of membrane
SPS	systemic progressive sclerosis
SPT	skin prick test
SPVR	systemic peripheral vascular resistance
SQ	subcutaneous; status quo
Sq CCa	squamous cell carcinoma
SR	sedimentation rate; side rails; system review; sinus rhythm; secretion rate; smooth-rough
S&R	seclusion and restraint
SRBC	sheep red blood cells; sickle red blood cells
SRBOW	spontaneous rupture of bag of waters
SRD	service-related disability; sodium-restricted diet
SRF	somatotropin-releasing factor
SRH	signs of recent hemorrhage
SRIF	somatotropin-releasing inhibiting factor
SR/NE	sinus rhythm, no ectopy
SRU	side rails up
ss	one-half
SS	saline solution; social service; signs and symptoms; Social Security; saliva sample; soapsuds; sum of squares; super-saturated
S&S	signs and symptoms; support and stimulation
SSA	Social Security Administration; salicylsalicylic acid; Sjögren's syndrome antigen A
SSCA	single shoulder contrast arthrography
SSD	source to skin distance
SSDI	social security disability income
SSE	soapsuds enema; saline solution enema; systemic side effects
SSEPs	somatosensory evoked potentials
SSKI	saturated solution of potassium iodide
SSOP	Second Surgical Opinion Program
SSS	sterile saline soak; scalded skin syndrome; structured sensory stimulation

ST	sinus tachycardia; skin test; slight trace; subtotal; surface tension; speech therapist; semitendinosus: straight; stomach; split-thickness; stress testing
stab	polymorphonuclear leukocytes in nonmature form
staph	staphylococcus
Staph aur	*Staphylococcus aureus*
stat	immediately
STB	stillborn
STD	sexually transmitted diseases; skin test done
STG	split-thickness graft
STH	somatotropic hormone; subtotal hysterectomy; soft tissue hemorrhage
STK	streptokinase
STNM	surgical-evaluative staging of cancer
strep	streptococcus
STS	serologic test for syphilis
STSG	split-thickness skin graft
subq	subcutaneous
SUD	sudden unexpected death
SUI	stress urinary incontinence
SUID	sudden unexplained infant death
SUN	serum urea nitrogen
SUP	superior; supinator
supp	suppository
SV	sigmoid volvulus; seminal vesical; single ventricle; stroke volume; severe; snake venom; subclavian vein
SVC	superior vena cava
SVD	spontaneous vaginal delivery
SVL	severe visual loss
SVPB	supraventricular premature beat
SVPC	supraventricular premature contraction
SVR	supraventricular rhythm; systemic vascular resistance
SVT	supraventricular tachycardia
SW	social worker; stab wound; spiral wound; stroke work
SWD	short wave diathermy
SWI	stroke work index; surgical wound infection
Sx	signs; symptoms; surgery
sym	symptoms; symmetrical
syr	syrup
SZ	seizure; schizophrenia

T

T	temperature; tablespoon; tender; tension; thoracic; testicles; time; tumor
t	teaspoon
T+	increased tension
T−	decreased tension
T$_{1/2}$	half-life
T$_3$	triiodothyronine
T$_4$	thyroxine
T−7	free thyroxine factor
TA	therapeutic abortion; toxin-antitoxin; traffic accident; temperature axillary
T&A	tonsillectomy and adenoidectomy
TAA	total ankle arthroplasty; thoracic aortic aneurysm; tumor-associated antigen
tab	tablet
TAB	tablet; therapeutic abortion
TAF	tissue angiogenesis factor
TAH	total abdominal hysterectomy; total artificial heart
TAL	tendon Achilles lengthening; total arm length
TAM	teenage mother; toxoid-antitoxoid mixture
TAO	thromboangiitis obliterans
TAPVD	total anomalous pulmonary venous drainage
TAR	thrombocytopenia with absence of the radius; treatment authorization request
TARA	total articular replacement arthroplasty
TAT	tetanus antitoxin
TB	tuberculosis; total bilirubin; total base; total body; tubercle bacillus
TBA	to be absorbed; to be added; to be admitted; testosterone-binding affinity
TBB	transbronchial biopsy
TBC	tuberculosis
TBF	total body fat
TBG	thyroxine-binding globulin
TBI	total body irradiation; traumatic brain injury
T bili	total bilirubin
tbl	tablespoon
TBM	tuberculous meningitis; tubule basement membrane; tracheobronchomalacia

TBNA	treated but not admitted; total body sodium; transbronchial needle aspiration
TBPA	thyroxine-binding prealbumin
TBR	total bed rest
TBSA	total burn surface area
tbsp	tablespoon
TBV	total blood volume; transluminal balloon valvuloplasty
TC	throat culture; true conjugate; Trauma Center; tissue culture; to contain; total capacity; total cholesterol
T/C	to consider
T&C	type and crossmatch; turn and cough
TCA	tricuspid atresia; terminal cancer
TCABG	triple coronary artery bypass graft
TCAD	tricyclic antidepressant
TCC	transitional cell carcinoma
TCDB	turn, cough, and deep breath
TCID	tissue culture infective dose
TCM	transcutaneous monitor; tissue culture media
TCMH	tumor-direct cell-mediated hypersensitivity
TCNS	transcutaneous nerve stimulator
TCOM	transcutaneous oxygen monitor
TD	tetanus-diphtheria; tardive dyskinesia; travelers diarrhea; thoracic duct; tone decay; total disability; treatment discontinued
TDF	thoracic duct fistula; thoracic duct flow; tumor dose fraction
TDM	therapeutic drug monitoring
TDN	transdermal nitroglycerin
TE	trace elements; tennis elbow; tracheoesophageal; tooth extracted; threshold energy; total estrogen
T&E	trial and error
TEA	total elbow arthroplasty; thromboendarterectomy
TEC	total eosinophil count
TEE	transesophageal echocardiography
TEF	tracheoesophageal fistula
TEG	thromboelastogram
tele	telemetry
TEM	transmission electron microscopy
TEN	toxic epidermal necrolysis; Total Enteral Nutrition
TENS	transcutaneous electrical nerve stimulation
TEP	tubal ectopic pregnancy; thromboendophlebectomy

tert	tertiary
TET	treadmill exercise test; tetanus
TF	tube feeding; to follow; total flow; tetralogy of Fallot; transfer factor; tubular fluid; tactile fremitus
TFA	total fatty acids
TG	triglycerides; thyroglobulin; toxic goiter
TGA	transposition of the great arteries; transient global amnesia
TGS	tincture of green soap
TGT	thromboplastin generation test
TGV	thoracic gas volume
TH	thrill; total hysterectomy; thyroid hormone
THA	total hip arthroplasty
THC	transhepatic cholangiogram
THE	transhepatic embolization
THR	total hip replacement
TI	tricuspid insufficiency
TIA	transient ischemic attack
TIBC	total iron-binding capacity
tid	three times a day
TIE	transient ischemic episode
TIG	tetanus immune globulin
tinct	tincture
TIT	*Treponema* immobilization test; triiodothyronine
TJ	triceps jerk
TKA	total knee arthroplasty
TKNO	to keep needle open
TKO	to keep open
TKR	total knee replacement
TL	tubal ligation; trial leave; team leader; total lipids; time lapse; time-limited
TLC	tender loving care; total lung capacity; thin-layer chromatography
TLD	thermoluminescent dosimeter; tumor lethal dose
TLNB	term living newborn
TLV	total lung volume
TM	trademark; tympanic membrane; temperature by mouth; tumor; transmetatarsal
T&M	type and crossmatch
TMET	treadmill exercise test
TMJ	temporomandibular joint
TMR	trainable mentally retarded
TMST	treadmill stress test
TMTC	too many to count

TN	team nursing; temperature normal; normal intraocular tension; true negative
TNB	term newborn
TND	term normal delivery
TNI	total nodal irradiation
TNTC	too numerous to count
TO	telephone order; transfer out; total obstruction
TOA	tubo-ovarian abscess
TOL	trial of labor
Tomo	tomography
TOP	termination of pregnancy
TOPV	trivalent oral polio vaccine
TORP	total ossicular replacement prosthesis
TOS	thoracic outlet syndrome
TP	total protein; temperature and pressure; true positive; thrombophlebitis
T&P	temperature and pulse
TPBF	total pulmonary blood flow
TPC	total patient care
TPE	total protective environment
TPH	thromboembolic pulmonary hypertension; transplacental hemorrhage
TPI	*Treponema pallidum* immobilization
TPM	temporary pacemaker
TPN	total parenteral nutrition
TP&P	time, place, and person
TPR	temperature, pulse, and respiration; total peripheral resistance; total pulmonary resistance
TPVR	total peripheral vascular resistance; total pulmonary vascular resistance
TQ	tourniquet
TR	time released; total response; trace; transfusion reaction
trach	tracheal; tracheostomy
TRC	tanned red cells
TRF	thyrotropin-releasing factor
TRH	thyrotropin-releasing hormone
TRI	trimester
TRIG	triglycerides
TRP	tubular reabsorption of phosphate
TS	test solution, transsexual; thoracic surgery; total solids; temperature sensitive
TSA	total shoulder arthroplasty
TSD	Tay-Sachs disease
T set	tracheotomy set
TSH	thyroid-stimulating hormone

tsp	teaspoon
TSP	total serum protein
TSS	toxic shock syndrome
TT	transtracheal; total time; thrombin time; tetanus toxoid
T&T	touch and tone
TTD	temporary total disability; tissue tolerance dose
TTO	to take out
TTR	triceps tendon reflex
TTVP	temporary transvenous pacemaker
TUR	transurethral resection
TURBN	transurethral resection bladder neck
TURP	transurethral resection of prostate
TV	*Trichomonas vaginalis*; tidal volume; trial visit
TVC	total volume capacity; timed vital capacity; triple voiding cystogram; true vocal cord
TVF	tactile vocal fremitus
TVH	total vaginal hysterectomy
TVP	transvenous pacemaker; transvesicle prostatectomy
TVSC	transvaginal sector scan
TVU	total volume of urine
TW	tap water; test weight
TWD	total white and differential count
TWE	tap water enema
TWG	total weight gain
Tx	treatment; traction; therapy
T&X	type and crossmatch
Ty	type

U

U	unit; unknown; upper; urology
UA	umbilical artery; uric acid; urinalysis; uterine aspiration; upper arm; upper airway; uncertain about
UAC	umbilical artery catheter
UAO	upper airway obstruction
UAT	up as tolerated
UAVC	univentricular atrioventricular connection
UBF	unknown black female
UBI	ultraviolet blood irradiation
UBM	unknown black male

UBW	usual body weight
UC	ulcerative colitis; unchanged; urine culture; uterine contraction; umbilical cord; unconscious; urethral catheterization
U&C	usual and customary; urethral and cervical
UCD	usual childhood diseases; urine collection device
UCG	urinary chorionic gonadotropin
UCHD	usual childhood diseases
UCI	urethral catheter in; usual childhood illnesses
UCO	urethral catheter out
UCR	usual, customary, and reasonable
UCS	unconscious; unconditioned stimulus
UCX	urine culture
UD	urethral discharge
UDC	usual diseases of childhood
UDO	undetermined origin
UE	upper extremity; undetermined etiology; under elbow
UES	upper esophageal sphincter
UFA	unesterified fatty acids
UFF	unusual facial features
UFFI	urea formaldehyde foam insulation
UFO	unflagged order
UG	urogenital
UGI	upper gastrointestinal series
UH	umbilical hernia; upper half
UI	urinary incontinence
UIQ	upper inner quadrant
UK	unknown; urokinase
UL	upper lobe
U/L	upper and lower
U&L	upper and lower
ULN	upper limits of normal
ULQ	upper left quadrant
UM	unmarried
umb	umbilicus
UN	urea nitrogen
ung	ointment
UNK	unknown
UNOS	United Network for Organ Sharing
UO	undetermined origin; urinary output
UOQ	upper outer quadrant
UP	upright posture
U/P	urine-plasma ratio
UPJ	ureteropelvic junction
UPOR	usual place of residence

UPPP	uvulopalatopharyngoplasty
UPT	urine pregnancy test
UR	utilization review; upper respiratory
URI	upper respiratory infection
url	unrelated
urol	urology
URQ	upper right quadrant
URTI	upper respiratory tract infection
US	unit secretary; ultrasonic; ultrasonography
USB	upper sternal border
USG	ultrasonography
USH	usual state of health
USI	urinary stress incontinence
USN	ultrasonic nebulizer
USO	unilateral salpingo-oophorectomy
USP	United States Pharmacopeia
UTD	up-to-date
ut dict	as directed
UTF	usual throat flora
UTI	urinary tract infection
UTO	upper tibial osteotomy
UTZ	ultrasound
UUN	urine urea nitrogen
UV	ultraviolet; urine volume; umbilical vein; urinary volume
UVA	ultraviolet A light; ureterovesical angle
UVB	ultraviolet B light
UVC	umbilical vein catheter
UVJ	ureterovesical junction
UVL	ultraviolet light; umbilical venous line
UVR	ultraviolet radiation
U/WB	unit of whole blood
UWF	unknown white female
UWM	unknown white male; unwed mother

V

V	vein; vision; voice; five; vomiting; vagina; volume
v	volt; very
VA	Veterans Administration; visual acuity; vacuum aspiration
VAC	ventriculoarterial connections
vag	vaginal; vagina
VALE	visual acuity, left eye

VAP	venous access port
VAR	variant; variation
VARE	visual acuity, right eye
VAS	vascular
vasc	vascular
VB	viable birth; venous blood
VBAC	vaginal birth after cesarean
VBG	venous blood gas
VBL	vinblastine
VC	vena cava; vital capacity; vocal cords
VCG	vectorcardiogram
VCR	vincristine; video cassette recorder
VCT	venous clotting time
VCU	voiding cystourethrogram
VD	venereal disease; vapor density
V&D	vomiting and diarrhea
VDA	visual discriminatory acuity
VDG	venereal disease-gonorrhea
vdg	voiding
VDH	valvular disease of the heart
VDL	visual detection level
VDRL	Venereal Disease Research Laboratory
VDS	venereal disease-syphilis
VDT	video-display terminal
VE	vaginal examination; visual efficiency
VEA	ventricular ectopic activity
VEB	ventricular ectopic beat
VEE	Venezuelan equine encephalitis
vent	ventricular; ventral
VEP	visual evoked potential
VER	visual evoked response
VF	visual field; vocal fremitus; ventricular fibrillation
V Fib	ventricular fibrillation
VG	ventricular gallop; vein graft; very good
VGH	very good health
VH	Veterans Hospital; vaginal hysterectomy; viral hepatitis; vitreous hemorrhage
VHD	valvular heart disease
VI	volume index
vib	vibration
VIP	very important person; voluntary interruption of pregnancy
VIS	vaginal irrigation smear
VIT	vital; vitamin
vit cap	vital capacity
VL	left arm (electrode)
VLBW	very low birth weight

VLDL	very low density lipoprotein
VLH	ventrolateral nucleus of the hypothalamus
VM	voltmeter
VMA	vanillylmandelic acid
VMH	ventromedial hypothalamus
VMR	vasomotor rhinitis
VN	visiting nurse; virus-neutralizing
VNA	Visiting Nurses' Association
VO	verbal order
VOD	vision, right eye
vol	volume
VOL	voluntary
VOR	vestibular ocular reflex
VOS	vision, left eye
VOU	vision, both eyes
VP	venous pressure; venipuncture; volume-pressure; ventricular-peritoneal; vice president
V&P	ventilation and perfusion; vagotomy and pyloroplasty
VPA	valproic acid
VPB	ventricular premature beat
VPC	ventricular premature contraction
VPDs	ventricular premature depolarizations
VPL	ventro-posterolateral
VPR	volume pressure response
VPRC	volume of packed red cells
VQ	ventilation-perfusion
VR	right arm (electrode); venous return; ventilation ratio; verbal reprimand; ventricular rhythm; valve replacement; vascular resistance; vocal resonance; vocational rehabilitation
VRI	viral respiratory infection
VRL	ventral root, lumbar
VRT	ventral root, thoracic; variance of residence time
VS	vital signs; very sensitive; vaccination scar; verbal scale; venisection; volumetric solution
vs	against; voids; vibration seconds
VsB	bleeding in the arm
VSBE	very short below elbow (cast)
VSD	ventricular septal defect
VSOK	vital signs normal
VSR	venous stasis retinopathy
VSS	vital signs stable
VSV	vesicular stomatitis virus

VT	ventricular tachycardia; tidal volume
V&T	volume and tension
VTE	venous thromboembolism
VTEC	verotoxin-producing *Escherichia coli*
VV	varicose veins
V&V	vulva and vagina
V/V	volume to volume ratio
VVD	vaginal vertex delivery
VVFR	vesicovaginal fistula repair
V/VI	grade 5 on a 6 grade basis
VVOR	visual-vestibulo-ocular-reflex
VW	vessel wall
VWD	von Willebrand's disease
VWM	ventricular wall motion
VZ	varicella zoster
VZIG	varicella zoster immune globulin
VZV	varicella zoster virus

W

W	water; white; weight; wife; week; widowed; watt
W+	weakly positive
w/	with
WA	when awake; while awake; wide awake
W or A	weakness or atrophy
WAF	weakness, atrophy, and fasciculation; white adult female
WAIS	Wechsler Adult Intelligence Scale
WAM	white adult male
WASS	Wasserman test
WB	whole body; whole blood; weight bearing; well baby
WBC	white blood cell; white blood count
WBCT	whole blood clotting time
WBR	whole body radiation
WBS	whole body scan
WC	white count; ward clerk; will call; whooping cough
WCC	white cell count
WD	well-developed; wet dressing; well-differentiated
W/D	withdrawn; warm and dry
WDWN	well-developed, well-nourished
WEE	Western equine encephalitis

WF	white female
WFI	water for injection
WFL	within functional limits
WHO	World Health Organization
WI	walk-in
WIA	wounded in action
WID	widow; widower
WISC	Wechsler Intelligence Scale for Children
wk	week; weak; work
WL	waiting list; work load
WM	white male; whole milk
WMF	white middle-aged female
WMM	white middle-aged male
WMP	weight management program
WN	well-nourished
WND	wound
WNL	within normal limits
wo	without
WO	written order; weeks old
W/O	water in oil; without
WOP	without pain
WPW	Wolfe-Parkinson-White
WR	Wasserman reaction; weakly reactive; wrist
WS	ward secretary
Ws	watts-second
wt	weight; white
W/U	workup
WV	whispered voice
W/V	weight-to-volume ratio
W/W	weight-to-weight ratio
WWAC	walk with aid of cane

X

X	times; ten; cross; break; removal of; start of anesthesia; crossmatch; except; xanthine
X+#	xiphoid plus number of fingerbreadths
X3	orientation to time, place, and person
XC	excretory cystogram
X&D	examination and diagnosis
X2d	times two days
XDP	xeroderma pigmentosum
Xe	xenon
XeCT	xenon-enhanced computed tomography
X-ed	crossed